Population Family Health and Development

Edited by

Tukutau Taufa
&
Caroline Bass

University of Papua New Guinea Press

Port Moresby

1993

Published by:
University of Papua New Guinea Press & Bookshop
P. O. Box 413
UNIVERSITY PO
NCD
Papua New Guinea
Tel: 675 + 326 7281 or 326 7675
Email: upngbooks@gmail.com

This book was originally published as a 2 volume set in 1993. This edition has been reprinted in 2013 as a single volume.

ISBN 978-9980-87-902-8

Cover design: Robert Sheridan
Original logo design: Vincent Tomaur

Papers presented at and arising from the 19th Waigani Seminar, University of Papua New Guinea, 16 - 22 June 1991

Population, Family Health and Development

Volume 1

These Volumes are dedicated

to our Patron

the late Ms Margaret Nakikus

TABLE OF CONTENTS

ACKNOWLEDGEMENTS

We gratefully acknowledge the financial assistance of our donors, The Australian High Commission, The World Bank, SPAFH with funding from USAID, IPPF, UNICEF, UNFPA, Air Niugini, the Bank of Papua New Guinea, the Post and Telecommunication Corporation, Ramu Sugar, and the Summer Institute of Linguistics.

Thanks are due to the hardworking 19th Waigani Seminar Organising Committee, our Patron Mrs Margaret Nakikus, Treasurer John Vince, Deputy Chairman N.G. Patil, and Committee Members Homolpi Warom, Arai Pula, Beatrice Avalos, John Shadlow and Eleina Butuna. Many thanks also to our technical editors H.G. Mannur, Beatrice Avalos, John Shadlow and Lance Hill, and to Aoare Lomai.

Our Special thanks go to Philomena Boden for the enormous amount of work she has put into word processing this entire publication. Her dedication and skill have been invaluable in the production of these volumes.

Tukutau Taufa
Caroline Bass

OPENING ADDRESS BY THE RT HON RABBIE L NAMALIU

Thank you for the privilege of officially opening the Waigani Seminar, which this year, has as its theme "Population, Family Health and Development."

This is a very timely and appropriate subject for a gathering as important and influential as the Waigani Seminar to address.

The relationship between people and development has been inadequately researched, and addressed, in the past in Papua New Guinea. I am delighted to say this is changing very rapidly and productively indeed. No where is that change more evident than in the comprehensive National Population Policy which I will outline during the course of my address this morning.

The resource development era we are entering presents us with both challenges and opportunities we will never face, or have, again. If our generation is to ensure that this and future generations of Papua New Guineans fully enjoy the benefits of this development, we must plan for, and ensure, our human resources are managed well. Any delay or neglect in this process will squander a chance which will never come our way again. That is why an integrated, comprehensive human development policy is so vital at this time.

A soundly based National Population Policy sets the foundation of our development process. To meet its great objectives, a National Population Policy must be much more than just a plan to reduce the population growth rate. That is but one small objective of a much more complete plan. The overall policy is not merely to reduce population growth......it is to improve the quality of life of all our people.

The National Population Policy, which I want to use this excellent occasion to detail, includes strategies to improve Maternal and Child Health, to improve Primary Health Care Services, to improve the status of women, and to improve both urban and rural living conditions, to mention just some of the key elements.

My government is concerned to ensure that people can expect to not only live longer, but also live better. The impact of past health care services has already been reflected by increases in the average life expectancy at birth. A child born in the 1990's can expect to live an average of over 50 years. Only 20 years ago, the âverage child could expect to live 40 years. While these are impressive achievements, we can do even better. One of the goals of the National Population Policy will be to ensure that the children of the future can look forward to an even longer, more satisfying, life span.

In the area of fertility, our situation is similar to that in population growth rate. Papua New Guinea has a total fertility rate of 5.4 per woman, which is moderate by Third World and Melanesian standards.

However, our success in recent decades in significantly reducing infant and child mortality levels, and increasing life expectancy, means that even if we are to lower our total fertility levels, population growth will still continue for several decades to come.

In such a situation, a strong Family Planning Programme is necessary, and it is necessary <u>now.</u>

My government is conscious of these trends, and their likely effect on the supply and demand for basic socio-economic services. We also want to ensure that the low priority given to population ends, and that there is the fullest consideration of the linkages between population, and development, at <u>all</u> levels of planning.

There are some unique problems in both launching, and maintaining, the momentum of a National Planning Policy.

Our people like to see policies and programmes that bring immediate and material benefits. A population policy, unlike other socio-economic policies, takes time to generate returns, its benefits are not immediately obvious, though they are substantial in the long-term. Population Policy programmes therefore need to start immediately, if we are to realise the benefits as soon as possible.

The history of the development of a population policy for Papua New Guinea has been a somewhat chequered one. After an initial false start in 1978, a cabinet decision in 1987 directed the Department of Finance and Planning to convene an expert committee on population policy, and establish a population planning and co-ordination unit. A National Advisory Committee on population policy was formed from relevant government, non-government and private groups. A draft guideline was prepared by the Committee which was adopted for the Government's National Population Policy, while the National Advisory Committee on Population Policy worked on details.

The National Advisory Committee on Population Policy submitted a detailed policy to the government in January this year.......and it was approved by cabinet just a month later.

In addition to formally approving a comprehensive policy, cabinet has approved the establishment of a National Population Council, and directed the Department of Health and Provincial Governments to be actively involved in the planning and implementation of the National Population Policy.

The fundamental aim of the policy is to achieve sustainable development in order to ensure our citizens attain and enjoy a standard of living and quality of life commensurate with human dignity and aspirations.

The policy is broadly based and multi-sectoral. It would be beyond the financial or manpower capacity of a single government, or non-government agency, to implement all the programmes envisaged.

Sectoral programmes that fall in line with Departmental areas of responsibility will be assigned to each agency for implementation. Programmes will have priorities to ensure the desired results are achieved, and the Department of Finance and Planning will play a lead role in co-ordination.

A wide range of very valuable work has already been done in a number of sectors that effect population. Our aim is to strengthen these programmes and co-ordinate them so we can achieve our set objectives.

The policy concentrates on three key areas - Health, Education, and Migration and Urbanisation.

In addition, rural agricultural development and the equitable distribution of basic services are seen as effective means of deterring rural-urban migration.

In the area of health care, previous and existing plans and programmes have been aimed at improving the welfare of the people through better primary health care, clinical services, ante natal care, family planning, safe drinking water and so on. The new policy seeks to continue, and significantly accelerate and upgrade, the improvements which have been achieved. The policy will ensure greater energy and resources are directed to these tasks in the future.

Preventive rather than curative health care, especially among women and children, will enjoy a high national priority.

Family planning activities will be both strengthened and expanded. They will play a lead role in reducing growth rates, as well as serving as a means to reduce maternal and child mortality. Families and couples who want to use contraceptives to plan and control birth will be assisted to do so. Contraceptive users will have access to family planning services and information to make informed decisions.

However, and I want to stress this, none will be forced to utilise contraceptives, and for those who choose not to use this means, alternative approaches will be made available.

We recognise that family planning services are an important avenue for widening women's opportunities. They enable women to exercise greater control over decisions affecting their daily lives.

That is why family planning services and information will be integrated with maternal and child health care, nutrition, family health education, and income and employment generating opportunities for women.

In the area of education, basic education is recognised as not only the key to integral human development, but also for its indirect contributions to population and development objectives.

Raising the level of education for women has been widely recognised as not only proper from the standpoint of equal opportunity, but also as a prime factor in reducing overall fertility levels. But it is equally important that increased educational opportunities for women will increase their employment opportunities, as well as their status, both of which are goals my government strongly supports.

The meeting of basic needs requires equal access for males and females to education, employment, small scale business activities, and numerous other areas.

In view of the unacceptably low status of women, and the close link between status and population and development strategies, much energy will have to be devoted to ensuring that women do realise the benefits to which they are entitled.

The youth of our nation are also key players in the population policy. The younger generation will become active contributors to population growth over the next decade or so. We must prepare them to develop rational and responsible attitudes to parenthood. To ensure this happens, family life education, family welfare and related issues will be included in the school curricula.

For the out of school population, both youth and adult, non-formal education programmes will also include family life education and family and community welfare components.

Our existing womens and youth organizations will be called on to play a much greater role because of their extensive community networks. They must strengthen their base, and their management and organisation, to play that wider role.

A key part of a successful population policy is public awareness. Our lessons from the past in this area have taught us that family planning and population issues must be treated with great care and sensitivity. General awareness campaigns leading to better-informed decisions on family planning, population and development goals will be given priority.

When we talk about an informed public, the issue of literacy must be considered. It is an important element of population policy, and our policy gives great emphasis to adult literacy programmes to improve public awareness.

In Papua New Guinea today, a major concern is the movement of people, especially school leavers, from rural to urban communities. Rural to urban migration has been linked to many of the law and order problems we have today.

However, the problem also lies with distorted accommodation costs, wage structures, and lack of income earning opportunities in rural areas.

The policy seeks to address the issues of shortages of housing, land use, and a lack of vital services to accommodate urban population growth.

At the same time, regional development policies relating to industry location must be fostered to achieve balanced economic and population distribution.

Rural agricultural development and diversity is also being expedited to deter urban migration.

No population policy can succeed without good information systems for realistic and factual planning. Conduct and survey data only become available every five or ten years. Improvements in existing data systems, and new sources, are needed to ensure that up to date and totally reliable information is used in population planning policies.

Research will also play an important role. Research and studies are to be action-oriented to identify prevailing levels and patterns of change which can be transformed into policy programmes.

An efficient institutional framework is being set up to enable these policies to be implemented. A National Population Council, comprising relevant ministries, with myself as Chairman, will be established by legislation.

The Council will be responsible for co-ordination, policy approval and programming. Technical details and routine co-ordination will be the responsibility of a Technical Committee, appointed by the Council, and drawn from national, provincial and non-government agencies. I want to stress the absolute importance of provincial government, and the non-government sector, giving their full commitment to helping to implement population policy programmes.

The structure, when in place, will give greater political commitment from the top and enhance the widest possible participation.

A small Population Planning and Co-ordination Unit will be located in the Finance and Planning Department to serve as a secretariat to both bodies.

I am confident the approach we are taking will bring the best results, and will do so without delay, and without non-productive cost.

The Policy is the work of many people, and many organisations. While they are too numerous to mention individually, I want them to know their work is appreciated, and it will continue to be appreciated in the future.

Before I conclude, I do want to thank the international donor and funding community, and overseas governments, who are giving generous support to the Population Policy and Programme, and to this Seminar.

I thank The World Bank, The Australian Government, through the High Commissioner here in Port Moresby, UNFPA, The South Pacific Alliance for Family Health, The IPPF, the ILO, and UNICEF, for their generous support to this important endeavour, an historic step along the road to sound development for Papua New Guinea, and for supporting the 1991 Waigani Seminar which dove-tails in with our Population Policy and Programme.

Such broad and on-going international support is greatly appreciated by my Government, and the organisers of this Seminar.

KEYNOTE ADDRESS BY CLIFFORD GILPIN

**Chief, Population and Human Resource Division,
Country Department for Indonesia, PNG and Pacific Islands,
The World Bank**

Honourable Prime Minister, distinguished seminar participants, Ladies and Gentlemen, it is a great pleasure for me to be here in Papua New Guinea to address this distinguished audience on a topic that is challenging mankind: the need to stabilize population growth in harmony with responses to many other challenges such as widespread poverty, high infant and maternal mortality, illiteracy, unemployment and environmental degradation. The Waigni Seminar on "Population, Family Health and Development", which marks the official launch of the PNG Population Policy, will no doubt provide a unique opportunity for a rich dialogue on the best approaches to implement population programmes beneficial to Papua New Guinea. Indeed, the comprehensive population policy adopted by the Government will enable the extension of family planning services and access to contraceptive information both to ensure benefits to individual families in terms of lower infant and maternal mortality, and to improve living conditions in the country, by helping to moderate the rate of population growth.

On behalf of the World Bank, I wish to congratulate the Government of Papua New Guinea for having taken this important step at a point where action programmes to deal with the issues of high fertility and other attending challenges can make the difference in terms of development prospects for this country in the early part of the twenty first century.

THE WORLD BANK AND POPULATION

It is not always widely known that the Bank has been actively involved in supporting population programmes for more than 20 years. The Bank began to discuss population issues systematically in the late 1960s. In 1970, the Bank, together with UNFPA and other donor agencies supported the setting up of the National Family Planning Coordinating Board in Indonesia and assisted a number of countries in other regions to address this problem. Why did the Bank become involved? For two reasons:

a) because it believed that the high rates of population growth of many developing countries were a serious impediment to their development and especially to their attempts to reduce poverty;

and, b) because it was recognized that there are very significant individual health and human rights benefits in making contraception readily available to individual couples.

In the 1980s, the Bank has also become increasingly concerned about the impact rapid population growth can have on the environment especially when combined with certain non demographic factors. For example, when agricultural lands do not produce sufficient yields to support the growing populations, farmers are forced to bring marginal lands, erosion-prone hillsides, semi-arid savannas and tropical forests, under cultivation leading to deforestation and desertification. This can have disastrous effects on the ecosystem and biodiversity. In PNG you are fortunate to be the home of not only the famous Bird of Paradise, but also of many other unique species. The opportunity to preserve these treasures is still available to you, something that many other places on earth have already foregone. Although population pressure is not always the main culprit of environmental destruction, it almost always exacerbates the problem.

While the Bank and the international community has been long aware of the negative effect that rapid population growth tends to have on development, in particular in resource poor countries, lately, in the 1990s, it has become increasingly clear how population growth interacts with development. Based on a wealth of research evidence and country experience, there is now broad consensus that investments in people, in education, health, nutrition and the socio-economic role of women, are pivotal to individual productivity, and individual productivity translates into macro-economic growth.

As the demand for investment in people escalates because of rapid growth in human numbers, governments are constrained in their ability to promote human development and policy makers are confronted with difficult choices between competing, yet complementary, priorities for development. Rapid population growth weakens the macro-economic performance by making it more difficult to finance per capita investments in education and infrastructure that ensure sustained economic growth. Moderating the rate of population growth makes it more possible for governments to meet competing investment needs and facilitates the development of human productive capacity.

High fertility is not only a macro-economic issue. It has also extremely important implications at the family level, in particular for mothers and their children already born, their nutritional status, access to health care and education, employment opportunities and status in the family. Family planning, as an aid to help women to minimize pregnancy and birth risks, and couples to maximize the well-being of their families, is therefore an important social service recognized as a human right by the international community and most individual countries. Responding to the needs of couples, and especially women, to control excessive fertility contributes to individual and social well-being and benefits in particular the poor, who are the first to lose out when services cannot keep pace with population growth. Lower fertility, fewer births, spaced at longer intervals, not too early or too late, substantially improves the health of both mothers and children.

The World Bank, concerned with long term development issues, clearly has to give high priority to population issues in the context of human development in all its aspects, including prominently, poverty alleviation and the protection of the environment. From a modest initial support, in the 1960s, for education and health programmes, the Bank has moved to the point, in the 1990s, of placing human resources development in all its aspects at the top of the development agenda and as one of the Bank's highest priorities for assistance.

Before addressing the issues in population, health and development facing Papua New Guinea and the Pacific, let me share with you a broad picture of the world's and Asia's population dynamics and the way in which the Bank, as well as the United Nations and many other donors and organizations working in development, have tried to assist in addressing these issues.

WORLD POPULATION DYNAMICS

The demographic record to date is well known: the world population has doubled from 2.5 billion in 1950 to over 5 billion today, with over 85% of this growth occurring in developing countries. Every year, about 90 million people are added to the world's population. Although fertility in developing countries is declining, about 85 percent of the LDC population is still growing above replacement level and the overall growth rate is two percent per year. Two percent may appear to be a small number, but in terms of population growth, is very high. If that rate were to continue for just over three decades, the population of the developing world would double from 4 to 8 billion. Fortunately, changes are taking place in developing countries at a rapid pace. Improvements in quality of life brought about by progress in literacy and schooling (particularly among girls), lower infant and child mortality and improved food availability, have helped reduce fertility, significantly assisted by widespread family planning programmes. Over 85% of the developing country population live in countries which have adopted policies to reduce rates of population growth. In special studies undertaken by the Population Council it has been found that around one third of the fertility decline may be attributed to family planning. However, the 1990's represent a very special turning point and challenges in the world's demographic transition: if the medium population projections of the United Nations are to be realized, the number of users of contraception must increase by 40 percent, from 460 million at the present time, to 640 million in the year 2,000 (i.e. in the next decade). Because of very high past fertility, the number of women of reproductive age will increase by 25 percent in this period. To compensate, the proportion of couples contracepting must increase substantially if fertility is to fall to the projected levels.

POPULATION ISSUES IN ASIA AND THE PACIFIC

Asia and the Pacific take a prominent place in the current state of population dynamics and their participation in efforts to reduce fertility is crucial. Over half of the world's 5 billion people live in Asia, and this region contributes more than half of the annual population growth of the globe. Due to this large concentration, what happens in Asia will largely determine the overall trends in world population. Although the major global effects of population growth will be contributed by the very large countries e.g. China, India, Indonesia, because people live in communities and within country frontiers, with very limited possibilities for migration transfers, the adverse effects of rapid population growth should be a matter of concern for all countries, large and small.

There are few common threads in Asian demography; indeed the diversity is so great that it is not possible to define an Asian demographic profile. There are marked differences between Eastern and South Asian countries regarding factors such as age at marriage, duration of breastfeeding and the use of contraception. To quote just one indicator of heterogeneity: the contraceptive prevalence rate varies from over 60% for countries well advanced in the demographic transition such as China, Korea and Thailand. While at the other end of the spectrum, the contraceptive prevalence rate can be measured in single figures. PNG and most of the Pacific Islands belong to the latter category.

Public policy can and has helped to reduce fertility through promoting increases in the age of marriage and duration of breastfeeding, but experience from countries that have made fast progress on fertility reduction has shown that family planning is and remains the main effective option for reducing fertility levels. As has been demonstrated by the family planning programmes of Indonesia, Thailand and Korea, the stronger the population programme effort, the more impact the programme will have. A vigorous population programme requires long term, sustained commitment by the leadership of a country at the highest level of government, involvement of the religious authorities, the support of the women's movement, and easy access to quality family planning services, including full information and counselling for the large majority of the population.

PAPUA NEW GUINEA AND THE PACIFIC ISLANDS

Fertility in the Pacific, remains very high, between 6 and 7 children per woman, and population growth is between 2 and 3 percent. The 1990s will be critical for decelerating population growth and for determining the ultimate size of the stationary populations. Even if replacement fertility were to be reached tomorrow, i.e. not more than two children per woman, the population would continue to grow, at a decreasing rate, for another 60 to 70 years because of the momentum for further growth inherent in the young age structure of the societies. Replacement level fertility is a long way off!

In Papua New Guinea, the effects of unrestrained fertility will place an enormous demand on resources as the country strives to develop. Population projections show, assuming constant fertility and a gradual improvem ent in life expectancy, (which are not entirely unrealistic assumptions), that by the year 2015 the population of the country would be 7.4 million, and later in the 21st century would stabilize at about 11 million, almost tripling its current size. If, however, PNG intensifies its effort and maintains a more than moderately strong commitment to its population policy, matched by equally strong programme effort, population growth could come down faster and earlier, and the ultimate population size could be about two million smaller. But much more significant for the country's development and its people's welfare would be other benefits obtaining from lower fertility, to which I wish to refer next.

1. The benefits of slower growth. During the process of demographic transition, more immediate benefits are to be reaped. Foremost and all important is the effect on women's health. Pregnancies which occur too early, too close, too often and too late, often place women's lives in danger. Women with a moderate number of children born at appropriate intervals and at the right

maternal age can better contribute to a harmonious family life, and develop their potential in the work force and society. Maternal mortality, which is only the tip of the iceberg hiding unknown amounts of disability and morbidity, is unacceptably high in Papua New Guinea, with large variations between different parts of the territory. During this seminar, a session is dedicated to women's health, and we will hear specifics on the preventable suffering still going on in Papua New Guinea. Drawing attention to the facts is the first step in seeking a remedy. Family Planning helps to reduce the risk factors in childbearing and, together with simple maternal and improved obstetric care, can dramatically and immediately reduce the waste in female lives.

2. Education. More education for women is one of the strongest, though slow acting, factors in reducing fertility. In all countries, women who have completed primary school have fewer children than women with no education, and everywhere the number of children declines (often substantially) as the education of mothers increases above the primary school level. The differences can be as large as four children between the highest and lowest educational groups. But any changes of this nature are slow to come about, since educational gains will only have effects in the fertility of the next generation. All the more reason, therefore, to act now concerning educational policies, particularly favoring the enrollment of girls. In fact, despite the expansion of primary and secondary education since Independence, the participation of girls in Papua New Guinea is still relatively low.

3. Women's Status. The status of women is a phrase covering many social and economic characteristics that effect women's lives. In other countries it has been found that among the causes of women's ill health and mortality, as well as of high fertility, their low status is a major contributing factor. The reproductive period is particularly stressful and puts at risk women's lives. Availability of health and family planning services is only one element in any efforts to enhance women's health conditio ns and lower fertility. Improvement of women's sta tus is an essential ingredient which may be encouraged by the Government with appropriate policies. In PNG, the recent adoption of a national policy on the status of women testifies to the Government's goal to improve the status of women.

CONCLUSIONS

I have listed here many important topics concerning population and family planning that will no doubt be discussed in depth in the following days, and will hopefully provide a good framework to the PNG Government for placing in motion the implementation of the enunciated population policy. There are in Asia and elsewhere many good examples of what works and doesn't work in population and family planning, and the Government has already shown keen interest in learning from other experiences. The record is good for fertility reduction in island territories although there is only limited scientific evidence of why this may be so. The record is full of success stories: Taiwan and Singapore in the early years of family planning, followed by Sri Lanka and Indonesia, and outside Asia, Mauritius and Jamaica. But limits in territory are not the only factors in those successful stories of fertility reduction. All the other contributing factors mentioned here have no doubt played a significant role; education, women's health and status, age at marriage and most prominently, good family planning services.

In the field of population and family planning, difficult challenges lie ahead, for donors as well as governments. For the development assistance agencies it will be important to:

a) significantly increase the financial assistance for population programmes which is necessary if governments are to achieve the 40% increase in contraceptive use by the year 2000 implied by the UN medium population projections;

b) carefully assess the lessons of experience from countries which have already successfully made the demographic transition, and assist in the dissemination and application of these lessons to other countries seeking to achieve the same transition; and

c) ensure effective coordination of assistance between the assistance agencies. To that effect, the World Bank is working closely with UNFPA, the Asian Development Bank and other international and bilateral agencies in the planning of population programme assistance.

For the Papua New Guinea Government, the official launch today of the National Population Policy is only a first, although essential, step: this stage must be followed by the development of appropriate strategies and their effective implementation. I am confident you can achieve these next steps, in line with the many other examples of the present Government taking bold and aggressive initiatives, including the increased attention to investments in health and education and the protection of the environment through the Tropical Forests Action Plan.

Papua New Guinea has now embarked on the challenging path of slowing down the pace of population growth. The World Bank, as well as other donors stand ready to help.

I have the pleasure to hand over the floor to the participants for what I trust will be very fruitful discussions.

Thank you very much.

A KEYNOTE ADDRESS BY MR SAAD RAHEEM SHEIKH,

CHIEF ASIA AND THE PACIFIC DIVISION, UNITED NATIONS POPULATION FUND

UNFPA is honoured to be invited to this important Forum of the 19th Waigani Seminar which is held in the context of a very unique region in terms of its ecological characteristics as well as its cultural, social and economic systems. Our cooperation with the countries of this region goes back many years, and in looking at developments in the field of population over the last few decades it is evident that much progress has taken place. Internationally, there is now increasing awareness of the need to balance population and resources as well as to protect the environment to achieve sustainable development. It is also evident that governments are increasingly considering population needs in their overall development strategies. In this context, I am pleased to note the remarkable efforts of the Pacific countries of the region and wish to congratulate their governments for taking a leading role in the adoption of population policies and initiation of population programmes that are interlinked with programmes in health, education, housing and employment. Indeed, we are confident that it is only through such integrated programmes that the objective of sustainable development can be achieved.

In terms of identifying future directions, towards the attainment of population goals and objectives, the "International Forum on Population in the Twenty-First Century", held in Amsterdam in 1989, with participants from 79 countries, including Papua New Guinea and Fiji, in its Declaration clearly identified several basic requirements. These are:

- strengthening of political commitment;
- development of national strategies and programmes;
- acceleration and expansion of resource mobilization;
- strengthening of the role and status of women;
- strengthening of the quality, effectiveness and outreach of family planning and maternal and child health programmes and services in both the public and private sector;
- heightening of community awareness and participation at all levels in the formulation and implementation of programmes and projects based on priorities and needs expressed by the women and men involved;

- intensification of international co-operation in the sphere of population activities, especially directed and adapted to the specific conditions, particularly socio-cultural conditions, of recipient countries.

These recommendations received support from the United Nations General Assembly as well as the OECD's Development Assistance Committee. Further, DAC members, in a high level meeting in 1990, agreed that slowing population growth to permit sustainable development should be one of the major priorities in development cooperation in the 1990s and it was strongly felt that new initiatives are vitally needed, both nationally and internationally. In this context UNFPAA was identified as the major coordinating agency for population activities. Coordination in the population field has gained much importance as countries begin to implement more complex programmes, and as the number of donors active in this field have increased, as have the resources available. UNFPA works closely in partnership with WHO, ILO, ESCAP, UNESCO, FAO and UNDP in order to jointly deliver population programmes. We are also moving into active collaboration with the World Bank and the Asian Development Bank.

UNFPA is in its third decade of existence and is ready to meet formidable challenges that lie ahead. Indeed, UNFPA has recently instituted a comprehensive programme review and strategy development (PRSD) exercise to ensure an analytical and critical approach to population planning. It is with great pleasure that I inform you of the successful completion of such an exercise in the South Pacific region in March this year. The PRSD exercise consisted of a complete review of past experiences, an assessment of new and emerging needs and a list of recommendations for future action in terms of developing overall national and regional strategies. The exercise covered all major sectors in relation to population concerns including health, planning, education, communication, women and environment. Mr Chairman, permit me to share with you briefly some of the major findings of the mission.

Although there are many variations in countries of this region, there appear to be broad similarities as well. The review of the health sector identified various problem areas that need to be addressed. A common feature among most of the Pacific countries is high fertility levels and population growth rates which appears to range between 2% in Fiji, to 3.5% in Solomon Islands and 4.2% in Marshall Island. Although in some regions population growth rates are extremely low and even negative, this is largely due to contraceptive prevalence rates and high maternal and infant mortality rates. We have observed alarming figures particularly for some of the Melanesian countries. In some regions of PNG, maternal mortality rates are estimated to be one of the highest in the world. Further, we find that high fertility levels, combined with the decline of the mortality rate, have resulted in recent decades, in a very young population, 50% of which is under 20 years old. This has far reaching consequences for many of the already fragile sectors such as education, labour and health services. Also evident is a growth in teenage pregnancies.

It was encouraging to note that almost all countries of the region have adopted the primary health care approach, in which the provision of family planning is an integral part of its basic approach to health care. For the vast majority of the population, primary health care centres are the first referral institution in case of health care need. Yet it was found that most centres tend to be by-passed and under-utilized because they are inadequately staffed and lack medical supplies. It is clear that a major effort is needed to improve the services at the primary level. Areas of priority include upgrading the knowledge and skill of health workers, increasing community participation at health centres, promotion of child spacing, identification of pregnancies at risk, improvement in the distribution of contraceptives, and increased health education activities.

In reviewing the situation with regard to population policy, it was found that significant progress had been made in the last decade. Although not all countries have adopted a population policy, nearly all have, in their National Development Plans, identified specific issues relating to population trends and potential effects. The institutional arrangements for implementing population programmes, such as National Coordinating Committees or Population Development Units need to be further developed and supported. It was also found that the lack of adequately trained personnel has inhibited progress in policy formulation, integrated planning, and data collection, analysis and research. It was emphasized that the development of national and regional skills should be of high priority.

At a more basic level, is the need to have appropriate and accurate data and information. In this context much progress is evident. All countries in the region have carried out their censuses as part of the 1990 round of cesnsuses. These have provided essential information. The data could, however, be of greater use if certain issues are addressed; such as achieving consistency and comparability of data among countries, processing and publishing data with minimum time lag, and improving national capabilities to evaluate and analyze the data. Also identified is the need to improve upon civil registration systems, and the conducting of sample surveys.

With regard to population education, in recent years most countries have acknowledged its benefits as an intervention strategy in addressing population problems. However population education projects have been limited in scope, substance and delivery, as they were planned on an ad hoc basis and without an overall IEC framework. Hence the emphasis has been on the formal system, especially in curriculum and institutional materials development for secondary schools and in-service teacher training. There is a need to expand population education into primary school curricula, particularly in countries where there is a high drop-out rate after primary schooling. Population education should be reconceptualized in order to reflect new developments and emerging population-related social concerns and more innovative materials and methods need to be developed.

In the non-formal sector, which can play a vital role in support of population programmes, it was found that although there is a wide range of population IEC activities in the South Pacific. The need is to develop a more comprehensive strategy for population communication activities and programmes and appropriate infrastructure, including human resource development and the production of communication materials, for a wide spectrum of target groups, such as youth, women, policy-makers and planners, community development and health-care workers. The two most important channels of communication in reaching the target population in this region would appear to be the radio network and community-based outreach networks. These organizations are doing impressive work in the field of health and development, but need to be sufficiently mobilized for population IEC activities. Finally, it was emphasized that at all levels, the training of personnel such as curriculum developers, trainers, teachers, field workers, and other communicators, should be given high priority to achieve the desired effectiveness of population education programmes.

These are some of the issues identified by the PRSD mission in collaboration with the national governments of the South Pacific. We are pleased to inform you that the formal report will shortly be published and we hope to projectize its recommendations expeditiously. The importance of population as a dimension of development has been recognized. There is a need to adopt a multi-sectoral approach to programme development towards achieving common objectives of socio-economic development.

I would like to thank and congratulate the organizers of this seminar, for the excellent arrangements and for giving me the opportunity of addressing this important meeting.

KEYNOTE ADDRESS BY MR V. T. PALAN

Regional Director, International Planned Parenthood Federation, East South East Asia and Oceania Region

It is with great pleasure that I am able to address this 19th Waigani Seminar on behalf of International Planned Parenthood Federation (IPPF).

IPPF is not, I think, well known in the Pacific, although it now operates in over 130 countries of the world, including eight Pacific countries, and is the world's leading voluntary family planning organization. It works to promote and support family planning services internationally and to educate people and governments about the benefits for the whole family, particularly mothers and children, of spacing and planning births.

IPPF was founded in 1952 in Bombay by the volunteer leaders of national organizations dedicated to family planning. The International Office has always been in London. It is registered as a British Charity and in 1977 it was incorporated by Act of Parliament.

IPPF's policies are formulated and agreed by representatives of its member Family Planning Associations. These Associations elect representatives to Regional Councils which in turn elect representatives to the Central Council. This determines IPPF policies and directs the Federation's work. Every three years a Members' Assembly reviews the role of IPPF and considers the way its objectives can best be accomplished.

On behalf of its members, the Federation seeks active support for family planning at national and international levels, campaigning for policy and legal changes which will encourage the provision and voluntary use of family planning services. This advocacy work is carried out by member Associations and at a regional and international level through Parliamentary groups, through links with the media and through a publications programme.

It is for this reason that IPPF has supported this Waigani Seminar on Population, Family Health and Development in the form of a grant of US$30,000.00.

The relationships between Population, Family Health and Development, as they relate to family planning is well known. When the means are available to enable couples to plan their families properly, the health and survival of women and children improves and so overall family health and community well being is enhanced.

Similarly, a balance between human numbers, human needs and the natural resources on which we all depend is a necessary condition of human happiness, prosperity and peace.

I am told that there is plenty of fertile land in Papua New Guinea, but while this may be the overall situation, I strongly suspect that there are families, and villages, which suffer land shortages, when there are too many sons to share too little land.

And, on a slightly different note, I have also been told that all children in PNG are loved and cared for, if not by their natural mother, then by grandparents or an aunty and uncle. But yesterday morning I was approached in Boroko by a young, I might say grubby young boy, who was begging for money. Was he a wanted and loved child? We must face the facts that times are changing, and populations and ensuing problems are growing.

Within East and South East Asia and Oceania Region, which has a total population of 1.7 billion or nearly one third of the world's population, PNG has the highest Maternal Mortality Rate with figures like 1000/100,000, or one out of every hundred mothers, as compared with Hong Kong with only 4 per 100,000.

The Patron of the Seminar and Patron of PNG Family Planning Association, said during her opening address at the Pacific Islands Planned Parenthood Affiliation's Council Meeting held recently in Port Moresby, that the family planning acceptance rate among married women in PNG is less than 5%. This might be compared to 74% acceptance for women in China. Similarly, the Crude Birth Rate is 44.5% in Solomon Islands compared to 10.8% in Japan. The Population Growth Rate in Solomon Islands is 3.47% (highest in the Pacific) and 0.39% in Japan (the lowest in the world).

The government of Papua New Guinea recognizes this problem, and has recently adopted a National Population Policy which includes in its objectives:

i. Slowing down the population growth rate by reducing fertility through shortening women's fertility span by promoting educational opportunity and the use of contraceptives.

ii. Promoting understanding of population dynamics in relation to social and economic development among decision makers and opinion leaders at national, provincial and local levels, and among the population at large.

iii. Expanding family planning information, education and services.

Included in the third point is a commitment that by 1995, 90% of all Aidposts will provide family planning services. But to simply provide services is not enough. What, for example, of the problem of male Aid Post Orderlies not being able to discuss the intimate details of family planning with female clients? Or the problem, that women are most often the acceptors of contraceptives, but it is the husband who normally makes the decisions.

There is a tremendous need for information, education and motivation, or as we in the family planning business call it, IEM services. IEM services not only for the general public so they can make rational choices in planning their families, but also training for all these Aid Post Orderlies and other health related workers. This is an immense undertaking in itself, without considering the logistics of providing actual services deliver; for example, how to keep all these Aidposts supplied with contraceptives.

Your Prime Minister, in his closing address to the PIPPA Council Meeting (the same meeting which his wife opened), recognized the problem when he said.

> ".....we are increasingly recognizing that governments alone cannot achieve the kind of progress that is necessary in these areas without the direct involvement and support of non-government organizations."

Volunteer, or non-government organizations, have emerged in recent years to be one of the most effective and influential channels and means of promoting population and development programmes and objectives.

For the past twenty years there has been official universal acceptance that access to family planning information and services is a basic human right. Although still denied to millions of men and women, this right was endorsed by the one hundred and fifty seven governments which participated in the International Conference on Human Rights, in 1968. It has since been repeatedly restated in international forums with increasing specificity, making it clear, for instance, that this is a right of individuals as well as parents, and of the young as well as those in established conjugal unions.

The human right to family planning is slowly beginning to find expression in national constitutions. It has called into question much archaic legislation such as the French law of 1920, now abrogated by France and several countries in Africa which were its former colonies. After much debate, Canada amended its Criminal Code in 1969 to legalize family planning and five Latin American countries - Ecuador, Mexico, Peru, Guatemala and Brazil - have declared family planning and responsible parenthood as constitutional rights.

This right is fundamental to the establishment of equal rights for men and women since it underscores the right of women to control and manage their own fertility, thus enabling them to enjoy other human rights, for example, the right to good health. The momentous Alma Ata Declaration on Primary Health Care in 1978 identified family planning as an essential component of health care.

The United Nations Convention on the Elimination of All Forms of Discrimination Against Women (CEDAW) requires member states to eliminate discrimination against women and promote their right to health care, including family planning.

Governments which are signatories to international instruments and have ratified conventions such as CEDAW have an obligation to offer all their citizens family planning information and services.

This obligation is more often honored in theory than in practice, because, as in other social sectors such as education, resources to do so are inadequate, or because lack of commitment and conviction about family planning persists. This applies even in countries where family planning is an acknowledged constitutional right, underscoring the gap that must be closed before right becomes reality.

Government attitude has perhaps been ambivalent in the Pacific Islands where the formulation of national population policies began only quite recently. In several Pacific countries, the term "Family Planning" is still considered unacceptable through its associations with limiting family size, although the promotion of child spacing is officially encouraged.

Governments, being sensitive to public opinion, naturally shy away from being seen as actively trying to limit the number of children a couple, or community, should have, even though this is not necessarily the prime focus of family planning programmes.

This is where voluntary agencies, like IPPF can assist. But we must then address the criticism that a large, multinational agency may not be sensitive to the unique local situation or needs of a small Pacific country.

A major characteristic of the IPPF structure is a network of independent, indigenous, national family planning associations. Each member country of IPPF, including the eight Pacific countries, have their own Family Planning Association which is based on a volunteer structure which brings together a number of individuals from a variety of backgrounds, who set the overall policy objectives for their FPA. The necessary staff are then employed to carry out these policies.

IPPF then supports those FPAs who choose to become members of IPPF through cash grants for projects and administration costs as well as for contraceptives and other commodities required for the programmes. The only real conditions for membership in IPPF are that the constitution of the FPA contain certain basic conditions such as the right of every individual to make a free choice, there can be no coercion in the IPPF system, and that they are engaged in activities which support the four constitutional objectives of IPPF, namely:

* Advance the education of the world's peoples in family planning and responsible parenthood.

* Preserve and protect the good health, both mental and physical, of parents, children and young people, through promoting and supporting effective family planning services.

* Educate people in the demographic problems of their own communities and of the world.

* Stimulate appropriate research into all aspects of human fertility and its regulation and to make known the findings of such research.

An example of the type of support which IPPF gives the Pacific FPAs is the Basic Essential Clinic Standards project. A consultative group of experts has met and has established the minimum standards which Pacific family planning clinics should maintain. A Minimum Essential Clinic Standards manual is being produced, along with laminated display posters, for use by Pacific FPAs. Once the manual has been field tested, it will be made available to other NGO and government agencies. Also, later this year, a family planning consultant will visit those Pacific FPAs which operate clinics to ensure that there is adequate training to be able to maintain these minimum standards.

In the Pacific, due to the unique geographical conditions of the region, the eight member FPAs have joined together to form the Pacific Islands Planned Parenthood Affiliation or PIPPA. The main objectives of PIPPA are:

* To contribute towards the preservation and protection of the health, both physical and mental, of parents, children and young people of the Pacific Islands through the promotion of education in responsible parenthood and by supporting effective, voluntarily-accepted family planning services.

* To promote the exchange of information and stimulate new programmes through the organization of conferences, meetings and other means.

* To strengthen member organizations and encourage the establishment of organizations in countries where none exist.

The member organizations are Cook Islands Family Welfare Association, Family Planning Association in Fiji, Family Planning Association of Papua New Guinea, Solomons Islands Planned Parenthood Association, Tonga Family Planning Association, Tuvalu Family Health Association, Vanuatu Family Health Association and Western Samoa Family Health Association.

In the medium term the FPA members of PIPPA will focus on strengthening family planning in the Pacific through the following strategies.

Service Delivery: The coverage and accessibility of FP services will be increased through an expansion of clinic and in particular community-based and commercial distribution networks to reach the rural communities.

The range and quality of contraceptive, health and IEM services will continue to be improved with more support for the development of monitoring, evaluation and training.

IEM: Programmes for the dissemination of accurate information about FP methods will be strengthened through the expanded use of the media and personnel.

The needs of young people for population, FLE and sex education will be met through an expanded programme for those both in and out of school.

The "Training of Trainers" such as teachers and youth workers in the content and process of FLE will increase the capacity of FPAs in this area.

Advocacy: FPAs will continue to work with the grassroots and political leaders in their countries to raise awareness of the contribution of FP to social and economic development, and to support the formulation of nation population policies. The formation of FPAs in the remaining Pacific countries will be supported through PIPPA and the work of the Regional Bureau.

<u>Resource Development</u>: Recruitment and training of more grassroots volunteers, particularly women and young people, will see further development and programme expansion.

PIPPA will be seeking additional sources for external donor funding to finance the expansion of the Pacific FP programme.

<u>Management and Organizational Development</u>: This will be encouraged and supported by the Regional Bureau to improve the capacity of the FPAs to implement high quality, cost-effective programmes.

The way in which each FPA chooses to implement these objectives will vary according to preference and country situations. For example, the Family Planning Association of Fiji concentrates primarily on the production of IEM materials whereas Tonga uses part-time village level workers who combine lessons in traditional weaving with family planning discussions.

Western Samoa combines a parasite eradication programme with their family planning activities and are considering expanding this to include such community health programmes as pit latrines.

CONCLUSION

The problems are well known, the solutions have been identified, all that remains is the collective will to make the necessary resources available.

In conclusion, I would like to quote the Secretary General of IPPF, Dr Halfdan Mahler who said, when speaking in Japan;

> "I would hope that in the '90s when we mention rationales like human rights, health and development rationales, that we would add the moral rationale to try to help those hundreds of millions of women who already now want possibilities to make each and every child a wanted child.
>
> We know that the resources are perfectly within the capacity of both developing and industrialized countries and know that those involved in FP are the ones who are taking the moral high road and not those who oppose and thereby deny women and families their vital democratic right to have the number of children they can take good care of."

DEMOGRAPHIC TRENDS AND POPULATION CHANGES IN THE PACIFIC

Each of the Papers presented in this book touch in some way on fertility, mortality and other population issues. This Section looks quite specifically at demographic trends in the region from various perspectives, ranging from the Pacific Islands to studies of small communities within Papua New Guinea.

Geoffrey Hayes compares population statistics for Papua New Guinea with data from 39 other lower middle income countries. He claims that, in comparison with these countries, Papua New Guinea has a relatively low population growth rate, and that this is not a function of the use of modern contraceptives. **David King** also discusses the relatively slow growth of both the total population of PNG and its towns during the 1980s. He describes patterns of urbanisation in Papua New Guinea and the increasing primacy of the major towns.

The **National Statistical Office** gives an overview of population trends in Papua New Guinea, looking at Census Statistics from as early as 1919, and **H.N. Shankar** provides a similar picture of Fiji with particular emphasis on differences between the two major ethnic groups.
Cherry Galo describes basic population trends in the Solomon Islands and Ministry of Health activities directed towards introducing Family Planning to the population.
Richard Taylor et al describe mortality patterns and identify factors which affect the health status of the populations of Pacific Island countries, while
Carol Jenkins looks at demographic changes within Papua New Guinea, with particular reference to the incidence of sexually transmitted diseases and their effect on fertility.

In two studies on a more micro level, **Deborah Lehmann** et al look at major events which have affected demographic trends in Tari in the Southern Highlands of PNG over the past sixty years. **Faridah and Rod Tilbury** discuss urban migration from the isolated Mt Brown area of Papua New Guinea and its effect on that community.

This Section comprises an excellent balance of Papers, which in combination give us a fascinating demographic picture of the Pacific region.

....

JOHN SHADLOW
Technical Editor
Geography Department
University of Papua New Guinea

THE DEMOGRAPHIC SITUATION IN PAPUA NEW GUINEA AND ITS POLICY IMPLICATIONS: AN INTERNATIONAL PERSPECTIVE

GEOFFREY HAYES[1]

INTRODUCTION

Among the social sciences, demography and economics are distinctive for their strong emphasis on quantification and statistical analysis. Attempts to understand the interaction between demographic and economic systems therefore involves a substantial exposure to statistics produced by the quite distinctive methodologies of these two disciplines. Indeed, some interpretations of the relationship between population and economic development see the issue simply as a race between two rates of growth: the rate of population increase on the one hand, and the rate of growth in Gross National Product on the other. This approach to the problem is appealing in its simplicity, but like many other uses of statistics it can be quite misleading (Huff 1954).

Like other scientific facts, demographic and economic statistics do not speak for themselves: their meaning and significance must be interpreted from some perspective. Furthermore, it cannot be assumed that only one perspective is possible; not only are there competing scientific paradigms in the population-development field (as in any other area of science), but the meaning or significance of a statistic may vary according to whether policy choices or other issues are at stake. Similarly, it is important to acknowledge that population change affects different interest groups in a population in different ways. Rapid population growth, for example, may be beneficial for a business class interested in maintaining the lowest possible cost of labour power, but workers' representatives may prefer a lower rate of growth in order to reduce competition in the labour market in the longer term and to maintain or increase wage rates. Viewed as a mediating force between groups, or as a manager of physical and human resources, the state has a special role to play in framing population issues and defining problems, but in this respect the state is merely one interest group among others--albeit often the dominant one.

[1] Department of Geography
University of Papua New Guinea

From a scientific viewpoint, the most important use of statistics is in the formulation or testing of scientific theories or models. Although some theoretical issues will be discussed in this paper, the primary aim is to place some of the often-quoted statistics on the demographic situation in PNG into a comparative international perspective. Such a perspective should promote a better understanding of what features of PNG's demographic situation can be considered typical of Less Developed Countries (LDCs) as a group and what features are unique--or at least distinctive. As the Pacific Islands region has increasingly attracted the attention of the international population agencies in recent years, a tendency to over-generalize from other world regions has become apparent. However, universalistic models based on such rough-cut categories as "the Third World", may seriously distort the demographic and economic realities of the region, and provide a misleading guide for policy formulation. This is especially problematic in the case of PNG which, as this paper argues, has a number of features not commonly found elsewhere in the developing world--or in other countries of the Pacific Islands region.

The paper also attempts to draw attention to the wide variation in the demographic characteristics of PNG's provinces and regions. Any attempt to formulate, or implement, public policies relating to population factors in development should take these internal variations into account as well.

POPULATION GROWTH IN PNG SINCE 1966

The size of the total population and its annual growth rate are the most commonly reported demographic statistics, both for individual countries and the world population in aggregate. Although it is useful to know the growth rate for a single year, or a small range of years, such a statistic only becomes truly meaningful as part of a time-series. Demographic change occurs slowly by comparison with the unstable fluctuations of economic systems. In those European societies which became unified nation-states in the 17th and 18th century, or in such transplanted European societies as the United States and Canada, historical series are available for 200 years or more, and such data-sets can reveal a great deal about the role of population in societal development. In the Pacific Islands region, the longest series go back only to the turn of this century, while in PNG, the earliest reliable growth rates for the country as a whole only date back to the mid 1960s. National level censuses were conducted in PNG in 1966, 1971, 1980 and 1990, resulting in population totals of 2.2, 2.5, 3.0, and 3.7 million persons respectively (Table 1). Thus, between the first national census in 1966 to the most recent in 1990, the population of PNG has increased by approximately 1.5 million persons. These figures imply an average annual growth rate over the 1966-90 period of 2.2 percent (Table 1).

Trends in the population growth rate

As figure 1 shows, the growth rate of PNG's total population (citizens and non-citizens) has remained at 2.1 percent per year on average for the past two intercensal periods (i.e., for almost two decades), whereas during the intercensal period 1966-71, the growth rate averaged 2.6 percent. The growth rate has therefore been declining since the mid-1960s, but this decline seems to have levelled-off in the past decade.

Some observers have suggested that the real population growth rate in Papua New Guinea during the last decade is higher than indicated by the census counts. A report to a Committee of the Australian Parliament prepared by the National Centre for Development Studies (NCDS 1989,3) claimed that the present growth rate was above three percent. Some international agencies have also reported rates above 2.5 percent (United Nations 1985; United Nations, ESCAP 1988; Kane and Lucas 1986). The basis on which these higher rates of growth have been estimated is not always made clear, but they generally derive either from the population projections prepared by the National Statistical Office following the 1980 census, or on United Nations projections.1 Since all population projections are based on assumptions, the selection of a specific population projection out of a set is necessarily a subjective procedure, and the possibility of error caused by professional or other biases is considerable. The use of projections to determine what the growth rate should be, in the absence of empirically based studies of what it actually is, is a questionable statistical procedure.

Independent verification of the intercensal growth rate is difficult to obtain in the absence of a reliable birth and death registration system in Papua New Guinea, but indirect estimation of birth and death rates based on 1966, 1971, and 1980 census data, give results generally consistent with what the census counts themselves show--as indicated in Table 2.

---

1 The figure given in United Nations ESCAP (1988) was derived from the Medium Variant of United Nations projections. The figure cited by Kane and Lucas (1986) appears to have been taken from U.S. Census Bureau sources.

While the time periods to which the percentage growth rates shown in Table 2 apply do not correspond precisely to the intercensal periods for which the rates in Table 1 were calculated, they do suggest similar rates of natural increase as the census counts themselves. The exception is the 1966-71 period which, according to the data in Table 1, had an average annual growth rate of 2.6 percent, while the 1966 census estimates suggested a rate of natural increase of only 2.2 percent annually. Both of these figures could be correct if there was a significant net inflow of international migrants during the intercensal period. For the other periods, it is reasonable to assume that international migration has made no net contribution to population growth. Because the methods used to obtain the results shown in Table 2 are subject to various errors (e.g., due to mis-statement of age), one cannot state with absolute certainty that the census results are confirmed, but there is no gross inconsistency between the two sets of data, and there is no reason to question that they were independently arrived at.[2]

The possibility of error in census counts must obviously be acknowledged. It is highly unlikely that any of PNG's censuses achieved full coverage of the entire population;[3] but this does not mean that the growth rates calculated from the census data are necessarily invalid. This conclusion would only follow if it were possible to reliably measure the undercount for each successive census, and to show that the undercount in any one census was higher or lower than the census preceding it, i.e., that there was a <u>relative</u> undercount. If the size of the undercount were known for only one census, it would only be possible to estimate the accuracy of the subsequent census if reliable birth, death, and migration statistics for the intercensal period were available. Unfortunately this is not the case in Papua New Guinea; although international migration figures are probably of reasonable accuracy, birth and death statistics are incomplete.

Regional variations in population growth

The other main conclusion which can be drawn from Table 1 and Figure 1 is that there is considerable variation in population growth rates, and their trends through time, between PNG's regions. In broad terms, the Islands and South Coast regions have similar patterns of change over the past two decades (a decline during the 1971-80 period followed by an increase in the 1980-90 period). The North

---

2 The two sets of data would not be independent if the methods used to produce the estimated birth and death rates had been selected because they produced results consistent with the intercensal growth rates. Inspection of the sources shown in Table 2 provide no reason to believe that this was the case.

3 Indeed, the 1966 and 1971 censuses did not aim at full coverage in the rural areas where sampling methods were used. Full coverage was attempted only in urban areas.

Coast and the Highlands regions, on the other hand, show a more consistent downward trend. Because the latter two regions together account for 63 percent of the total population, the national pattern of change is obviously affected by them and follows a similar--if less distinct--pattern.

The most notable and perhaps unexpected feature of Figure 1 is the jump in the growth rate in the South Coast and Islands regions in the 1980-90 intercensal period (by 44 percent in the former and 25 percent in the latter) compared to the previous intercensal period. The most likely explanation for this is a further decline in the crude death rate in these regions since 1980 accompanied by little change in the crude birth rate; but until the results of the 1991 Demographic and Health Survey (to be carried out by the National Statistical Office) are available this is a matter of speculation.

INTERNATIONAL PERSPECTIVES ON POPULATION GROWTH IN PNG

Accepting that PNG's overall population growth rate is presently around 2.1 percent annually, how does this compare with other countries, world regions, or the global average? Some summary statistics for various categories of countries and the world as a whole for the mid-1980s are presented in Table 3. It will be seen that, while PNG's growth rate is above the world average of 1.7 percent, it is otherwise unexceptional. Indeed, PNG's growth rate is identical to the average for LDCs during the first half of the 1980s, and is below the rate for the least developed countries during this period. PNG also falls well below the current rate of growth in Africa (3.0%) and is about half the growth rate in Kenya (4.3%)--the highest current growth rate of any nation-state (United Nations 1990, 174).4

Recent articles in PNG newspapers have claimed that PNG's population growth rate is "amongst the highest in the world", and this has been repeated by some high Government officials.5 The information presented in Table 3 suggests that such a statement is inaccurate, or at least misleading. If we accept that the rate of growth is around 2.1 percent annually, then PNG's growth rate is identical to that of the less developed countries as a group and to the Pacific Islands region as a whole.

---

4 It is worth noting that Kenya has had a government-sponsored family planning programme since the 1960s but this has had little impact on fertility rates (Frank and McNicoll 1987).

5 The statement appears to have originated from the National Statistical Office. See *Post-Courier*, 1 May 1991.

Criteria for international comparison

Such broad-based comparisons as above are useful only up to a point. What is perhaps a more interesting question is how PNG compares with countries with similar socio-economic characteristics? The answer to this question obviously depends upon what constitutes a "similar" country. The usual criterion employed by demographers working in the Pacific region is a geographical/cultural one whereby PNG is compared with other Pacific Island countries, or more specifically, with its near "Melanesian" neighbours. Indeed, demographers have frequently used the demographic parameters of Solomon Islands and Vanuatu as standards against which the validity of estimates for PNG might be judged on the grounds that all three are Melanesian in culture. What this approach fails to acknowledge is that "Melanesia" is by no means a unified cultural area. For example, neither Solomon Islands nor Vanuatu has more than one third of its population living in a highlands region as does PNG. Both the Solomon Islands and Vanuatu are predominantly Oceanic cultures, similar certainly to the Islands region of Papua New Guinea, but dissimilar in some demographically important respects from the Highlands cultures of the interior of the PNG mainland.

Furthermore, it makes little sense to compare PNG with the Pacific Islands average, since, as the largest population in the region (63 percent of the total), it makes the greatest contribution to regional averages, so this is virtually comparing PNG with itself. Comparing PNG with the other Pacific Island countries as a group is also problematic: with the possible exception of Fiji, all Pacific countries other than PNG contain small populations; the population of PNG's smallest province (Manus) is larger than eight Pacific Island countries or territories, and if PNG's most populous provinces were nation-states, they would make up eight of the top ten countries in the region after Fiji and Solomon Islands. These considerations suggest that while Pacific-wide comparisons are useful to a degree, in the case of PNG other bases of comparison may be more appropriate and revealing.

Lower Middle Income Countries

An alternative comparative reference employed in this paper is an economic one, namely the group of countries classified by the World Bank as "Lower Middle Income" in the early 1980s and having populations of one million population or more (World Bank 1984). This income group includes countries with a Gross National Product (GNP) per capita of between $US450 and $US1,600 in the early 1980s. With a GNP per capita of $US820 in 1982, Papua New Guinea falls about in the middle of this range. For comparative purposes, Fiji has been added to the group--even though its population does not reach the one million mark--since it fits into this income class and is the next largest to PNG in the Islands region.. In total there were 39 countries in this income category in the early 1980s with an aggregate population of 670 million. Some basic demographic and other socio-economic indicators have been compiled in Table 4 from which most of the data discussed in following sections have been derived.

It is clear from Table 4 that very few countries in this income range had an annual population growth rate below PNG's. Only Thailand (2.0%), Lebanon (2.0%) and Cuba (1.0%) had lower growth rates while all the remaining countries had higher rates. The average for the group as a whole was 2.5 percent. From this perspective, PNG's growth rate is exceptional only insofar as it is somewhat below average for countries at a similar economic level. The truly exceptional countries in the group are Cuba (1.0%), at the low end of the scale, and Zimbabwe (4.2%) at the other extreme.

IMPLICATION OF PNG'S GROWTH RATE FOR DEVELOPMENT

It does not, of course, follow from the discovery that PNG is a rather average developing country in demographic terms that concern about the rate of growth can therefore be dismissed; it merely provides a basis for rejecting the more extremist characterizations of PNG's demographic situation which have appeared in the popular press and elsewhere.

Assessing the implications of a particular population growth rate for a country's economic development or general social welfare is a difficult matter. Statistical approaches usually emphasize the exponential nature of population growth, with the "doubling time" of a population becoming shorter as the rate of growth increases. Thus, a population growing continuously at 2.1 percent will double in 33 years, whereas a population growing at 3.5 percent will double in 20 years. The inference is often drawn from this that such periods represent the time during which existing social and economic infrastructure and trained personnel will also have to be doubled (schools and teachers, hospitals and doctors, roads, ports, etc.). Such an approach naturally leads to consideration of whether the social and economic institutions of a country are capable of responding to such rapidly increasing demands--usually with pessimistic conclusions. The validity of such an inference depends on three assumptions: (1) that the rate of growth will continue at its current level; (2) that the existing infrastructure is unable to absorb further numbers; (3) that the current population size is such that no further economies of scale, or other efficiencies, are possible. Whether these assumptions are valid (especially 2 and 3) requires careful analysis of the institutional characteristics of the particular country in question.

Another important concept in this context is the notion of "population momentum". This refers to the tendency of a population to keep on growing well beyond the point when the average couple is merely replacing itself. This phenomenon is caused by the fact that in populations in which fertility rates have recently declined from high levels, a high proportion of the population is in the reproductive age groups. Consequently, the absolute number of new members being added to the population will tend to decrease slowly, or possibly increase, before eventually declining--even though fertility rates have declined to low levels. The concept of population momentum can be given mathematical expression in terms of a multiplier referring to the total amount a population is likely to grow before achieving zero, or near zero, population growth (Chesnais 1990; World Bank 1984, 254). Here too, however, such statistics can only be derived from assumptions regarding the length of time which is likely to pass before fertility rates decline to replacement levels. Moving that time closer to the present may be one of the objectives of population policy, thus reducing the ultimate size that the population will reach before stabilizing. How urgent a matter this is from an economic point of view depends upon the size that the population has already attained relative to the present economy of the country or its future prospects. An assessment of the latter quite obviously goes beyond purely quantitative questions or strictly demographic factors.

In the PNG case, the concept of population momentum can be illustrated by the increase in the numbers being added to the population between the last intercensal period and the one preceeding it. Between 1971 and 1980, about 58,000 persons were being added (net) per year, while in the recent intercensal period (1980-90) the annual increment increased to 68,400. In the past decade, then, the total increase was about 684,000 persons--equivalent to the 1981 population of Fiji. If the population growth rate remained at 2.1 percent per year through to the end of the century, the number of persons being added to the population per year would increase to about 86,000, and would reach 100,000 by about 2003. At an annual increment of 100,000 persons per year, the population of PNG would be growing by one million persons per decade.

These numbers provide a more intuitively meaningful grasp of the implications of a particular growth rate than does the rate itself. Similarly, it seems intuitively unlikely that PNG could continue to absorb an additional one million persons per decade while simultaneously increasing the level of living per capita. It should be acknowledged, however, that the perceived inability of PNG to absorb such numbers is only partly a function of the numbers themselves, but also relates to the low level of administrative and managerial capacity within the state bureaucracy, even to maintain a reasonable level of services to the current population.

In order to offset population momentum and to stabilize the numbers being added each year to no more than the 1980-90 average (68,400), PNG's population growth rate would need to decline to about 1.7 percent during the next decade--a reduction of about 19 percent over the current rate. If it is assumed that a reduction of this magnitude is also dependent upon the quality and quantity of government services (e.g., family planning) a similar skepticism is probably justified.

DETERMINANTS OF POPULATION GROWTH IN PNG: INTERNATIONAL COMPARISONS

National level

For policy and other purposes, it is important to acknowledge that the same population growth rate can result from various combinations of birth and death rates, and that these combinations change through time. Figure 2 has been constructed to show birth and death rates separately--along with the population growth rates which result from their combination--for the group of lower middle income countries listed in Table 4. For comparative reference, the birth and death rates for the world population in aggregate, Australia and New Zealand, and Sweden, have been added to the graph.

The extremes in the global demographic situation are represented on this figure by Sweden with zero population growth (determined by a birth rate and death rate both around 10 per 1,000), and Zimbabwe at the other extreme with annual growth above 4 percent. Among the lower middle income countries (i.e., excluding Australia/New Zealand and

Sweden), Papua New Guinea falls somewhat below the mean growth rate. PNG's particular combination of birth and death rates is identical with its nearest western neighbour, Indonesia, and similar to Peru and Egypt. In terms of the overall growth rate, only Lebanon and Thailand had a lower rate than PNG, due in each case to both lower death and birth rates.

Another conclusion which can be drawn from Figure 2 is that while PNG's death rate is average for this group of countries, its birth rate is below average, thus producing a lower than average growth rate. In a sense, then, what needs to be explained about PNG is why its birth rate is low relative to its death rate (with the exception of Zimbabwe, all the countries with a higher death rate also have a higher birth rate, and in some cases substantially so). It is perhaps also worth reflecting on why PNG's birth and death rates in the early 1980s were identical to those of Indonesia, its nearest Southeast Asian neighbour. That these two countries would have similar death rates is not particularly surprising in view of the low levels of per capita incomes in both places, but the similar birth rate is somewhat puzzling. In recent years, Indonesia has instituted a reputedly highly successful family planning programme, and this is evident in the high proportion of married women employing some form of contraception (53 percent according to Table 4). In PNG, the proportion of married women using contraception is said to be around 6 percent (Muirden 1982); yet the birth rate is the same as Indonesia's.[6] One hypothesis which might be inferred by such figures is that the proportion of the population using contraception is not the primary determinant of a country's birth rate--at least not among lower middle income countries. This hypothesis is examined further below.

In comparative terms, PNG's demographic situation would seem to fit about mid-way between African countries (with high birth and death rates), and Latin American and Asian countries with generally lower birth and death rates. On balance, however, it is closest to the Asian/Latin American pattern.

Provincial variations

In the previous discussion of regional variations in population growth rates in PNG, the rates of growth referred to were based on enumerated populations at the various census points; thus inter-provincial and international migration were included as causes of growth. In this section we refer only to rates of *natural increase*-

6 Survey data collected in 1980 by Agyei (1988) suggests that 13.1 percent of rural women and 20.8 percent of urban were currently using modern forms of contraception, but the sample appears to have been biased in favour of women with more than primary education (McMurray 1985, 11).

-the balance of births minus deaths--thus the direct effects of migration are excluded. The wide variation in rates of natural increase between provinces is clearly evident from Figure 3, but it is also clear that provincial rates are largely a function of the region to which the province belongs. Thus, the Islands provinces other than Manus all fall at the high end of the range with growth rates between 2.7 and 3.5 percent, while the Highlands provinces are clustered at the low end of the range with rates of natural increase ranging downwards from 1.8 to 1.3 percent.

The same data are superimposed upon a map of PNG in Figure 4, which shows two distinctive geographical patterns. The first pattern is an east-west one: that is, no province to the west of Central Province has a growth rate above 2.4 percent, and no province to the east of Central Province has a growth rate below 2.5 percent. The second geographical pattern is a concentric one: the low growth rate provinces (below 2.0%) are clustered in the Highlands interior; the medium growth (above 2.0% and below 3.0%) provinces are--with some important exceptions--located on the north and south coasts, while high rates (3.0% and above) are found in the two Islands provinces of West New Britain and North Solomons.

An understanding of the socio-economic determinants of these variations requires, first of all, a breakdown of their demographic determinants, i.e., birth and death rates. This has been done in Figure 5 which shows the extremely wide variation between provinces in the two rates, and the absence of a clear general relationship between them. Actually, regression analysis suggests that there is a weak negative relationship (R2=0.11) between the crude birth rate and the crude death rate. This relationship is shown by the regression line plotted on the same data in Figure 6. The implication here is that to the extent that there is any relationship between these variables, among PNG's provinces higher birth rates tend to be associated with lower death rates. In countries undergoing demographic modernization (the "demographic transition") this relationship is normally positive, i.e., higher birth rates are associated with higher death rates. In PNG the relationship--although quite weak--is in the opposite direction, .

The main point here is that in Papua New Guinea provincial variations in the rate of natural increase cannot be explained by one of its determinants alone. That is, the variation between the provinces is not a function of a similar birth rate accompanied by varying death rates--or vice versa. Rather, both birth and death rates vary seemingly independently of each other. The extreme combinations are probably represented by West Sepik Province on the one hand with a high death rate and a moderate birth rate, and the North Solomons Province on the other with a high birth rate and a low death rate.

An explanation of the socio-economic determinants of these provincial level variations in natural increase is beyond the scope of this paper, but some hypotheses for further investigation can be suggested. The condition most in need of explanation is the association of high mortality and low fertility in the Highlands, West Sepik Province, and, to a lesser extent, Gulf Province. High mortality in these areas is perhaps a function of the low level of development combined with a physical environment conducive to high rates of infectious disease, as well as presenting substantial obstacles to the delivery of health services. The Highlands provinces were also the last in PNG to be contacted by more technologically advanced societies; thus, education and general literacy levels remain low compared to the coastal and Island provinces.

Some of these factors may also explain the low levels of fertility found in the low-growth provinces. Venereal disease in females may have resulted in a significant proportion of women of child-bearing age suffering from secondary sterility.7 The lower level of development and relatively slow pace of socio-cultural change will also have left intact many traditional institutions, practices, and beliefs which have kept fertility at relatively low levels in the past. It is also possible that the low female life expectancy (40-45 years) in these provinces may have had some depressing affect on fertility because many women's reproductive lives will have been cut short by their premature death; but this is unlikely to be a major factor.

FUTURE DIRECTIONS?

Given the short history of census-taking in PNG, it is difficult to describe recent population trends, let alone predict future patterns of change in the population with any confidence. As a technical matter, it is certainly not difficult to project a population forward into the future on the basis of *assumptions* about what the future trends in births, deaths, and international migration might be; this is simply a mathematical procedure made increasily easy to carry out with the advent of powerful microcomputers. It is also not difficult with the aid of such computers to show populations growing very rapidly to enormous sizes and impossible densities within a few generations. Such simplistic methodologies are more often employed for ideological than for scientific reasons; as devices for convincing the naive that a population "explosion" is

7 Dr Glen Mola, personal communication. Also see the paper presented at the Waigani Seminar by Dr Deborah Lehmann.

imminent, such projections can be effective elements in population "education" programmes, but they have little bearing upon real planning decisions.

What is usually lacking from the projection approach is any systematic assessment of the *probability* that any of the assumptions might turn out to be true. In other words, to present a model, or theory, of how the population is likely to behave as a system. This is not an easy task since no single model of demographic evolution is generally accepted by demographers, and disagreement persists over some of the basic determinants of demographic change. One factor often pin-pointed to the exclusion of all others, is whether a country has a population policy and how effective it is if it has one. To some degree this is the approach taken by M.L. Bakker who prepared projections for PNG on the basis of 1980 census results (Bakker 1985). Of the five population "scenarios" prepared, three referred explicitly to potential policy approaches which might be adopted by the PNG government in the future: (1) Scenario "A" in which government would stress both family planning (lower fertility) and the quality of life (lower mortality); (2) Scenario "B", a "qualified pride in numbers" approach which would place less emphasis on family planning programmes than scenario A while retaining the emphasis on reduced mortality; (3) Scenario "E" in which government would encourage rapid decline in mortality while supporting measures to increase fertility. The rates of growth implied by each of these scenarios over the 1980-90 intercensal period were 2.2, 2.2, and 2.5 percent respectively.

We now know that none of these "scenarios" came to pass in that it was not until 1991 that an explicit population policy was officially announced by the government; thus policy (other than existing approaches to health and family planning) has had no effect on the population size up to 1990. In any case, it is possible to reject "Scenario E", since the 1990 census results (estimated population of PNG: 3.69 million) fell short of the 3.82 million expected under this set of assumptions. But it is also true that the 1990 count fell somewhat short of the total expected under scenarios "A" and "B" (3.70 and 3.73 million respectively) as well. On balance, however, the 1990 results were closer to what Bakker suggested could be expected under a moderate population policy (Scenario "A"), even though no such policy was in effect during the period.[8] Indeed, the recorded average annual growth rate for the 1980-90 period (2.1%) was slightly below the lowest rate suggested by the five projections carried out by Bakker (2.2%).

---

8 It is worth noting that in the short run (i.e., ten years) under Bakker's scenarios there is virtually no difference between the population expected under a moderate population policy, and under no policy at all.

With the advent of PNG's official population policy, it is now possible to assess the longer-term (1990-2000) plausibility of the projections prepared with 1980 demographic data. The pro-natalist scenario "E" can probably be dismissed as inapplicable, since there now appears to be a broad political consensus in PNG in favour of the reduction of fertility through stronger family planning programmes. While it is possible that future governments may back-track on this policy, the lack of controversy over the current policy,9 and the fact that it was initiated by the present opposition in Parliament and completed by their opponents, suggests that this is somewhat unlikely--unless some form of extra-Parliamentary opposition develops.

Scenario "B" also appears unlikely insofar as the idea that PNG as a nation needs more people to develop its natural resources seems to be in retreat as the early economic optimism of the post-independence period has waned. Certainly no significant public figure has pressed this argument in recent years. On the other hand, as Bakker indicated in discussing this scenario, there are likely to be many local groups which believe that larger numbers will increase their power over resources (especially land) viz-a-viz neighbouring groups, or will strengthen their demands for various government services, so a pro-natalist philosophy may persist in some less-developed areas. Whether such views will have a discernable effect on fertility rates in the face of government efforts in the opposite direction is uncertain, but seems unlikely--especially if substantial progress is made in the areas of female education.

Of the three projections, then, scenario "A" appears to be the most likely. It is consistent with the thrust of the current population policy, and with the population growth trend since 1980. If this projection turns out to be accurate, the growth rate would fall below 2.0 percent during the next five years (1990-95), and decline to 1.4 percent during the first decade of the next century. By 2015 the citizen population would reach 5.5 million and the annual growth rate would then be 1.2 percent. Looking again at Figure 5, the suggestion here is that by the year 2000, PNG as a whole would have a birth and death rate similar to where the Eastern Highlands Province was in 1980, and would continue to move downwards and to the left towards the one percent line as both fertility and mortality rates decreased.

Whether this scenario will come to pass is by no means certain, however. How much change is required in some provinces is apparent when one looks at the position of the

---

9 There has been public concern over the role of Depo Provera in the family planning programme, but generally speaking not over the goal of reducing fertility.

most modernized provinces in the country such as the National Capital District, East New Britain, and North Solomons Province. Substantial declines in fertility will be required in these provinces if the overall growth rate is to decline. On the other hand, declining mortality in the absence of declining fertility in the Highlands provinces could have a marked upward effect on the national growth rate, and more than offset any declines in fertility which might occur elsewhere. Since the Islands and South Coastal provinces only make up 37 percent of the total population, their impact on overall growth, even with high fertility, is much less than is the case for the North Coast and the Highlands, which collectively account for the remaining 63 percent.

Furthermore, fertility has probably reached a peak in the Islands region and it is reasonable to expect declines as the economic contradiction between high parity and the chances for upward social and economic mobility become increasingly apparent. In this sense, the Highlands and the North coast region may be the most important areas on which to focus population policy efforts.

POPULATION POLICY: DEVELOPMENT OR FAMILY PLANNING?

Obviously the demographic future of PNG depends on the determinants of demographic change and whether these are likely to change either as a result of economic development or government population policies. We can distinguish between two sets of views on what aspects of socio-economic change are crucial. One school of thought believes that economic development will bring down the population growth rate whether or not organized, government-sponsored, family planning programmes exist. This approach focusses mainly on the institutional or organizational context in which family-size motivations and goals are formed, and the structural conditions which produce wide disparities of wealth in developing countries. The other school of thought, prominent within the international technical assistance and family planning agencies, is that state-sponsored family planning programmes are both necessary and sufficient in themselves, regardless of the state or direction of development in the country, and regardless of the structural conditions of the economy and society. Thus, the "demand" for family planning services is assumed to exist but supplies and services are lacking or their costs are too high. There are various gradations of views which fall in between these extremes as well as approaches which attempt to combine aspects of the two. The following section considers the applicability of these views to the lower middle income countries (including PNG) and reviews some of the empirical data supporting each approach.

Economic growth and development

If the *level* of economic development (as measured by per capita income) determined the rate of population growth, we would expect to see a close association between these two variables across a range of countries. In the case of the lower middle income countries, this does not appear to be the case, as Figure 7 illustrates. The regression line suggests a very weak negative relationship between between the two variables (R2=0.06). While it is true that virtually none of the countries at the high income end of the range have growth rates above 3.0 percent, whereas several poor countries do, it is also true that some poorer countries have rates of growth substantially below countries at much higher income levels. (Papua New Guinea, Thailand, and Indonesia are good examples.)

The absence of a clear relationship between per capita income level and the rate of population growth is often mentioned in support of the argument that family planning programmes are more important than economic growth in bringing down the population growth rate. Thus, one might point to the fact that among the countries appearing in Figure 7, Indonesia and Thailand have the lowest population growth rates, while they have also had among the most vigorous family planning programmes in the Southeast Asia region. Unfortunately the rate of natural increase is not a good measure either of the success of family planning programmes or the effects of the level of living per capita on population growth. First of all, income per capita would affect both birth rates and death rates simultaneously, with off-setting consequences for the overall population growth rate. Thus, an increase in income per capita may tend to decrease the death rate faster than it decreases the birth rate, resulting in a higher growth rate. Second, some countries with very weak family planning programmes nevertheless have a relatively "low" rate of population growth. The situation of Papua New Guinea in this regard is interesting. Of the countries which are closest to it on Figure 7 in terms of per capita income and population growth (Thailand, Indonesia, Philippines and Egypt) all have had strong family planning programmes in the past, whereas PNG has had a weak programme. This raises the important question of why PNG's population growth rate should be similar to countries with strong family planning programmes, when its own programme is almost non-existent? One answer is that PNG has higher mortality. But while this explanation seems reasonable in the cases of Thailand, Philippines, and Egypt, it is not applicable in the case of Indonesia which has the same death rates as PNG. An obvious hypothesis is that fertility is kept down by a range of socio-cultural factors--such as prolonged breast-feeding (enforced by legal restrictions against bottle-feeding), long post-partum abstinence periods--as well as by high mortality and infectious disease rather than by the use of modern contraceptives provided by family planning programmes.

In order to eliminate the confounding effects of per capita GNP on mortality, it is necessary to look at the affect of economic development on fertility alone. Todaro (1981, 166) tested the hypothesis that per capita GNP was correlated with crude birth rates in 12 Less Developed Countries. Although there was a negative correlation between the two variables, it was very weak. I performed a similar regression analysis on the 32 countries in the lower middle income group using the Total Fertility Rate (TFR) as the measure of fertility. The results are shown in Figure 8 and suggest a much stronger (R2 = 0.38) inverse relationship than Todaro found in his smaller group of countries. There is little doubt, however, that the very wide range of TFRs in countries with per capita incomes between $US800 and $US1,000 has considerably weakened the general relationship, and it is clear that within this sub-group of countries the level of GNP per capita does not come close to explaining the average number of births per woman. What can be said with certainty is that countries with per capita GNP above $US1,300 (in 1982 values) do not have TFRs above 6; but there are apparently other ways to lower the TFR than simply increasing per capita GNP.

The position of PNG on Figure 8 suggests that relative to other countries in this income group, its TFR is slightly lower than it would be expected to be on the basis of its per capita GNP.

In attempting to explain the lack of a clear association between the level of development and fertility, Todaro (1981, 168) suggested that the distribution of income might be a more important variable than the actual level of per capita income, or its rate of growth. Todaro's analysis of the 12 Third World countries in his sample showed that countries with a more equal distribution of income do tend to have lower birthrates (Todaro 1981, 168), although the relationship is far from linear.[10] Unfortunately it was not possible to test this hypothesis among lower middle income countries as the required data were not available for more than a few cases.

The hypothesis has frequently been proposed that the key to reducing fertility rates, and thereby population growth, is a higher rate of economic growth.[11] Todaro (1981, 167) also tested this hypothesis with 12 Third World countries and found the relationship between crude birth rates and the rate of economic growth to be "tenuous" if such special cases of rapid economic growth as Taiwan and South Korea

---

10 I tested this relationship using the data provided by Todaro and found that $R^2 = 0.34$ with quite a large standard error.

11 This was the essence of the presentation by Professor Helen Hughes at the Waigani Seminar.

are removed from the sample. I also tested this hypothesis on lower middle income countries, again using the TFR as the measure of fertility rather than the crude birth rate. The results are shown in Figure 9 and it will be seen that there is a weak negative association ($R2 = 0.10$) between these variables, suggesting that in general the rate of economic growth is not a major determinant of fertility.[12] It is worth noting, however, that a number of countries which had relatively low fertility in relation to their level of GNP per capita (Indonesia, Thailand, and Egypt) were also among those which had recently experienced rapid economic growth (above 3.0% per year). Again, PNG's TFR was about where it would be predicted to be in relation to its rate of economic growth.

Todaro has also argued that higher rates of economic growth may be associated with fertility decline in those countries which distribute that economic growth such as to reduce the level of income inequality (Todaro 1981, 168). This is a plausible hypothesis but data were not available to test it among lower middle income countries.

It should be clear from the foregoing analysis that at least among lower middle income countries there is no simple relationship between population growth--or fertility taken alone--and either the level of GNP per capita or its rate of growth. Thus, policy approaches which assume that economic growth alone will bring about a fertility transition are probably mistaken. This does not mean that economic development is irrelevant to the process, only that economic growth--which is the quantitative rather than qualitative component of development--is inadequate by itself. It is possible, however, that GNP per capita must move beyond a certain threshold level before its relationship with fertility becomes strongly negative. There was a suggestion of this in Figure 8 with a much closer (negative) relationship being apparent between GNP per capita and total fertility at both the low and the high end of the income scale. Within the the income band US$700 to $US1,100 there is virtually no relationship between per capita GNP and fertility.

Fertility, Contraceptive use and family planning

The lack of a clearly deterministic relationship between development (as measured by GNP per capita or its rate of growth) and fertility rates should not be taken as unqualified support for the proposition that family planning programmes are the key variable in bringing about a fertility decline, since many other factors (culture change being a major one) would also need to be considered. In any case, it is extremely difficult to test the

---

12 The same regression was performed using the growth rate of GDP per capita rather than GNP with similar results.

relationship between fertility and family planning statistically since there is no single index of programme effort which is also independent of fertility outcomes (Ahlburg 1990). It is also difficult to distinguish those changes which are related to the programme itself and those which derive from general socio-economic change occurring simultaneously. What is not in doubt, however, is that fertility levels are to a considerable degree a function of the proportion of married women in a population who are (or whose husbands are) using some form of contraception. The correlation between these variables among the lower middle income countries is shown clearly in Figure 10.

A potential problem with the data on which Figure 10 is based is the strong possibility that the use of contraception is understated in countries where post-partum abstinence, or other traditional methods, are a significant means of spacing births, such as in Papua New Guinea. Indeed, "using" contraception is itself a complex variable which says nothing about the effectiveness of this use and the different motivations associated with it--including the motivation to *maximise* the number of surviving children by means of child-spacing (Hawkes and Charnov 1988). Papua New Guinea's position on Figure 10 is somewhat anomalous: of all the countries in which less that ten percent of married couples employ some form of contraception (other than PNG these are all African countries), PNG has the lowest Total Fertility Rate. This would still be true even if the data on contraceptive use in PNG understated actual use by two and a half times. To put this the other way around, given PNG's TFR of 5.4, the expected proportion of married couples using contraception would be about 25 percent, instead of the 6 percent normally reported.

The unusual position of PNG on Figure 10 can be interpreted in several ways. First, and most obvious, is the possibility that the statistics on contraceptive use in PNG are much understated. This also raises the further question of the definition of "contraception". The World Bank data include "abstinence" as a contraceptive method, but the figure cited for PNG probably excludes abstinence, withdrawal, or rhythm methods other than for those women who employed rhythm method after consultation with a health worker. It is worth noting that some sources have suggested that only 3 percent of couples in PNG currently use a contraceptive method (Department of Finance and Planning 1991, 18), rather than the 6 percent used in Figure 10. The 3 percent figure is probably based on the narrowest possible definition of what constitutes contraception or family planning, and, if correct, raises even more starkly the question of how the TFR in PNG is maintained at such a low level (relative to other lower middle income countries) in the virtual absence of modern contraception.

Another possible interpretation of PNG's situation is that the measurement of fertility is flawed and that actual fertility is much higher than indicated. This does not seem plausible in the light of the careful analysis of the 1980 census data on fertility carried out by Bakker (1986b).

The position of PNG is also interesting by comparison with Thailand and the Philippines (countries with similar per capita incomes) and Indonesia, which has a much lower per capita income. Since all of these countries have had organized, government-sponsored family planning programmes for some time, the suggestion is that the existence of these programmes is responsible for the high rates of contraceptive use. Such an interpretation would certainly be supported by the data shown in Figure 11. While contraceptive use is generally higher in those lower-middle income countries which had attained per capita incomes above $US1,300, there is an extremely wide range of rates of contraceptive use in countries between $US600 and $US800 per capita income. The clear anomalies here are Thailand and Indonesia with very high rates of contraceptive use (59% and 53% respectively). At the other extreme are the African countries of Nigeria, Cameroon, Ivory Coast, along with Papua New Guinea.

While the use of contraception is inversely related to total fertility rates, it does not follow that there is an equally clear relationship between the presence of a family planning programme and contraceptive use. As already mentioned, the missing link in the causal chain is the motivations related to use. The motivation to use contraception among married couples to limit family size (not just to space children) arises from the institutional milieu in which families are located. The presence of a family planning programme may have an independent effect on such motivations, but it is unlikely that this is particularly strong if social, economic and cultural conditions are conducive to large family size--as is the case in much of Africa (Caldwell and Caldwell 1987). Among the lower middle income countries, Zimbabwe is an example of a country which has had a family planning programme since the late 1970s, but although contraceptive prevalence rates increased with the introduction of the programme, fertility did not decline (Freedman 1987). As research in many countries, including Papua New Guinea (McDowell 1984), has shown, the desire for a large family may be economically rational from the viewpoint of parental security in old age as well as other goals related to family structures. Indeed, Agyei (1988) found that the majority of survey respondents in PNG desired at least six children at a time (1979) when the average woman in Papua New Guinea was having 5.4 children at the then-current age-specific fertility rates. McDowell's discussion of what would be an acceptable population policy to rural Papua New

Guineans (1988, 263) implies that "four or five children" would be sufficient to meet the genuine needs of the average rural family. With a TFR around 5, and considering that infant mortality rates remain high in many rural areas, there appears to be little objective basis for the large-scale adoption of modern family planning in PNG. This does not suggest the complete absence of a "demand" for family planning services, since women of above-average parity (and some below it) may well have preferred to have fewer children--not because the children were "unwanted" but because women freely acknowledge the inconvenience, stress, and risk of many pregnancies (McDowell 1988). However, in spite of the apparently obvious role that one would expect the use of modern contraceptives to play in ensuring wide birth intervals, empirical data collected elsewhere show that the proportion of births occurring after an interval of less than two years tends to increase as contraceptive prevalence rates increase (Bongaarts 1987). The reason for this may be that the use of modern contraception is accompanied by a decline in customary forms of child-spacing or family limitation, thus leading to higher fertility, or the two processes of change may simply offset one another leaving fertility about the same.

CONCLUSION

Comparing a country's population statistics with those of other, similar, countries is one way of making such statistics meaningful--although by no means the only way. This paper has used demographic and other data on 39 lower middle income countries in order to provide a perspective on PNG's demographic situation in the early 1980s, and to reflect on the likely direction of demographic change during the 1990s. At the same time, some consideration was given to the regional and provincial variations in birth and death rates. The following conclusions appear to be justified.

Although there are doubts about the accuracy of Papua New Guinea's censuses, the population growth rate appears to have changed little, if at all, during the past two decades. Around 1980, PNG's population growth rate was modest relative to its income class and similar to that for the less developed countries as a whole. The main reason for PNG's comparatively modest growth rate was its lower than average birth rate compared to countries with similar per capita incomes and rates of economic growth. PNG's birth rate was similar to that of several lower middle income Latin American counties, but the proportion of married couples employing contraception was closer to that of the much poorer African countries. PNG's lower birth rate was not, therefore, a function of the use of modern contraceptives, as in other countries, but was more than likely determined by socio-cultural and other factors not fully understood.

The birth and death rates for the country as a whole are the product of wide differences between regions. Thus, to the extent that PNG's overall birth rate is lower than might be expected, the reason can be found in the relatively lower fertility levels found in particular in the Highlands region.

The future prospects for population growth in Papua New Guinea are difficult to forecast, and an analysis of the relationship between economic growth, per capita income, contraceptive use, and fertility rates among the lower middle income countries provides no clear pattern which PNG might be expected to follow. Rapid economic growth does not necessarily bring down fertility, although there does appear to be a threshold point in the level of per capita income (about $US1,300 in 1982 values) above which continuing high fertility is rare. PNG's per capita GNP in 1990 remains well below this level, and is likely to remain there for some time--in spite of a potential mineral and petroleum boom expected in the mid-1990s. If economic growth is to have a depressing effect on fertility, its benefits would need to be shared widely.

While this study did not attempt to measure the relationship between the strength of family planning programmes and the use of contraceptives, it did show that there is quite a strong inverse relationship between the level of contraceptive use and the total fertility rate among lower middle income countries. Nevertheless, PNG occupied an anamolous position in that its total fertility rate was considerably lower than would be expected on the basis of the proportion of couples employing some form of contraception. Why this should be so is an important research topic with serious implications for the design and implementation of population policies. Should fertility rise in the populous Highlands and North Coast regions, while the death rate continued to decline, the overall result would be an increase in the national population growth--possibly to the rates currently found in Solomon Islands and Vanuatu. Such an increase would perhaps stimulate an interest in examining the likely effectiveness of current population policy approaches.

REFERENCES

Agyei, William 1988. Fertility and Family Planning in the Third World: A Case Study of Papua New Guinea. London: Croom Helm.

Ahlburg, Dennis 1990 Population Policies: Do They Work? Working Paper 90-02-1. Center for Population Analysis and Policy, University of Minnesota.

August, Clare Tabokom 1987 The Family Planning Association of Papua New Guinea: Further Comments, In The Ethics of Development: Papers from the 17th Waigani Seminar edited by Susan Stratigos and Philip J. Hughes. Port Moresby: University of Papua New Guinea Press.

Bakker, M.L. 1985 Population Projections for the Citizen Population of Papua New Guinea for the Period 1980 to 2015. Paper Prepared for Seminar on Population Growth and Its Implications. National Statistical Office.

1986a.The Mortality Situation in Papua New Guinea: Levels, Patterns, and Trends. Research Monograph Number 4. Port Moresby: National Statistical Office.

1986b.Fertility in Papua New Guinea: A Study of Levels, Patterns and Changes based on Census Data. Research Monograph Number 6. Port Moresby: National Statistical Office.

Bongaarts, John. 1987 Does Family Planning Reduce Infant Mortality Rates? Population and Development Review 13(2):323 -334.

Caldwell, John C. and Pat Caldwell. 1987 The Cultural Context of High Fertility in Sub-Saharan Africa. Population and Development Review 13(3):409-437.

Clunies-Ross, Anthony. 1984 Migrants From Fifty Villages. Boroko: Institute of Applied Social and Economic Research. Monograph No. 21.

Coale, Ansley J. 1986 Population Trends and Economic Development. In World Population and U.S. Policy: The Choices Ahead, edited by Jane Menken. New York: W.W. Norton.

Frank, Odile and Geoffrey McNicoll 1987 An Interpretation of Fertility and Population Policy in Kenya. Population and Development Review 13(2):209-244.

Freedman, R. 1987 The Contribution of Social Science Research to Population Policy and Family Planning Program Effectiveness. Studies in Family Planning 18:57-82.

Hawkes, Kristen and Eric L. Charnov 1988 On Human Fertility: Individual or Group Benefit? Current Anthropology 29(3):469-471.

Huff, Darrell 1954 How to Lie With Statistics. New York: W.W.Norton.

Kane, Peggy and David Lucas. 1986 An Overview of South Pacific Population Problems. Asia-Pacific Population Journal 1(4):3-16.

McDevitt, Thomas 1982 Trends and Differentials in Mortality, In Population of Papua New Guinea. New York and Noumea: United Nations ESCAP and South Pacific Commission. ESCAP/SPC Country Monograph Series No. 7.

McDowell, Nancy (ed) 1988 Reproductive Decision-Making and the Value of Children in Rural Papua New Guinea. Boroko: Institute of Applied Social and Economic Research. Monograph No. 27.

McMurray, Christine 1985 Recent Demography of Papua New Guinea. Working Paper No 85/5. Canberra: National Centre for Development Studies.

Muirden, Neil 1982 Family Planning Programmes, In Population of Papua New Guinea. New York and Noumea: United Nations ESCAP and South Pacific Commission. ESCAP/SPC Country Monograph Series No. 7.

National Centre for Development Studies. 1989 Australia's Relations with Papua New Guinea. Submission to the Joint Committee on Foreign Affairs and Trade. Canberra: NCDS.

Papua New Guinea, Department of Finance and Planning 1991 An Integrated National Population Policy for Progress and Development. Port Moresby: Department of Finance and Planning.

Papua New Guinea, National Statistical Office 1988 1980 National Population Census, Final Figures: National Summary. Port Moresby: National Statistical Office.

1991 1990 National Population Census, Preliminary Figures: Census Division Populations. Port Moresby: National Statistical Office.

Simon, Julian 1989 On Aggregate Empirical Studies Relating Population Variables to Economic Development. Population and Development Review 15(2):322-332.

South Pacific Commission 1985 Population 1983. Statistical Bulletin of the South Pacific No. 26. Noumea: South Pacific Commission.

1987 South Pacific Economies: Statistical Summary. No. 11, 1987.

Todaro, Michael P. 1981 Economic Development in the Third World. Second Edition. New York: Longman.

United Nations 1989a World Population Prospects 1988. New York: United Nations Department of Social and Economic Affairs.

1989b Statistical Yearbook for Asia and the Pacific. Bangkok: Economic and Social Commission for Asia and the Pacific.

1990a 1988 Demographic Yearbook. New York: United Nations Department of International Economic and Social Affairs, Statistical Office.

1990b Special Report: The Population Situation in the Least Developed Countries. World Population Monitoring 1989. Population Studies No. 113. New York: United Nations.

United Nations, ESCAP 1982 Trends and Differentials in Fertility, In Population of Papua New Guinea. New York and Noumea: United Nations ESCAP and South Pacific Commission. ESCAP/SPC Country Monograph Series No. 7.

1988 Population Data Sheet 1988. Bangkok: Economic and Social Commission for Asia and the Pacific.

World Bank 1984 World Development Report 1984. New York: Oxford University Press.

Table 1: PNG Population Change 1966-90*

Province	Census Year 1966	1971	1980	1990	Annual average growth rates 1966-1971	1971-1980	1980-1990	1971-1990	1966-1990
Western	61,860	70,898	78,575	108,705	2.73	1.13	3.25	2.25	2.35
Gulf	55,310	58,564	64,120	68,060	1.14	1.00	0.60	0.79	0.86
Central	146,331	193,837	116,964	140,584	na	na	1.84	na	na
NCD	na	na	123,624	193,242	na	na	4.47	na	na
Oro	58,575	66,514	77,442	96,762	2.54	1.67	2.23	1.97	2.09
Milne Bay	100,157	109,460	127,975	157,288	1.78	1.72	2.06	1.91	1.88
South coast	422,233	499,273	588,700	764,641	3.35	1.81	2.61	2.24	2.47
Southern Highlands	184,101	192,854	236,052	302,724	0.93	2.22	2.49	2.37	2.07
Enga	na	134,586	164,534	238,357	na	2.21	3.71	3.01	na
Western Highlands	291,142	211,456	265,656	291,090	na	2.51	0.91	1.68	na
Simbu	167,245	160,245	178,290	183,801	-0.86	1.17	0.30	0.72	0.39
Eastern Highlands	204,032	239,639	276,726	299,619	3.22	1.58	0.79	1.18	1.60
Highlands	846,520	938,780	1,121,258	1,315,591	2.07	1.95	1.60	1.78	1.84
Morobe	209,066	249,033	310,622	363,535	3.50	2.43	1.57	1.99	2.31
Madang	152,047	170,953	211,069	270,299	2.34	2.32	2.47	2.41	2.40
East Sepik	157,931	181,893	221,890	248,308	2.83	2.18	1.12	1.64	1.89
West Sepik	99,607	93,978	114,192	135,185	-1.16	2.14	1.69	1.91	1.27
North coast	618,651	695,857	857,773	1,017,327	2.35	2.30	1.71	2.00	2.07
Manus	20,679	24,866	26,036	32,830	3.69	0.51	2.32	1.46	1.93
New Ireland	50,298	59,543	66,028	87,194	3.37	1.14	2.78	2.01	2.29
East New Britain	109,930	113,750	133,197	184,408	0.68	1.73	3.25	2.54	2.16
West New Britain	44,192	61,515	88,941	127,547	6.61	4.05	3.61	3.84	4.42
North Solomons	72,479	96,363	128,794	165,000	5.70	3.19	2.48	2.83	3.43
Islands	297,578	356,037	442,996	596,979	3.59	2.40	2.98	2.72	2.90
Total	2,184,982	2,489,947	3,010,727	3,694,538	2.61	2.09	2.05	2.08	2.19

* The 1990 population of North Solomons Province was estimated on the assumption that 1971-80 natural increase of 3.5% continued but all non-North Solomons born were evacuated in 1990 and no new net in-migration occurred. Other assumptions could, of course, be employed.

Sources: Papua New Guinea, NSO (1988, 1991)

Table 2: Crude rates of natural increase based on indirect estimation methods applied to the 1966, 1971, and 1980 PNG censuses

	Census years		
Crude rates*	1966	1971	1980
Birth rate	43.1	38.0	34.2
Death rate	20.7	16.6	13.2
Natural increase	22.4	21.4	21.0
Population growth (%)	2.2	2.1	2.1

*Per 1,000 population

Sources: United Nations, ESCAP (1982, 54); McDevitt (1982, 75); Bakker (1986a, 82); Bakker (1986b, 131).

Notes: The 1971 birth rate has been estimated from data in Bakker (1986b) rather than from ESCAP (1982), since the latter source appears to have over-estimated the birth rate. The crude death rate has been taken from McDevitt (1982), although these estimates could also be questioned.

Table 3: Population growth in PNG in comparative perspective

Region/country	Annual rate of growth (percent)	Period
World	1.7	1985-90
Less developed countries	2.1	1980-85
Least developed countries	2.4	1980-85
Africa	3.0	1985-90
Kenya	4.3	1988
Latin America	2.1	1985-90
Southeast Asia	1.9	1985-90
Indonesia	2.1	1985-88
Philippines	2.4	1985-88
Pacific Islands	2.1	1982-87
Pacific Islands exc PNG	2.1	1982-87
PAPUA NEW GUINEA	2.1	1980-90
Australia and New Zealand	1.4	1985-90

Sources: South Pacific Commission (1987); United Nations (1990a, 1990b);

Table 4: Population data for lower middle income countries Ca 1982

GNP Rank From low to high	Country	Continent	Population (1982)	GNP Per capita	Land Area Km ^{2}	Persons per square kilometre	Birth Rate	Death Rate	Percent natural increase	Total fertility rate	Life expectancy at birth	Percent married women using Contraception
1	Sudan	Nth Africa	20,200,000	440	2,506,000	8	45	18	2.7	6.6	47	5
2	Mauritania	Nth Africa	1,600,000	470	1,031,000	2	43	19	2.4	6.0	45	1
3	Yemen PDR	Middle-East	2,000,000	470	333,000	6	48	19	2.9	6.9	46	na
4	Liberia	W. Africa	2,000,000	490	111,000	18	50	14	3.6	6.9	54	na
5	Senegal	W. Africa	6,000,000	490	196,000	31	48	21	2.7	6.5	44	4
6	Yemen Arab Rep.	Middle-East	7,500,000	500	195,000	38	48	22	2.6	6.8	44	1
7	Lesotho	Africa	1,400,000	510	30,000	47	42	15	2.7	5.8	53	5
8	Bolivia	S. America	5,900,000	570	1,099,000	5	43	16	2.7	6.3	51	na
9	Indonesia	SE Asia	152,600,000	580	1,919,000	80	34	13	2.1	4.3	53	53
10	Zambia	Africa	6,000,000	640	753,000	8	50	16	3.4	6.8	51	na
11	Honduras	Central America	4,000,000	660	112,000	36	44	10	3.4	6.5	60	27
12	Egypt	Middle-East	44,300,000	690	1,001,000	44	35	11	2.4	4.6	57	24
13	El Salvador	Central America	5,100,000	700	21,000	243	40	8	3.2	5.6	63	34
14	Thailand	SE Asia	48,500,000	790	514,000	94	28	8	2.0	3.6	63	59
15	PNG	Pacific	3,100,000	820	462,000	7	34	13	2.1	5.4	53	6
16	Philippines	SE Asia	50,700,000	820	300,000	169	31	7	2.4	4.2	64	36
17	Zimbabwe	Africa	7,500,000	850	391,000	19	54	12	4.2	8.0	56	15
18	Nigeria	Africa	90,600,000	860	924,000	98	50	16	3.4	6.9	50	6
19	Morocco	Nth Africa	20,300,000	870	447,000	45	40	15	2.5	5.8	52	19
20	Cameroon	W. Africa	9,300,000	890	475,000	20	46	15	3.1	6.5	53	2
21	Nicaragua	Central America	2,900,000	920	130,000	22	45	11	3.4	6.3	58	na
22	Ivory Coast	W. Africa	8,900,000	950	322,000	28	48	17	3.1	7.0	47	3
23	Guatemala	Central America	7,700,000	1130	109,000	71	38	9	2.9	5.2	60	18
24	Congo	Africa	1,700,000	1180	342,000	5	43	10	3.3	6.0	60	na
25	Costa Rica	Central America	2,300,000	1430	51,000	45	30	4	2.6	3.5	74	65
26	Peru	S. America	17,400,000	1310	1,285,000	14	34	11	2.3	4.5	58	41
27	Dominican Republic	Caribbean	5,700,000	1330	49,000	116	34	8	2.6	4.2	62	42
28	Jamaica	Caribbean	2,200,000	1330	11,000	200	27	6	2.1	3.4	73	55
29	Ecuador	S. America	8,000,000	1350	284,000	28	37	8	2.9	5.4	63	34
30	Turkey	Middle-East	46,500,000	1370	781,000	60	31	9	2.2	4.1	63	38
31	Tunisia	Nth Africa	6,700,000	1390	164,000	41	34	9	2.5	4.9	61	41
32	Colombia	S. America	27,000,000	1460	1,139,000	24	29	7	2.2	3.6	64	49
33	Paraguay	S. America	3,100,000	1610	407,000	8	31	7	2.4	4.2	65	36
34	Angola	Africa	8,000,000	na	1,247,000	6	49	22	2.7	6.5	43	na
35	Cuba	Caribbean	9,800,000	na	115,000	85	16	6	1.0	2.0	75	na
36	Korea (North)	Asia	18,700,000	na	121,000	155	30	7	2.3	4.0	64	na
37	Lebanon	Middle-East	2,600,000	na	10,000	260	29	9	2.0	3.8	65	na
38	Fiji	Pacific	715,375	na	18,272	39	30	5	2.5	3.3	63	na
Total			670,315,375	840	20,970,272	32	37	12	2.5	5.0	57	na

Source: World Bank (1984) Note: na = 'not available'. Data for Mongolia not included in table for lack of space.

Figure 1 Intercensal growth rates by region 1966-90

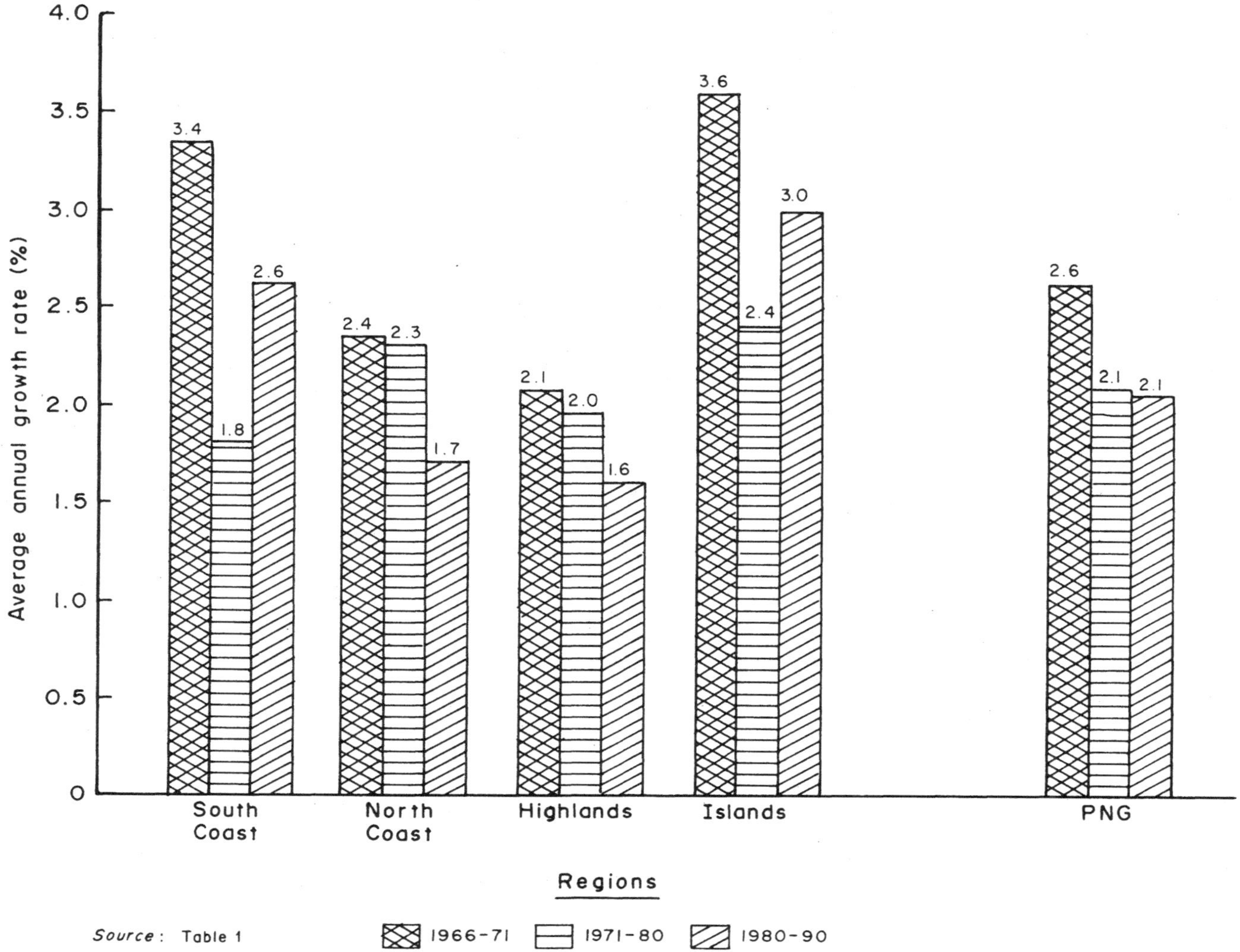

Source: Table 1

Figure 2 Birth, death and population growth rates of lower middle income countries, 1980-85 (of 1.0 million population or more)

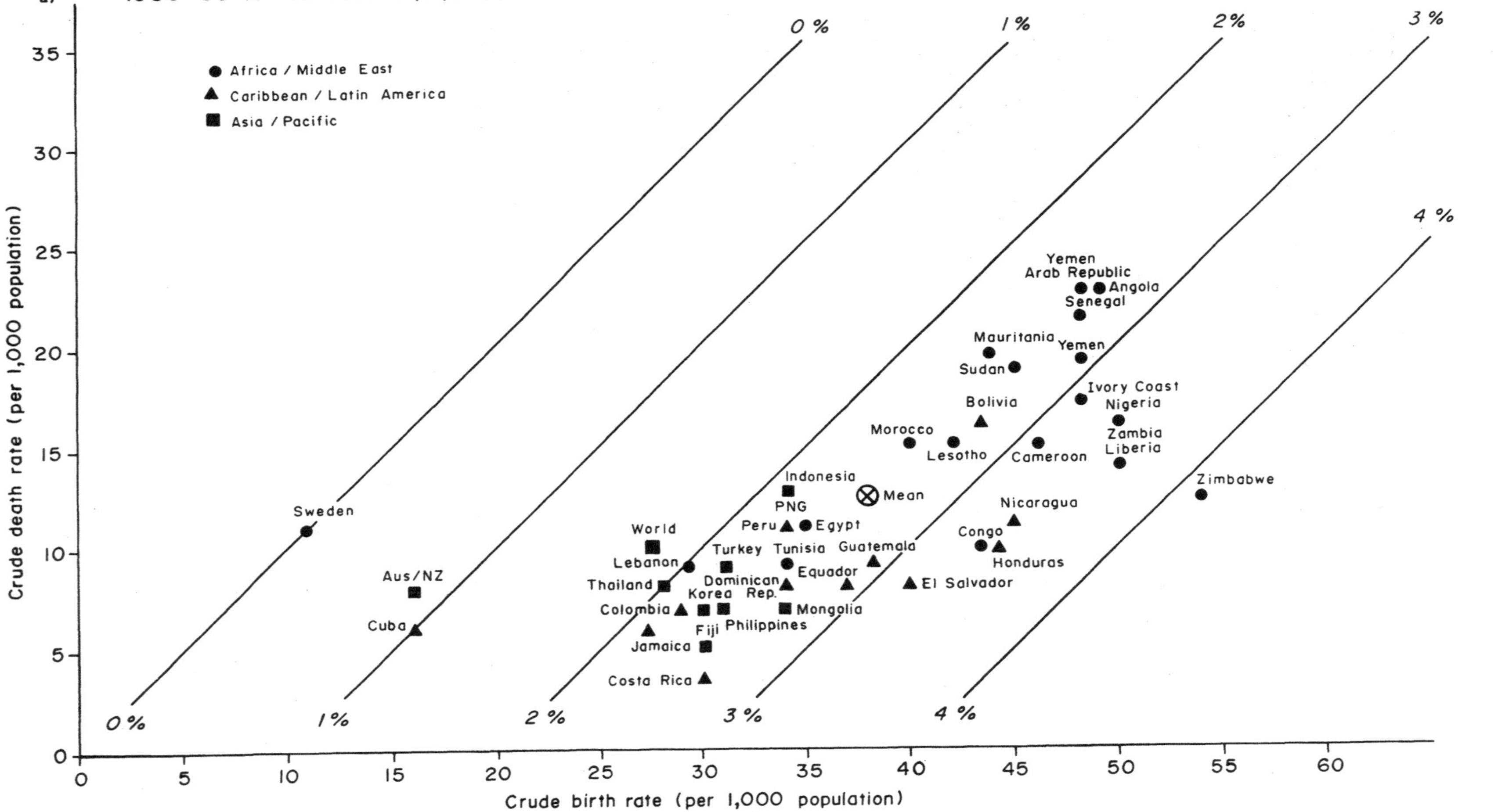

Source: Table 4

Note : See Table 4 for list of countries

Figure 3 Rate of natural increase (%) by province 1975-80*

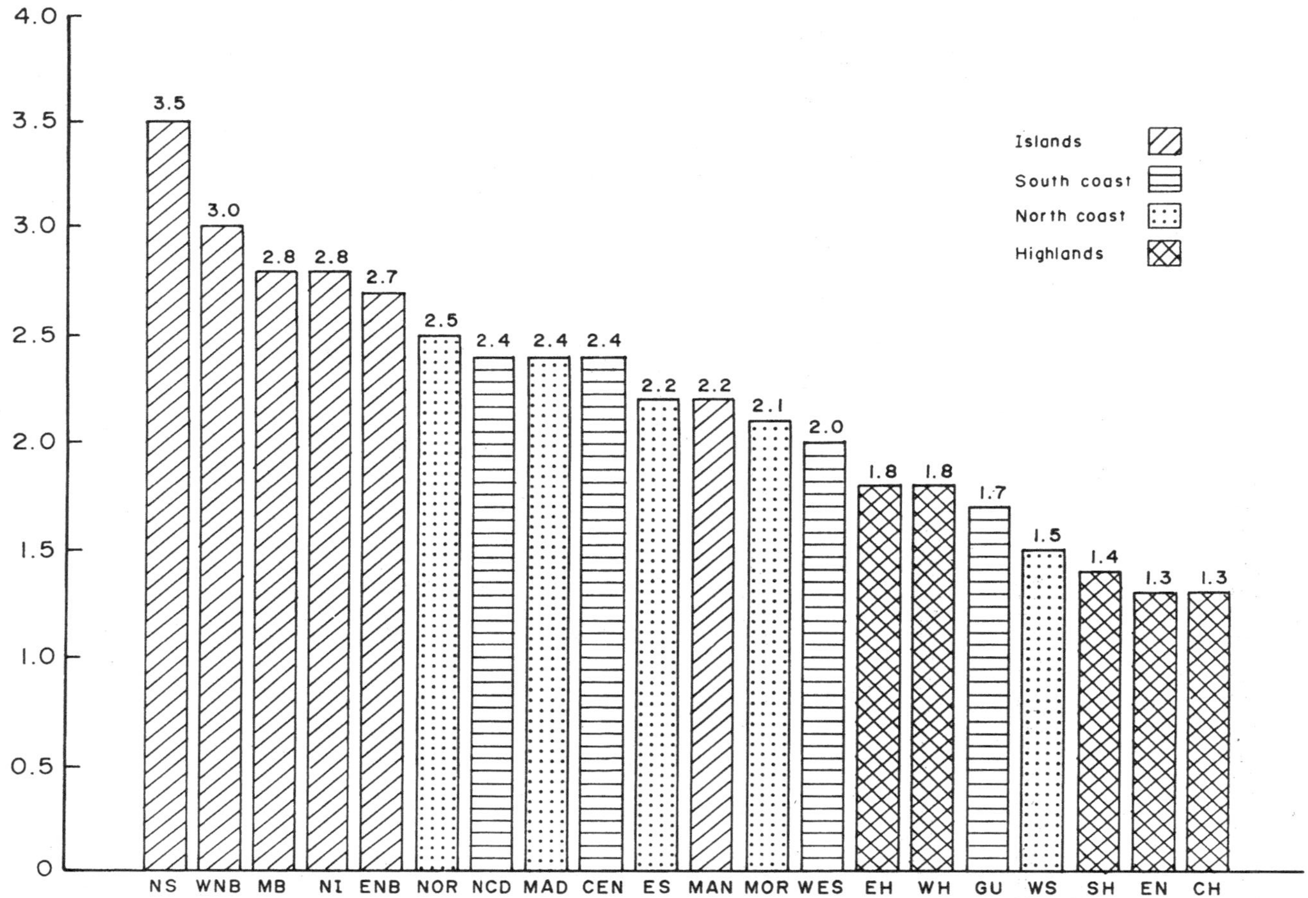

* Standardized on population of PNG 1980

Source: Calculated from Bakker (1986a; 1986b)

Figure 4 Rates of natural increase by province 1975-80: geographical patterns.

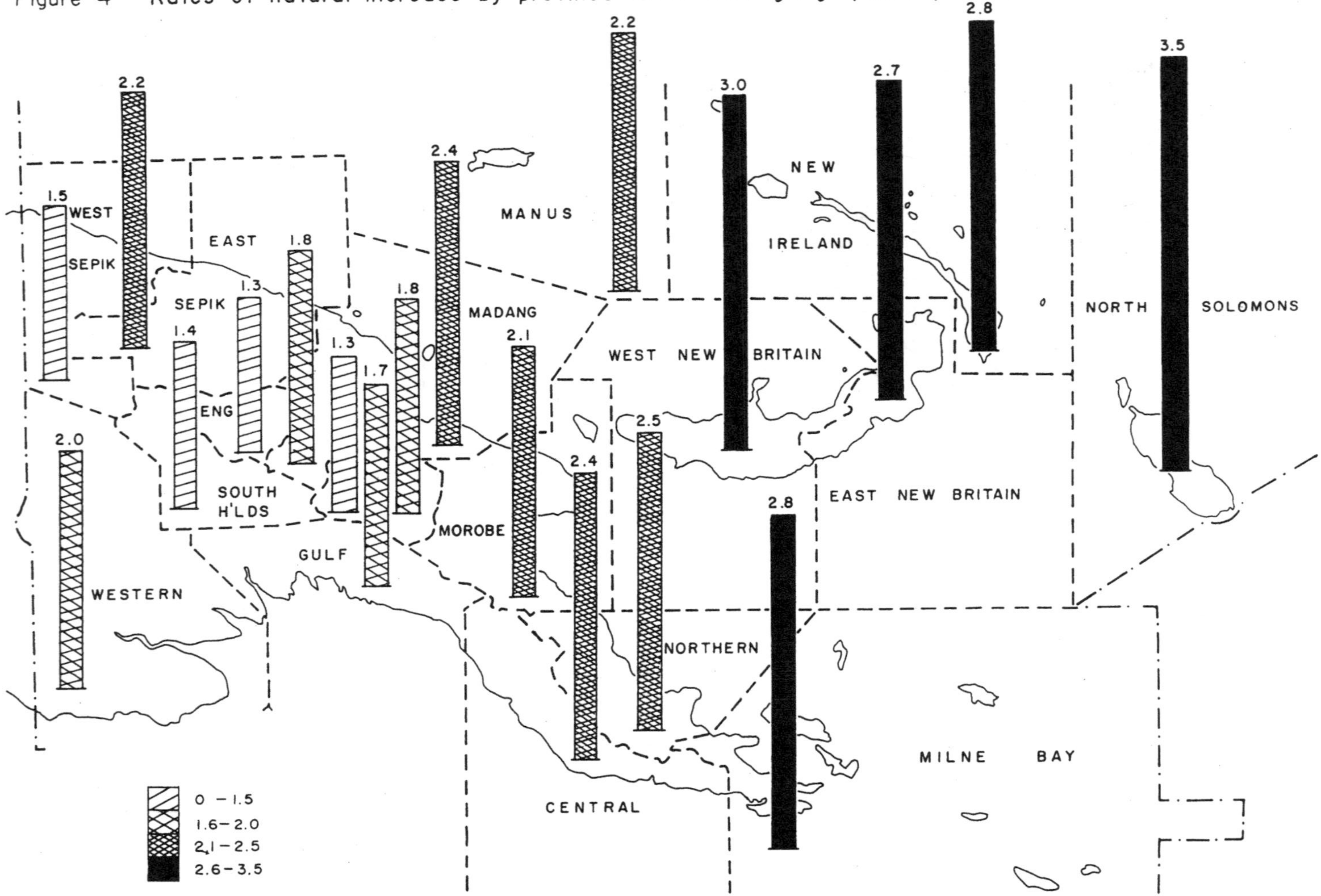

Source: Calculated from Bakker (1986a, 1986b)

Figure 5 Birth, Death and natural increase rates by province, 1980.

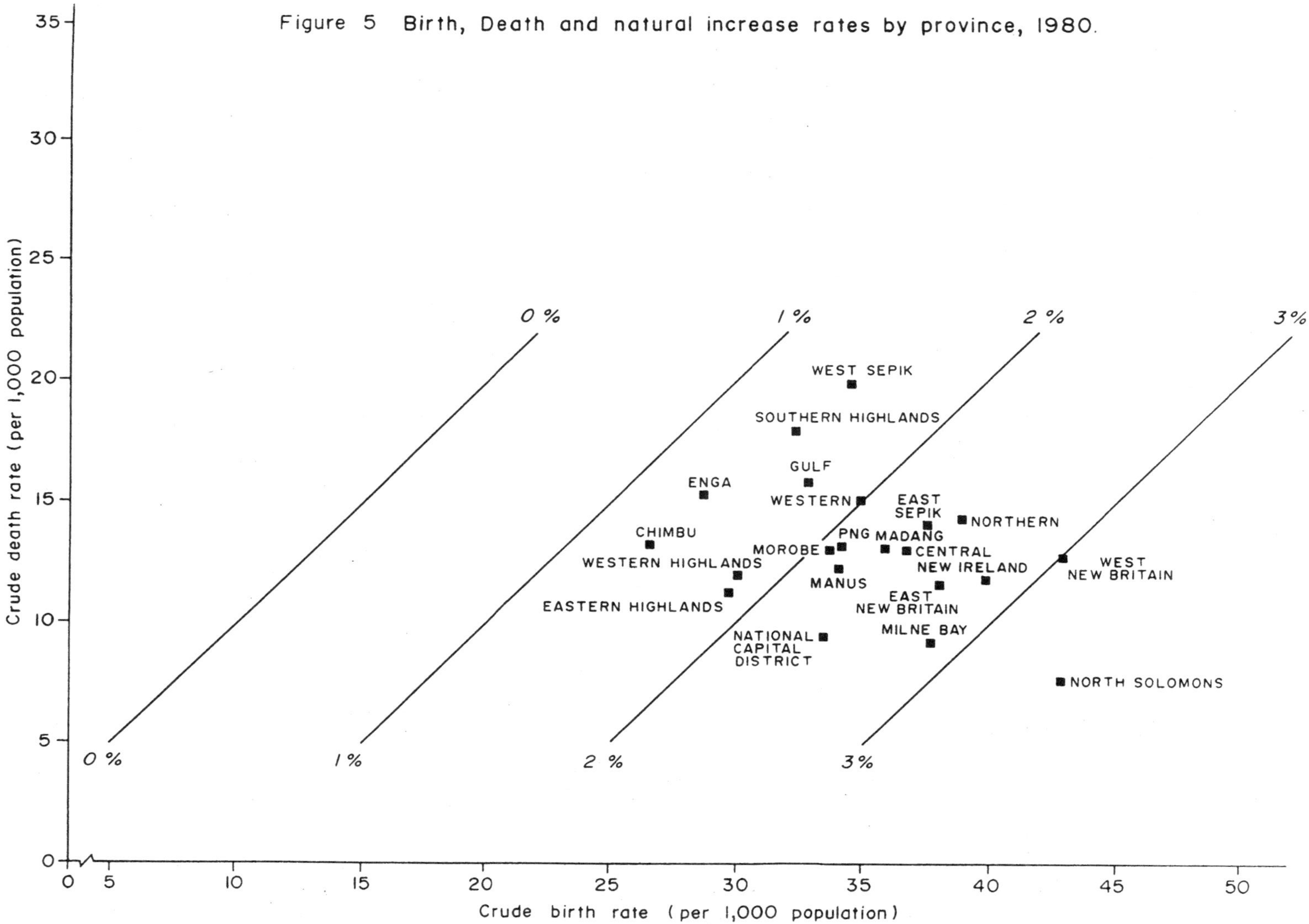

Source : Calculated from Bakker (1986a; 1986b)

Figure 6 **Relationship between birth rates and death rates by province, 1980.**

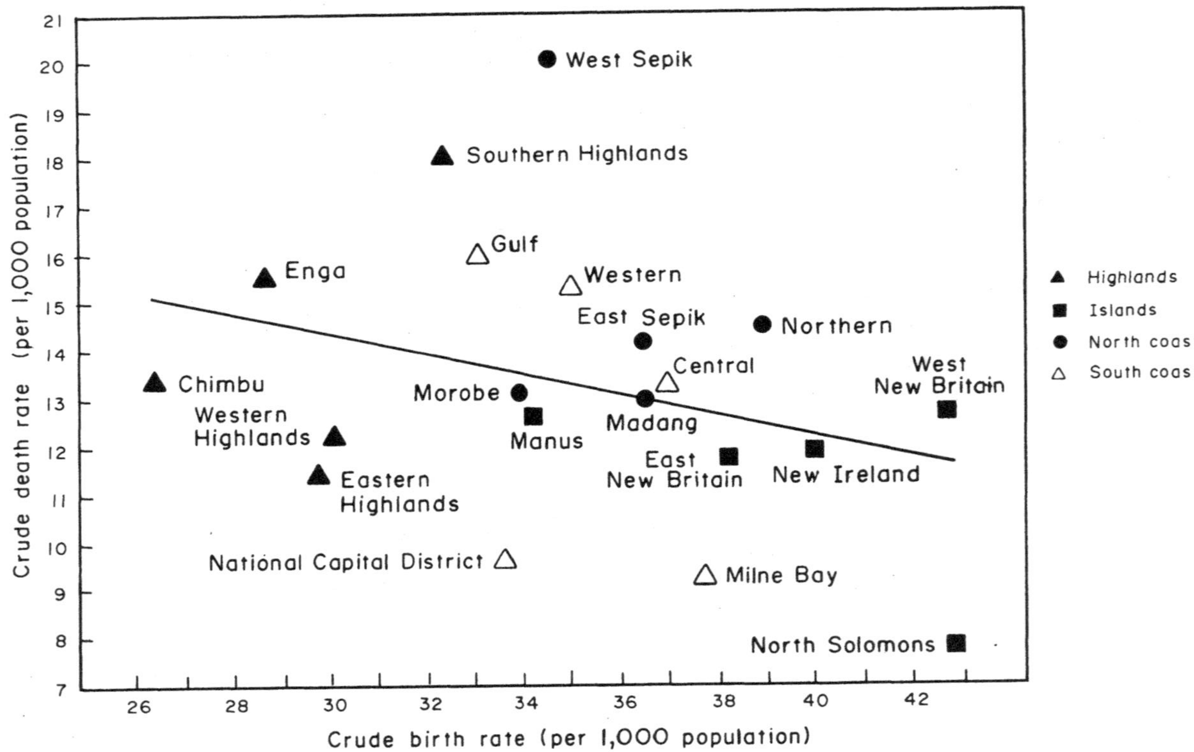

Source : Calculated from Bakker (1986a; 1986b)

Figure 7 **Relationship between rate of natural increase and GNP per capita (Lower-middle income countries)**

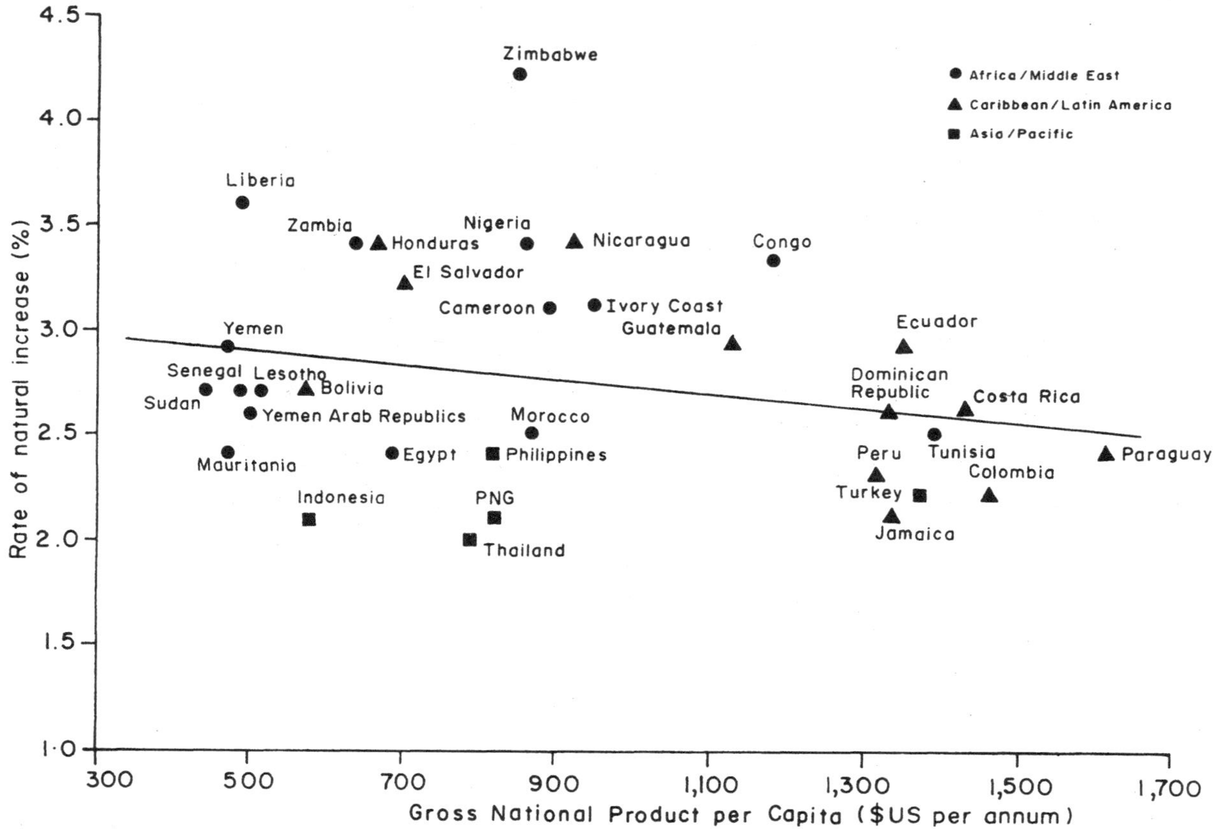

Source : Table 4

Figure 8 Relationship between GNP per capita and total fertility rate.

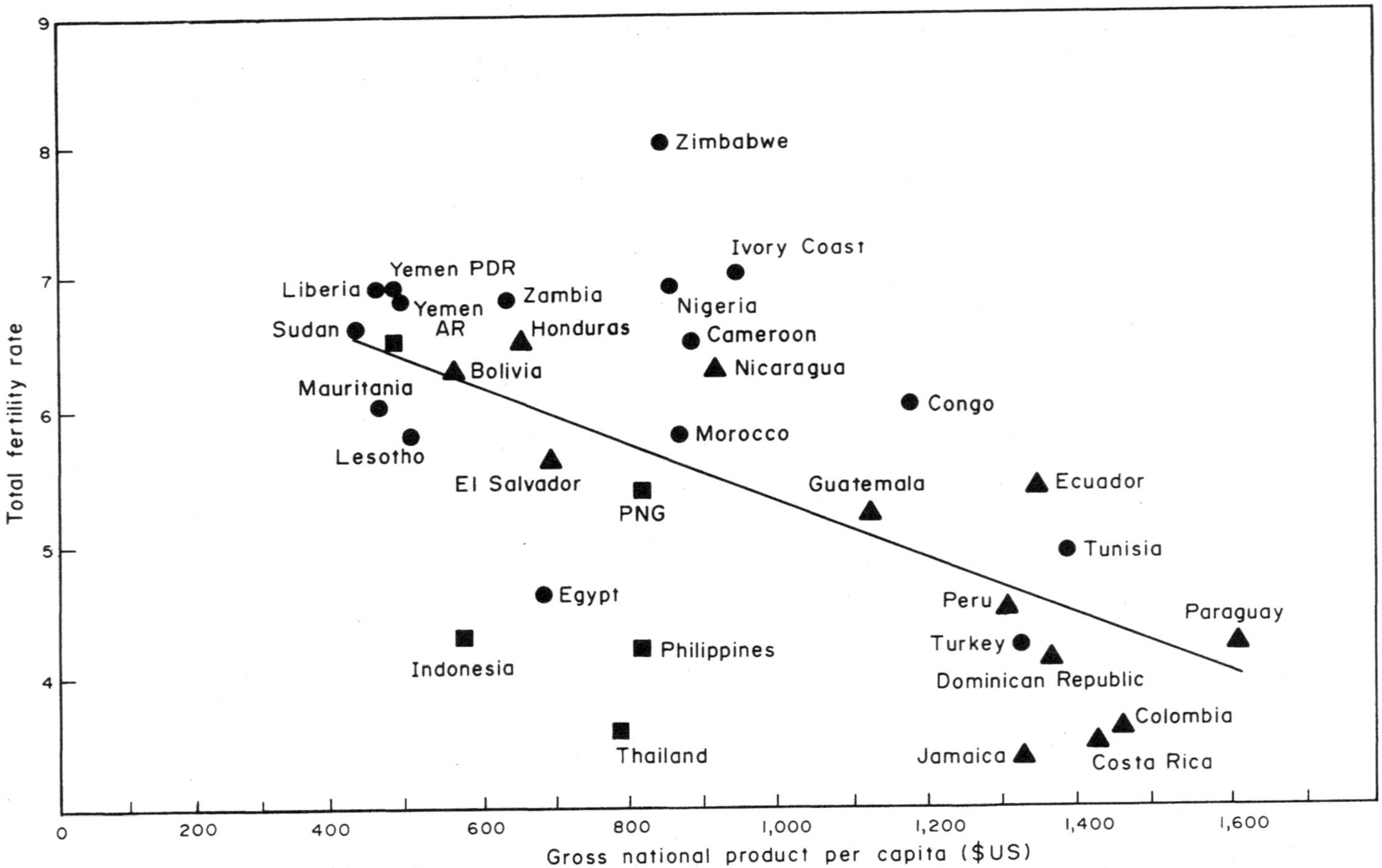

Source : Table 4

Figure 9 Rate of growth in GNP per capita and total fertility rate

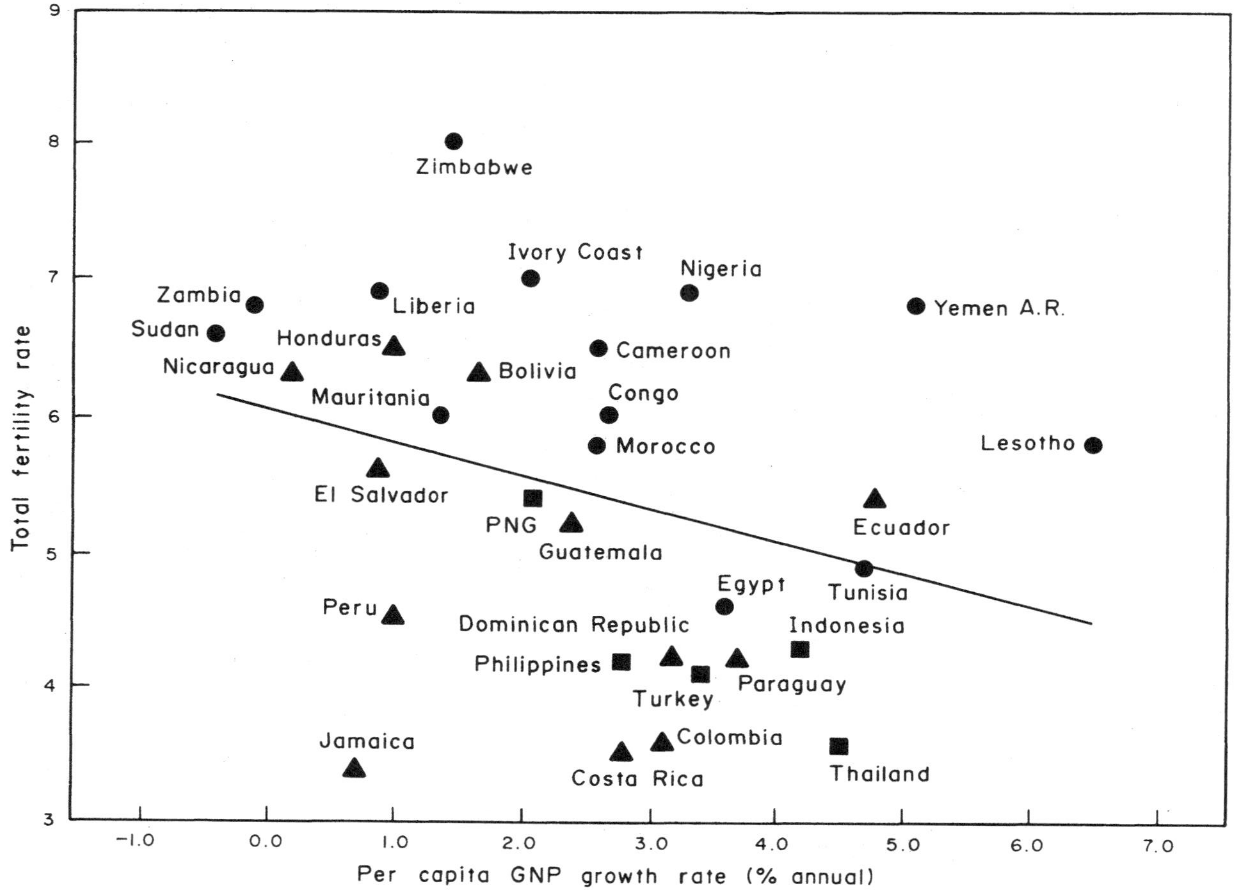

Source: World Bank (1984)

Figure 10 Relationship between total ferlility rate and contraceptive use (Lower - middle income countries ca 1980)

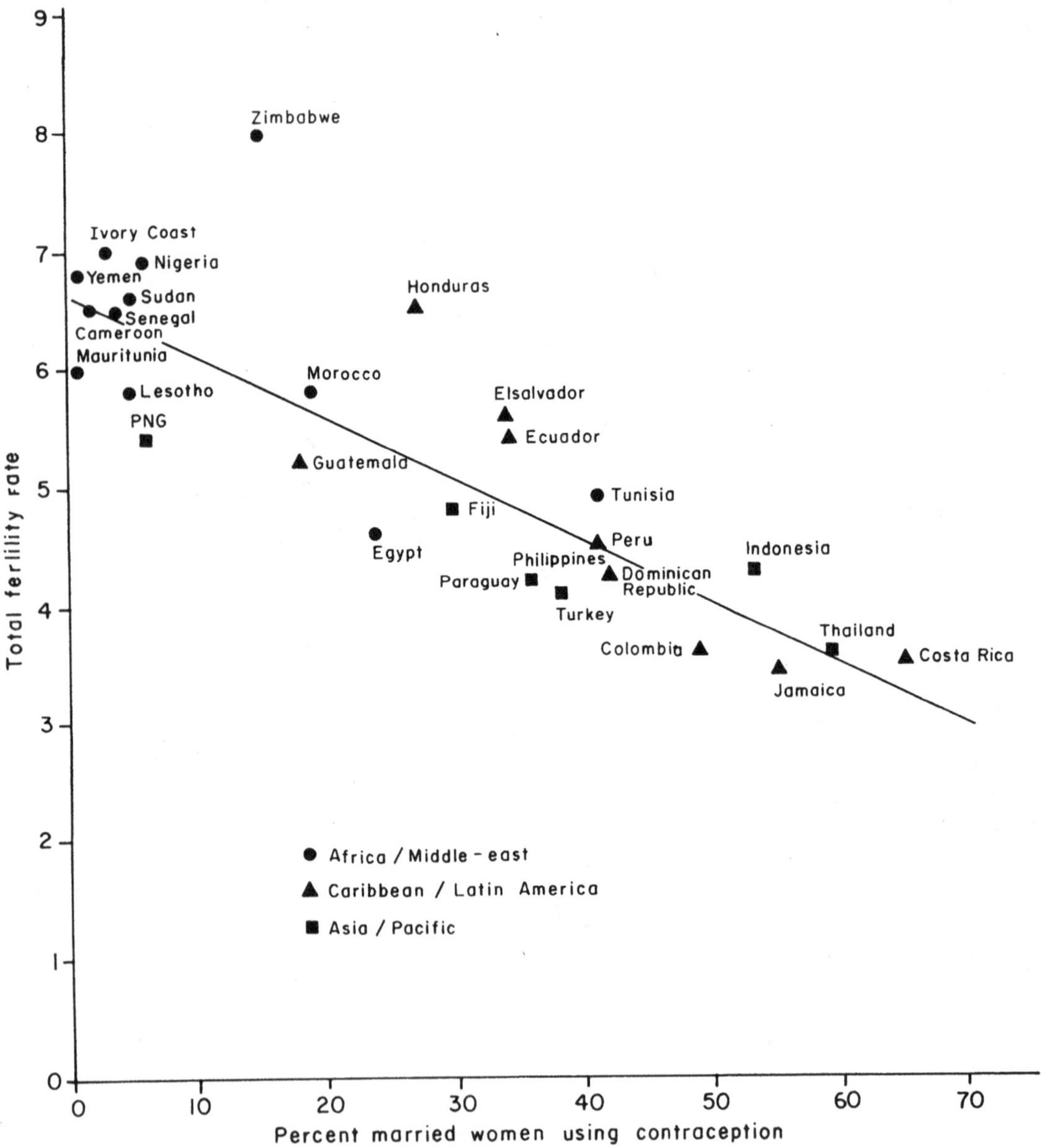

Figure 11 Relationship between GNP per capita and percent married women using contraception.

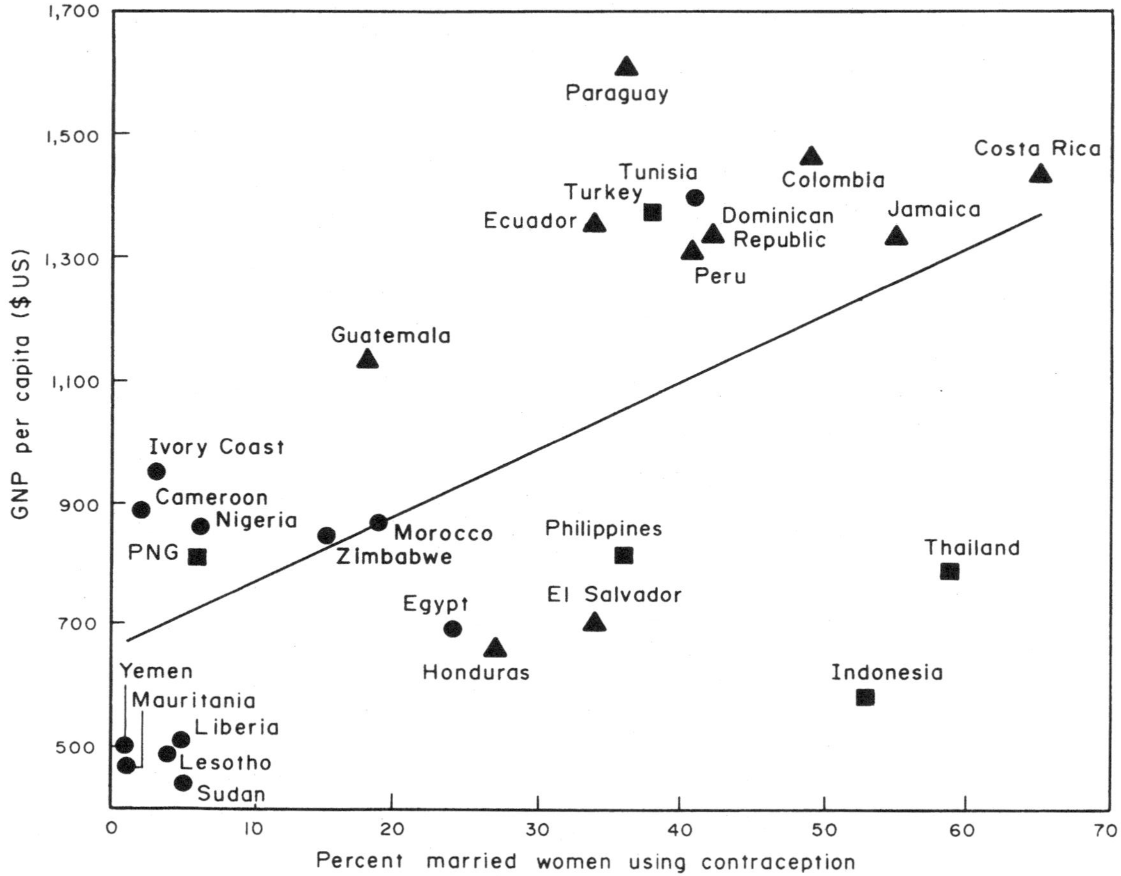

Source: Table 4

URBANIZATION IN PAPUA NEW GUINEA: TRENDS FROM 1966 TO 1990

DAVID KING[1]

The preliminary figures of the 1990 census suggest that both the total population of Papua New Guinea and its towns have grown more slowly than we might have anticipated during the 1980's. Each census has been analysed with qualifying remarks about the level of undercounting, with adjustments and re-classifications adding further confusion. I anticipate that the 1990 census will be no different, with upward revisions of population totals and rates of growth making later alterations to initial estimates of growth and change. If Papua New Guinea's population has only grown at 2.1% a year since 1980, that is a positive benefit to the country in its struggle to develop. However, there are problems with the census data that must be faced before any attempt is made to analyse the trends in urban growth.

The most urbanised province in 1980 has not been included in 1990. In 1980 112,172 North Solomon Islanders lived in Papua New Guinea, of whom 108,726 were resident in their province of birth. It can reasonably be assumed that most of these people plus their offspring born in the 1980's are still resident in the province, while most of the balance of 16,738 non-North Solomon Islanders, and their post 1980 offspring are no longer in the province. Thus there are variable base levels from which to compute an estimate of the province's population now. While the country as a whole grew at 2.1%, the rate of increase in North Solomons by 1980 was the highest in the country; a rate that was partially caused by in-migration to the mine, but was additionally the result of the highest rate of natural increase in the country. It is likely that the events of the last two years have reduced fertility as well as increasing mortality, especially amongst infants. Consequently upper and lower estimates of the North Solomons' population in 1990 show a wide variation.

[1] Senior Lecturer in Geography, James Cook University of North Queensland

As a result of the crisis in North Solomons it is likely that urban populations in the province have declined absolutely. Certainly Panguna appears to have become a ghost town, while the services and functions of most other centres are minimal or non-existant. It can be assumed that all centres in the province have dropped considerably in the rank size list, but some may still be urban centres of a sort. Some of the people who have left North Solomons have moved to other towns in Papua New Guinea and may represent a part of a future reconstructed urban system in North Solomons. Thus where they have inflated the population of a town, such as Rabaul, a comparison of population and growth rates is to some extent artificial.

A more serious difficulty lies in reconciling the urban household survey of the mid 1980's with the 1990 census figures. Recent estimates of high rates of urban growth and migration in Papua New Guinea have been based on the high rates of increase indicated by the survey. The discrepancy is illustrated in Table 1, below.

TABLE 1. COMPARISON OF 1980 AND 1990 CENSUS FIGURES AND THE 1986 URBAN HOUSEHOLD SURVEY.

	1980 Census	**1986 UHS[1]**	**1990 Census**
Port Moresby	118,424	175,612	190,117
Lae	61,617	84,533	80,655
Wewak	19,890	32,601	23,224
Goroka	18,511	25,350	17,855
Daru	7,127	8,256	8,490
Ambunti	1,505	2,139	1,251
KAPL	20,505	32,094	

Note: 1. UHS - Urban Household Survey took place between late 1985 and early 1987. It was a stratified sample in Port Moresby and random in the other towns, except Daru which was a complete census. The totals have been derived from estimates based on the survey results.

2. Generally the same areas are compared, except for Ambunti, where the urban boundary was extended for the UHS, while the 1990 boundary is not known.

3. KAPL stands for Kieta, Arawa, Panguna and Loloho

Source: NSO - 1980 and 1990 censuses and UHS Preliminary Population Estimates.

It is clear from Table 1 that either something is wrong or that the pattern of urbanization has been very strange. It is unlikely that the pattern of migration has been rapidly into the towns, or that it has been followed either by a flow outwards or in the case of the capital a dramatically reduced rate of increase. While the state of the economy in the early 1980's might have prompted an increased migration rate, improvement in the late eighties was followed by the downturn that resulted from the Bougainville crisis. It is extremely improbable that large numbers of people returned to the rural sector in the late 1980's.

Either the 1986 Urban Household Survey was a severe over-estimate of the rate of growth, or the 1990 census represents a severe undercount. It is possible that both of these occurred and that the rate of urbanization in response to the recession may have been greater in the early 1980's than later in the decade.

What is most probable is that these figures form a starting point: base data of where the country is at. However it is most unlikely that undercount revisions will inflate the census figures into a high growth scenario. The data indicate continued moderate, steady growth, as shown in Table 2.

TABLE 2. URBAN AREAS OF PAPUA NEW GUINEA: POPULATION AND RANK SIZE 1990.

Rank	Town	Population	Growth rate %	Expected Population	% of Expected Population
1.	N.C.D[1]	194,295	4.6	-	-
2.	Lae	80,655	2.7	97,147	83.0
3.	Madang	27,057	2.4	64,765	41.8
4.	Wewak	23,224	1.6	48,574	47.8
5.	Hagen/Kag.	18,977	2.1	38,859	48.8
6.	Goroka/Bi.	18,368	-0.1	32,382	56.7
7.	Rabaul/Nonga	18,186	2.0	27,756	65.5
8.	Pop./Higaturu	12,299	2.8	24,287	50.6
9.	Daru	8,490	1.8	21,588	39.3
10.	Kimbe	8,363	6.1	19,429	43.0
11.	Gusap	8,304	-	17,663	47.0
12.	Vanimo	7,908	9.9	16,191	48.8
13.	Bulolo	7,421	1.0	14,946	49.6
14.	Kavieng	6,486	3.4	13,878	46.7
15.	Alotau	6,435	4.1	12,953	49.7
16.	Mendi	6,192	4.0	12,143	51.0
17.	Loreng/Lomb	5,804	1.3	11,429	50.8
18.	Tabubil	4,670	-	10,794	43.3
19.	Biala/Kapiura	4,527	-	10,226	44.3
20.	Wau	4,268	6.2	9,715	44.9

21.	Kiunga	4,000	11.0	9,252	43.2
22.	Kundiawa	3,987	-0.8	8,832	45.1
23.	Kainantu	3,692	-0.2	8,448	43.7
24.	Aitape	3,686	0.9	8,096	45.5
25.	Kokopo	3,151	3.8	7,772	40.5
26.	Yonki	2,817	-	7,473	37.7
27.	Aiyura/Ukarumpa	2,479	4.0	7,196	34.4
28.	Balimo	2,264	7.4	6,939	32.6
29.	Wabag	2,047	3.0	6,700	30.6
30.	Mosa	1,598	-	6,476	24.7
31.	Angoram	1,404	-2.7	6,268	22.4
32.	Ialibu	1,353	-	6,072	22.3
33.	Baimuru	1,337	7.6	5,888	22.7
34.	Buluma	1,314	-	5,715	23.0
35.	Ambunti	1,251	1.9	5,551	22.5
36.	Kerevat	1,212	3.0	5,397	22.5
37.	Porgera	1,174	-	5,251	22.3
38.	Kerema	1,152	1.5	5,113	22.5
39.	Maprik	1,129	0.1	4,982	22.7
40.	Bereina	1,074	6.3	4,857	22.1
41.	Kerowagi	1,003	-1.7	4,739	21.2
42.	Kwikila	983	-0.4	4,626	21.2
43.	Banz	925	0.1	4,518	20.5
44.	Namatanai	872	1.5	4,366	20.0
45.	Malalaua	872	0.4	4,366	20.0
46.	Tari	815	2.8	4,224	19.3
47.	Sogeri	792	-3.6	4,134	19.2
48.	Tapini	786	3.6	4,048	19.4
49.	Kupiano	768	-2.1	3,965	19.4
50.	Bwagaoia	748	2.7	3,847	19.4
51.	Bogia	748	-0.1	3,847	19.4
52.	Finschhafen	741	-0.2	3,736	19.8
53.	Minj	730	-2.0	3,666	19.9
54.	Laiagam	692	-2.1	3,598	19.2
55.	Ihu	690	2.5	3,533	19.5
56.	Samarai	662	-2.6	3,470	19.1
57.	Kandrian	637	0.3	3,409	18.7
58.	Losuia	594	0.3	3,350	17.7
59.	Kokoda	545	-	3,293	16.6
60.	Mumeng	490	-0.5	3,238	15.1
61.	Chuave	472	-4.3	3,185	14.8
62.	Saidor	467	-0.7	3,134	14.9
63.	Wapenamanda	444	2.1	3,084	14.4
64.	Kikori	438	-5.4	3,036	14.4
65.	Mutsing/Kaiapit	424	-1.9	2,989	14.2
66.	Hoskins	393	-	2,944	13.3
67.	Lakuramau	386	-	2,900	13.3
68.	Tufi	349	-	2,857	12.2
69.	Esa'ala	332	1.3	2,816	11.8
70.	Taskul	218	-	2,776	7.9
Mean of largest 15 towns					51.3
Mean of all urban places					30.3

Note 1: National Capital District includes the Central Province adjacent C.D. of Goldie River Urban (population in 1990 was 1,053. In 1980 it was part of Hiri District with 913). Similarly other functionally connected urban C.D.s have been included with their "parent" urban areas: Mt.Hagen/Kagamuga, Goroka/Bihute, Rabaul/Nonga, Popondetta/Higaturu, Lorengau/Lombrum, Biala/Kapiura, Kokopo/Vunapope, Aiyura/Ukarumpa. Kaiapit headquarters has relocated to Mutsing, which is sometimes referred to also as Kaiapit.

Note 2: North Solomons towns are unranked and unenumerated. They are Kieta/Arawa/Loloho, Panguna (which appears to have ceased to exist as a town), Buin, Sohano/Buka Passage, Tinputz, Wakunai.

Note 3: Other central places (existing since 1966 or earlier) are as follows: Pomio, Talasea, Telefomin, Lumi, Miak, Henganofi, Okapa, Baiyer River, Kompian, Kandep, Simbai, Pangia, Nipa, Koroba, Kagua, Rabaraba, Magarida, Woitape. These places have district or sub-district functions, but have populations below 500.

Source: National Statistical Office, 1990 Census Preliminary Figures.

Table 2 has grouped some settlements that have previously been counted as one place even though the preliminary figures of the 1990 census had separated them. This is because they had been counted as one place in 1980 and in 1971. In the case of Arawa and Panguna this had seemed fairly illogical, but all other joint settlements are functionally linked as one place. The following tables use the same grouping, so that the number of central places has increased only slightly.

However, as the 1990 census has included some central places that have less than 500 people, Table 2 also lists, in note 3, other functionally central places, some of which may include rural peripheral settlements that boost their populations to over 500.

The growth rates for the period 1980 to 1990 are for the comparable areas as they are identified from the preliminary figures. Further analysis of boundaries etc. may adjust the details of these figures, but will probably not alter the general trends. Thus Table 3 below, compares the overall urban proportions for all Papua New Guinea's censuses.

TABLE 3. URBAN GROWTH 1966 TO 1990

	1966 census	1971 census	1980 incl.NSP	1980 excl.NSP	1990 excl.NSP
National Pop.	2,150,300	2,435,400	3,010,727	2,881,933	3,529,538
Total Urban Population	103,600	285,016	395,713	370,223	536,860
% Urban	4.8	11.7	13.1	12.8	15.2

Source: NSO

Without North Solomons, and even if there has been an undercount, both the total number and proportion of the population of Papua New Guinea living in urban areas has increased. The rate of increase is slower than in earlier decades, and even if the natural increase in towns were the same as for the rest of the country, most of the urban population increase in most central places would be the result of natural increase, rather than in-migration. Bakkers analysis of the 1980 census indicated that fertility and natural increase levels were much higher in the urban than the rural sector. Thus it can be concluded from the slower rate of urban growth indicated by the 1990 preliminary figures that urban natural increase is contributing more people to urban growth than in-migration. This trend was noticeable from the 1980 figures.

At an earlier point of urbanisation most population increase came from migration (Jackson 1976). Port Moresby's dramatic 12.2% annual growth rate between 1966 and 1971 added 34,659 people, 6,932 a year on average, while the slower 4.6% increase of NCD between 1980 and 1990 added 70,671 at a mean of 7,067 a year. In the 1960's and 1970's all towns expanded rapidly from small bases, as urbanisation got under way from a small base. While Port Moresby (NCD) has maintained its pace of increase the smaller towns have not. Between 1966 and 1971 the total urban population added a mean of 36,301 a year. After 1980 the total urban population (excluding North Solomons towns) only increased by a mean of 16,664 a year. Furthermore most of the late 1960's 36,301 would have been migrants, while most of the 1980's 16,664 would have been the addition of children born in the towns. Thus the indication is that migration to the urban areas has decreased markedly. The fact that the fall off in migration is so great would also support the notion of a considerable undercount. While an undercount would apply to the rural sector as much as to the urban, any inflation of the figures would leave the urban proportion basically the same, but greater totals would increase the number of migrants to a more likely level.

If urban areas have a mean rate of natural increase between 2.5% and 3.0% a year, as suggested by Bakker, then more than 50% of their growth would have been from natural increase. Thus only 8,000 or fewer migrants would have been added to all of the towns of Papua New Guinea each year throughout the 1980's. Yet several completely new towns, principally Tabubil, Gusap (at Ramu Sugar) and the oil palm towns were added entirely from migration during this period.

However, despite the difficulties of reconciling the lack of migration, the small towns are uniformly stagnating or declining. During the early phases of urbanisation, all central places attracted migrants. Since 1971, and most probably since Independence, these small places have received no further inputs and few have grown at rates above the mean national natural increase. Of the 41 small towns with less than 2,000 people, 15 actually declined and only 7 grew at rates above the national mean. Usually these places expanded because of a specific input, such as a high school or similar service. There are 8 completely new towns, 2 mining, 5 agricultural and 1 a service town, while existing places like Kiunga and Hoskins have experienced rapid expansion in relation to the same developments. It is most unlikely that these places have diverted more than a minimum number of migrants. They either drew population from existing towns, especially in the case of the mining settlements, or attracted agricultural pioneers, many of whom probably would not have been potential urban migrants.

As a consequence of these trends, the largest towns have pulled gradually ahead of the smaller, and the Capital has increased its primacy in relation to all other towns. Tables 2, 4 and 5, and the figures, all illustrate aspects of size and rank relationships. The expected population is based on the rank size rule that was initially devised by Zipf and developed by Berry as a tool for measuring and predicting the expected size of central places in an urban hierarchy. Very simply it predicts a population size based on the size of the largest place in the system, divided by the rank of each individual smaller place. While many modifications have been made to the rank size rule, it has been used in its simplest form here, because only total population figures are available and the data base for functions and occupations etc. is not totally reliable. However, it should be pointed out that Walsh (1983) did a number of analyses of various aspects of the 1980 urban census data to measure the urban hierarchy as illustrated by rank size relationships. As well as ranking towns by the size of their total population, he also ranked them by the size of their workforce in different sectors and type of employment. While individual towns varied from the general population curve, all of his graphs showed a similarity of shape that justifies use of the total population figures as representative of the hierarchy.

The rank size curve (a straight line on log log graph paper) shows the expected populations based on the size of Port Moresby (NCD). The divergence from the expected line indicates the relationship of the different levels of places to one another and to the capital. The three graphs illustrate the increasing primacy of Port Moresby in relation to the other larger towns. While Lae and Moresby have maintained an approximate expected relationship, the other large towns have slipped, parallel, but smaller than expected. The rest of the places in 1971 (similar to 1966, Jackson 1977) were grouped in decreasing steps. By 1980 these smaller places had begun to diverge from the stepped pattern. The 1990 rank size illustrates an increase in the divergence away from expected size.

For each of the three censuses the percentage divergence from the expected population was calculated for each town, and is expressed as a proportion of each town's expected population. In 1971 the mean proportion of all towns of the expected population, was 54.3%. By 1980 this mean had fallen to 40.8% and by 1990 it has reached 30%. More important than the actual rank size rule is this total measure that allows comparison of different census totals. The decline from 54 to 30% is a measure of increasing primacy.

However, increasing primacy is dependent upon differential migration rates, thus suggesting that people may actually have been leaving towns that are lower in the hierarchy for those which are higher, especially Port Moresby and Lae. This will be an interesting area for further research on the final census figures. Again this would also suggest that there have been more in-migrants than the moderate growth rates indicate.

Table 4. Urban Areas of Papua New Guinea: deviation from rank size expected population.

Rank	Town	Expected pop.	1971 % of expected	Rank	Town	Expected pop.	% of expected
1.	Pt.Moresby	-	-	24.	Kimbe	3,188	36.8
2.	Lae	38,254	101.2	25.	Kwikila	3,060	37.7
3.	Rabaul	25,502	104.0	26.	Kiunga	2,943	37.8
4.	Madang	19,127	87.2	27.	Maprik	2,834	38.1
5.	Wewak	15,301	98.1	28.	Wabag	2,732	39.4
6.	KAPL	12,751	128.6	29.	Aitape	2,638	39.2
7.	Goroka	10,930	110.4	30.	Kerowagi	2,550	40.4
8.	Mt.Hagen	9,563	118.5	31.	Sogeri	2,468	41.0
9.	Daru	8,501	67.6	32.	Banz	2,391	41.7
10.	Popondetta	7,650	58.7	33.	Ambunti	2,318	42.7
11.	Loreng/Lomb	6,955	62.2	34.	Balimo	2,250	34.0
12.	Bulolo	6,376	62.8	35.	Minj	2,186	34.0
13.	Kavieng	5,885	56.1	36.	Buin	2,125	34.2
14.	Kerema	5,465	48.6	37.	Laiagam	2,068	33.4
15.	Alotau	5,100	49.0	38.	Bogia	2,013	33.7
16.	Mendi	4,782	52.1	39.	Kikori	1,962	34.1
17.	Kundiawa	4,500	52.9	40.	Bereina	1,913	35.0
18.	Angoram	4,250	50.8	41.	Baimuru	1,866	35.7
19.	Kainantu	4,027	52.7	42.	Tapini	1,822	36.3
20.	Kokopo	3,825	53.9	43.	Losuia	1,779	35.1
21.	Samarai	3,643	53.5	44.	Tari	1,739	34.7
22.	Wau	3,478	55.0	45.	Miak	1,700	34.5
23.	Vanimo	3,326	56.5				
Mean - top 14 towns			82.3%	Mean all towns			54.3%

Source: NSO 1971 Papua New Guinea Census
Note: KAPL stands for Kieta, Arawa, Panguna and Loloho.

The mean proportion of the largest towns from the expected rank size population has also dropped considerably. In 1971 the largest towns between rank 1 and 15 were 82.4% of the expected populations. By 1980 they had dropped to 68.6% and by 1990 were only 51.3%. Increasing primacy has affected these places as well as the smaller centres, but not to the same extent.

Table 5. Urban Areas of Papua New Guinea: deviation from rank size expected population.

Rank	Town	Expected Pop. (1980)	% of expected	Rank	Town	Expected pop.	% of expected
1.	Pt.Moresby	-	-	29.	Kerowagi	4,275	27.8
2.	Lae	61,994	99.5	30.	Sogeri	4,133	27.6
3.	Madang	41,329	51.6	31.	Maprik	4,000	28.0
4.	KAPL	30,997	67.2	32.	Balimo	3,875	28.6
5.	Wewak	24,798	78.8	33.	Ambunti	3,757	27.4
6.	Goroka	20,665	91.0	34.	Kwikila	3,647	27.9
7.	Mt.Hagen	17,713	86.7	35.	Kupiano	3,543	26.7
8.	Rabaul	15,498	96.6	36.	Banz	3,444	26.7
9.	Popondetta	13,776	67.6	37.	Minj	3,351	25.9
10.	Daru	12,399	57.7	38.	Kerevat	3,263	27.4
11.	Bulolo	11,272	60.3	39.	Buin	3,179	27.6
12.	Loreng/Lom	10,332	51.0	40.	Samarai	3,100	27.1
13.	Kimbe	9,538	49.1	41.	Laiagam	3,024	28.6
14.	Kavieng	8,856	51.6	42.	Malalaua	2,952	28.4
15.	Alotau	8,266	52.1	43.	Kikori	2,883	28.3
16.	Kundiawa	7,749	55.5	44.	Finschhafen	2,818	26.8
17.	Mendi	7,293	56.6	45.	Bogia	2,755	27.7
18.	Kainantu	6,888	55.3	46.	Namatanai	2,695	27.6
19.	Kerema	6,526	51.4	47.	Chuave	2,638	27.9
20.	Aitape	6,199	54.3	48.	Baimuru	2,583	25.9
21.	Vanimo	5,904	51.7	49.	Kandrian	2,530	24.5
22.	Wau	5,636	42.1	50.	Tari	2,481	24.7
23.	Kokopo	5,391	40.7	51.	Bereina	2,431	24.1
24.	Angoram	5,166	35.4	52.	Losuia	2,384	24.1
25.	Aiyura/Uk.	4,960	34.0	53.	Bwagaoia	2,339	24.4
26.	Wabag	4,769	31.8	54.	Tapini	2,296	23.7
27.	Buka	4,592	33.0	55.	Ihu	2,254	24.2
28.	Kiunga	4,428	30.1	56.	Mumeng	2,214	23.5
				57.	Kaiapit	2,175	23.7
				58.	Saidor	2,138	23.4
Mean - top 15 towns		68.6%		Mean of all towns		40.8%	

Source: NSO 1980 Papua New Guinea Census
Note: KAPL stands for Kieta, Arawa, Panguna and Loloho.

For comparison equivalent rank size figures for Fiji are also included. Having only 15 towns, the separate means for the Papua New Guinean towns present a shart contrast. Although Fiji has only a quarter of Papua New Guinea's population it has a much higher urban population. The 227,025 urban dwellers in 1986 formed 39% of the population. This is not surprising, given the large landless Indian Fijian population. Also because of the smaller size of the country it may be expected that there will be fewer towns and greater emphasis placed on the capital.

However, Fiji is the only other Pacific nation, besides Papua New Guinea, that supports an urban hierarchy. A comparison of table 6 and the Fiji rank size curves, with the census data for Papua New Guinea, shows that Suva is a very strongly primate city.

Table 6. Urban Areas of Fiji: deviation from rank size population.

1986				1976			
Rank	Town	Expected Pop.	% of expected	Rank	Town	Expected Pop.	% of Expected
1.	Suva	-	-	1.	Suva	-	-
2.	Lautoka	70,636	55.3	2.	Lautoka	58,913	49.0
3.	Lami	47,091	35.5	3.	Nadi	39,276	33.1
4.	Labasa	35,318	46.8	4.	Labasa	29,427	44.0
5.	Nadi	28,255	53.9	5.	Nausori	23,565	54.4
6.	Nausori	23,546	59.4	6.	Ba	19,638	46.7
7.	Ba	20,182	50.8	7.	Vatukoula	16,832	38.2
8.	Vatukoula	17,659	27.1	8.	Rakiraki	14,728	25.5
9.	Sigatoka	15,697	30.1	9.	Sigatoka	13,092	27.8
10.	Rakiraki	14,127	23.8	10.	Levuka	11,783	23.5
11.	Levuka	12,843	22.5	11.	Navua	10,712	24.0
12.	Savusavu	11,773	24.4	12.	Savusavu	9,819	23.4
13.	Navua	10,867	25.5	13.	Tavua	9,064	23.7
14.	Tavua	10,091	22.1	14.	Korovou	8,416	3.4
15.	Korovou	9,418	3.6				
Mean all towns			34.3%	Mean all towns			32.1%

Source: 1976 and 1986 Fiji censuses

The primacy of Suva has been advantageous to Fiji's attempts to industrialise. The basis of Fiji's development has been to boost the economic sectors. Decentralisation has played a very small part in government policy. In Papua New Guinea, on the other hand, decentralisation and the attendant expenditure of provincial government, has been of primary importance. Even though the 1980's saw some of the enthusiasm for provincial government diminish, there has been an underlying attempt to keep services and functions out in the provinces as much as possible. The diminution of primacy has been a positive government policy since Independence, even when some governments have shifted emphasis marginally away from decentralisation.

When compared to Fiji's hierarchy, the urban system of Papua New Guinea is still extensive and regionalised. However it must be acknowledged that government policy has probably only slowed down an otherwise inevitable trend towards primacy. Before decentralisation became government policy urbanization was already boosting the small centres. There was least primacy at the beginning of the urban trend, in the 1960's. Subsequently, as government has attempted to spread services, the largest places, especially Port Moresby, have pulled away from the smaller centres, which have probably already played their part in pioneering development in Papua New Guinea.

Thus although the 1990 preliminary census figures suggest that the rate of urbanisation is slowing down, primacy is increasing inexorably, and urban problems will also increase. Not only is it necessary to boost spending on urban services to counteract urban problems, it is time that the towns are recognised for their development potential. Rather than trying to slow their remorseless growth by doing nothing to improve urban centres, it is time to harness their growth, to create jobs for their large unemployed populations and to let the largest places lead development.

REFERENCES

Bakker, M. 1983. "The 1980 Census: some problems encountered in the analysis of demographic data." Yagl Ambu. 10.3 UPNG.

Berry, B & Garrison W. 1958. "Alternative explanations of urban rank-size relationships." Annals of the Association of American Geographers. Vol 48.

Bureau of Statistics. 1988. Population Census 1986. Suva.

Chandra R. 1980. Urbanization in Fiji: 1966 - 1976.

Harding J. 1982. Urban Growth 1966 - 80. Research Monograph Number 1. NSO, Port Moresby.

Jackson R. 1976. An Introduction to the Urban Geography of Papua New Guinea. Geography Department Occasional Paper Number 13. UPNG.

King D. 1981. "Preliminary results of the 1980 Census of Papua New Guinea." Australian Geographer. PNG Scene No. 22. Vol. 15.2. Sydney.

National Statistical Office. 1988. Preliminary Population Estimates: Urban Household Survey 1985-87. Port Moresby

National Statistical Office. 1991. Preliminary Figures: 1990 National Population Census. Port Moresby.

Walsh A. 1983. "Up and Down the PNG Urban Hierarchy." Yagl Ambu 10.3. UPNG.

Rank Size Relationships of Urban Areas
Papua New Guinea 1971

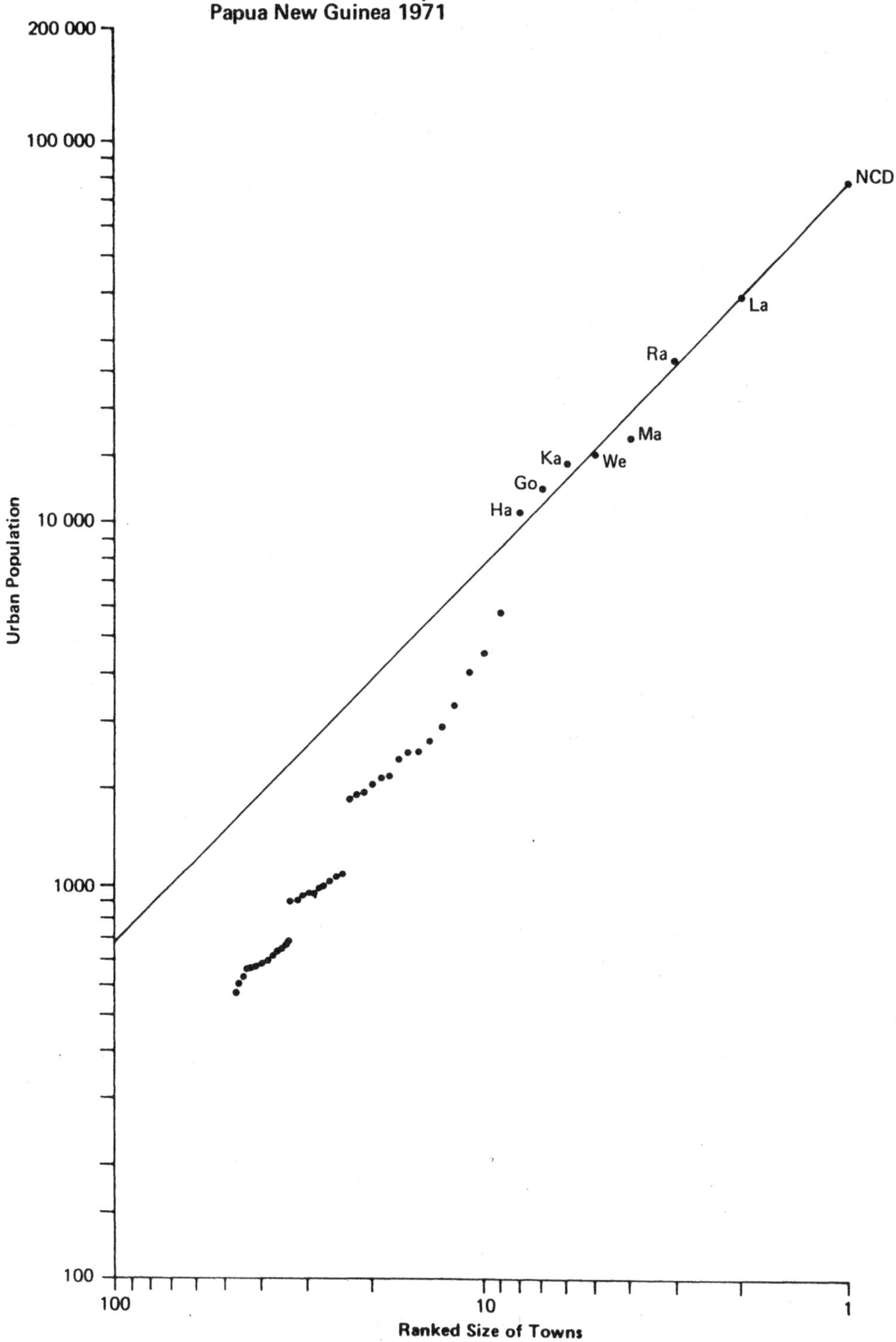

Source: Papua New Guinea 1971 Census, National Statistical Office.

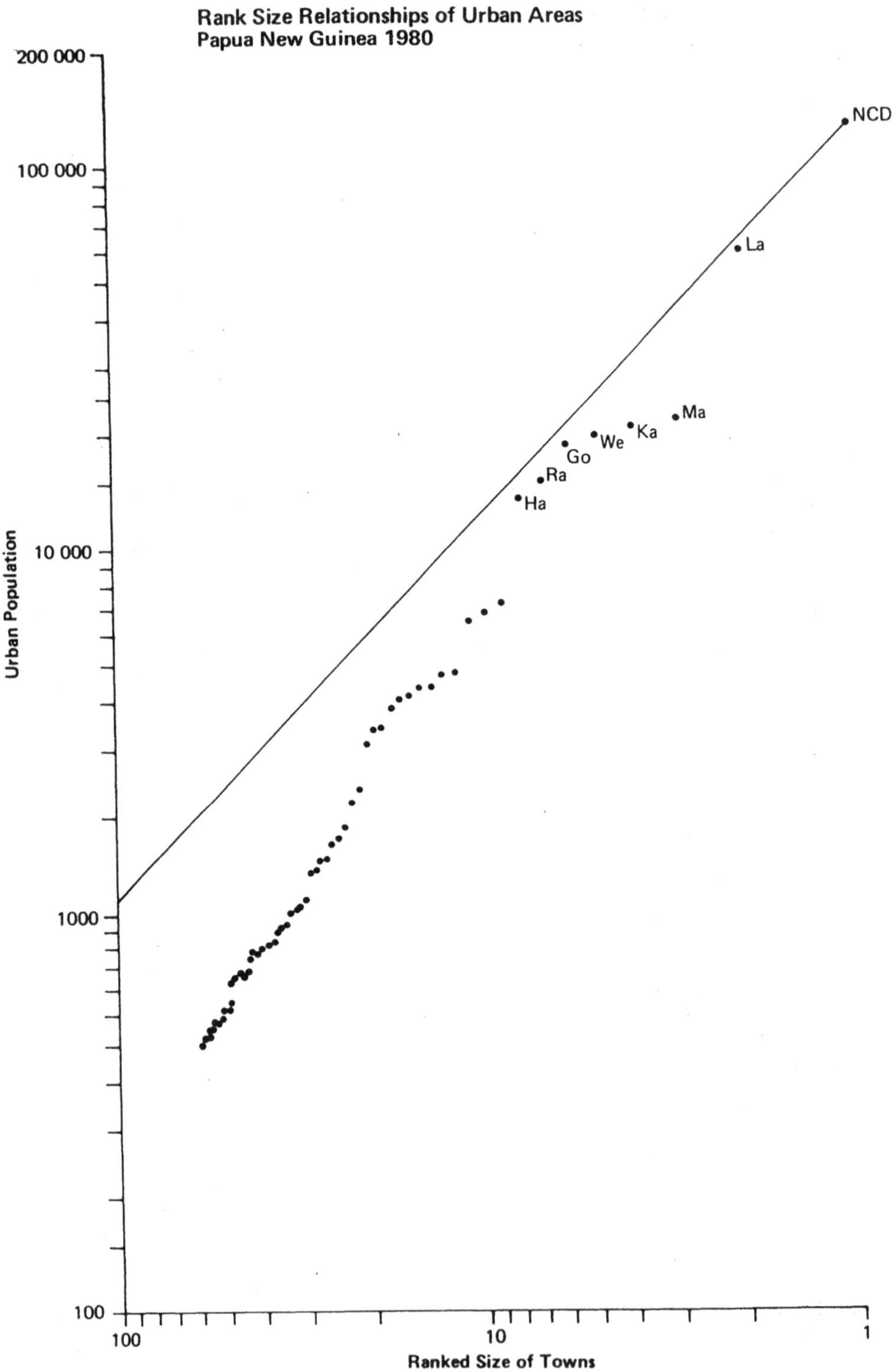

Source: Papua New Guinea 1980 Census, National Statistical Office.

Rank Size Relationship of Urban Areas
Papua New Guinea 1990

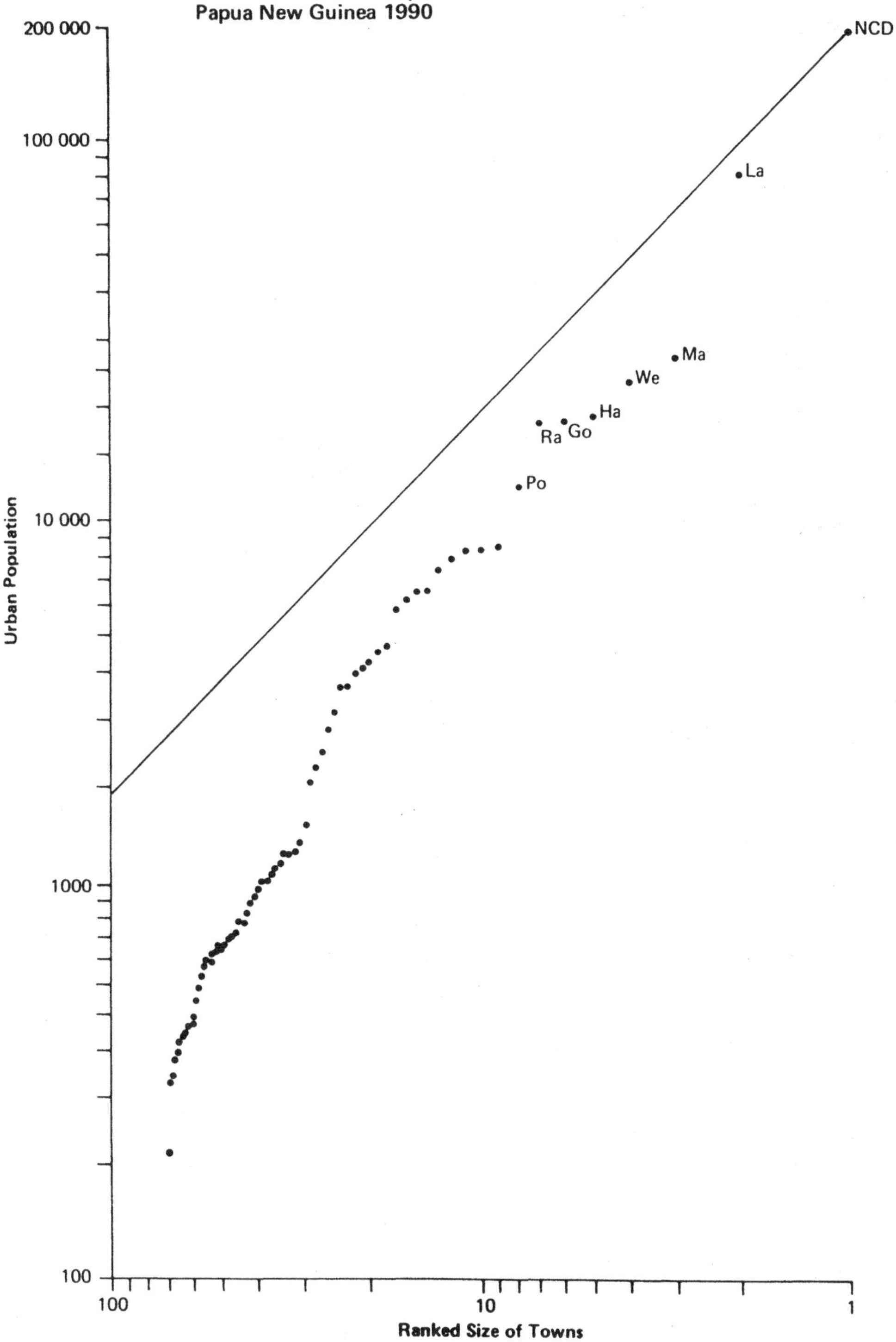

Source: Papua New Guinea 1990 Census, Preliminary Figures, National Statistical Office.

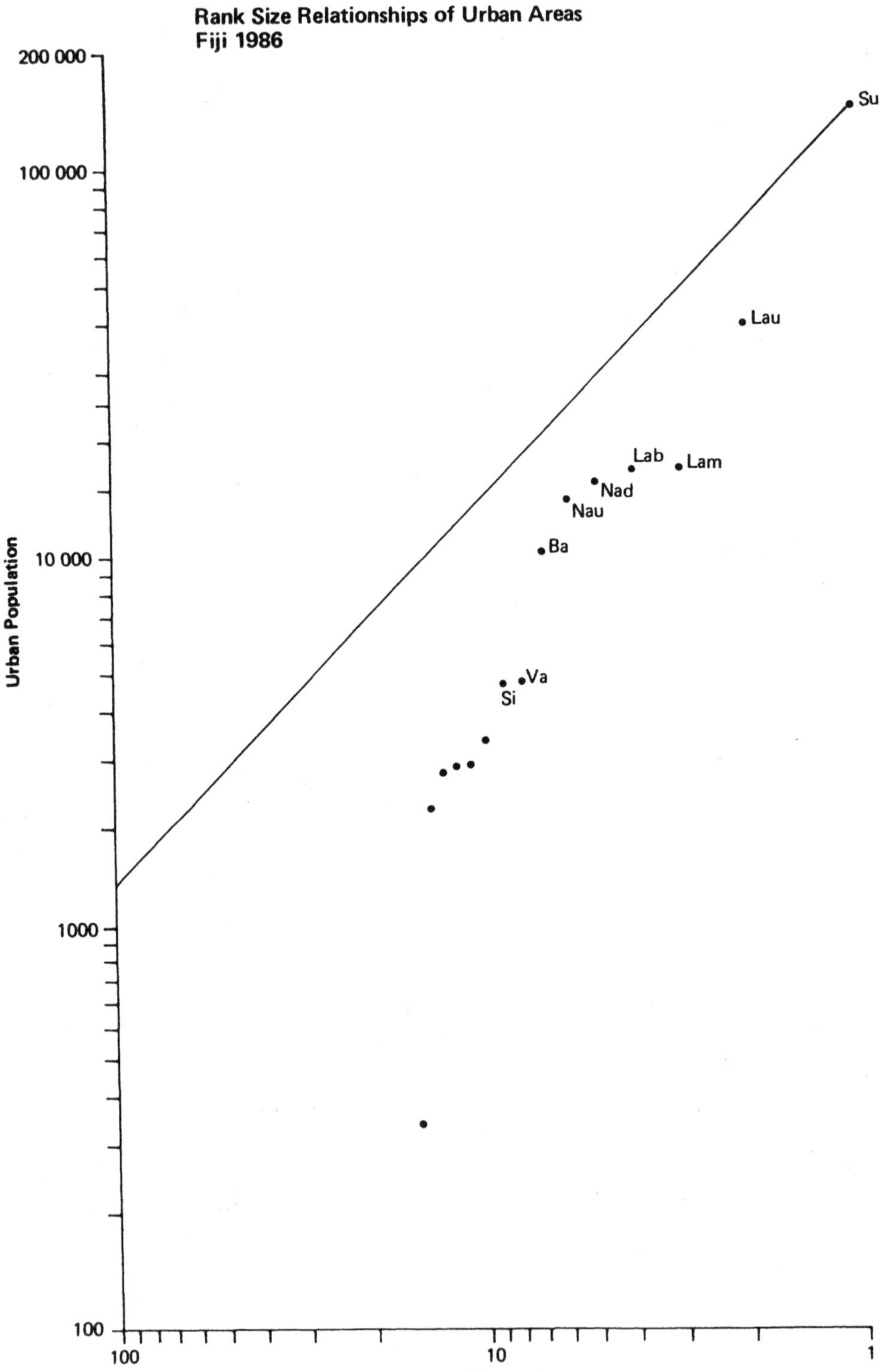

Source: Fiji 1986 Census, National Bureau of Statistics.

Rank Size Relationships of Urban Areas
Fiji 1976

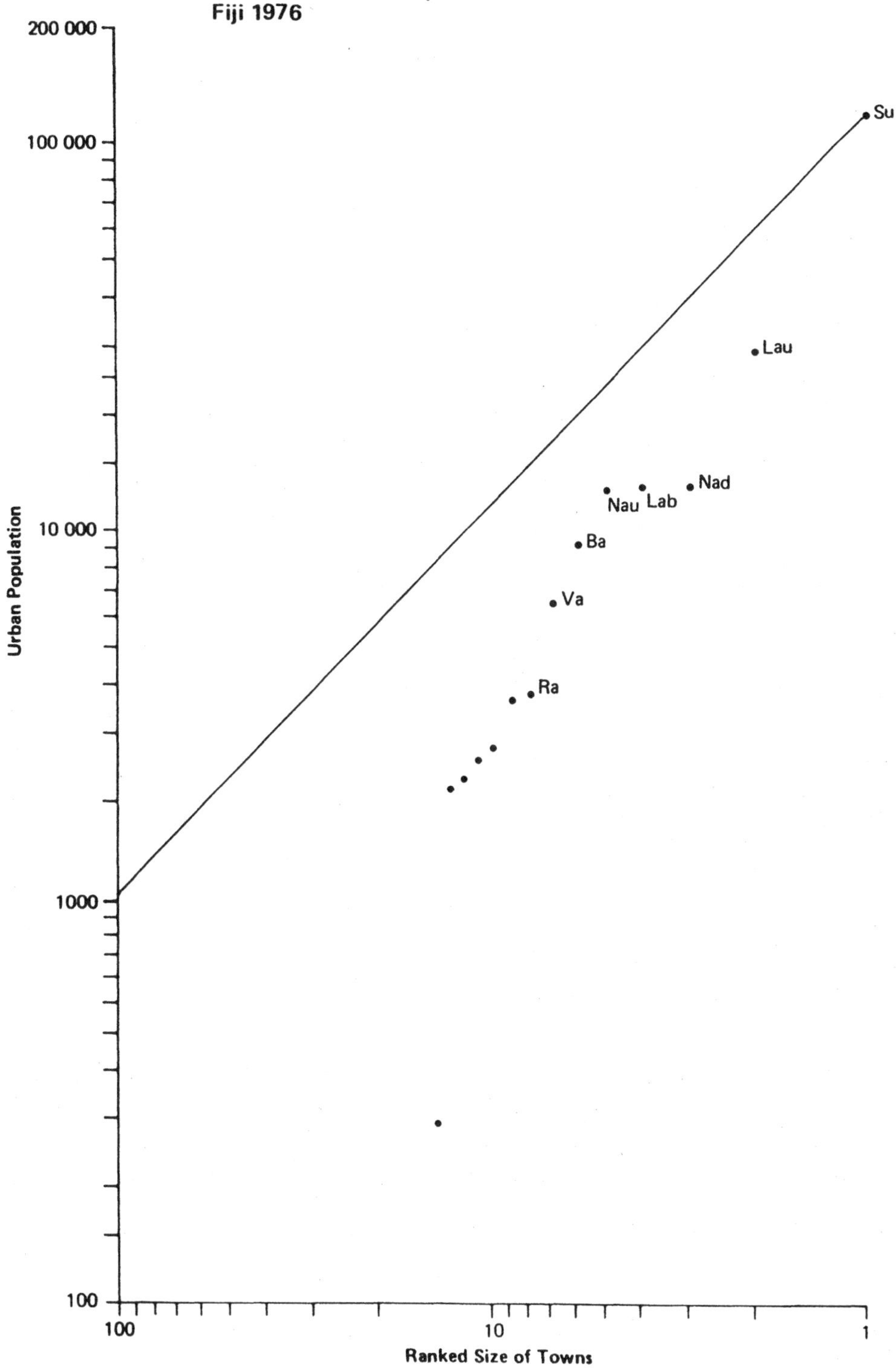

Source: Fiji 1976 Census, National Bureau of Statistics

DISEASE AND DEMOGRAPHIC CHANGE IN PAPUA NEW GUINEA

CAROL JENKINS[1]

INTRODUCTION

This paper will focus on the demographic evidence for the effects of diseases which have a marked effect on fertility, i.e. gonorrhoea, chlamydia and other causes of pelvic inflammatory disease in women and reduced spermatogenesis in men. Historically, in several geographical regions, such as New Ireland during the war years and the southeastern coast of West New Guinea several decades earlier, low levels of fertility were thought to be associated with the introduction of sexually transmitted diseases (STDs). In the latter case, further detailed investigations showed that the high proportion of barren women could not be attributed to the disease in question, which was donovanosis (Vogel and Richens 1989). In the former case, widespread use of penicillin in 1954 for the control of gonnorhoea led to a rapid doubling of the total fertility rate (Ring and Scragg 1973). In the 1966 census, Morobe and Milne Bay districts reported lower fertility than expected. In these areas also the possibility of infection as the underlying factor contributing to lowered fertility was suspected (van de Kaa 1971). Interpretation, however, was always complicated by suspicions of underreporting of births, especially by older women. In more remote areas where STDs were not considered to be a problem, studies produced differing results. Among the Breri people of the lower Ramu Valley, Stanhope (1970) found that only 3% of couples remained childless throughout life, but Serjeantson (1975) found that 9.3% of married women over 40 years old never bore a child in Kiunga, Western Province. Secondary infertility was not addressed in either study.

While the level of family planning usage in Papua New Guinea has not risen over the past few decades, and may even have dropped, especially in rural areas, the prevalence of STDs has risen markedly. Reported cases of gonorrhoea nationally rose from 7005 in 1979 to 11,183 in 1983. In 1973 Sterly wrote that syphilis had been introduced into the highlands after the construction of the Highlands Highway only four years previously. The first case was treated in Goroka in 1969.

1 Papua New Guinea Institute of Medical Research

Successful yaws eradication campaigns of the prior decades had prepared the nation's populations for the invasion of syphilis. Several hospital-based medical studies documented high proportions of both tubal occlusion in females and absent or reduced spermatogenesis in males (Kariks and McGovern 1971; Campbell and Roberts-Thomson 1974). Studies of both female in-patients (Rooke 1982) and out-patients (Mola 1983) conducted in Port Moresby have demonstrated that at least 15% of the former and 48% of the latter who present for gynaecological treatment have pelvic inflammatory disease, most of which can be accounted for by Neisseria gonorrhoea and Chlamydia trachomatis. By 1984 a review of trends in STDs showed that the incidence rates of gonorrhoea and syphilis were 32/1,000 and 11/1,000, representing an eighteen-fold increase over 1972 (Lombange 1984). Recently published health department statistics report incidence rates for gonorrhoea of 10/10,000 in 1969 increasing to 69/10,000 in 1986 (Department of Health 1991). While statistical accuracy is compromised by underreporting and poor data management, there is little doubt that the rates of incidence and prevalence have been increasing rapidly. The interpretation, therefore, of current fertility levels, in particular where they appear to be lower than expected, is confounded by rising levels of infertility secondary to infection and some unknown level of usage of family planning.

STUDY AIMS AND POPULATIONS

Over the past two decades, few studies of specific populations have been conducted which would allow for a closer examination of the components of demographic change. The purpose of this paper is to examine selected components of fertility and infertility in a coastal, highland and fringe highland region from data collected in the 1980s by the Papua New Guinea Institute of Medical Research. All populations in this study are situated in Madang Province and exemplify various levels of exposure to the influences of modernization. Table 1 summarizes the characteristics of these samples.

METHODS

Sampling procedures were somewhat different in each area, but irregularities were controlled in later statistical procedures. The mixed North Coast and Amele populations were enumerated and random sampling procedures were therefore possible. A random sample of approximately one-third of all women, stratified by age group in ten year intervals between ages fifteen and eighty were selected. An alternative woman was selected for each in case the first woman was unreachable. Demography division staff from the PNGIMR were trained to conduct reproductive history taking. Each spouse change was recorded and birthdate documentation sought for all women and their children. In the event of no written documentation, event calendars were used to estimate the date of birth to the nearest year. Among the Gende, reproductive histories were collected during walking patrols to all Gende villages. Birthdates and marriage dates were provided by the Catholic Church records. Reproductive histories of Hagahai women were collected by the author in 1985 and have been updated until present. The data presented represent the situation current at the end of 1990.

Estimated trends in fertility were examined using the method of intercensal averaging of age-specific fertility rates for hypothetical cohorts (Zlotnik and Hill 1980). Cohorts were reconstructed for 1984, 1974 and 1964 among the North Coast, Amele and Gende populations. Infertility was estimated by the method known as Subsequent Infertility as developed by Larsen and Menken (1989). Unmarried women were excluded in these analyses.

RESULTS

Table 3 presents an overview of the fertility trends for these populations. Fertility appears to be declining over the decades. The likelihood of a real demographic transition, entailing deliberate family size control through the use of family planning seems remote. The best estimates of usage rates for rural populations places the proportion of users at 6% (Muirden 1982). Table 4 presents the results of an analysis of age-specific infertility rates, including both primary and secondary infertility, compared to data from the World Fertility Survey on several African populations (Larsen and Menkin 1989). Rates of age-specific infertility among the Gende, in whom we may safely assume negligible levels of contraceptive use, fall between those of Sudan and Cameroon. Larsen and Menken's demonstration of the insensitivity of their method to low levels of contraceptive use suggests that the method has comparable usefulness in Papua New Guinea.

Contraceptive use is likely to be very low in all of these samples. The health centre for the Gende provided no contraceptives. For the Hagahai, high levels of secondary infertility are therefore presumably due entirely to infection. Although health personnel report no signs of STDs among the Hagahai as yet, serological evidence of chlamydia does exist. It is assumed that chlamydia is far more widespread in the more exposed populations of Papua New Guinea.

Age-specific infertility rates among the coastal populations suggests relatively high rates of pelvic inflammatory disease. The Amele have the lowest infertility rates, followed by the North Coast Catholic women. Access to health care best explains these differences. Contraceptive usage is likely to be very low among all of these rural women.

DISCUSSION

The data presented here suggest that, under the present level of contraceptive use in Papua New Guinea, downward trends in fertility cannot be taken to indicate the beginnings of demographic transition, but must be viewed as most likely due to rising levels of infection-derived infertility. Infertility levels in the study populations are as high or higher at each age group as those in Sudan. In this study's rural populations, primary sterility is not yet at levels as high as those in some parts of Africa, but such levels have been found elsewhere in Papua New Guinea and require further study. Overall, secondary infertility appears to play the larger role in dampening fertility rates. Without better data on contraceptive usage and continuance, it is admittedly difficult to assess the exact degree to which infection is lowering fertility. It is clear, however, that the rise in prevalence rates of gonorrhoea far outstrip the rise, if any, in contraceptive usage in rural areas over the past few decades. Evidence of fertility decline reported for the 1980 census in the most urbanized areas of the nation may well reflect both rising STDs and rising contraceptive use.

The demographic evidence presented here has implications for future family planning programmes as well as the AIDS epidemic in Papua New Guinea. Despite factors such as lowered age at menarche which may contribute to increased fertility, in specific areas, fertility is dropping. Further research which will document the true community-level prevalence of STDs among both men and women in relation to contraceptive use is urgent. Most importantly, such research must be linked with behavioural studies allowing for a fuller explanation of the cultural and health service delivery factors contributing to the changing levels of fertility and infertility in Papua New Guinea.

TABLE 1: CHARACTERISTICS OF STUDY POPULATIONS

POP	LOCATION	SIZE	SAMPLE N	YEAR SAMPLED	AGE RANGE	TYPE SAMPLE
AMELE	N.COAST	6800	560	1984	15-80	RANDOM 28 VILLAGES
GENDE	HIGHLAND	5600	561	1984	15-80	EVER MARRIED 31 VILLAGES
MIXED	N.COAST	15,000	1493	1984	15-80	RANDOM 71 VILLAGES
HAGAHAI	FRINGE	272	80	1985-1990	15-55	ALL

TABLE 2. MORTALITY ESTIMATES BASED ON CHILD EVER-BORN METHOD FOR MOTHERS 25-30 YEARS OLD.

POP	IMR	TODDLER MORT RATE	LIFE EXPECT AT BIRTH
AMELE	68	12	65.4
N.COAST	70	13	64.9
GENDE	98	24	58.8
HAGAHAI	217	100	36.7

TABLE 3. INTER-SURVEY AVERAGE COHORT PARITY AND TOTAL FERTILITY FOR RECONSTRUCTED CENSUSES OF STUDY POPULATIONS

	NORTH COAST		AMELE		GENDE	
Age Group	1964-1974	1974-1984	1964 1974	1974-1984	1964-1974	1974-1984
			AVERAGE COHORT PARITY			
15-19	0.223	0.746	0.277	0.571	1.000	0.333
20-24	1.409	1.678	1.309	1.775	1.349	1.180
25-29	3.019	3.281	3.360	3.095	3.061	1.626
30-34	4.568	4.785	4.634	4.775	4.156	2.899
35-39	6.112	5.811	5.456	5.873	5.755	3.741
40-44	6.416	6.493	6.180	6.426	6.136	4.539
45-49	7.839	6.682	8.456	6.658	7.311	5.713
			TOTAL FERTILITY			
ALL	7.84	6.73	8.51	6.70	7.36	5.75

TABLE 4 PROPORTION SUBSEQUENTLY INFERTILE, SI(5), ESTIMATED FOR NORTH COAST, N.COAST CATHOLIC, N.COAST LUTHERAN, AMELE, AND GENDE POPULATIONS COMPARED TO SUDAN AND CAMEROON

Age Group	North Coast	N.C.Catholic	N.C.Lutheran	Amele
20-24	0.10	0.08	0.11	0.10
25-29	0.15	0.13	0.16	0.13
30-34	0.36	0.29	0.33	0.29
35-39	0.55	0.56	0.56	0.50
40-44	0.76	0.72	0.77	0.77
Sample Size	867	319	548	324
Year	1984	1984	1984	1984

	Gende	Hagahai	Sudan*	Cameroon*
20-24	0.10	0.18	0.09	0.17
25-29	0.22	0.21	0.14	0.26
30-34	0.33	0.53	0.27	0.38
35-39	0.54	0.68	0.44	0.51
40-44	0.77	0.82	0.71	0.69
Sample size	455	62	2228	4468
Year	1983	1990	1982	1983

* Source: Larsen and Menken (1989)

REFERENCES

Campbell G R, and Roberts-Thomson K (1974) Infertility in the Highlands.

Department of Health (1991) Papua New Guinea National Health Plan 1990-1995. Port Moresby: Papua New Guinea Department of Health. Papua New Guinea Med. J. 17 (4): 347-353.

Karike J, and McGovern V J (1971) Impaired spermatogenesis and tubular fibrosis in Niugineans: A post-mortem study. Pathol. 3:13

Larsen U, and Menken J (1989) Measuring sterility from incomplete birth histories. Demography 26: 185-201.

Lombange C (1984) Trends in sexually transmitted disease incidence in Papua New Guinea. Papua New Guinea Med. J. 27 (3/4): 145-158.

Mola GDL (1983) Pelvic inflammatory disease in Port Moresby. Papua New Guinea Medical Society Mini-Symposium, Port Moresby.

Muirden N (1982) Family planning programmes. In Population of Papua New Guinea. Country Monograph Series No. 7.2. New York/Noumea: United Nations/South Pacific Commission, pp. 117-129.

Ring A, and Scragg R (1973) A demographic and social study of fertility in rural New Guinea. J. Biosoc. Sci. 5:89-121.

Rooke PW (1982) Pelvic inflammatory disease in Port Moresby General Hospital. Papua New Guinea Med. J. 25: 29-32.

Serjeantson S (1975) Marriage patterns and fertility in three Papua New Guinean populations. Human Biology 47:399-413.

Stanhope J M (1970) Patterns of fertility and mortality in rural New Guinea. New Guinea Res. Bull 34:24-38.

Sterly J (1973) Social context of epidemic syphilis in the Chimbu District, New Guinea. Ethnomedizin II:3/4:311-328.

Van de Kaa D J (1971) The Demography of Papua New Guinea's Indigenous Population. Phd Thesis, Australian National Univ, Canberra.

Vogel L C, and Richens J (1989) Donovanosis in Dutch South New Guinea: History, evolution of the epidemic and control. Papua New Guinea Med. J. 32:203-218.

Zlotnik H, and Hill K (1981) The use of hypothetical cohorts in estimating demographic parameters under conditions of changing fertility and mortality. Demography 18:103-122.

DEMOGRAPHIC TRENDS IN TARI, SOUTHERN HIGHLANDS PROVINCE, PAPUA NEW GUINEA

D LEHMANN[1], J VAIL[2], I D RILEY[3], D R CROCKER[2]

INTRODUCTION

The work of the Tari Research Unit (TRU) in health and demography is highly germane to the theme of the 19th Waigani Seminar; hence, in this paper we would like to give broad consideration to the work of the Unit, while two specific studies are reported elsewhere in this volume (Hughes, 1991; Vail, 1991).

In October this year the Tari Research Unit will be 21 years old. The Unit was set up in the Tari Basin in the Southern Highlands Province of Papua New Guinea (PNG) by Riley primarily to determine the burden of disease (particularly pneumonia) and to evaluate interventions aimed at reducing mortality (Riley, 1979). However, the demographic base maintained throughout the Unit's life provides a unique opportunity to examine demographic trends in a population experiencing rapid social change. Most of the data presented here are for the period 1970-1984. More recent data are currently being analysed in detail.

The usefulness of the demographic base maintained by TRU has in the past been recognised by many researchers in different fields. There have been studies on land-use, soil fertility, nutrition, anthropology and health. Bryant Allen is preparing a monograph incorporating the findings of many of the studies carried out in Tari before 1985. The demographic base has also been used to validate two indirect methods of mortality estimation (Alto, 1991 in this volume; R Bhasin, T Smith and S Rogers, in preparation).

[1] Papua New Guinea Institute of Medical Research, PO Box 60, Goroka, Eastern Highlands Province, Papua New Guinea.

[2] Tari Research Unit, Papua New Guinea Institute of Medical Research, PO Box 35, Tari, Southern Highlands Province, Papua New Guinea.

[3] Tropical Health Program, Faculty of Medicine, University of Queensland, Herston, Qld 4006, Australia.

The Tari Basin lies approximately 6 degrees south of the equator and is inhabited by the Huli people who live between 1500 and 1800 metres above sea level in scattered homesteads surrounded by deep ditches; traditionally men and women live separately. Annual rainfall is approximately 2500 mm and temperature varies between 10°C and 25°C daily, with little seasonal variation. Table 1 lists the most important events over the past 60 years which are relevant to the process of modernization in Tari.

METHOD OF DEMOGRAPHIC SURVEILLANCE

The method of demographic surveillance has been described in detail elsewhere (Riley, 1979; Lehmann, 1984). The population under surveillance includes all people who claim affiliation to clans included in the area under surveillance, irrespective of whether they are permanently resident in the area or not. Reporters are affiliated to the clans which they monitor and have at least primary school education. They collect information on pregnancies, births, deaths, migrations and marriages on a monthly basis. Until now it has been necessary to use male reporters which is not optimal for obtaining accurate information about events occurring during pregnancy, childbirth and the neonatal period. Since many Hulis are not necessarily resident on their own clan ground, fortnightly meetings of all reporters are important to exchange information about events occurring outside individual reporters' areas. All data are collated monthly by office staff. In the event of death, a mortality clerk interviews relatives to obtain information on symptoms which occurred prior to death. Any additional information available from the health services is also used to ascertain the cause of death. Cause of death is coded by an epidemiologist according to a classification of symptom complexes developed by one of us (IDR).

RESULTS

The total population under demographic surveillance in 1977 was 24,000 and in 1990 32,000. Riley (1979) reported a crude death rate (CDR) of 12/1000/annum for the period 1971 - 76. Subsequently the CDR rose to 15/1000/annum between 1977 and 1983 (Lehmann, 1984). Life expectancy at birth between 1978 and 1982 was 51 for females and 50 for males (Lehmann, 1984), much the same as Riley (1979) found in the early '70s. Bhasin, Smith and Rogers (in preparation) calculated life expectancies over the period 1977 to 1989 as 52.0 and 53.6 years for males and females, respectively. The annual growth rate has consistently been in the order of 2.2%. Between 1977 and 1990 there has been little change in the crude birth and death rates apart from 1980 when the CDR rose to 23/1000/annum as a result of an influenza epidemic which affected all age groups. This epidemic may in part explain why the CDR was higher between 1977 and 1983 than in the early 1970s; since 1981 the CDR has been relatively steady around 12/1000/annum. It is noteworthy that mortality rates for pneumonia and chronic lung disease were also higher between 1977 and 1983 than previously reported (Lehmann, 1984; Riley, 1979).

Between 1980 and 1984 the crude birth rate was 34/1000/annum (Lehmann, 1984), the same as during the early 1970s (Riley, 1979). Other measures of fertility did not change either over the same period; the average completed family size was 4.7. Preliminary analysis suggests that there has not been a marked increase in fertility over the past decade.

Between 1980 and 1984, the mean birth interval between a livebirth and a subsequent birth was 36 months (D Lehmann, unpublished data) which suggests that the Huli were still adhering to traditional customs forbidding intercourse in the immediate postpartum period and for a long time afterwards while women are lactating. However, the mean birth interval was only 22 months between a stillbirth and a subsequent birth; the birth interval is also likely to be shortened following the death of a child in the first year of life. To avoid the stress on women of frequent pregnancies in close succession, we must find ways of promoting the utilisation of maternal and child health services which are already in existence and also identify ways of improving the quality of these services.

INFANT MORTALITY

Riley (1979) estimated infant mortality rates for the period 1920-71 by collecting data on outcome of pregnancies and survival of offspring as part of a retrospective fertility survey of a random sample of 774 women. For the periods 1972-74 and 1980-83, infant mortality rates have been determined directly from demographic surveillance (Figure 1). There was a dramatic decline in the infant mortality rate over 50 years before 1972. The most rapid decline was following derestriction in 1962. It was only then that a major extension of health services was possible in areas some distance away from the government station. We attribute the rapid decline in infant mortality (particularly post-neonatal mortality) to the availability of penicillin to treat pneumonia, which accounts for half of all infant deaths. The decline in mortality took place at a time when there were no socio-economic changes in Tari other than the provision of rural health services. Infant mortality has not declined further (and in fact the post-neonatal mortality rate has risen slightly) during the 1970s and 1980s; once mortality has fallen to a certain level, it may be necessary to provide other interventions in addition to basic health services to reduce mortality further. On the other hand, the emergence of bacteria which are partially resistant to penicillin, the increased transmission of viral infections (e.g. measles) as a result of the increased mobility of the population, and possibly a decline in the quality of health services, may also explain why infant mortality has not declined further.

CAUSE OF DEATH

In order to plan and evaluate interventions aimed at reducing mortality, it is necessary to know what illnesses kill people and what the cause-specific mortality rates are. Table 2 shows the proportion of all deaths in different age groups caused by a selection of diseases between 1977 and 1983 (Lehmann, 1984). Pneumonia accounts for more than half the deaths in children under 1 year of age and one-third of all deaths in the 1-4 year age group, and respiratory diseases (chronic lung disease and pneumonia) account for more than 40% of deaths among those aged 45 years or more. Gastroenteritis and dysentery are important causes of death among toddlers. Injuries were the most important cause of death in young adults, with very high rates of suicide among females and homicide among males and females (Barss, 1991). It is noteworthy that Riley (1979) reported only 2 deaths from measles between 1971 and 1976 while there were 48 deaths from measles between 1977 and 1983 (Lehmann, 1984).

IMPACT OF SPECIFIC INTERVENTIONS

Three interventions (a pneumococcal vaccine trial, pigbel immunisation and oral rehydration programmes) have had an impact on childhood mortality in Tari. They provide examples of how the demographic base has been used to evaluate innovative methods of disease control as well as programmes established by the Division of Health of the Department of Southern Highlands Province. Furthermore these interventions suggest that we may see a marked reduction in childhood mortality in the near future if these and other planned interventions are successfully implemented on a wider scale.

1. PNEUMOCOCCAL VACCINE TRIAL

In the highlands of PNG, pneumonia accounts for a high proportion of deaths. Therefore we will only succeed in reducing overall childhood mortality through interventions aimed at reducing mortality from pneumonia. The pneumococcus accounts for approximately half of bacterial pneumonias in the highlands of PNG (Shann et al, 1984, Barker et al, 1989). A randomised placebo-controlled trial of polyvalent pneumococcal vaccine took place in Tari between 1981 and 1985 among children aged 4 months to 5 years (Riley et al, 1986). During the trial period, pneumonia mortality fell by half in the 1-4 year age group (Lehmann, 1984). There were less than half the number of deaths attributed to pneumonia as the sole cause of death among children who received the vaccine compared to the placebo group (Riley et al, 1986). In the vaccinated group, there were no deaths due to pneumonia alone among children more than 12 months of age (D Lehmann et al, unpublished data). Total mortality was 30% lower in the vaccine than the placebo group (Riley et al, 1986). Unfortunately, this polyvalent pneumococcal vaccine does not prevent death in children aged less than 9 months who are at greatest risk of dying of pneumonia. However, new vaccines are currently being developed and the possibility of passive immunisation of young children by vaccinating pregnant women is under investigation.

Immunisation against pneumonia could result in a marked reduction in childhood mortality in PNG in the not-too-distant future. Of course this is dependent firstly on whether vaccines will be available at prices which we can afford and secondly on the successful delivery of vaccine to rural areas.

2. **PIGBEL**

Previously pigbel was the commonest cause of death in children aged 5-14 years in some areas of the highlands (Davis, 1984). Pigbel vaccine has been provided throughout the highlands to children attending MCH clinics since 1980 or 1981. Following the introduction of pigbel vaccine in Tari there has been a dramatic reduction in mortality from this disease (Lawrence et al, 1990).

3. **ORAL REHYDRATION PROGRAMME**

In Tari, we were also able to demonstrate a significant decline in mortality from diarrhoea following the introduction of a province-wide oral rehydration programme (Frankel and Lehmann, 1984). Sadly, since 1983, problems in the implementation of the programme have resulted in a renewed increase in diarrhoea mortality (Rogers, 1988).

MIGRATION

During the 1960s and 1970s, young Huli men were recruited through the Highlands Labour Scheme to work on plantations in coastal areas (Harris, 1977) and many stayed away from Tari for several years. Few women travelled outside Tari at that time. More recently, particularly since the completion of the Highlands Highway in 1981, both Huli men and women have travelled extensively to other parts of the highlands. During the 1980s more than 40% of young adult males were absent from Tari at any particular time (D Lehmann, unpublished data). People no longer stay away from Tari for prolonged periods but make frequent short excursions. Between 1980 and 1984, the total number of migrations rose 3-fold, but in view of the brief periods spent out of Tari, the actual number of people absent from Tari at any particular time changed little over the same period (D Lehmann, unpublished data).

A large number of Hulis have thus been exposed recently and rapidly to the outside world and a non-traditional society. The benefits of frequent travel in and out of Tari include the potential of participating in a cash economy, the import of goods to Tari and experience of the new world. However, on the negative side, movement of Hulis, other Papua New Guineans and expatriates in and out of Tari has resulted not only in a dramatic increase in the incidence of sexually transmitted diseases, but also in the import of viruses such as measles and influenza to which people might not otherwise have been exposed. Previously, the bachelor cult and then the long-term migration to plantations on the coast meant that men did not marry until they were perhaps 10 years older than women. With the present short-term migration pattern of both men and women as well as the tendency of men to take their wives with them out of Tari for longer periods of time, men are likely to marry earlier and start having children at a younger age.

COMMENT

During the 1970s and early 1980s, we did not see dramatic changes in overall mortality and fertility rates. However, there have been major social changes in Tari during the past decade. One might speculate that overall fertility has not risen as a result of the increased incidence of sexually transmitted diseases and hence secondary infertility. It is likely that in the years to come mortality will decline (as a result of increased utilisation of health services and the availability of new vaccine to prevent childhood deaths) but the birth rate is unlikely to fall at an equivalent rate. At present rates of mortality and fertility there will be twice as many people living in Tari within 30 years, and the central part of the Tari Basin is already one of the most densely populated areas in PNG. We must urgently consider ways of dealing with the rapid changes occurring in Tari which may also be relevant to many other parts of PNG. These include:

1. implementing some of the measures to improve soil fertility and increase crop yields recommended by Wood (1985);

2. providing equitable opportunities for education and good health;

3. providing adequate family planning services. This has frequently been expressed as a felt need by women in Tari but not always been shared by Huli men (Frankel, 1982). At the same time, means of preventing sexually transmitted diseases must be available to both men and women.

ACKNOWLEDGEMENTS

We would like to thank some of the many people who have helped prepare the data included in this paper. First and foremost we would like to thank the Hulis who have been so tolerant of our frequent intrusions on their personal lives and all the reporters, reporter supervisors and office staff of the Tari Research Unit. Tony Mount and Steve Tulloch assisted in data management, programming and analysis. Drs L Clarke, J Hohnen, M Hohnen, W Alto and R Crittenden and Mr M Mauludu provided support and advice to members of the Tari Research Unit.

REFERENCES

Alto W. Measurement of Child Mortality in Association with a multi-purpose birth certificate programme in the Southern Highlands Province of Papua New Guinea. 1991 Proceedings from the 19th Waigani Seminar.

Barker J, Gratten M, Riley I, Lehmann D. Montgomery J, Kajoi M, Gratten H, Smith D, Marshall TF de C, Alpers MP. Pneumonia in children in the Eastern Highlands of Papua New Guinea: a bacteriologic study of patients selected by standard clinical criteria. J Infect Dis 1989; 159:348-352.

Barss PG. Health impact of injuries in the highlands of Papua New Guinea: a verbal autopsy study. DSc thesis, Johns Hopkins University, Baltimore, 1991.

Davis MW, ed. Pigbel. Necrotising enteritis in Papua New Guinea. Papua New Guinea Institute of Medical Research Monograph No. 6. Goroka: Papua New Guinea Institute of Medical Research, 1984.

Frankel S. Family health services and the organization of health care in Tari. An evaluation prepared for the Southern Highlands Project. Mendi, Southern Highlands Province: Media Unit, 1982.

Frankel SJ, Lehmann D. Oral rehydration therapy: combining anthropological and epidemiological approaches in the evaluation of a Papua New Guinea programme. J Trop Med Hyg 1984: 87:137-142.

Harris GT. Labour supply and economic development in the Southern Highlands of Papua New Guinea. In: May RJ, ed. Change and Movement. Readings on Internal Migration in Papua New Guinea. Canberra: Australia National University Press, 1977.

Hughes J and Dyke T. Barriers and bridges to the spread of sexually transmitted diseases amongst the Huli of the Southern Highlands Province of Papua New Guinea. 1991, Proceedings from the 19th Waigani Seminar.

Lawrence G, Lehmann D, Anian G, Coakley CA, Saleu G, Barker MJ, Davies M. The impact of active immunisation on enteritis necroticans in Papua New Guinea. Lancet 1990; 2:1165-66.

Lehmann D. Tari Research Unit. Final report for the Southern Highlands Rural Development Project. Mendi, Southern Highlands Province: Media Unit, 1984.

Riley ID. Pneumonia in Papua New Guinea. A study of the effects of western medicine upon disease in a developing country. MD thesis, University of Sydney, 1979. 369pp.

Riley ID, Lehmann D, Alpers MP, Marshall TF de C, Gratten H, Smith D. Pneumococcal vaccine prevents death from acute lower respiratory infections in Papua New Guinean children. Lancet 1986; 2:877-881.

Rogers S. Oral rehydration therapy: review of a programme in the Southern Highlands Province of Papua New Guinea. MFCM dissertation, Faculty of Community Medicine, United Kingdom, 1988.

Shann F, Gratten M, Germer S, Linnemann V, Hazlett D, Payne R. Aetiology of pneumonia in children in Goroka Hospital, Papua New Guinea. Lancet 1984; 2:537-541.

Vail J. Impact of the Mt Kare goldrush on people in the Tari District. 1991, Proceedings from the 19th Waigani Seminar.

Wood AW. The stability and permanence of Huli agriculture. Department of Geography, University of Papua New Guinea and Southern Highlands Rural Development Project Occasional Paper No. 5. Mendi, Southern Highlands Province: Media Unit, 1985.

Table 1. Historic events related to modernization in Tari

1934	Fox brothers came through Tari
1935	J Hides and LJ O'Malley patrol
1938-40	Patrols by I Champion and others
1938	J Taylor and JR Black stayed in Hoiebia during Hagen-Sepik patrol
1952	Patrol post set up in Tari
1954	First health patrol
1955+	Different missions arrived in Tari
1961-62	Tari/Koroba area declared 'under administration control'
1960s & '70s	Huli men recruited to work on plantations in coastal areas through Highlands Labour Scheme
1970	Tari Research Unit, Tari High School, Dauli Teacher's College established
1981	Completion of Highlands Highway linking Tari to Mendi, Mount Hagen etc
1982+	Oil exploration in vicinity of Tari
1987-90	Mount Kare goldrush
1990-	Development of Hides gas field south of Tari to provide power to Porgera gold mine

Table 2. Proportion of all deaths at varying ages caused by a selection of diseases (1977-83)

CAUSE	AGE (YEARS)				
	≤1	1-4	5-14	15-44	45+
Pneumonia	53%	34%	21%	11%	19%
Chronic lung disease	-	-	-	8%	24%
Gastroenteritis/ Dysentery	5%	22%	21%	2%	6%
Measles	4%	5%	-	0.8%	0.9%
Neonatal/ Congenital	21%	1%	-	-	-
Accidental injury	1%	6%	12%	20%	3%
Total deaths	**235**	**289**	**109**	**325**	**1365**
Mortality rate/1000/annum	**68**	**18**	**2**	**5**	**47**

URBAN MIGRATION FROM THE MOUNT BROWN AREA OF THE INLAND RIGO DISTRICT OF CENTRAL PROVINCE, PAPUA NEW GUINEA

F E TILBURY[1] AND R N TILBURY[2]

INTRODUCTION

The Ago people of Mt Brown number about 2000 in total, with a shared language and customs. As is usual in other parts of Papua New Guinea, a few surrounding villages also speak the Ago language, in addition to their own, due to intermarriage over many years. The Ago people are currently located in twelve main villages in the Mt Brown area of inland Rigo in the Central Province of Papua New Guinea, approximately 100km due east of Port Moresby. Although close to the capital it is categorized in the remotest 5% of the country by the Health Department, mainly due to its rugged mountainous terrain. Access to the area is limited, it being about two days walk from the end of a four-wheel-drive road at Wiga. An airstrip was opened in 1988 serviced by a third level airline (Douglas Airways), however, after only 18 months the airline closed and now flights into Mt Brown are by charter only.

The Ago people are traditionally patrilineal and polygynous. Slash and burn (swidden) shifting agriculture provides the basic diet of kaukau (sweet potato), yam, taro, bananas, sugar cane, aibika and other greens, which is supplemented by pandanas fruit, wild mangoes, other tree fruit, prawns, eels, wild pigs, cuscus, cassowary and domestic pigs. Intensive subsistence cultivation, in a shifting pattern, provides a plentiful supply of food.

Due to its remoteness, development in the area has been slow and irregular. The missionaries first opened a school in the area as far back as 1953 (1, 2) where the lessons were given by the resident pastor himself. Other villages opened mission schools at different times when they could afford to pay for a pastor. The mission schools taught only lower primary and they came and went depending on the availability of pastors. The people's initial ambivalence to the mission schools (3), which saw villagers sending their children to hide in the bush or telling them to act slow when the missionaries first came, in fear that the children would be

1 Department of Anthropology, Sociology and Social Work
The University of Papua New Guinea

2 Chemistry Department, The University of Papua New Guinea

taken away to school, very quickly changed to enthusiasm for education. In fact, one of the most stated reasons for migrating from Mt Brown is the unreliability of the village school. In 1979 the first government school opened in the area in the village of Homenomu. The furthest walk to the school is about 6 hours, but some students stay at the school returning to their villages for the weekend. This school has since been struggling to stay open due to teachers not wanting to stay. At present two classes (grades 3 and 4) are offered with a total enrolment of 21 or only 13.2% of the children of school age (10-19 years of age) residing in the area. this compares to over 53% of this age group schooling just two years ago (1989) when four classes (grades 1, 2, 5 and 6) were being offered.

Health services were also initially established by the missionaries on a limited basis and in the 1960s the government established two aidposts in the area(4). Currently there are still two aidposts in the area each with an aidpost orderly but there are always difficulties in maintaining any stock of basic medicines. They are located within 4 hours walk of the furthest village but responsibility is not well defined. This has lead to loss of life as recently as 1988 when a woman fell off a cliff and was bleeding heavily. A villager rushed to the aidpost (4 hour walk) but was turned back and told that the other aidpost was responsible for the woman's village. So he rushed to the other aidpost whose orderly also insisted that he was not responsible for the woman's village - by the time responsibility was determined the woman had died.

Coffee was introduced (5) in many of the villages in the area in the 1960s, but by 1964 all but one village had given up and neglected their crops due to the difficulty in reaching markets (5). This was also compounded by a coffee eradication programme (4) in the area in 1965 due to coffee rust. That the area was suitable for coffee growing was evidenced by the fact that after its attempted introduction it was found growing wild but unfortunately unsuitable for use. It is now being grown on a small scale, with adequate training. However, the people still require a government subsidy to transport it to market. Other cash crops such as chilli and cardamon have been sucessfully grown in the area since the early 1970s but there is still difficulty in transporting the produce to market.

Trade stores have also come and gone on a regular basis in most villages in the area since about 1966 (6), but once again obtaining stocks has proved difficult. In 1989 one trade store was burnt down by its owner out of frustration and in protest after not being able to get some supplies. There are currently four trade stores operating in the area. Other facilities in the area include three sports fields and six religious centres.

The purpose of this paper is to examine the rate and extent of migration of the Ago people and to study the effects that this has had on individual and village life and how it is effecting the culture of the people. The Ago people were selected for this study because the population was small enough to include the majority of the people in the study and yet large enough to provide adequate statistics for wider applicability. A limitation on the study is that the applicability of the results to people of other areas, who may not have experienced the same difficulties, and hence not had the same degree of pressure to migrate.

METHODOLOGY

The difficulty of defining migration in Papua New Guinea has been noted by Young (7). We have defined migration as an absence from the rural village for a period greater than six months and with the intention of setting up residence. Simpler definitions have been used (8, 9) but the period of stay (one month, and three months as used in kiap times, respectively) is far too brief to give any real indication of whether a person has migrated or is just visiting. It is common practice for the Ago villagers from Mt Brown to 'visit' relatives or friends in Port Moresby and rural non-villages (RNVs) for periods extending to several months.

The basic data, such as name, age, sex, clan, religious denomination, family size, marital status, education and migration experience, have been acquired by a survey of the total population of ten villages. This survey was carried out in April 1989. Follow up interviews were also carried out in April 1990 and April 1991. In addition, a further 188 Ago migrants living in Port Moresby and several rural non-villages were interviewed.

HISTORICAL PERSPECTIVE OF THE MIGRATION OF THE AGO PEOPLE

Although the Ago people's first contact with Europeans was during the First World War there had only been limited contact until the Second World War and village life had remained relatively undisturbed between the wars. Government patrols had visited the area in 1935 and again in 1943 but spent less than four days in the Ago villages. Several men were recruited to work on nearby plantations, but generally there were more than enough willing workers from closer areas of Rigo so that the patrols did not usually need to recruit from this area and only about 20 men had worked on the plantations prior to 1945. It was not until early in 1945, just a few months before the end of the war, that major contact was made in the form of recruitment by Government Officers. Almost 100 young men (18-30 years of age) were taken to act as carriers for the war effort. This would account for 57% of the total population of Ago men in this age group today, but it would be expected to be an even higher percentage of the population in 1945. Surviving war carriers interviewed in the village say that in fact all of the strong young men from each village were taken at that time. The Ago men were used to carry supplies for the army and also to carry the injured back to their base camps. The first Ago man to see the smoke from, and hear, a machine gun being fired escaped that same night from the army camp and made his way back to his village. So horrified was he with what he saw, that he told the other villagers his story and assured them that none of the other men would ever return. Fortunately, the war ended soon after this episode and nearly all of the young men were returned to their villages after a few months absence. This was the first large movement of people from the area.

Migration to Plantations and Towns of the Central Province

The government patrols had appointed village councillors and policemen from within each village and increased contact was maintained with the Government station at Rigo after the war. Around 1950 the first (voluntary) migration of the Ago people took place when four men came to Rigo to ask for permission from the Government to go to work on the plantations. They were taken by boat from Gabagaba to Port Moresby and then out to surrounding plantations (such as the Doa and Mariboi estates). By 1953 about 25 young Ago men were working on various plantations throughout what is now the Central Province, and by 1960 this figure had reached 100. Table 1 shows the rate and number of Ago people migrating to Port Moresby and the plantations and small towns (rural non-village (RNV) migration) of the Central Province by five-yearly intervals since 1950, as well as the cumulative totals. This estimated data is based on government patrol reports and several independent informants.

Table 1: Number and Percentage of Ago Migrants in Rural Non-Villages and in Port Moresby by Five-Yearly Intervals since 1950

Period	1951-55	56-60	61-65	66-70	71-75	76-80	81-85	86-90
Rural Non-Village								
Number migrated	40	60	150	-50	50	50	50	50
% of Village Population	2.4	3.6	9.4	-3.6	4.3	4.8	5.3	5.9
Total Number of Migrants	40	100	250	200	250	300	350	400
% of Total Popn Migrated	2.4	5.9	14.7	11.8	14.7	17.6	20.6	23.5
Port Moresby								
Number migrated	0	10	40	300	50	50	50	100
% of Village Popn	0	0.6	2.5	21.4	4.3	4.8	5.3	11.8
Total Number of Migrants	0	10	50	350	400	450	500	600
% of Total Popn Migrated	0	0.6	2.9	20.6	23.5	26.5	29.4	35.3
Total								
% of Total Popn Migrated to RNVs and Port Moresby	2.4	6.5	17.6	32.4	38.2	44.1	50.0	58.8

This first phase of migration was almost exclusively restricted to young strong unmarried men. The few who were married almost always left their wives back in the village. The intention at this time was not to stay on the plantations permanently but just to earn some money to buy goods for themselves and their extended families in the village and then return to the village. During the 1960s the trend changed and many of the unmarried men working on the plantations went back to the villages only to marry and return to the plantations with their wives. Also with small communities being established on the plantations, it now became much easier for married men to go to work on the plantations and to bring along their immediate family. This trend has also been noted by Levine and Levine (10) and Dakeyne (11) for the Highlands and northern Papua regions, respectively. This trend would partly account for the upsurge in migrants to RNVs in the 1961-65 period shown in Table 1. This five-year period saw almost 10% of the total village population migrating to the RNVs.

With the advent of formal education of the Ago people in the 1950s some were able to obtain semi-skilled work in the small towns in the Rigo and nearby areas. With the growth of these small towns in the 1960s there were also more employment opportunities for unskilled workers. These factors could also help to explain the larger rate of migration in the early 1960s. The growth of the small towns brought with it new markets for the sale of local produce. However, the distance and the difficult access to the Mt Brown region prevented the Ago people from directly participating in these markets from their home villages. For those who were working on nearby plantations or in the towns, the markets offered an additional source of income if they could grow their own gardens. This also made the migration to RNVs more attractive for spouses and families, since they could then tend the gardens while the men were working.

Table 1 shows an overall decrease in the number of migrants in RNVs in the period 1966-70. There are probably two main reasons for this overall decline. Firstly, there was a decline in plantation employment from the late 1960s, and secondly, Port Moresby became much more accessible around this time and may have attracted those who became unemployed on the plantations. An additional factor may have been a greater rate of migrants returning to their home villages after the initial upsurge in migration in the early 1960s.

From 1970 through to the present there has been a steady increase in the number of migrants in RNVs, approximately 4-6% of the total village population every five years. During this period, however, many of the plnatations were closed or drastically reduced their operations and hence would not account for many new migrants, and in fact this should have lead to a fall in the number of migrants due to loss of employment. The movement to small towns could have compensated for the decline in migration to the plantations but it would not have accounted for the overall steady increase over this period if the plantation migrants returned to their villages. A most interesting development took place at this time on the plantations. Since many families had joined the men on the plantations in the 1960s and had planted gardens, small villages modelled on their home villages had emerged on the plantations. When the plantation closed these poeple found that there were obvious advantages in staying in their new village rather than returning to Mt Brown, the main one being that they were close to markets so that they still had a steady income which would not have been available to them in their home village.

One example of these new villages is Sivigoro, located on the outskirts of Kwikila. It has many of the advantages of urban life, being close to the Kwikila market which provides an average family income of K50 per fortnight from the sale of produce, readily available goods in town, as well as easy access to Port Moresby. It also retains many of the stated advantages of village life, such as 'free' food, water and housing, and no set working hours. One major disadvantage is land ownership. In the case of Sivigoro, the plantation was sold back to the original landowners in 1973 and the landowners tried to chase the new settlers off their land but were not successful. An agreement was finally reached whereby the landowners tax the Ago people for the use of their land. It was noted that a degree of integration of the Ago people and the landowners has already developed with the formation of one large village and some inter-marriage.

Migration to Port Moresby

In the late 1950s a track was made between Rigo and Port Moresby and the first Ago man to migrate to Port Moresby came by this track in 1958 and obtained employment in Port Moresby as a domestic servant. The journey meant sleeping out for at least two nights on the track between Rigo and Port Moresby and there was a real danger of being attacked by other village people along the way, because the Ago people were very different from the coastal peoples. For this reason only about ten Ago men had come to Port Moresby for work by 1960. Two significant developments occurred in the early 1960s. Firstly, in 1960 an Australian man married to a coastal lady started the first transport service from Kwikila to Port Moresby, to bring people's produce to market and also for passengers. Secondly, in 1961 two American men discovered copper around the Wiga area and extended a rough road built during the war from Kwikila to Buka to Wiga for use by trucks. Incidentally, after the completion of the road, the men began digging for the copper and almost immediately dug up a recently buried man from Wiga, whereupon the villagers chased them out and soon after they left the country.

These two developments meant Port Moresby was now much more accessible and the 1960s saw the greatest level of migration of the Ago people with over 20% of the total village population migrating to Port Moresby in the period 1966-70 (Table 1). As mentioned earlier, however, a portion of these migrants would have come from the RNVs instead of directly from the villages. During the 1970s and most of the 1980s the level of migration was fairly constant (ca.5%) but had slowed significantly from the 1960s level. The 1970s also saw a rise in the number of migrants returning to the village, so there must also have been an increase in the actual number of migrants but this not evident in Table 1 since it only shows the net migration. The main areas of employment for those who came to Port Moresby in the 1960s were shopkeepers, drivers, labourers and domestic servants.

Table 1 shows that the rate of migration to Port Moresby has doubled in the last five years to almost 12% of the total village population from a rate of about 5% for the previous 15 years. This is attributed to the recent opening of the airstrip which, despite the costs, is heavily used by many of the villagers, even now that flights into the area are by charter only.

RESULTS

Migration Experience of Resident Villagers

Table 2 compares the percentage of the population resident in the ten villages studied who have never migrated, with those who have returned to their village. It is seen that overall about one in every five villagers have had some migration experience. For the male population this increases to one in four, while for females it is only one in every eight.

Table 2 Total Population of Mt Brown Villages by Sex and Migration

	MALES		FEMALES		TOTAL	
	N	%	N	%	N	%
Never Migrated:	241	75.3	251	88.1	492	81.3
Returned Migrant:	79	24.7	34	11.9	113	18.7

When the age of the villagers is considered an interesting pattern emerges (Table 3). The general trends are firstly, as expected, very few of the children resident in the village have had migration experience (about 6% for either males or females), this level then doubles to about 13% for the 15-24 year age group (total), then increases to almost 34% for the next two age groups (25-44 years of age), and finally there is a further increase to about 40% for the above 45 year age groups. However, when sex is considered different trends are observed. Thus, the percentage of the male population that have had migration experience increases directly with age from 6% for male children through to almost 70% for the over 54 age group. While almost 70% of men over the age of 54 have had migration experience, only about 16% of women in this age group have. For females the peak of having had migration experience is at the age of 25-34 and not at the oldest age group as is the case for males. Even at the peak, less than 30% of the women have had migration experience. The data for female migration experience suggests that, for the women, migration is a relatively new phenomena compared to the men. Similar trends to the above were observed (8) for the Kilenge villages of West New Britain.

TABLE 3 Male, Female and Total Population of Mt Brown Villages by Age and Migration Experience

Age Group:	0-14	15-24	25-34	35-44	45-54	55+	Total
MALES							
Never Migrated:	93.6	80.6	58.8	50.0	44.4	31.2	75.3
Returned Migrant:	6.4	19.4	41.2	50.0	55.6	68.8	24.7
FEMALES							
Never Migrated:	93.3	92.5	72.1	82.9	93.7	84.2	88.1
Returned Migrant:	6.7	7.5	27.9	17.1	6.3	15.8	11.9
TOTAL							
Never Migrated:	93.6	86.8	66.2	66.2	62.8	60.0	81.3
Returned Migrant:	6.4	13.2	33.8	33.8	37.2	40.0	18.7

This data is suggestive of two interpretations. Firstly, it may indicate that the older a person becomes the more likely they will return to the village from a migration, or secondly, that the figures reflect the first large wave of migration from this area in the 1960s. These two interpretations, however, are not mutally exclusive and both may account for the trend to different degrees. The second interpretation is supported by the fact that the villagers aged above 44 years now would have been in the prime age group (16-30) for migration in the early 1960s. Since it was mainly the men who migrated at this stage then this would also explain the lower number of women with migration experience in these age groups. The trend also seems to support the claim of many of the Ago urban dwellers that they will eventually return to their village, be it due to termination of employment, their children completing their education, or land related issues.

Almost all of the resident villagers have visited Port Moresby and/or the RNVs and many do so on a regular basis. In April 1991 the extent of 'visiting' was examined and it was found that 22.3% of the total village population were absent at that time. Of these, 35.6% were visiting in Port Moresby while 63.7% were visiting in five different RNVs in the Central Province (one person was visiting in another province). The same is not true, however, for the Ago migrants visiting the villages. Although ties to the village are strong and it is always seen as home, it is surprising to note the infrequency with which visits back to the village are made. Ryan (12) also notes this. At the time of interviewing <1% of the total Port Moresby and RNV migrants were visiting the Ago villages. While this value may be higher in the December/January vacation period when migrant workers would be able to visit, of those interviewed many had not visited the villages for several years.

Effect of Migration on Village Population

Table 4 gives the breakdown of the population according to age and sex for the ten villages studies as of 1990 and compares this with previous census data (13) for the entire census division of Mt Brown. Unfortunately, the 1990 Census data collected by the National Statistical Office was not available at the time of writing. Data for the same ten villages could not be abstracted from previous census data due to village movements, formations, amalgamations, splits and at least one village having been missed out previously. The important point to note from Table is that the age distribution of the Ago population in 1990 did not differ significantly from that of the entire Mt Brown census division ten years earlier.

TABLE 4: PERCENTAGE POPULATION OF MT BROWN VILLAGES BY SEX AND AGE

	1980		1990	
	MALES	FEMALES	MALES	FEMALES
Age Group				
0-5 Years	9.7	9.1	9.9	7.4
6-17 Years	18.3	14.8	18.3	14.0
18-45 Years	15.6	17.9	18.7	20.3
46 + Years	7.8	6.8	5.3	6.0
Totals:	51.4	48.6	52.9	47.1
Total Number of Residents:	1813 = 100%		605 = 100%	
Resident Sex Ratio	106 : 100		112 : 100	
% Residents Under 18 Years	51.9		49.8	

It is estimated that the total Ago village population has fallen from 950 in 1980 to 700 in 1990 (corresponding to values of 820 in 1980 and 605 in 1990 for the ten villages studied). This represents a decrease of 26% in the population in just ten years. Table 1 indicates that this decline is not abating and thus it does not augur well for the survival of the Ago village system in the future.

Table 5 compares some population characteristics of the Ago villages for 1990 with the 1980 values (14) for urban areas and the country as a whole. These characteristics have been defined in accordance with Walsh (14). The two dependency ratios (youth and age) for the Ago villages are seen to lie between those of the urban areas and the country as a whole, while the corresponding child-woman ratio is lower than either the urban or national values. The latter indicates that there are marginally less infants (0-5 years) in relation to the number of women in the child-bearing age group (15-44 years) for the Ago villagers than in Papua New Guinea generally. All these factors are suggestive of a stable population. The only negative aspect in Table 5 is the lower sex ratio of the Ago villages for the adult population (15-44 years). The value is less than either the towns or the country as a whole and being under 100 indicates that there are more females than males in the adult Ago population. This is despite the excess of male to female residents in the total population as shown in Table 4.

TABLE 5: DEMOGRAPHIC COMPARISONS OF AGO VILLAGES WITH URBAN AREAS OF PAPUA NEW GUINEA AND THE COUNTRY AS A WHOLE

	Child-Woman Ratio	Dependency Ratios Youth	Age	Sex Ratio (M/F) 15-44 years
Apo Villages	724	744	57	91.0
Papua New Guinea	772	810	69	109.8
Papua New Guinean Towns	791	711	18	153.5

Thus the migration of the Ago people has had a two fold effect on the village population. Firstly, despite the Ago village population being relatively stable, migration has caused a 'hole' in the adult male population in the villages. This may also be a factor in the lower child-woman ratio in the Ago villages compared to the whole of Papua New Guinea as indicated in Table 5. Although overall the fall in the adult male population may only be a minor consideration, due to the large variation between villages it may be a major factor in the stability of some villages. For example, in one village where the adult sex-ratio has fallen to just 42.9 it would already be exerting considerable pressure on the survival of the village. Secondly, and most importantly, the sheer numbers of the Ago migrating is causing a rapid decline in the village population. At current levels of migration, the population of the Ago villages could vanish within the next 40 years.

Effect of Education on Migration

Table 6 gives the percentage of village residents who have had any formal education by decades and their average grade achieved. It is seen that overall 36% of the village population have had some schooling; however, a further 29% of the population had not yet achieved the normal school age (10 years of age). Hence 51% of the population above school age had had some formal education. It is interesting to note that 39.5% of all village residents with some education were still attending school in the area in 1989, but that this figure had dropped to under 9.6% by 1991 due to the difficulties in keeping teachers at the school. Hence very few are able to complete primary schooling or to go on to secondary school.

This is evidenced by the fact that although the percentage of the 'not at school' population aged ten years and over with some schooling is more than double the national average (14) (39.0%) compared to 18.2%), the percentage reaching secondary education is only one-twelfth the national value (14). Of those who had attended school the average grade achieved was only 3.6, but for those who had stopped their schooling the average grade was 4.0.

TABLE 6: EDUCATION OF RESIDENT AGO VILLAGERS BY AGE AND SEX

Age Group:	0-10	11-20	21-30	31-40	41-50	51-60	61+	Total
TOTAL								
Population	182	159	90	69	57	29	19	605
% of Total	30.0	26.3	14.9	11.4	9.4	4.8	3.1	100
No. Educated	5	100	46	35	30	3	0	218
% Educated	2.7	62.9	51.1	50.7	52.6	10.3	0	36.0
Average Years of Schooling	1.2	3.2	4.9	3.7	3.0	3.3	0	3.6
MALES								
% Educated	3.8	68.9	75.0	72.4	62.2	25.0	0	43.8
Average Years of Schooling	1.3	3.4	5.9	4.6	3.4	3.3	0	4.0
FEMALES								
% Educated	1.3	55.1	35.2	37.5	35.0	0	0	28.1
Average Years of Schooling	1.0	2.8	3.4	2.3	2.0	0	0	2.7

The difference in proportion of males to females with some education is highlighted in Table 6. The data tends to indicate that there has only been advances made in the education of women recently, in the last ten years. Prior to this (ca. 1950-80) about one-third of all the women were being educated compared to more than two-thirds of the men. In addition, none of the women resident in the village between 50 and 60 years of age had any schooling compared to 25% of the men in this age group. This last fact should not be surprising though, since people in this age group would have been schooling prior to the 1950s which was before the advent of the mission school in the Mt Brown area. Thus they would have been required to leave their village to attend the nearest school and at this early stage only the males would have been allowed to go. As is common throughout Papua New Guinea, not only were fewer women educated but even those who managed to get to school did not attend for as long as the men. The average grade achieved by the women who had previously attended school was 2.9 compared to an average of 4.5 for the men. The variation of number of years of schooling with age for both males and females is shown in Table 6.

Although the data is limited, the percentage educated and the education level of migrants, as well as returned migrants, is greater than for those who have always lived in the village. In addition, almost 90% of the Ago people with post-primary education are currently living outside of the Ago villages and a further 4% are returned migrants. Thus it seems clear that education is a major determinant of migration.

Circular Migration

Tables 1-3 show that of the total Ago population, 58.8% are currently living outside of the Ago villages (35.3% in Port Moresby and 23.5% in RNVs), a further 7.7% have previous migration experience and are now living in the villages, and the remaining 33.5% have always lived in the villages. This means that less than 12% of all migrants have returned to stay in the village, while 88% have remained in Port Moresby and the RNVs. Therefore for the Ago people the propensity to migrate (8) is high (58.8% - the proportion still absent from the villages), while the degree of circular migration is very low (8.3% - the proportion of returned migrants).

The inverse relationship between the propensity to migrate and circular migration (8) and its relationship to geographic location in coastal regions (giving a pattern of high migration and low circular migration), a relationship questioned by Van Groningen (8), is also contradicted by the data presented. Being an inland region one would expect to find a high degree of circular migration, and low propensity to migrate and yet the opposite trend is reported. A far better measure would be access to facilities - one might expect high circular migration for villages which have easy access to education, health and income earning facilities, and high migration for villages which do not have easy access to such facilities.

The basic "push-pull" model (8) which explains circular migration by pointing to economic and social push or pull factors (economic pull from the city and social push from the village for migration, and vice versa for remigration) can be used to some extent to explain why the people migrate, but fails to explain the lack of remigration due to the social push from the city (pressure from wantoks on unemployed people to return to the village) and economic pull of the village (on those who find the cost of living in Port Moresby too high). It also fails to explain the second major reason for migration, viz the search for a good education.

DISCUSSION

Reasons for Migrating

In other developing countries a move to the city is, for many, their only chance for survival (15). This is not the case in most parts of Papua New Guinea, where subsistence crops are abundant for the population size and no-one is threatened with starvation. Urban migration then becomes a question of relative poverty. According to King (16) urbanization is a habit-forming luxury to which people in Papua New Guinea are not yet addicted. As with many other Western habits it appears the addiction has now taken hold, at least for parts of the population, and the search for 'something better', which the towns supposedly have, is becoming increasingly strong and widespread.

Others (10, 17) have found rural migrants' reasons for moving to towns include the desire for new experiences, the wish to avoid traditional obligations and the dullness of village life, the desire to earn money, the desire for better or further education, the attraction of better services, land pressure, the lack of rural money-making opportunities and more.

Very few of the Ago migrants have a level of education or technical skills which makes them appropriate for the urban workforce, in contrast to Dakeyne's (11) subjects who, although comparatively close neighbours to the Ago people, have had a much longer experience of contact. There were only 11 people (6%) of those interviewed who fall into the category of semi-skilled - e.g. carpenters, a bricklayer, a printer, a plumber, a laboratory technician, a cook and a taxi-driver. Yet those with any education still come in the hope of getting unskilled work. There were no adult Ago women in formal employment in Port Moresby at the time of interviewing.

A portion of the informants were asked why they had come to town. By far the most common reason given was in order to find work so as to earn some money to buy goods. For the women, the majority migrated not through their own volition but because they were to marry a man who had migrated or because their husband was migrating or because their husband, who had migrated and left them in the village, had found employment. Skeldon (9) also finds that female migration is associated with movement of families rather than single women looking for work. A secondary reason was in order to get a good education for their children, a factor also noted by Smith (18). No-one stated that land pressure or the excitement of urban surroundings were reasons to migrate. One informant stated that other people come to town because they are too lazy to make gardens or are frightened of custom (it is assumed this means sorcery).

Reasons for Remaining in Urban Areas

Reasons for remaining in town appear to be based on the short term. Several informants said they stayed in town to attend literacy school (started by the Baha'i community of Port Moresby in 1991). Many women stay because "my husband is here". A few stay for their children's education. One had lost his traditional land through absence from his home village and felt that he could not return because he has no land to pass on to his sons. The majority of the men stated that they stayed because of their employment and of those only a few said that they would return to the village if they became unemployed. Many did say, though, that if they could not find any employment then they would return to the village. However, it was also reported in the villages that often, especially among the young adult migrants, when a migrant returned to their village after working in Port Moresby or in RNVs they left again within about six months to seek further employment.

The pull of the city is strong. One informant bemoaned the fact that even when given the money to return to the village, the unemployed stay on, using up the money and still expecting accommodation. There seems to be a double-think among urban settlers which keeps them in Port Moresby and yet maintaining (in many instances very strongly) that 'the people' should go back to the village.

Skeldon (9) states that "the forces controlling the movement of people are the result of a complex interplay between economic and social variables". As pointed out by Strathern (19) the usual explanations for why people have migrated involve very general comments, such as for goods/money, or education. Behind these general explanations is always a more specific individual reason for leaving the village. These may include such things as the death of a spouse, parent or child, the fear of sorcery over a particular incident (Koroma (20) also notes this reason), the failure of an economic enterprise such as a cash crop or trade store, or being taunted by others who have been to the city.

The stated reason is usually the general one, but a little probing reveals the underlying cause. The general reasons (10, 17) apply to all people who live in remote rural communities - generally, all would benefit from a move to the city in terms of material, physical and educational well-being. However, only those who have some other private spur to action actually go.

Conroy (21) expands on Hutton's (22) three levels of explanation of labour migration in Africa, and these can be applied to Papua New Guinea. The basic explanation is economic - the difference between earning opportunities in the village as compared to the urban centre. This factor is important for the Ago people because there are very few economic opportunities at their place of origin due to transport difficulties and the lack of other developments. Attempts have been made to join the cash economy while remaining in the village, i.e. the building of trade stores, planting of cash crops, and building the airstrip, but the problems of transport have proved insurmountable. The second explanation is the "perception of relative deprivation" - as stated, the realization of relative poverty where, though a person has enough to eat, they do not feel that they have enough of everything else. The third explanation is the 'last straw' or final factor which is often the personal reason people eventually give for their move.

The first two levels of explanation bring up economic questions behind migration. Several authors (21,23,24) suggest that the probability of finding employment in the urban centre influences people's decisions about whether to migrate. The Todaro (23) model suggests that the main factors influencing such a decision are the expected wage differential (a comparison of one's possible rural earnings with urban earnings) combined with the probability of finding employment. In Papua New Guinea the second factor would seem to be undermined by the migrant stock variable, the unquestioned satisfaction of one's needs while looking for work by a wantoks who are already established in towns. It also fails to address the eternal optimism of the migrants who are sure that they will find employment. Ryan (12) has also noted this trend - the flood of migrants continues despite their knowledge of the difficult employment situation in Port Moresby, because new migrants know they will be supported.

This factor also neutralizes the distance factor deterrent. Proximity as a factor for migration takes on an interesting aspect when one looks at the remoteness of Mt Brown. The cost of air travel would deter migrants (as it does in the Highlands) but the fact that it is possible to walk to Wiga and then get road transport to Port Moresby means that distance is not an important factor deterring migration.

The expected wage differential is an important factor drawing the Ago people to the city. In the village one can expect to make about K50 per month per family from cash crops. In the city the average wage among the Ago people is K100 - K200. The wage difference is therefore real enough. However people do not add the extra costs of living in town to this, although these are a very common cause for complaint. This is another case of double think - one comes to town to earn money, a lot more money than can be earned in the village, but one uses all the money earned on the extra costs of maintaining an urban lifestyle. Strathern (25) has noted this for Hagen migrants in Port Moresby. One would actually end up with more money in the village, where there is nothing to spend it on.

The 'bright lights' theory, the notion that people are drawn to town by the vibrant, exciting aura of the place which has been transmitted by those who have been in town or who have heard of it through others, has been questioned by some authors. For the Ago people, and other Papua New Guinean urban migrants, the pull of the 'bright lights' is as much a factor for migration as the economic reasons. It is not stated as a reason for coming, but is evidenced in the things people say about why they like living in the city, as well as in the prestige afforded to those who have lived in the city, regardless of whether they have gained any conspicuous material wealth. Baxter (26) also notes this among the Orokaivan temporary migrants.

Baxter (26) found that Orokaivans living in Moresby generally neither plan to return home in the near future, nor do they "see their living conditions as being oppressively bad, while most regard them as being indisputably better than village living conditions". Many of the Ago people have the same perception. When quizzed on what the major problems of urban life are, rather than discussing the 'rascal' threat, or the lack of work, or the difficulty of finding land for gardening, or the lack of housing, most people simply stated that the lack of money and high prices, as well as the expectations of wantoks (both those in the city and those back in the village), were the only real problems they feel. The 'rascal' problem is apparently a luxury issue which is only on the minds of the urban elite. Several said there were no problems in living in the city.

It may be that the phenomenon of the 'ambivalent townsmen', observed by Levine and Levine (10), is changing, and that people are becoming reconciled to the problems of urban living and are increasingly vocal about its advantages rather than disadvantages, as the Levines predicted.

Reasons for Remaining or Returning to the Village

Of the returned migrants who are currently living back in the village a majority said they had returned due to land-related problems - either fears that their land would be taken over by someone else due to their absence, or that it was not being looked after properly, or because their parents had died and they were needed to tend the land. Others had returned for economic reasons - they could no longer afford to feed their increasing families in Port Moresby. One youth returned after his arm had been broken in a PMV accident - for him Port Moresby was definitely a bad place!

Those who had never migrated also gave land as the major reason they stayed - no-one to look after it, fear of someone taking it, pride in being there to keep the village looking nice. Others held fears about living in the city - they would be killed by rascals or in a traffic accident, or would get into trouble. However they all felt that it was good that some Ago people are in Port Moresby since the migrants can send back money and goods and food, and will look after any visitors from the village.

Urban migration has influenced not only the way the Ago people live when they are in town, it has also affected relationships and traditions of people still in the village. The use of cash and material goods brought and sent back to the village are obvious changes. Traditions such as clan exogamy and village endogamy have changed. In the village this has been necessitated by the extent of migration in order to preserve the village numbers. Parents no longer choose their children's partners, and the people complain of unmarried girls getting pregnant. As noted by other authors, and by the early patrol reports (5), traditional leadership patterns have changed with the older, wiser men having to compete with the young, educated and city-wise men. Polygyny is being practised less and less (only 4 of the adult male villagers (<3%), all of whom were over 40 years of age, were polygynous at the time of this study compared to around 25% in the 1940s, and none of the urban dwellers interviewed were polygynous). Family relationships are changed by children being sent to stay with relatives in Port Moresby to attend school. Apparently they also get a different sort of education in the use of alcohol, marijuana and gambling, according to the urban informants. Another change which has occurred through the increasing tendency to educate girls, as well as boys, is the tendency for men to marry less-educated women - a slowly decreasing category.

CONCLUSIONS

The Mount Brown region is one of the latest areas to come into contact with European 'development' (11, 12, 26, 27). Due to its remoteness, contact was delayed. The rapidity with which the migration process has taken place is all the more alarming since it has been only over a 30-40 year period. As mentioned earlier, if migration continues at the current level it may be reasonable to ask who will be left in Mt Brown in 40 years' time. Although the rate varies according to certain external factors such as job recruitment, transportation and so on, there is a steady outmigration from the area. This trend will need to be addressed by policy makers in this country.

We cannot stop educating people for fear that they will then migrate to cities. Making education more rurally relevant may help, but it would seem that the curiosity that an enquiring mind develops and the vision of 'something better' that those who go to school emerge with, make people want to experience the novelty of urban life. The task then is perhaps not to discourage people from coming to urban centres, but to create a larger number of smaller urban areas which have all the facilities that attract migrants, but which would be easily accessible to rural people.

The lack of 'step migration' to small rural towns in Papua New Guinea is a major constraint on rural development, according to Young (28). The people who come to town are those who want 'development', people who need encouragement- not discouragement, people for whom the urban pull is irresistible.

In 1970 it was noted (29) that the problems of urban housing are small and easily fixed in Port Moresby compared to other developing countries' cities, but that the urban migrants must be seen as permanent rather than transitory. The 1979 Waigani Seminar (30) confronted the problems of urbanisation. Skeldon (9) found that migration is increasing, it is increasingly urban orientated, and time spent outside the home village area is increasing. Morauta (27) warned of the preference of people to live in towns rather than their home villages, who are raising children who know nothing of village life. Twenty years on, the problems of urban housing have not been solved but are still not insurmountable. Our data indicates that the move to towns is continuing as access gets easier, and obviously the urban planners will have to address this issue more seriously.

REFERENCES

1. Rigo Patrol Report No. 7/1956-57, Rigo Sub-District Office, Central District, Territory of Papua New Guinea.

2. L Gray, Sinabada - Woman Among Warriors, Joint Board of Christian Education, Melbourne, 1989, p. 115.

3. Ibid., p.111.

4. Rigo Patrol Report No. 3/1965-66, Rigo Sub-District Office, Central District, Territory of Papua New Guinea.

5. Rigo Patrol Report No. 6/1964-65, Rigo Sub-District Office, Central District, Territory of Papua New Guinea.

6. Rigo Patrol Report No. 1/1966-67, Rigo Sub-District Office, Central District, Territory of Papua New Guinea.

7. E.A. Young, "Population Mobility in Agarabi/Gadsup Eastern Highlands Province", in R.J. May (ed.), Change and Movement, Australian National University Press, Canberra, 1977. pp. 173-202.

8. D.H. van Groningen a Stuling, "Migration of the Kilenge: A Village Study", Yagl-Ambu, 7 (2), 1980. pp. 33-46.

9. R. Skeldon, "Internal Migration" in R. Skeldon (ed.), The Demography of Papua New Guinea, IASER Monograph 11, 1979. Ch. 7.

10. H.B. and M.W. Levine, Urbanization in Papua New Guinea: A Study of Ambivalent Townsmen, Cambridge University Press, Cambridge, 1979.

11. R.B. Dakeyne, "Labour Migration in Papua New Guinea: A Case Study from Northern Papua", in R.J. May (ed.), Change and Movement, Australian National University Press, Canberra, 1977. pp. 155-161.

12. D. Ryan, "Toaripi in Port Moresby and Lae", in R.J. May (ed.), Change and Movement, Australian National University Press, Canberra, 1977. pp. 147-154.

13. Final Figures: Provincial Summary (Central Province), 1980 National Population Census, National Statistical Office, Papua New Guinea, 1983.

14. A. C. Walsh, Migration and Urbanization in Papua New Guinea, 1980 National Population Census Research Monograph No. 5, National Statistical Office, Papua New Guinea, 1987.

15. G. Breese (ed.), The City in Newly Developing Countries, Prentice-Hall, London, 1972. Ch. 35.

16. D. King, The Small Towns and Outstations of Papua New Guinea, Geography Department Occasional Paper (New Series) No. 3, University of Papua New Guinea, 1983

17. R.G. Ward, "Internal Migration and Urbanization in Papua New Guinea" in R. J. May (ed.), Change and Movement, Australian National University Press, Canberra, 1977. pp. 27-51.

18. G. Smith, "Urban Pressures on Education in the Central District of Papua", Papua New Guinea Journal of Education, 7(1), 1971. pp.34-54.

19. M. Strathern, "The Disconcerting Tie: Attitudes of Hagen Migrants Towards Home", in R.J. May (ed.), Change and Movement, Australian National University Press, Canberra, 1977. pp. 247-266.

20. J.F. Koroma, "A Study of the Bundi People in Urban Goroka", in R.J. May (ed.), Change and Movement, Australian National University Press, Canberra, 1977. pp. 203-215.

21. J.D. Conroy, Urban Growth and Unemployment in Papua New Guinea, IASER Discussion Paper No. 16, 1977.

22. C.R. Hutton, "Rates of Labour Migration", in J. Guglar (ed.), Urban Growth in Sub-Saharan Africa, Nkanga 6, Makerere Institute of Social Research, 1971.

23. M.P. Todaro, "A Model of Labour Migration and Urban Unemployment in Less Developed Countries", American Economic Review, 59, 1969. pp. 138-148.

24. D. Gupta, "Growth Pole Theory and Urban Growth in Papua New Guinea", in R. Jackson, J. Odongo and P. Batho (Eds.), Urbanisation and its Problems in Papua New Guinea, 1979 Waigani Seminar Proceedings, University of Papua New Guinea, 1980. pp. 118-128.

25. M. Strathern, "No Money on Our Skins", New Guinea Research Bulletin No. 61, Australian National University, 1975.

26. M.W.P. Baxter, "Orokaiva Rural-Urban Contacts and Attitudes", in R.J. May (ed.), Change and Movement, Australian National University Press, Canberra, 1977. pp. 162-172.

27. L. Morauta, "Malalauas in Port Moresby", in R.J. May (ed.), The Urban Household Survey: Town Profiles, IASER Monograph 12, 1979. Ch. 2.

28. E. Young, "The Small Highlands Towns - Kundiawa, Kainantu and Minj", in R.J. May (ed.), The Urban Household Survey: Town Profiles, IASER Monograph 12, 1979. Ch. 7.

29. J. V. Langmore and N.D. Oram, "Port Moresby Urban Development", New Guinea Research Bulletin No. 37, Australian National University, 1970.

30. R. Jackson, J. Odongo and P. Batho (Eds.), Urbanisation and its Problems in Papua New Guinea, 1979 Waigani Seminar Proceedings, University of Papua New Guinea, 1980.

TEACHING DEMOGRAPHY TO MEDICAL STUDENTS

K J PATAKI-SCHWEIZER[1]

This paper is derived from teaching demography to medical students at the University of Papua New Guinea (UPNG) over the past two decades, given some semesters when other colleagues have done it. My interest in the subject has continued over this time and I wish to share some observations and thoughts, for certain patterns and issues emerge which are interesting and worth attention.

The question of literacy has been of major concern in Papua New Guinea (PNG) as for any developing country and more recently, for some developed ones where poverty, isolation or eroding administration has affected education. Less articulated is the question of formal numeracy or, ability to work with numerically-presented information. This normally is seen to start in the primary grades, and continues through high school into tertiary education. Often it is included (or presumed) within that broader area termed science. There has been a great deal of concern and criticism, some of it justified and much of it unfair concerning the quality of education in Papua New Guinea at primary and secondary level, if not for tertiary students in the areas of the sciences. (I will make some comments apropos of this at the end of the paper.) These concerns have clear relevance for demography and related disciplines such as statistics.

The medical programme at the UPNG is taught by the Faculty of Medicine and is divided into four broad areas, each with a department: Basic Medical Sciences (formerly Human Biology), Clinical Sciences, Community Medicine (formerly Social and Preventive Medicine) and Pathology. There is ongoing debate about whether these four core areas are a better or worse approach to medical education, given specialization and information availability with their stimuli for academic fission. History will no doubt decide the relative wisdom of our Faculty founding fathers in the middle-late 1960s, although curriculum integration for the final level of graduation is something to be particularly desired. With respect to mathematical teaching in the Faculty, our department does a good deal of it directly or indirectly including required courses in statistics, demography, epidemiology and behavioural science plus fieldwork over a four-year period and after an introductory science year on the main campus; at present there is pressure for expansion to six years. Table 1 outlines our departmental programme.

[1] Department of Community Medicine
University of Papua New Guinea

TABLE ONE

	Semester 1	Semester 2
YEAR II	Introduction to Behavioural Science	Medical Statistics Demography Block* Field Studies Week
YEAR III	Principles of Epidemiology and Health Care	Infectious Diseases Environmental Health Block
YEAR IV	Medical Ethics	------------------
YEAR V	------------------	Occupational Health Block Malariology Block Regional and Rural Health **

* includes Field Exercise

** includes 4-week provincial field programme

Table Two outlines the Demography Block as it is presently structured. It is taught during the second semester in the second year of studies as part of the semester-long course in Medical Statistics and Demography. Given the increasing demand for time within the Faculty, Demography occupies four weeks of a 17-week semester which also includes an intensive Field Studies Week on health status in a selected village (see Table One). Together with the first-semester course in Behavioural Science, these four sections form an integrated introductory sequence with a cumulative final grade.

TABLE TWO

DEMOGRAPHY BLOCK

Week 1	Introduction: Demographic Behaviour
	Demographic Concepts and Terms
	Demographic Statistics
	Computational Exercises
Week 2	Demographic Status and Trends: PNG, South Pacific and World.
	FIELD EXERCISE
	Analysis of Field Exercise
	Presentation of Field Exercise
Week 3	Contraception
	Family Planning
	Computational Exercises
Week 4	Block Revision
	Assessment

One can report with fair assurance that our students enjoy both statistics and demography, to make the strong distinction. In fact, they often want more demography, quite likely an artifact of the shorter exposure well this side of any learning-curve saturation. They are particularly responsive to actually doing the calculations and determining vital statistics for themselves, even for the admittedly very crude rates they can approximate from their field exercises. I would note though that with the 25-40 students doing that exercise each year over the years, we have computed village Rates of Natural Increase starting at 2.1/1000 in 1977, the first year of the exercise and slowly increasing to 2.5-2.8/1000 at present. These rates also include expected anomalies of negative growth for villages with major outmigration and high transient activity (e.g., -5.8/, -7.0/, and -10.0/1000) or growth spurts (8.0/, 10.0/ and 14/1000), to be expected at these low sample sizes and indicative of local population dynamics in Papua New Guinea.

The students show a strong interest in Family Planning and in the actual methods of contraception available and/or used, both modern and traditional. "Traditional" is used here in the broader sense given the many ways of cultures in the world, and certainly in Papua New Guinea with some 750 formal languages. More extreme world examples of control such as female sub-incision, infibulation and castration are also discussed and placed in cultural perspective. Overall, the response to this section of the block is one of great if shocked attention followed by strong vocal interest.

And what of their difficulties in the course? There are those involving specific questions about numerical computation and certain concepts, in particular Birth Interval, Age-Specific Fertility Rate and Total Fertility Rate. But the more challenging, I believe are in numerico-mathematical functions including:

1) difficulty with <u>rates</u> (x per y) and <u>reciprocals</u> (y: 1/x, x: 1/y)

2) difficulty with <u>ratios</u> (x to y, y to x)

3) difficulty with <u>percentages</u> (crossing two domains; exceeding 100%)

4) difficulty with <u>scale</u> (e.g. giving the PNG population as 300 thousand or 30 million, or the world as 500 million)

5) difficulty with quantifying <u>time</u>-frames (immediate, short-, medium-, long-term).

These would appear to work back to earlier education and probably more than that, although such difficulties may well be shared cross-culturally as part of sapient learning. One recalls the interesting work by Lancy and his group in the late 1970s through the PNG Department of Education on traditional counting systems, and the influence of enculturation which we have all undergone in our respective identities,(1), (2). If one's early and formative years occur in a local world which itemizes phenomena in terms of e.g., a base-2 system, or -3, -4, -5, -15, -20 AND "1" (a continuous body-parts tally system) as exist in PNG rather than our own base-10*, so much a part of western scientific thought, this would be an additional cognitive factor in the formal learning process for a traditionally-enculturated student. Furthermore, a basic awareness of conception, contraception, spacing and related morbidity and mortality is very likely inculcated or latent within the particular cultural nexus of the individual. One would not overemphasize these related factors but simply mention them in the context of this paper. Meanwhile, it is evident that our students enjoy working with vital statistics in demography and with theoretical and applied demographic concepts, do so quite acceptably by and large, and are very interested in contraceptive methods.

The recent (June 1991) introduction of a National Population Policy for Papua New Guinea signals the beginning of a programme which requires demographic awareness and particularly so for involved professionals. Accordingly, the incorporation of this subject through teaching at whatever scale of time and detail takes on a increased importance. Therefore, a final comment can be made: it has been said by some that "those that can, do, and those that can't, teach". Concerning this intemperate dichotomy plus national concerns about family planning, reproductive decision-making, a major increase in STD, the emergence of HIV and in the larger context of a continuing population growth that cuts more and more into national goals and potentials, it is evident that all of us must deal with the didactics of demography whether in class, health programmes, research, clinical advice, media or marketing.

* Rudimentary base-10 counting systems are also present in Papua New Guinea, e.g. the Ponam language in Manus Province.

As Papua New Guineans well know, there are two sides to any exchange, including that of information, and one must respect this basic reciprocity. Accordingly, with particular respect to this country and the concerns of this paper, one would assert the reverse of the above shibboleth: "those that can't" will do whatever, whilst "those that can" will and must teach. Such effort is timely and it is needed.

REFERENCES

1. Lancy, D.F., ed. The Indigenous Mathematics Project. Papua New Guinea Journal of Education, Special Issue, Vol. 14, 1978

2. Pataki-Schweizer, K.J. Notations on education and culture. In Towards a Philosophy of Teacher Education for the University of Papua New Guinea, J. Weatherhead, ed. Waigani: UPNG Printery, 1977, pp. 44-47

MORTALITY IN PACIFIC ISLAND COUNTRIES CIRCA 1980 IN RELATION TO SOCIOECONOMIC, DEMOGRAPHIC, HEALTH SERVICE AND OTHER VARIABLES

RICHARD TAYLOR[1]

NANCY DAVIS LEWIS[2]

TIM SLADDEN[3]

INTRODUCTION

The demographic and health transitions that are occurring in developing countries are associated with profound changes in disease incidence, and have important implications for development priorities, disease control programmes and therapeutic services. Coale (1973) noted that traditional societies often experience high fertility and mortality both of which fall during transition to low levels now observable in industrialised populations.[1] Transition is usually characterised by a period of rapid population growth since fertility decline often lags behind mortality decline. Influences that determine high mortality appear to be less resistant to modernisation than those maintaining high fertility. Transition is also characterised by a change in the main causes of morbidity and mortality from infectious and respiratory disease to a pattern dominated by non-communicable disease and accidents.[2]

Scattered across the Pacific are some of the globe's smallest nations and territories (Figure 1). Seven Pacific Island countries (PICs) have fewer than 15,000 people, and only Papua New Guinea and Fiji have over 500,000 people. Fifteen of the twenty-one island groups are either independent, or internally self-governing in free association with a metropolitan power. Limited land area, scarcity of natural resources, small population size, and distance and isolation all pose serious problems for development. Both deep-sea commercial fishing and mining are high technology and capital intensive industries requiring dependence on outside investment and expertise.

We have recently reported data describing the health transitions occurring in PICs.[3] The entire transition spectrum can be observed, ranging from populations experiencing high mortality, with cause structures

[1] Associate Professor, Department of Public Health, University of Sydney
[2] Associate Professor, Department of Geography, University of Hawaii
[3] Research Assistant, Department of Public Health University of Sydney

dominated by infectious and respiratory disease, to those with low mortality, and cause structures dominated by non-communicable disease and "external" causes. The Pacific Island countries provide an opportunity to study contemporary health transitions by cross-sectional analysis using a comparative ecological method. This method has been used extensively in the past. Preston (1975) considers it to be preferable to comparing variation in the rate of change of health in relation to other indices.[4]

Several factors have been suggested as causes of past mortality declines in developed countries, and contemporary mortality declines in developing countries. These factors include economic development, technological and health care service advances, social development (especially education), and environmental and nutritional improvements. The relative importance of these factors may vary in different situations, however, there is consensus that they are all involved to some extent in the health transition.

This paper reports a cross-sectional, ecological analysis of the relationship of mortality with geopolitical, socioeconomic, health service and other variables in PICs. This approach has both the strengths and weaknesses of an ecological study. The aim is to identify significant correlates and determinants of health status, and catalysts of the current health transition in the Pacific Island context. Such information is relevant to overall development and aid policies, inter-sectoral activities aimed at improving health status, and disease control programmes in the Pacific region.

METHODS

A comparative, cross-sectional analysis of grouped data from various political jurisdictions in the Pacific Island region was performed. Mortality level (Table 1) and cause were the outcome factors of interest, and the study factors included a wide range of geopolitical, socioeconomic, demographic, health service and other descriptive variables as listed in Tables 2 and 3.

The strengths of ecological studies are that they provide an overview on a total regional level of what is actually taking place, including the degree of variability between different populations, and enable study of exposure variables over a wide range of intensity, and of exposure variables which only apply to groups. The weaknesses of ecological studies are the inter-correlation between variables, the inability to control for confounders, and the difficulty in obtaining data on all important variables which may cause a particular effect.

PIC mortality data relating to the late 1970s and early 1980s were obtained from a combination of sources including vital registration, censuses and population surveys.[3] Wherever possible direct death registration was used to derive life expectancy and mortality rate data. Indirect estimations were obtained from censuses and surveys when these data were deficient. Mortality data from different sources (e.g. vital registration and census) were cross-checked for consistency. Accuracy was also assessed by one of the authors (RT) who was familiar with most of the data collection systems deployed throughout the Pacific region. Wherever doubt concerning under-enumeration existed vital registration data was tested using the Brass growth-balance method,[5] and data were adjusted for under-reporting if necessary.

Because of variable under-reporting of death by cause, the cause structure of mortality was assessed using proportional mortality by major cause group only, for all ages and both sexes combined. The principal chapter headings from the International Classification of Diseases (ICD) code were used. Data were sometimes based on hospital deaths only, and may have been influenced by selection bias. We have previously provided detailed information on sources and accuracy of Pacific Island mortality data.[3]

Descriptive, socioeconomic, geopolitical, demographic and health service data were mainly obtained from the South Pacific Commission's (SPC) statistical summary for the year 1980, and other sources where these data were deficient. Only variables that were available for all PICs were included in the analysis. Categorical variables were generally assigned values of 0 or 1, but occasionally ordinal scales were used.

The general descriptive variables included were ethnicity, geographic island type and political status. The major Pacific ethnic groups were categorised (Melanesian, Polynesian and Micronesian), plus data was obtained for Fiji Indians, New Caledonian Europeans, and non-Chamorro inhabitants of Guam. Countries were classified as high islands (volcanic), atolls only, or a mixture of the two. For the political status variable, countries were classified as independent, independent-association status, or territories. This classification was objective, being accepted by all observers, including the countries concerned. However, a spectrum of political situations exists in the Pacific, with certain states on the border between these categories.

Economic variables included gross domestic product (GDP), imports, exports and foreign aid (all in Australian dollars at 1980 value). Aid was defined as total external assistance (bilateral and multilateral). Demographic variables included total population, proportion of the population less than 15 years (%) and population density (persons/km^2). Urbanisation was measured as the proportion (%) of the population in areas locally defined as being urban. Education was assessed from the proportion (%) of school-aged children at school. Health service variables were population per doctor and population per hospital bed, and malarious and non-malarious areas were also defined.

The majority of the statistical analysis was kept simple since multivariate methods using small numbers of cases and highly inter-correlated variables could be expected to be unhelpful. Univariate analyses were performed, relating mortality to individual study variables in a cross-sectional fashion. Scattergrams and correlation coefficients were derived to show associations between variables. Labelled scattergrams were particularly useful, providing information on countries that conformed to the typical pattern as well as ones that did not. Logarithmic transformation was employed to obtain more linear relationships for some demographic and economic variables, and a power transformation (x^5) was used for the education variable. Transformations of mortality variables by either logarithmic or logit methods were unhelpful.

For some analyses countries were grouped according to certain categorical study factors (political status and malaria). The average life expectancy for each group was calculated, and then adjusted for certain confounding factors using analysisof covariance (SPSS, ANOVA package). Such adjusted univariate method of analysis was useful in assessing the influence of political status and malaria in the presence of considerable inter-correlation.

Stepwise, linear regressions of dependent mortality indices, and independent descriptive variables were performed, with and without inclusion of the political status variable. Beta (B) coefficients, R^2, and changes in R^2 were calculated for each variable added into the equation. This method of analysis was generally unhelpful and produced some unrealistic results, probably because of the small number of cases, relatively large numbers of variables, influence of outliers, and degree of inter-correlation between variables.

RESULTS

Table 1 gives estimated life expectancies at birth in each PIC for males and females separately, and for both sexes combined (represented in Figure 2). For the indigenous population groups, life expectancy was lowest in Melanesians, highest in Polynesians, and of intermediary length in Micronesians, with overlap between the three groups. Of the non-indigenous peoples, Fiji Indians had similar life expectancies to indigenous Pacific populations, but New Caledonian Europeans and non-Chamorros (Asians and Europeans) of Guam had the highest of any group. Melanesian ethnicity correlated negatively with both-sexes life expectancy at birth, and female life expectancy at birth and 15 years, and correlated positively with all age-specific mortality rates (Table 4). Melanesian ethnicity also correlated positively with proportional mortality from infection and perinatal conditions, and negatively with that from cardiovascular disease (Table 5).

Data for each of the descriptive variables are given in Tables 2 and 3. Correlation coefficients between descriptive variables and mortality indices are shown in Tables 4 and 5. No statistically significant associations of life expectancy or mortality indices with geographic island type were observed, although life expectancy was slightly, but non-significantly, negatively correlated with atoll countries.

Political independence correlated negatively with life expectancy (Table 4; Figure 3) and positively with mortality rates. It was also correlated positively with proportional mortality from infection, and negatively with that from 'external' causes (Table 5).

After political status, economic variables had the most influence on mortality (Table 4). GDP per capita correlated positively with life expectancy, although Nauru and Papua New Guinea were significant outliers as illustrated in Figure 4. Imports (and log imports) per capita correlated positively with all measures of life expectancy (Figure 5), except those for adult males ($\geq$15 years). Imports also correlated positively with proportional mortality from cancer and cardiovascular disease, and negatively with that from infection (Table 5). Aid per capita correlated positively with life expectancy for both sexes at birth, female life expectancy at birth and 15 years, and negatively with child and adult mortality.

Total population and (log total population) did not correlate with life expectancy. Population did however correlate with adult (15-64 years) mortality rates, and also with proportional mortality from perinatal conditions, but not other causes. The proportion of the population less than 15 years and population density both correlated negatively with life expectancy at birth. Urbanisation correlated positively with life expectancy at birth except for Nauru which was a significant outlier (a totally urbanised population with low life expectancy). Urbanisation also correlated positively with proportional mortality from 'external' causes and from cancer, but negatively with that from respiratory disease.

Higher proportions of school age children at school correlated positively with life expectancy and negatively with mortality rates. Figure 6 shows an apparent rise in life expectancy with increasing education (transformed education variable). Education correlated positively with proportional mortality from cardiovascular disease, and negatively with that from infection and perinatal conditions.

Doctor availability was related to almost all mortality indices. Population per doctor correlated positively with mortality rates, and negatively with life expectancy and proportional mortality from infections. Availability of hospital beds was not a significant variable in univariate analyses and did not correlate with any mortality indices.

Malarious countries (Papua New Guinea, Solomon Islands and Vanuatu) had lower life expectancies than non-malarious countries (Table 7). Malaria correlated positively with all mortality rate variables, and negatively with most life expectancy variables. It also correlated positively with proportional mortality from infections and from perinatal conditions, and negatively with that from cardiovascular disease. Observed differences in mean life expectancy between malarious and non-malarious countries actually increased after adjusting for socioeconomic variables.

With regard to political status, mean life expectancy in territories was approximately three years longer than in associated states, and ten years longer than in independent countries. Adjusting for demographic, health and socio-economic factors simultaneously, using analysis of covariance, removed most of the differences in mean life expectancy between countries grouped by political status. Models incorporating restricted numbers of variables also removed these differences.

Several descriptive variables were shown to be predictors of life expectancy and mortality rates in multiple linear (step-wise) regression analyses. Political independence was the most important explanatory variable for both-sexes and male life expectancy (at birth and 15 years), and for childhood and adult mortality rates.

DISCUSSION

In this study, data on mortality and socioeconomic, demographic and other descriptive parameters in Pacific Island countries have been collated from statistics produced by the countries themselves, the South Pacific Commission, and other regional and international agencies. Although these data are not infallible they provide the most complete record available, and give a reasonable overview of different PICs for comparative purposes. The sources and methods of adjustment of mortality data have been previously published.[3]

For an ecological analysis of grouped data, the number of cases is low (20 PICs in this study), and computed statistical parameters from correlation analyses, regressions and analysis of covariance may not reach levels of statistical significance. Some trends that do not appear to be statistically significant may be important, and atypical outlying cases can have strong effects on computed statistics producing spurious effects. Nevertheless, this data set comprises all Pacific Island countries; it is not a sample.

The data are average values for the various mortality and socioeconomic indices for each Pacific Island country. In reality, considerable heterogeneity exists within each country, particularly in New Caledonia and Fiji, where large sections of the population are comprised of different ethnic groups. In some but not all countries rural and urban lifestyles are very different. Large income differentials also exist between various sectors of the population in countries such as Papua New Guinea, New Caledonia, French Polynesia, Guam, etc. Although sex- and ethnic-specific life expectancy and mortality estimates are available, and some information on rural/urban mortality differentials exist, there are no group specific socioeconomic or descriptive data with which to correlate these data.

Inter-correlations between variables make it difficult to investigate causal associations between certain factors and mortality indices. Some study factors are proxies for other measured or unmeasured variables. Some study factors are intervening variables in the causal chain, and other may act as confounders.

The relation between macro-economic indicators and health status in developing countries is still debated, although there are consistent trends found in almost all studies. International cross-sectional ecological studies usually reveal an S-shaped relationship between life expectancy and per capita economic indices, such as a log GDP. Cumper (1981) observed a significant association of national income with lower infant mortality and higher life expectancy.[6] He concluded that increased income appears necessary for improvements in health status, but the proportion of national resources devoted to health services, efficiency of the use of these resources, foreign assistance, and per capita income also influence population health. He also observed that health status may be dissociated from economic indicators, particularly GDP per capita, since these indicators provide no information on distribution of income. An international comparative study by Preston (1975) estimated that growth in income accounted for 10-25% of the growth in world life expectancy from the 1930s to the 1960s.[4] Although Preston implies that the balance may be due to technical disease control measures, the social development hypothesis (particularly education) now has more currency.

In this study we found a correspondence between life expectancy and GDP, although both Nauru and Papua New Guinea were significant outliers with lower life expectancies than would be expected from their GDPs (Figure 4). In Papua New Guinea GDP per capita is not high but life expectancy remains lower than expected. Unequal income distribution partly accounts for this; more years of life may be lost by people with below average incomes than are gained by people with equivalent above average incomes. It may also be the case that a proportion of resource industry profits are sent overseas, and although they appear in the GNP, they are not accessible to the population. There may also be a disparity between economic and social development resulting in an inability to use available economic resources wisely. A similar situation exists in the wider international context for some of the oil-exporting countries.

Nauru has a very high per capita GDP, but a lower than expected life expectancy. Taylor and Thoma (1985) have shown that in this case, considerable mortality from accidents and diseases of modernisation are associated with high consumption expenditure in the absence of appropriate social and legal norms.[7] This situation resembles to some extent that observed in certain ethnic minorities in developed countries, such as Australian Aborigines. This may seem paradoxical, but Australian Aborigines have access to sufficient financial resources through welfare payments to consume large amounts of unhealthy products provided their spending on other living expenses are kept minimal.

Imports per capita reflect population spending power and contact with the outside world, and was the economic index best correlated with mortality data. Imports per capita correlated positively with most measures of life expectancy, and with a cause of death structure characteristic of urbanised countries - low infectious disease and high cancer and cardiovascular disease.

Aid per capita correlated positively with life expectancy (especially for females), and negatively with mortality rates. It is important to recognise that many Pacific countries are highly aid dependent, and aid as a proportion of GDP varies from 7% to 100%.

Proportional mortality from 'external' causes correlated positively and significantly with all economic indices, urbanisation and Micronesian ethnicity, and negatively with political independence. Motor vehicle accidents (MVAs) are probably responsible for many of these deaths. Wintemute (1985) showed that MVA related mortality correlates weakly but directly with economic development (GNP per capita), especially in less developed countries.[8]

It has been suggested by Grosse (1980) that social factors which affect health may operate through behaviour related to: infant feeding and child care, use of available health services, personal hygiene, fertility, and diet.[9] All these factors are associated with education (often measured by literacy), particularly of females. Social factors influence mortality decline, and may explain part of it independently of economic, health service or environmental factors. However, a minimum level of economic development may be necessary for such social factors to significantly affect health status.[4]

Pendleton & Yang (1985) found education to be an important predictor of mortality.[10] Caldwell et al's work (1975, 1979, 1983 & 1984) showed that mother's education especially, exerts a strong, independent influence on infant and child mortality.[11,12,13,14] Education may improve familial food distribution and use of health services, and cause other behaviour changes that give improved protection to the weakest and most vulnerable. Literacy rate is also an important predictor of mortality,[15,9] and a powerful explanatory factor of differential fertility.[16]

Certain countries and societies are outliers in relation to the standard international correspondence of mortality with economic indicators. Low mortality rates are associated with comparatively low GDP per capita in the People's Republic of China, Sri Lanka, Cuba, Costa Rica and also in the state of Kerala in South India. High literacy rates and policies favouring social equity are implicated as an explanation for the dissociation of the usual nexus between health and economy.[17] There are no countries in the Pacific in which health status is better than one might expect from economic indices.

In this study education was a significant positive predictor of life expectancy and negative predictor of mortality rates. This was particularly the case for women and infants. The proportion of the population under 15 years correlated inversely with life expectancy, probably because of the characteristic pyramidal age structure in the least developed countries. Proportion of the population less than 15 years correlated positively with proportional mortality from accidents, probably because of an intercorrelation with the size of the 15-25 year age group, which suffers considerable mortality from external causes. Urbanisation also correlated with proportional mortality from external causes, probably due to motor vehicle accidents (MVAs).

There is continued debate concerning the role of health services as determinants of health status. Mckeown (1976) concluded that health services contributed little to the mortality decline in Western Europe,[18] whilst Stolnitz (1955a,b) and Preston (1975) suggest that medical technology contributed greatly to the rapid mid-20th century mortality decline in certain developing countries.[19,20,4] The influence of socioeconomic and health service variables on mortality in developing countries were linked in Pendleton and Yang's study (1985),[10] but health services appeared to play a greater role for countries in early stages of demographic and health transition than those in later transition.

In this study the availability of doctors was correlated negatively with mortality rates and positively with life expectancy. There was no correlation between the provision of hospital beds and mortality indices. The reasons for these findings are not clear, however, the availability of doctors is intercorrelated with economic indices.

Melanesian ethnicity was a prominent indicator of high mortality, especially for females, although this was probably confounded by malaria and socioeconomic factors. The three Melanesian countries with the lowest life expectancies were also malarious, underdeveloped and independent, with large dispersed and rural populations. Within each ethnic group a spectrum of health status is observed that correlates with overall development.

Political status is a particularly difficult variable because it is the outcome of many inter-acting historical, geographic, strategic and cultural factors, and highly correlated with economic and social factors. In this study political status was a powerful predictor of life expectancy, but its effects could be removed by adjusting for demographic and socioeconomic factors.

Certain factors which may be determinants of adverse health status (such as malaria, low level of development and dispersed populations) may also be related to the progression to political independence. Significant ethnic admixtures with Europeans, as seen in French Polynesia and Guam, and high levels of migration to and from metropolitan countries (e.g. from Cook Islands and Niue to and from New Zealand) increase acculturation and may change health-related behaviours. These factors may be separate determinants of low mortality and also continued political attachment. Many newly independent nations experienced poor health status prior to independence, and several territories have had relatively good health status for sometime. The large proportion of Europeans in certain Island states, such as Guam and New Caledonia, reflects their territorial status, and also contributes to high life expectancy when this population is included in total country estimates.

Economic indices and education are probably intervening variables in the causal chain between political status and mortality. Political status has both direct and indirect effects on aid flows and investment, and is linked to the extent and quality of health services, particularly therapeutic and hospital services. Population and population density are difficult to interpret as variables since they may to some extent be direct causes, or effects, of political status, and may be linked to mortality through such associations. For example some small, densely populated, island states remain connected with larger metropolitan countries because they are easy to administer and have strategic value. Economic development resulting from connection with metropolitan countries also frequently promotes migration and urbanisation.

Malaria is an established determinant of high mortality rates, and various studies have shown that mortality decline accompanies malaria control. Gray (1975) studied post-war mortality decline in Sri Lanka which coincided with extension of health services, an anti-malaria campaign, nutrition improvements and economic development.[21] The anti-malaria campaign appeared to be responsible for an approximate 25% reduction in crude death rates, and accounted for most inter-provincial differences. Improvements in health services, nutrition, and the economy contributed indeterminately to mortality decline, though this has been debated.[22,23] In this study the presence of malaria was correlated with high mortality, and malarious countries had an average life expectancy 10 years lower than non-malarious countries. This difference could not be removed by adjusting for socioeconomic or demographic factors.

This study has explored the inter-connected influence of: political association with metropolitan countries, economic factors, education, demographic indices, endemic disease, and provision of health services on varying life expectancy and mortality rates in PICs. The extent of the health and demographic transitions in each island state can be determined from overall levels of mortality and the cause structure of mortality. As transition occurs, mortality drops and life expectancy increases; while less infectious and acute respiratory disease is observed, it is to varying extent replaced more by non-communicable conditions and 'external' causes of mortality. This process of replacement of one group of diseases by another may lead to a stagnation in the decline of mortality such as occurred in males in many industrialised countries during the 1950s and 1960s. In other instances an actual increase in mortality may occur; such as in male Nauruans[7] and Fiji Indians.[24]

In summary, the less developed Melanesian, malarious countries and dispersed atoll nations experienced higher mortality than other PICs, with higher proportional mortality from infectious disease. In general females had longer life expectancy than males. Certain Island states associated with metropolitan countries had relatively lower mortality, with higher proportional mortality from cardiovascular and other non-communicable diseases. Economic and education variables appeared to be intervening variables in this process, and various potential confounding influences were identified which are likely to be directly and independently associated with both political status and health status. However, despite the complexities, it is apparent that some Island states have been able to work out mutually beneficial continuing connections with metropolitan countries. Such associations are seen by these states as preferable to the stark realities of political independence with very small populations, little land, few natural resources, no migration opportunities and extreme geographic isolation.

The identification of factors significantly associated with health status in PICs should assist individual governments, as well as donor nations and regional and international aid organisations, to design and implement appropriate inter-sectoral development policies, for reducing morbidity and mortality in populations of small Pacific Islands states.

REFERENCES

1. Coale A. The demographic transition. International Union for the scientific study of population. International population Conference. Liege, Belgium. 1, 53-72, 1973.

2. Orman, A. The epidemiological transition, a theory of population change. Milbank Memorial Fund Quarterly 49, 509-538, 1971.

3. Taylor, R, Lewis, N D & Levy, S. Societies in transition: mortality patterns in Pacific Island populations. International Journal of Epidemiology 18, 634-646, 1989.

4. Preston, S. The changing relation between mortality and level of economic development. Population Studies 29, 231-248, 1975.

5. Brass, W. Methods of estimating fertility and mortality from limited and defective data. Population Centre, University of North Carolina, Chapel Hill, USA, 1975.

6. Cumper, G. National incomes and health: implications of some recent additions to the data. Journal of Tropical Medicine and Hygiene 84, 49-61, 1981.

7. Taylor, R & Thoma, K. Mortality patterns in the modernized Pacific island nation of Nauru. American Journal of Public Health 75, 149-155, 1985.

8. Wintemute, G. Is motor vehicle related mortality a disease of development? Accidents, Analysis and Prevention 17, 223-237, 1985.

9. Grosse, R. Interrelation between health and population: observations derived from field experiences. Social Science and Medicine 14, 99-120, 1980.

10. Pendleton, B. & Yang, S. Socioeconomic development and mortality levels in less developed countries. Social Biology 27, 220-229, 1980.

11. Orubuloye, I. & Caldwell, J. The impact of public health services on mortality: a study of mortality differentials in a rural area in Nigeria. Population studies 29, 259-272, 1975.

12. Caldwell, J. Education as a factor in mortality decline: an examination of Nigerian data. Population Studies 33, 395-413, 1979.

13. Caldwell, J., Reddy, P. & Caldwell, P. The social component of mortality decline: An investigation in South India employing alternative methodologies. Population Studies 37, 185-205, 1983.

14. Caldwell, J. Introductory remarks on interactions between health, mortality and development. In Mortality and Health Policy. International Conference on Population. United Nations, Department of Economic and Social Affairs, New York, 1984.

15. Krishnan, P. Mortality decline in India, 1951-1961: Development versus public health program hypothesis. Social Science and Medicine 9, 475-479, 1975.

16. Chang, H., Warren, R & Pendleton, B. Testing and clarifying a macro model of socioeconomic change and fertility. Sociol Biology 26, 30-50, 1979.

17. United Nations, Department of Economic and Social Affairs. Mortality and Health Policy. In International Conference on Population. New York, 1984.

18. Mckeown, T. The modern rise of population. Edward Arnold, London, 1976.

19. Stolnitz, G. A century of international mortality trends: I. Population Studies 9, 24-55, 1955.

20. Stolnitz, G. A century of international mortality trends: II. Population Studies 10, 17-42, 1955.

21. Gray, R. The decline of mortality in Ceylon and the demographic effects of malaria control. Population Studies 28, 205-229, 1975.

22. Frederiksen, H. Determinants and consequences of mortality trends in Ceylon. Public Health Reports 76, 659-663, 1961.

23. Meegama, S. Malaria eradication and its effects on mortality levels. Population Studies 21, 207-237, 1967.

24. Taylor, R, Sladden, T & Lewis, N D. Secular trends in mortality in Pacific Island populations 1940-1990, (in preparation, 1989).

FIGURES 3-6: KEY

AS	=	AMERICAN SAMOA
CI	=	COOK ISLANDS
FJ	=	FIJI
FP	=	FRENCH POLYNESIA
FS	=	FEDERATED STATES OF MELANESIA
GU	=	GUAM
K	=	KIRIBATI
MI	=	MARSHALL ISLANDS
NA	=	NAURU
NC	=	NEW CALEDONIA
NI	=	NIUE
NM	=	NORTHERN MARIANAS
PA	=	PALAU
PG	=	PAPUA NEW GUINEA
SI	=	SOLOMON ISLANDS
TN	=	TONGA
TV	=	TUVALU
V	=	VANUATU
WF	=	WALLIS & FUTUNA
WS	=	WESTERN SAMOA

Table 1. LIFE EXPECTANCY & INFANT MORTALITY IN PACIFIC ISLAND COUNTRIES, CIRCA 1980.

COUNTRY	Life expectancy at birth Male	Female	M&F	Infant Mortality (/1000)	Years Covered	Source of Estimate
MELANESIA						
New Caledonia						
Melanesians	(58.1)	(61.4)	59.6	39.3	1978-80	Vital registration
Europeans	(69.3)	(76.9)	72.5	8.5	1978-80	Vital registration
All	62.8	68.6	65.6	27.1	1978-80	Vital registration
Fiji						
Melanesians	62.9	65.1	64.0⁺	29.9	1981-83	(Ministry of Health)
Indians	60.2	63.9	62.1⁺	40.5	1981-83	(Death recording)
All	61.6*	64.5*	63.1	33.0	1981-83	(adjusted)
Papua New Guinea	48.7	50.7	49.6	76.5	1975-79	Census 1980
Solomon Islands	54.1	54.0	54.1⁺	52.5	1971-75	Census 1976
Vanuatu	56.2	53.7	55.0⁺	94.0	1974-78	Census 1979
POLYNESIA						
American Samoa	67.8	75.5	70.1	18.2	1978-82	Vital registration
Cook Islands	64.4	69.9	67.2⁺	28.5	1979-81	Vital registration
French Polynesia	(60.1)	(64.2)	61.9	56.9	1976-78	Vital registration
Niue	(64.1)	(69.7)	66.5	10.6	1978-82	Vital registration
Tokelau	-	-	-	37.0	1970-79	Vital registration
Tonga	(60.8)	(65.2)	62.8	40.7	1973-75	Census 1976
Tuvalu	56.9	60.1	58.5⁺	43.0	1974-78	Census 1979
Wallis & Futuna	61.5	63.6	62.9	49.3	1974-78	Vital registration
Western Samoa	60.6	66.1	63.1	33.0	1980-82	Vital statistics survey
MICRONESIA						
Federated States of Micronesia	(56.5)	(59.3)	57.8	45.2	1979-81	Vital registr (adjusted)
Guam						
Chamorros	(66.7)	(73.3)	69.5	13.4	1979-81	Vital registration
Others	(71.4)	(79.8)	74.9	13.2	1979-81	Vital registration
All	70.0	76.6	73.0	13.3	1979-81	Vital registration
Kiribati	50.3	53.8	52.1⁺	92.5	1973-77	Census 1978
Marshall Islands	(58.4)	(61.9)	60.0	44.8	1979-81	Vital registr (adjusted)
Nauru	48.4	60.5	54.5⁺	31.0	1976-81	Vital registration
Northern Marianas	62.5	71.1	65.9	26.4	1979-81	Vital registration
Palau	62.7	70.4	65.6	27.6	1979-81	Vital registration

Figures in brackets estimated from the both-sexes life expectancy, using a linear regression of the sex-specific and both-sexes life expectancy, in countries and ethnic groups for which these data are available (excluding Nauru).
*Average of two main ethnic groups.
⁺Average of male and female.

Source: Taylor et al (1989).

Table 2. DESCRIPTIVE AND SOCIOECONOMIC VARIABLES INCLUDED IN THE COMPARATIVE ANALYSIS (I). PACIFIC ISLAND COUNTRIES, CIRCA 1980.

COUNTRY	Major Ethnic Group	Island Type	Political Status Status	Year of Independence[+]	Population	Proportion of Population <15yrs (%)
MELANESIA						
New Caledonia	Melanesian/ European	High Islands	Territory	-	142 500	39
Fiji	Melanesian/ Indian	High Islands	Independent	1970	646 500	41
Papua New Guinea	Melanesian	High Islands	Independent	1975	3 060 000	43
Solomon Islands	Melanesian	High Islands	Independent	1978	235 000	48
Vanuatu	Melanesian	High Islands	Independent	1980	119 900	46
POLYNESIA						
American Samoa	Polynesian	High Islands	Territory	-	33 200	41
Cook Islands	Polynesian	Mixed[#]	Semi-autonomous	(1965)	17 400	42
French Polynesia	Polynesian	Mixed[#]	Territory	-	149 800	42
Niue	Polynesian	Atoll	Semi-autonomous	(1974)	3 200	46
Tokelau	Polynesian	Atolls	Territory	-	1 600	46
Tonga	Polynesian	High Islands	Independent	always	98 400	44
Tuvalu	Polynesian	Atolls	Independent	1978	7 600	34
Wallis & Futuna	Polynesian	High Islands	Territory	-	11 200	47
Western Samoa	Polynesian	High Islands	Independent	1962	156 000	48
MICRONESIA						
Federated States of Micronesia	Micronesian	Mixed[#]	Semi-autonomous	(1986)	79 500	46
Guam	Micronesian/ Others[*]	High Islands	Territory	-	107 000	35
Kiribati	Micronesian	Atolls	Independent	1979	59 900	41
Marshall Islands	Micronesian	Atolls	Semi-autonomous	(1986)	31 800	51
Nauru	Micronesian[**]	Atoll	Independent	1968	8 000	44
Northern Marianas Islands	Micronesian	High Islands	Semi-autonomous	(1985)	17 600	41
Palau	Micronesian	High Islands	Semi-autonomous	(1988)	12 400	40

[*] Asians
[**] Nauruans only
[#] Mixed = High Islands & Atolls
[+] Dates in brackets indicate official achievement of semi-autonomous status. Defacto semi-autonomous status has existed in various Micronesian states for some years before signing of the Compact of Free Association.

Source: South Pacific Economies 1981, Statistical Summary, South Pacific Commission, Nouméa, New Caledonia.

Table 3. DESCRIPTIVE AND SOCIOECONOMIC VARIABLES INCLUDED IN THE COMPARATIVE ANALYSIS (II). PACIFIC ISLAND COUNTRIES, CIRCA 1980.

COUNTRY	Pop. Density#	Urban-isation##	Education+	Economic Indices (per capita; A$) GDP	Imports	Exports	Aid	Health Indices Population per Doctor	Population /hosp bed	Malaria
MELANESIA										
New Caledonia	7	61	99	5 879	2 511	2 013	1 234	815	101	-
Fiji	35	37	93	1 698	870	433	47	2 233	354	-
Papua New Guinea	7	13	36	1 201	587	240	95	15 620	243	+
Solomon Islands	9	9	47	547	284	247	137	6 250	163	+
Vanuatu	10	18	71	639	378	209	325	5 327	153	+
POLYNESIA										
American Samoa	169	43	88	3 442	3 013	5 214	1 091	1 133	171	-
Cook Islands	74	27	99	983	1 177	222	520	1 053	114	-
French Polynesia	46	59	99	6 292	3 240	169	944	1 036	158	-
Niue	13	21	98	957	922	142	970	1 650	71	-
Tokelau	160	0	99	478	214	40	1 063	400	51	-
Tonga	141	26	96	526	356	78	134	2 865	299	-
Tuvalu	292	30	97	478	341	5	573	1 875	97	-
Wallis & Futuna	44	0	87	805	495	0*	676	2 700	77	-
Western Samoa	54	21	88	723	384	62	135	2 768	224	-
MICRONESIA										
Federated States of Micronesia	113	46	89	810	237	64	660	3 313	244	-
Guam	197	91	88	3 700	4 050	1 500	381	1 214	527	-
Kiribati	854	36	85	384	326	44	287	1 953	196	-
Marshall Islands	176	60	86	915	313	209	498	3 975	294	-
Nauru	348	99	95	20 000	1 473	9 400	0	700	24	-
Northern Marianas Islands	37	94	98	3 014	3 184	2 386	1 857	1 036	209	-
Palau	25	63	95	1 515	683	1 427	1 147	1 033	134	-

#Population density (persons/km²)
##Proportion of the population residing in urban areas (%)
+Proportion of school age children at school (%)
*Designated as 1 for the purposes of logarithmic transformation
Economic indices are in 1980 Australian dollars.

Source: South Pacific Economies 1981 Statistical Summary, South Pacific Commission, Nouméa, New Caledonia.

Table 4. CORRELATION COEFFICIENTS BETWEEN MORTALITY INDICES AND DESCRIPTIVE AND SOCIOECONOMIC VARIABLES. PACIFIC ISLAND COUNTRIES, CIRCA 1980.

Variable	Life expectancy (years): at birth			at 15 years			Mortality Rates (per 1000): Infant	child	child	Adults
	all	males	females	all	males	females	<1yr	1-4yr	5-14yr	15-64yr
Melanesian+	-0.60*	-0.47	-0.66**	-0.51	-0.33	-0.61*	0.59*	0.61*	0.68**	0.69**
Micronesian+	-0.23	-0.34	-0.10	-0.33	-0.45	-0.14	0.07	0.00	-0.01	-0.05
Polynesian+	0.36	0.37	0.32	0.39	0.39	0.33	-0.26	-0.21	-0.29	-0.26
Atolls+	-0.30	-0.39	-0.22	-0.37	-0.44	-0.29	0.03	0.04	0.19	0.19
High Islands+	0.22	0.29	0.18	0.28	0.34	0.23	-0.05	0.01	-0.06	0.04
Mixed Atolls/High Islands	0.06	0.07	0.03	0.07	0.07	0.03	0.03	-0.08	-0.16	-0.27
Political status@	0.68**	0.67**	0.65**	0.66**	0.60**	0.64*	-0.43	-0.58*	-0.67**	-0.72**
Independent+	-0.67**	-0.66**	-0.66**	-0.60	-0.53*	-0.61*	0.51*	0.66**	0.79**	0.80**
Semi-autonomous+	0.26	0.23	0.28	0.13	0.09	0.18	-0.33	-0.40	-0.49	-0.46
Territory+	0.50	0.51	0.46	0.54*	0.51	0.51	-0.24	-0.33	-0.37	-0.44
Population	-0.45	-0.42	-0.44	-0.47	-0.38	-0.48	0.35	0.33	0.49	0.58*
(log) Population	-0.34	-0.24	-0.40	-0.26	-0.10	-0.36	0.40	0.41	0.38	0.41
Population <15yrs (%)	-0.33	-0.28	-0.36	-0.38	-0.28	-0.43	0.22	0.09	0.05	0.15
Urbanisation (%)	0.31	0.16	0.45	0.19	0.07	0.42	-0.37	-0.42	-0.28	-0.34
Population density (km^2)	-0.31	-0.39	-0.24	-0.25	-0.30	-0.17	0.33	0.39	0.37	0.23
(log) Population density	-0.62*	-0.48	-0.72*	-0.55	-0.29	-0.73**	-0.05	-0.04	-0.05	-0.12
Education (%)	0.62*	0.52*	0.66*	0.59**	0.40	0.67**	-0.54*	-0.61*	-0.64**	-0.75**
Education#	0.57*	0.45	0.62*	0.51	0.31	0.61*	-0.58*	-0.62*	-0.56*	-0.64*
GDP/capita	-0.07	-0.25	0.08	0.22	-0.50	0.05	-0.21	-0.25	-0.13	0.09
(log) GDP/capita	0.29	0.14	0.41	0.14	-0.12	0.37	-0.41	-0.49	-0.20	-0.24
Imports/capita	0.62*	0.55*	0.66*	0.57*	0.42	0.68**	-0.44	-0.50	-0.41	-0.46
(log) Imports/capita)	0.62*	0.53*	0.69**	0.55*	0.35	0.69**	-0.48	-0.54*	-0.39	-0.46
Exports/capita	0.07	-0.11	0.24	-0.12	-0.40	0.18	-0.33	-0.32	0.02	0.01
(log) Exports/capita	0.26	0.16	0.38	0.10	-0.10	0.34	-0.37	-0.42	-0.12	-0.16
Aid/capita	0.52*	0.50	0.55*	0.47	0.42	0.53*	-0.38	-0.47	-0.58*	-0.62*
(log) Aid/capita	0.45	0.42	0.49	0.43	0.36	0.49	-0.35	-0.43	-0.53*	-0.60*
Malaria+	-0.60*	-0.47	-0.66**	-0.51	-0.33	-0.61*	0.59*	-0.61*	0.68**	0.69**
Population/doctor	-0.62*	-0.53*	-0.66**	-0.60*	-0.42	-0.68**	0.54*	0.55*	0.59*	0.70**
(log) Population/doctor	-0.62*	-0.48	-0.72	-0.55	-0.29	-0.73**	0.57*	0.63*	0.49	0.62*
Population/hospital bed	0.24	0.29	0.18	0.28	0.34	0.20	-0.06	-0.07	-0.16	-0.13

#Power transformation (x^5)
*p<0.05;
**p<0.001
+Categorical variable (0,1)
@Ordinal variable (1,2,3)
Economic indices in 1980 Australian dollars.

Table 5. CORRELATION COEFFICIENTS BETWEEN MORTALITY INDICES AND DESCRIPTIVE AND SOCIOECONOMIC VARIABLES. PACIFIC ISLAND COUNTRIES, CIRCA 1980.

	Proportional Mortality by Cause (%):					
Variable	Infections	Cancer	Cardiovascular Disease	Respiratory Disease	Accidents	Perinatal Conditions
Melanesian+	0.66**	-0.47	-0.63**	-0.39	-0.48	0.68**
Micronesian+	0.20	0.00	-0.12	-0.31	0.53*	0.03
Polynesian+	-0.43	0.12	0.34	0.19	-0.20	-0.32
Atolls+	0.06	-0.36	-0.17	0.19	0.08	0.00
High Islands+	-0.06	0.12	0.04	-0.15	-0.03	0.19
Mixed Atolls/High Islands+	0.01	0.30	0.16	-0.04	-0.06	-0.26
Political status@	-0.58*	0.48	0.37	-0.02	0.40	-0.48
Independent+	0.57*	-0.46	-0.39	-0.06	-0.51*	0.42
Semi-autonomous+	-0.19	0.11	0.16	0.16	0.39	-0.03
Territory+	-0.44	0.39	0.26	-0.10	0.17	-0.43
Population	0.44	-0.27	-0.33	0.43	-0.43	0.12
(log) Population	0.45	0.01	-0.23	-0.11	-0.38	0.08
Population <15yrs (%)	0.38	-0.34	-0.43	0.28	0.14	0.13
Urbanisation (%)	-0.31	0.53*	0.48	-0.56*	0.58*	-0.23
Population density (/km²)	0.24	-0.12	-0.18	-0.32	-0.05	-0.11
(log) Population density	-0.14	0.23	0.20	-0.44	0.19	-0.27
Education (%)	-0.71**	0.49	0.70**	-0.36	0.39	-0.58*
Education#	-0.73**	0.42	0.71**	-0.11	0.25	-0.52*
GDP/capita	-0.06	0.18	0.20	-0.31	0.47	-0.20
(log) GDP/capita	-0.32	0.45	0.45	-0.34	0.55*	0.35
Imports/capita	-0.55*	0.62*	0.63*	-0.33	0.31	-0.36
(log) Imports/capita)	-0.55*	0.57*	0.65**	-0.29	0.34	-0.38
Exports/capita	-0.17	0.17	0.22	-0.27	0.63*	-0.12
(log) Exports/capita	-0.28	0.42	0.38	-0.12	0.52*	-0.09
Aid/capita	-0.55*	0.22	0.37	0.10	0.38	-0.18
(log) Aid/capita	-0.47	0.25	0.29	-0.01	0.53*	-0.25
Malaria+	0.66**	-0.47	-0.63*	0.39	-0.48	0.68**
Population/doctor	0.68**	-0.44	-0.61*	0.42	-0.48	0.38
(log) Population/doctor	0.75**	-0.45	-0.66**	0.16	-0.45	0.44
Population/hospital bed	-0.05	0.42	0.20	-0.33	-0.09	-0.10

#Power transformation (x^5)
*p<0.05;
**p<0.001
+Categorical variable (0,1)
@Ordinal variable (1,2,3)
Economic indices in 1980 Australian dollars.

Table 6. MEAN LIFE EXPECTANCY AT BIRTH BY POLITICAL STATUS, UNADJUSTED AND ADJUSTED FOR CERTAIN DESCRIPTIVE AND SOCIOECONOMIC VARIABLES. PACIFIC ISLAND COUNTRIES, CIRCA 1980.

	Mean Life Expectancy at Birth (both sexes) (years)#					
Variable	Independent (a) (n=9)	Semi-Autonomous (b) (n=6)	Territory (c) (n=5)	Difference (c-a)	Difference (b-a)	Significance of difference (a),(b) & (c) p
UNADJUSTED	57.0	63.8	66.7	9.7	6.8	<0.01
ADJUSTED FOR SINGLE VARIABLES						
Population (R^2=0.55)	57.6	63.3	66.3	8.7	5.7	<0.05
Population Density (R^2=0.05)	57.2	63.6	66.5	9.3	6.4	<0.01
Imports (log) (R^2=0.56)	58.2	64.0	64.3	6.1	5.8	ns
Aid per capita (R^2=0.49)	57.3	63.6	66.5	9.2	6.3	ns
Population per doctor (log) (R^2=0.56)	58.1	63.3	65.3	7.2	5.2	<0.05
Education (power transformed) (R^2=0.59)	58.0	62.7	66.1	8.1	4.7	<0.05
Malaria** (R^2=0.59)	58.1	62.9	65.8	7.7	4.8	<0.05
ADJUSTED FOR CERTAIN VARIABLES						
Population, Population Density, Imports, Education & Malaria (R^2=0.80)	61.2	61.9	61.4	0.2	0.7	ns
ADJUSTED FOR ALL VARIABLES*						
(R^2=0.85)	61.1	62.2	61.3	0.2	1.1	ns

#Excluding Tokelau
**Considered either as a covariate (values 0 or 1), or as a factor (0,1)
*Adjusted for (log) imports per capita, (log) population per doctor, education (power transformation = x^5), aid per capita, population, population density & malaria.

Table 7. MEAN LIFE EXPECTANCY AT BIRTH BY MALARIA STATUS, UNADJUSTED AND ADJUSTED FOR CERTAIN DESCRIPTIVE AND SOCIOECONOMIC VARIABLES. PACIFIC ISLAND COUNTRIES, CIRCA 1980.

	Mean life expectancy at birth, both sexes (years)			
	Malaria present (n=3)	Malaria absent (n=17)	Difference	Significance of difference
Unadjusted	52.9	63.0	10.1	ns
Adjusted* (R^2=0.81)	51.4	63.2	11.8	ns (p=0.06)

*Adjusted for: imports per capita (log), aid per capita, population, population density, education (power transformation = x^5), population per doctor (log).

THE PACIFIC ISLANDS

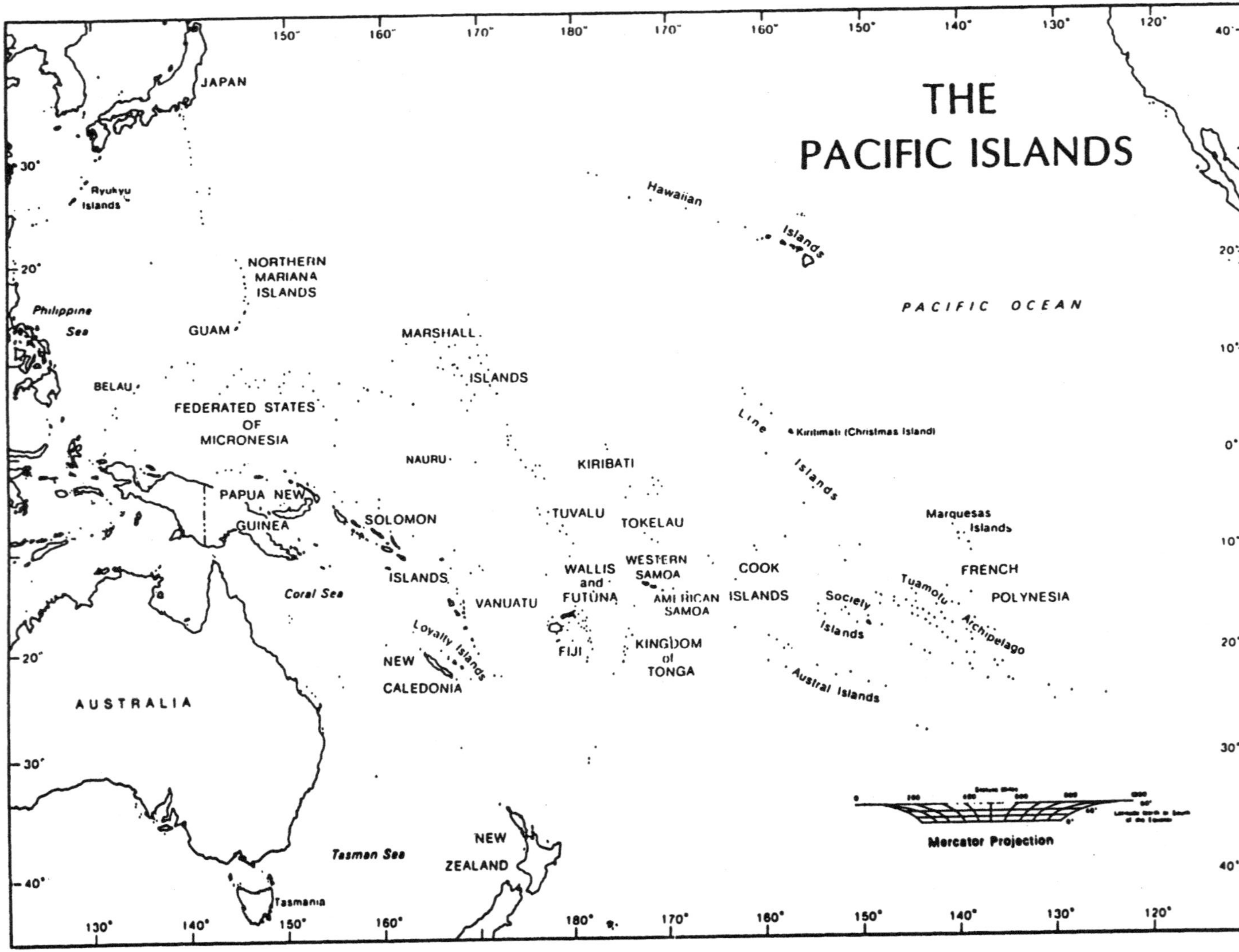

FIGURE 2.

EXPECTATION OF LIFE AND ETHNICITY
PACIFIC ISLAND COUNTRIES, CIRCA 1980

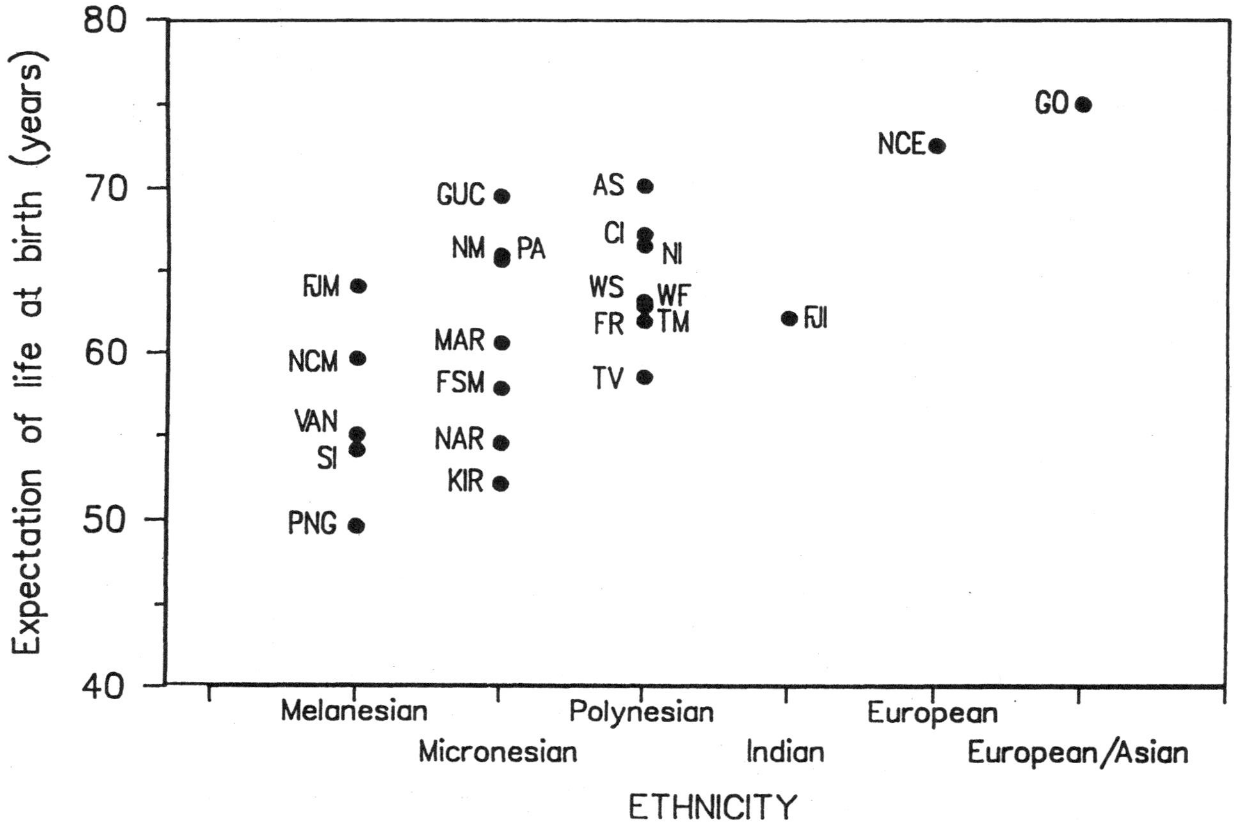

KEY

AS - American Samoa
CI - Cook Islands
FJI - Fiji Indians
FJM - Fiji Melanesians
FR - French Polynesia
FSM - Federated States of Micronesia
GO - Guam others
GUC - Guam Chamorros
KIR - Kiribati
MAR - Marshall Islands
NAR - Nauru
NCE - New Caledonia Europeans
NCM - New Caledonia Melanesians
NI - Niue
NM - Northern Marianas
PA - Palau
PNG - Papua New Guinea
SI - Solomon Islands
TV - Tuvalu
TM - Tonga
VAN - Vanuatu
WF - Wallis & Futuna
WS - Western Samoa

rt01

FIGURE 3.

EXPECTATION OF LIFE AND POLITICAL STATUS
PACIFIC ISLAND COUNTRIES, CIRCA 1980

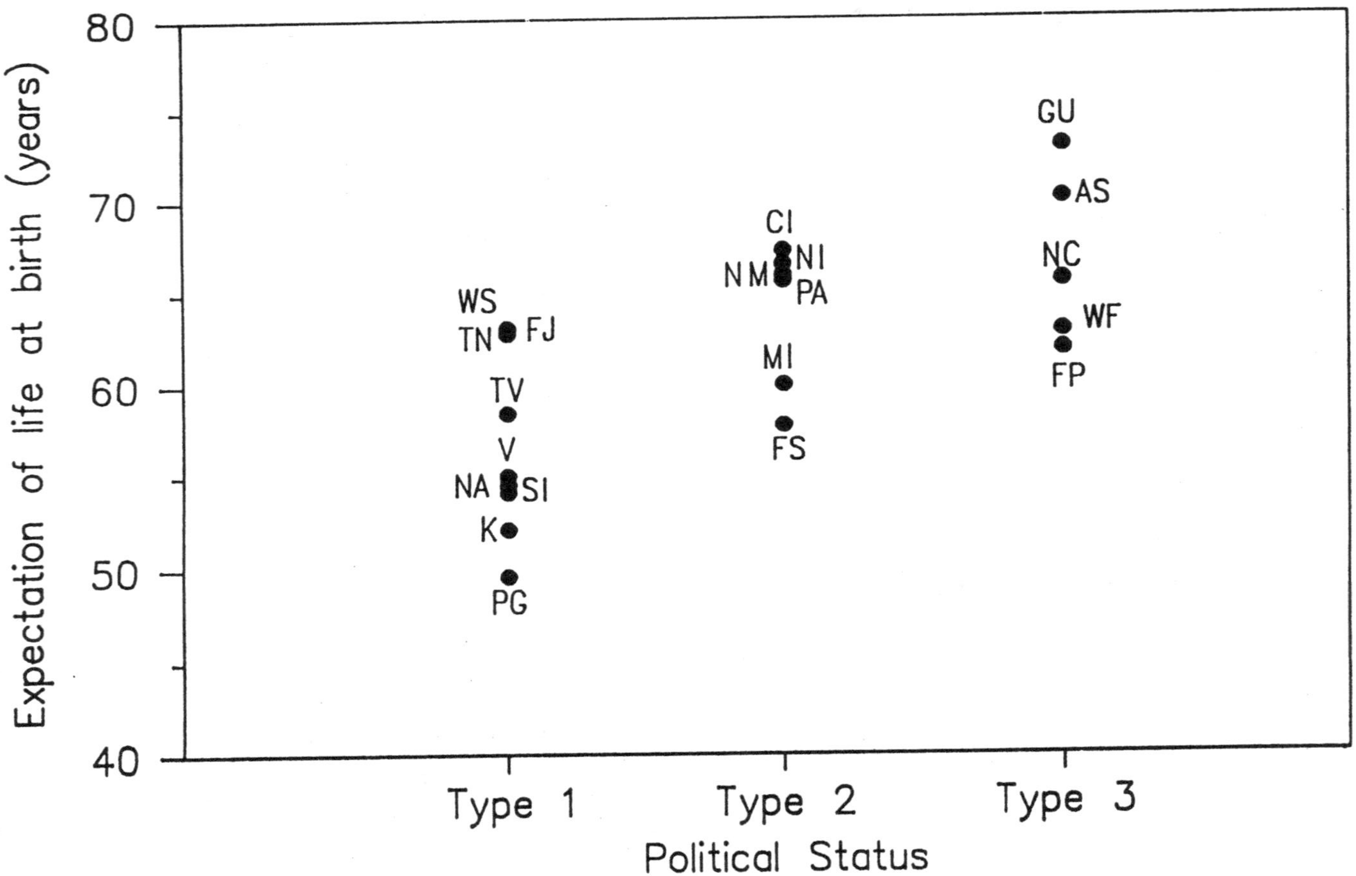

INDEPENDENT SEMI-AUTONOMOUS TERRITORY

rt36

FIGURE 4.

EXPECTATION OF LIFE AND GROSS DOMESTIC PRODUCT, (GDP)
PACIFIC ISLAND COUNTRIES, CIRCA 1980

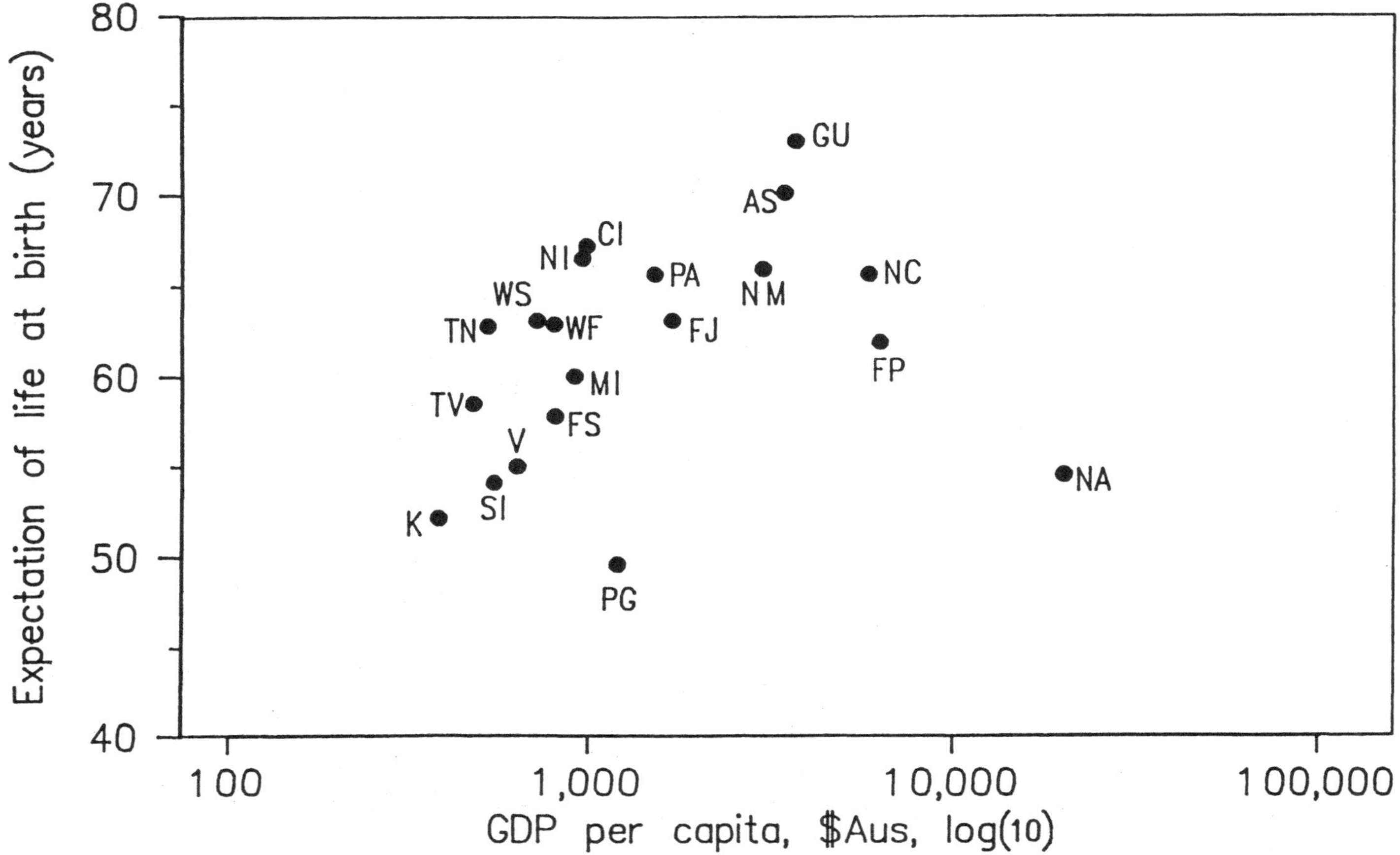

EXPECTATION OF LIFE AND IMPORTS PER CAPITA
PACIFIC ISLAND COUNTRIES, CIRCA 1980

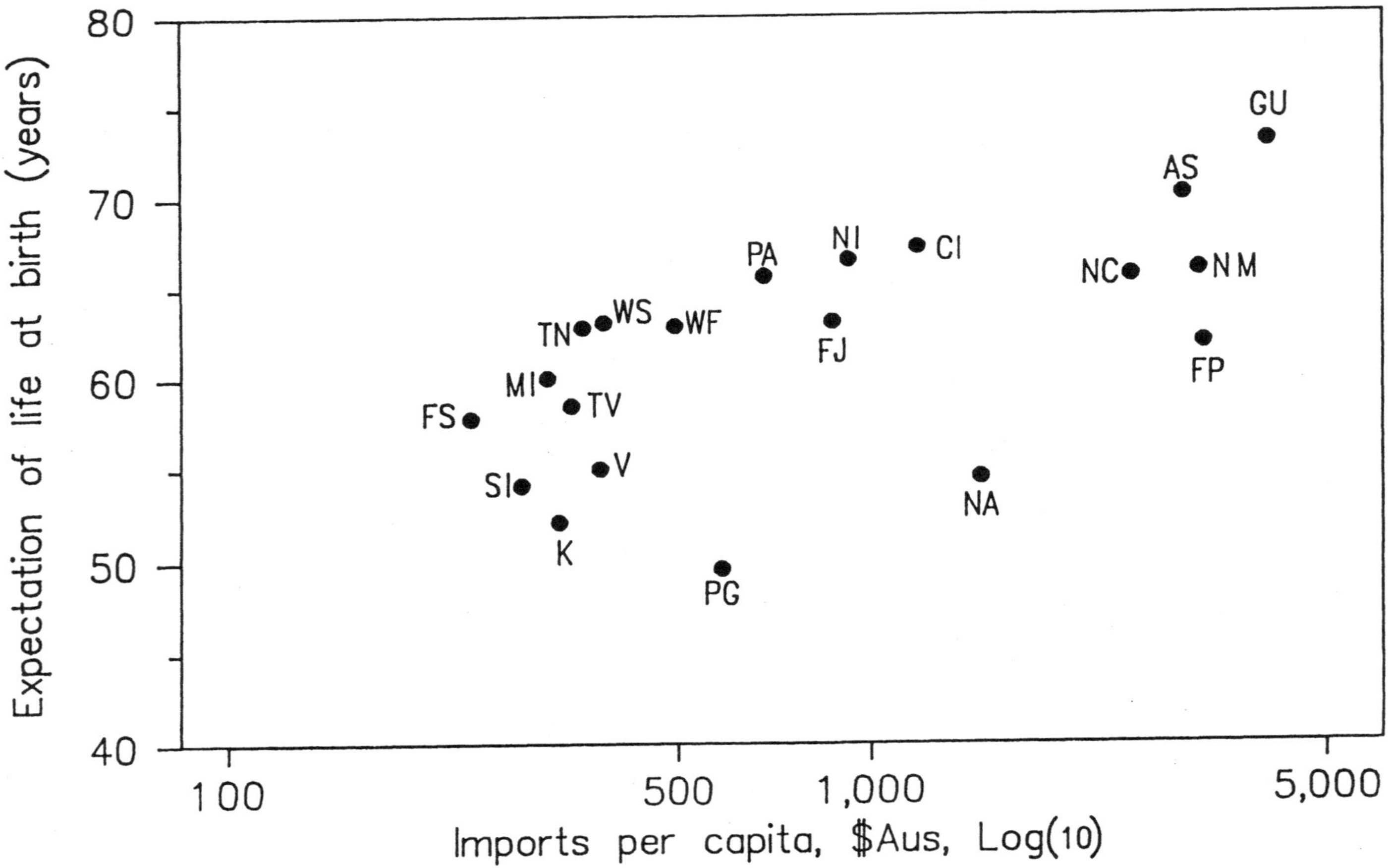

RT05

FIGURE 6.

EXPECTATION OF LIFE AND EDUCATION
PACIFIC ISLAND COUNTRIES, CIRCA 1980

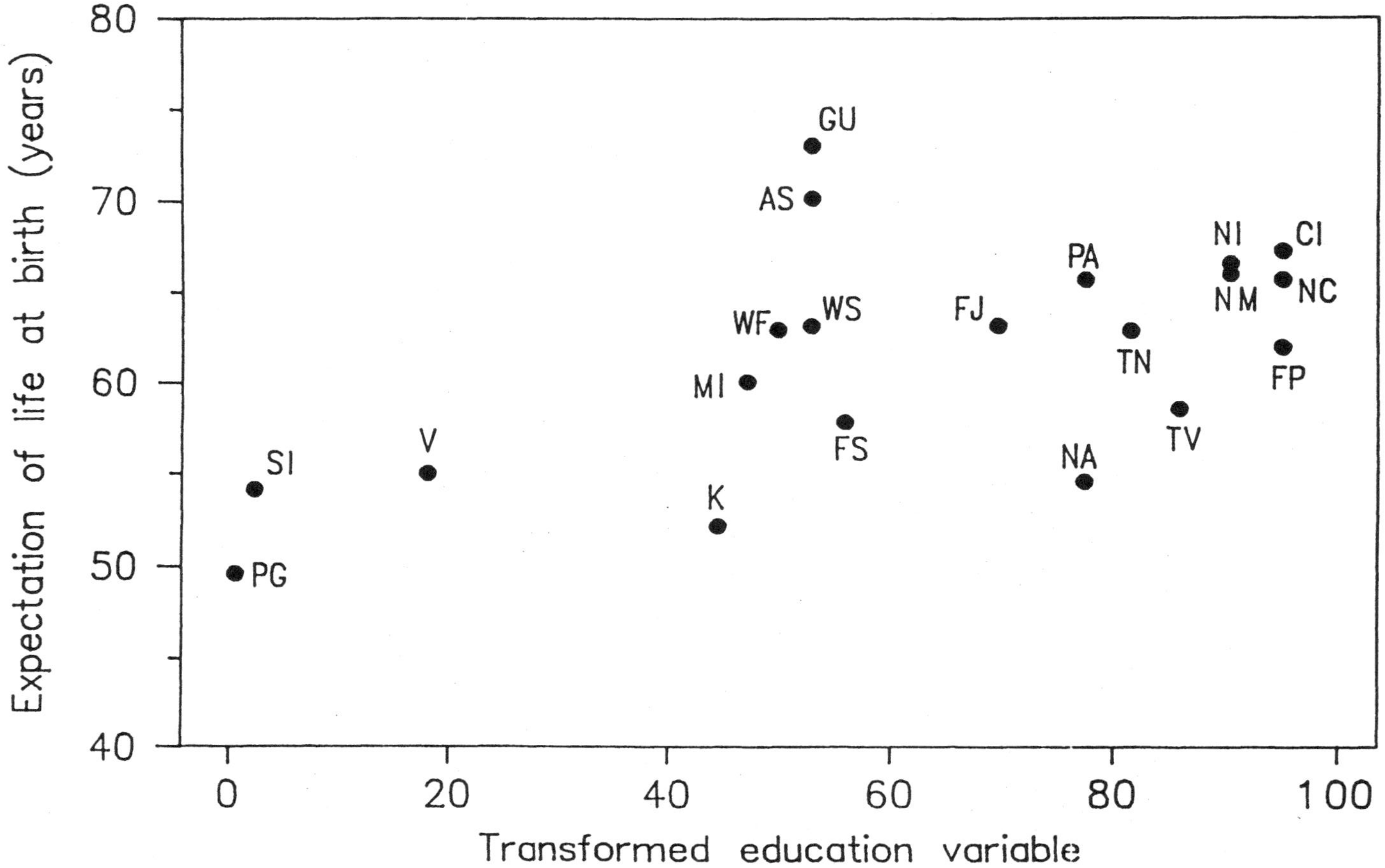

POPULATION TRENDS IN PAPUA NEW GUINEA

NATIONAL STATISTICAL OFFICE[1]

INTRODUCTION

The Paper is presented in two parts. Part I deals with population growth rates based on available population estimates for some parts of the country, and population data collected in the population censuses of Papua New Guinea since 1966. In Part II of the paper, only a brief overview of the available natural increase rates of population has been made. No discussion has been made in the paper on the causes and/or causal effect of the inrease or decrease of population for the country as a whole, or for rural and urban areas or provinces.]The effect of inter-provincial migration on the growth rates of provinces has also not been considered in the paper.

PART I - POPULATION GROWTH RATES

Depending on the availability of population data and their reliability, the discussion in this part is divided mainly into two periods viz., pre-second world war and post-war periods.

PRE-SECOND-WORLD-WAR POPULATION GROWTH

Population data collection is a relatively recent activity in Papua New Guinea compared to other third world countries. The collection of population data began in the New Guinea Region in 1914 and in the Papua Region in 1919. But the data were not collected for all parts of these regions. They were collected for a few island groups of the New Guinea Region and for the areas under government control or some influence in the Papua Region. Some of the population enumerated by the taxation and medical censuses are reproduced below for some selected years.

1 Department of Finance and Planning, Waigani, Papua New Guinea

TABLE 1 - TOTAL ENUMERATED POPULATION, NEW GUINEA, 1914 - 1940 (1)

Year	Total Enumerated Population including indentured labour	Annual Growth Rate (percent)	Annual Growth Rate 1914 - 1940 (Percent)
1914	152,075	-	
1920	166,721	1.53	
1925	257,551	8.70	
1930	400,067	8.81	5.66
1935	478,843	3.59	
1940	662,724	6.50	

TABLE 2 - TOTAL ENUMERATED POPULATION, PAPUA, 1919/22-1936/37 (2)

Year	Total Enumerated Population including indentured labour	Annual Growth Rate (percent)	Annual Growth Rate 1922 - 1937 (percent)
1914/22	162,531	-	
1931/32	157,962	-0.28	2.20
1934/35	224,908	11.78	
1936/37	230/962	1.33	

The collection of population data seems to have been disrupted in the Papua Region during the Second World War period as no population data are available for that period and up to 1949. Population data for some island districts of the New Guinea Region are available for the period 1940 - 50 to indicate the population loss due to war as given below.

TABLE 3 - POPULATION OF SOME ISLAND DISTRICTS OF NEW GUINEA, 1940 -1950(3)

Island District	Population including indentured Labour			Annual Decrease (Percent)
	1940	1950	Loss 1940-50	
Bougainville	51,010	41,191	9,819	
New Britain	91,403	80,285	11,118	
New Ireland	41,703	34,953	6,750	
Manus	14,314	12,587	1,727	
TOTAL	198,430	169,016	29,414	1.6

POST-WAR POPULATION GROWTH

The post-war population figures for Papua and New Guinea as collected during routine counts by the Department of District Administration (DDA) are given below for some selected years. These figures share some of the weaknesses of the pre-war figures but they are more representative for the country as a whole.

TABLE 4 - TOTAL INDIGENOUS POPULATION OF PAPUA NEW GUINEA, 1950, 1966(4)

Year ended 30 June	Total Population ('000)	Annual Growth Rate (%)	Annual Growth Rate 1950-1966 (%)
1950	1,440		
1955	1,690	3.20	2.56
1960	1,880	2.13	
1965	2,118	2.38	
1966	2,170	2.42	

As the two parts of Papua New Guinea, viz. New Guinea and Papua were administered by two different colonial governments before the Second World War, the collection of population data was also done differently with varying, incomplete coverage. Thus these two sets of data are discussed separately for each region without attempting any unification for the whole country. As can be seen from Table 1, the population of the New Guinea Region increased more than two fold (2.40 times) in ten years between 1920 and 1930 and 1.66 times in the decade up to 1940. This shows a doubling of population every 12 years in the New Guinea Region during the period up to 1940.

But the population increase in the Papua Region was much slower at about 2.20 percent per annum during 1919 - 37, which implies about 32 years to double the initial population.

Although complete population data are not available for any region of Papua New Guinea for the period 1940-50, the figures available for 4 island districts of New Guinea (Table 3) show that about 15% of the population were lost during the period due to the Second World War and its after-effects.

The total population of Papua New Guinea as a whole as collected in the DDA routine census was 1.44 million in 1950. The population figures available from the same source up to 1966 are given in table 4 above which shows that the population of PNG grew from 1.44 million in 1950 to 2.17 million in 1966 giving an annual increase of about 2.56 per cent over the period of 16 years. The first country-wide census of population taken in 1966 however shows a slightly lower population at 2.15 million which gives a growth rate of about 2.51 percent per annum during the 1950-66 period.

The breakdown of population of Papua New Guinea by urban - rural and citizen - noncitizen classifications for all the censuses since 1966 are preliminary and do not include the population of North Solomons Province where the census could not be taken for political reasons. The non-citizen population of the 1990 census is an estimate based only on non-citizen population of NCD. To facilitate the computation of population growth rate between the 1980 and 1990 censuses, the population figures for 1980 excluding North Solomons province have also been presented in Table 5. As the non-citizen population varied significantly between censuses due to the recruitment policy of the government of the period, this component of the population is shown separately in Table 5 and intercensal population growth rates are presented separately for citizen population only and for total population including non-citizens in Table 6 below.

TABLE 5 - TOTAL POPULATION, BY RURAL/URBAN AND CITIZEN/NON-CITIZEN, 1966-1990, PAPUA NEW GUINEA.

Year	Area	Citizen	Non-citizen	Total
1966 (30/6)	Rural	2,046,672	10,268	2,056,940
	Urban	103,645	24,401	128,046
	All areas	2,150,317	34,669	2,184,986
1971 (30/6)	Rural	2,203,636	9,981	2,213,617
	Urban	231,773	44,545	276,318
	All areas	2,435,409	54,526	2,489,935
1980 (30/9)	Rural	2,612,510	5,086	2,617,596
	Urban	365,547	27,584	393,131
	All areas	2,978,057	32,670	3,010,727
1990 (11/7)	Rural	2,995,726	3,600	2,999,326
	Urban	524,311	16,400	540,711
	All areas (1)	3,520,037	20,000 (2)	3,540,037
1980 (30/9) excluding NSP	Rural	2,506,872	4,838	2,511,710
	Urban	345,679	24,544	370,223
	All areas (3)	2,852,551	29,382	2,881,933

(1) The 1990 census figures are preliminary based on a hand count and do not include the population of North Solomons Province where the census could not be taken for political reasons.

(2) The figures for the non-citizen population of 1990 census could not be arrived at yet. These figures have been estimated based on the non-citizen population of NCD only, which is 7,444 for 1990 census and was 11,195 in 1980.

(3) As the 1990 census figures do not include the population of North Solomons Province, the 1980 census figures excluding North Solomons Province have also been presented for comparability.

TABLE 6 - INTERCENSAL POPULATION GROWTH RATES, 1966 - 1990, PAPUA NEW GUINEA

Year	Citizen Population Only		Total Population Including Non-Citizens	
	Population	Annual Growth Rate (%)	Population	Annual Growth Rate (%)
1966 30 June	2,150,317	-	2,184,986	-
1971 30 June	2,435,409	2.49	2,489,935	2.61
1980 30 Sept	2,978,057 2,852,551(1)	2.17	3,010,727 2,881,933(1)	2.05
1990(1) 11 July	3,520,037 3,550,000(3)	2.15 2.24	3,540,037(2) 3,570,000(3)	2.10 2.19

(1) Excluding population of North Solomons Province for comparability.

(2) Based on the estimate of non-citizen population made in foot-note 2 of Table 5.

(3) Enumeration in missing CUs of some provinces is still underway and it is expected that the total population in these CUs may be up to 30,000. This population estimate includes these 30,000 persons.

An estimate of total population of Papua New Guinea as a whole for any time before the Second World War is not feasible, as population data was collected only for a few parts of the country by different colonial governments. But from the fragmentary data that are available for the two parts of the country, viz. New Guinea and Papua, it is evident that population growth was spectacular at about 5.7 per cent per annum in the New Guinea region and very moderate at about 2.2 percent per annum in the Papua region. However, the population of the New Guinea region included a significant number of indentured labourers, and the Papua region faced an out-migration of labour.

During the 1940s when the Second World War was actively fought in various parts of Papua New Guinea, the collection of population data was disrupted in most parts. But from the data collected in island districts of New Guinea (Table 3) it is apparent that there was a loss of about 15% of the population due to war, which gives a population decline of about 1.6 percent annum during the period 1940-50.

After a very fast growth of population of over 4 per cent per annum before the Second World War and a decline of population (about 1.6%) due to war, the first estimate of total population of Papua New Guinea is available for the year 1950, which stood at 1.44 million. This population figure is largely enumerated, but also includes an estimated part of 31.1%. Taking this as the first base population of Papua New Guinea, it is observed that the citizen population of PNG doubled itself in 30 years by 1980, with an annual growth rate of about 2.4%. The intercensal annual growth rate during this whole period 1940-90 appears to have decreased successively from about 2.56% during 1950-66 to 2.15% during 1980-90. It must, however, be mentioned that the 1990 population census figures are yet to be finalized, including the population of numerous missing CUs in some provinces. When the enumeration is complete, it is estimated that the total population of PNG may be about 3.724 million including North Solomons Province. The citizen population growth rate between 1980-90 will have increased to 2.24% per annum, excluding North Solomons Province.

RURAL AND URBAN POPULATION GROWTH

As population data by rural and urban classifications are available only since the 1966 census, the growth of rural and urban populations are presented separately in Table 7 for the citizen population only for the intercensal periods between 1966 and 1990 censuses. The urban population in the first population census of PNG in 1966 was only about 5.86 per cent of the total population. But it increased abruptly to about 11.1% of the total population in the 1971 census. This more than doubling of the urban population in 5 years produced an annual increase of urban population of 16.1% during 1966-71. The population growth rates in the later two inter-censal periods, viz. 1971-80 and 1980-90, were not as spectacular as that in the previous intercensal period (1966-71) and they seem to have slowed down gradually. These abrupt and spectacular urban population growths had influenced the rural population to grow at much slower rates of below 2 per cent per annum during the inter-censal periods. While the growth of urban population (which is only about 15% of the total population in the 1990 census) seemed to have decreased over the intercensal periods 1966-90, the growth rate of the rural population (which is about 85 per cent of the total population) increased gradually from about 1.5% to about 1.9% over the intercensal periods 1966-90. This suggests a continuous increase, although of little magnitude, in the future growth rate of the rural population of Papua New Guinea.

TABLE 7 - INTERCENSAL GROWTH RATES OF CITIZEN POPULATION, RURAL AND URBAN, PNG, 1966-90

Year	RURAL		URBAN	
	Population	Annual Growth Rate (percent)	Population	Annual Growth Rate (percent)
1966 (30 June)	2,046,672	-	103,645	-
1971 (30 June)	2,203,636	1.48	231,773	16.10
1980 (30 Sept)	2,612,510 2,506,872(1)	1.84	365,547 345,679(1)	4.93
1990 (11 July)	2,995,726(2) 3,025,000(3)	1.82 1.92	524,311(2)	4.26

(1) Excluding population of North Solomons Province to make them comparable with the 1990 population.

(2) Based on the estimate of non-citizen population made at foot-note 2 of Table 5.

(3) Includes 30,000 persons with reference to foot-note 3 of Table 6.

CITIZEN POPULATION GROWTH BY PROVINCE, 1966-90

The citizen population growth rates of PNG as a whole declined gradually from 2.5% per annum during the intercensal period 1966-71 to 2.2% per annum during the intercensal period 1980-90. But this continuous decline in the population growth rates was not experienced in all the provinces. It was only in seven provinces, Gulf, Central, Western Highlands, Eastern Highlands, Morobe, East Sepik and West New Britain, that a continuous decline in the annual growth rates took place between these intercensal periods. Three provinces, Southern Highlands, Madang and East New Britain, had a continuous increase in population growth rates between these intercensal periods. Decrease in the growth rates between the first two intercensal periods and increase in the growth rates between the last two intercensal periods were experienced in seven provinces, Western, NCD, Milne Bay, Northern, Enga, Manus and New Ireland. The reverse order of an increase in the growth rates between the first two periods and a decrease in the growth rates between the last two periods took place in two provinces, Chimbu and West Sepik. It may be noted that the population of Chimbu and West Sepik Provinces was lower in the 1971 census compared to the

1966 census, giving negative population growth rates during 1966-71. These growth rates, however, increased during 1971-80 and fell again during 1980-90.

The population growth rate during 1966-71 varied widely in the provinces around the national growth rate of 2.49% per annum. They varied from a negative growth rate of -1.18% in West Sepik to a growth rate of 6.51% in West New Britain Province. The variation in the growth rates of provinces was not so wide (varying from a minimum of 0.65% to a maximum of 4.05%) during the 1971-80 period. The variation, however, increased during the 1980-90 period.

As the 1971 population figures were adjusted upward for under-enumeration, the growth rates shown for 1966-71 and for 1971-80 may not be accurate estimates of the actual growth rates. This problem can be avoided if growth rates are calculated for the period 1966-80. However, the period is so long that short term fluctuations in the growth rate are lost and only an average growth rate over the relatively long period of 14 years is available. These growth rates during 1966-80 are also given in Table 8 for comparison.

COMPARABILITY OF POPULATION FIGURES BETWEEN CENSUSES

The population figures given in Table 4 for the period 1950-65 were mainly subject to increased coverage of enumerated population in the census as the years passed by, besides other methological weaknesses. While the estimated population in the 1950 census was about 31.1% of the total population, this proportion decreased to 1.2% in the 1965 census taken by the Department of District Administration. Thus the comparability of the census figures increased with the increase in the enumerated population of the censuses over the passage of time.

In the 1966 and 1971 nation-wide censuses, the population figures were subject to sampling errors for the vast rural population in addition to other methodological and operational problems faced in these censuses. Moreover, the 1971 census figures were adjusted upward for under-enumeration. The 1980 population census was the first census taken on a full count basis but other methodological aspects were similar to those used in the previous censuses. The 1990 census, although similar to the 1980 census in fully enumerating the population, differed from the previous one in some methodological and operational aspects as mentioned below.

The 1990 census used a single coverage rule of defacto enumeration, i.e. persons who were present in the household "last night" were counted in the census for both urban and rural areas. This was slightly different from the coverage rule used in the 1980 census for rural areas, where persons who usually lived in the village were counted in the village unless they had spent the previous night in an urban area or a rural non-village.

The enumeration period was a week in both urban and rural areas in the 1990 census whereas it was a long period of 2-3 months in the rural areas in the 1980 census. A large number of enumerators (more than 15,000) and supervisors (about 5,000) were recruited locally and trained for the enumeration of population in the 1990 census compared to less than 5,000 enumerators and supervisors used in the 1980 census, mostly as members of rural patrol teams.

PART II. NATURAL INCREASE RATES OF POPULATION

The second part of this paper briefly attempts to provide an overview of movements in the rate of natural increase as a result of changes in the birth and death rates prevailing in the country during the following time periods:

Prior to the 1966 census
Since the 1966 census

1. NATURAL INCREASE RATES PRIOR TO 1966 CENSUS

To go back into the distant past and try to estimate the trend of natural increase would be misleading, since the data for such estimates were never collected on a national or regional scale. Although some efforts were made to collect information on vital rates during the post-war period, there were considerable doubts about the quality of the data.

During the early 1960's an attempt to estimate the natural growth rate for the country as a whole was carried out by Vines through an epidemiological sample survey he conducted in three regions, covering 1,000 people in each region. His calculations showed an overall rate of natural increase of 1.35 percent, from the combination of a crude birth rate of 30.4 and crude death rate of 16.9 per 1,000 population. This estimate seemed unacceptably low compared to an average annual growth rate of 2.2 percent estimated based on data from DDA for the same period 1961-66.

Van de Kaa pointed out that Vines' estimated "birthrate of 21.6 for the Highlands region seems too low to be plausible and it is inconsistent with proportion of children under 10 years old reported at the time. Consequently Vines' estimates are of limited assistance and cannot yield a confirmation of earlier findings"(5). Further work on estimating the rate of natural increase was carried out by the Bureau of Statistics (now NSO) based on DDA data but using different approaches.

The result produced by the Bureau of Statistics showed an estimated rate of natural increase of 2.22 percent for PNG as a whole. This seems to be much in accord with the 2.2 percent produced for the 1961-66 period and to support it strongly.

2. NATURAL INCREASE RATES SINCE 1966 CENSUS

The discussion on this will be based on data presented in Table 9.

Since the 1966 census, attempts have been made to estimate vital rates to form a basis for estimating the rate of natural increase. An analysis of 1966 census data produced by Van de Kaa for PNG as a whole showed that while fertility remained high at around 40/1000, the death rate had declined steadily to 18.1, resulting in a rate of natural increase of 2.2 percent. At regional level, the rates varied considerably. At the extreme was The Island Region, which had a CBR in excess of 43/1000, but recorded the lowest death rate, resulting in an exceptionally high rate of natural growth. The lowest growth at the regional level was the Highlands, with 1.8 percent. However, at provincial level, the variation may be even greater, as suggested by Van de Kaa in his analysis of 1966 data.

The 1971 census does not yield any data for meaningful comparison to be produced at any level. However it was observed by Rafiq (1979) and McDevitt (1979) that while fertility increases between 1966 and 1971 were observed in most provinces, fertility decline was noted in some of the provinces, such as Central, Morobe and Manus, as well as in Chimbu and Enga, where land shortage is keenly felt(6).

A detailed analysis of 1980 census data by Martin Bakker(7) provided a very useful picture of demographic transition occurring since 1966. For the country as a whole, fertility experienced some decline to about 34.2/1000, while mortality experienced a dramatic decline down to 13.2/1000 population. This change produced a natural growth rate of 2.1% for the same period, a slight drop since 1966. The urban-rural comparison shows a huge growth rate for urban areas at 2.9 percent compared to 1.97 percent for rural areas. At the regional level, the CBR for the Islands continued to remain around 40/1000 population, while CDR had dropped very low to 10.5/1000. This yielded a rate of natural increase of about 3.0%, which was the highest for any region of PNG during the period.

Using the 1980 data, projections were made for 1990. The estimated CBR was 34.7 and CDR 12.2 per 1000 population. At the regional level, some declines were expected in all regions. Notable decline in fertility was projected for the Highlands, with a rate of increase at around 1.5 percent. Despite a further drop in the mortality rate, the Islands region would continue to maintain its position as a high population growth area. Bakker (1986) provided figures for the provinces showing the highest fertility rate in PNG was recorded in the New Britain Provinces, where TFR was in excess of 6.0 children per woman.

3. OTHER CONSIDERATIONS

While the rate of natural increase has experienced some fluctuation between 2.0 percent and 2.2 percent for the country, the TFR and IMR have both shown declining trends since 1966.

According to Van de Kaa, the IMR for the period prior to 1966 may have been in the vicinity of 200/1000 live births. In 1966, the IMR recorded for the country as a whole was 135/1000, which declined by almost 50.0 percent to 72/1000 live births in 1980. A further decline is expected to 1990 reaching a level of 52/1000 live births. Similar trends can be observed in the regions. Most regions are experiencing and will continue to experience a fast decline in infant mortality rates.

The TFR for the country as a whole declined very little from 5.5 in 1966 to 5.4 in 1980. It has been projected to decline to about 5.1 in 1990; however, to what extent this assumption is valid only remains to be seen. What one can conclude on the basis of data presented so far is that, despite drops experienced over the years, fertility will continue to remain persistently high in PNG for some time.

CONCLUDING REMARKS

As a series of population growth rates are not obtainable based on reliable population estimates for the pre-war period, no conclusive trend of population growth rates can be drawn for that period. However, population estimates available for the Islands Region of Papua New Guinea indicates a very high population growth rate for the pre-war period, when population was doubling about every 15 years. This was, however, not the case for the Papua Region, which was losing its adult population on account of migration of indentured labour to the New Guinea Region. This high growth of population cannot be supported by any available data on natural increase rates of population for that period. There was a loss of some population during 1940-50 due to the Second World War and its after-effects. The population appears to have grown at an annual rate of about 2.6 percent during 1950-65 which is strongly supported by the available natural increase rate of 2.2 percent for the period. During the following 5 years, or the first intercensal period of 1966-71, the growth rate slowed down slightly to 2.5% per annum, and fell further to 2.2 percent during the 1971-80 intercensal period. The last intercensal period of 1980-90 did not record any fall, but a slight rise in the annual growth rate of the citizen population of PNG. These annual growth rates of population are supported by the natural increase rates of population of PNG over the period.

One striking feature of the growth of citizen population of Papua New Guinea is that its rural population growth rate has always been on the rise since 1966-71, from an annual rate of 1.48% to 1.92% during 1980-90, whereas the urban population growth rate has been declining from a very high rate of about 16% to a moderately high rate below 4% per annum.

Wide variation prevails between the provinces in the level and decline of annual population growth rates. The annual population growth rate during 1980-90 was the lowest at 0.32% in Gulf Province and the highest at 5.25% in NCD. They are generally higher in the Island Provinces (around 3%) and the lowest in the Highlands Provinces.

TABLE 8 - CITIZEN POPULATION GROWTH RATES BY PROVINCES, 1966 - 1990, PNG

PROVINCE	POPULATION				Annual Growth Rate (percent)			
	1966	1971	1980	1990(1)	1966-71	1971-80	1966-80	1980-90
Western	61,424	70,339	78,337	108,543	2.71	1.16	1.71	3.34
Gulf	55,077	58,273	63,843	67,934	1.13	0.99	1.04	0.64
Central	134,693	175,515	116,361	140,174	5.29	2.87	3.72	1.90
N C D	(2)	(2)	112,429	187,760	(2)	(2)	(2)	5.25
Milne Bay	99,161	108,528	127,725	157,118	1.81	1.76	1.78	2.12
Northern	57,967	65,918	77,097	96,528	2.57	1.69	2.00	2.30
Southern Highlands	183,635	192,047	235,390	302,127	0.90	2.20	1.74	2.55
Enga	289,452	131,816	164,270	238,177	3.41	2.38	2.75	3.80
Western H/lands	(3)	211,456	264,129	291,991	(3)	2.40	(3)	1.03
Chimbu	166,923	159,729	178,013	183,613	-0.88	1.17	0.45	0.32
Eastern H/lands	201,978	236,752	274,608	299,156	3.18	1.60	2.16	0.88
Morobe	204,370	240,930	305,356	360,159	3.29	2.56	2.82	1.69
Madang	149,986	168,212	209,656	269,337	2.29	2.38	2.35	2.56
East Sepik	156,406	180,149	220,872	247,584	2.83	2.20	2.42	1.17
West Sepik	99,141	93,479	113,849	139,339	-1.18	2.13	0.97	2.07
Manus	20,232	24,356	25,859	32,710	3.71	0.65	1.72	2.40
New Ireland	49,334	58,507	65,675	86,942	3.41	1.25	2.01	2.87
East New Brtn	104,887	108,238	130,730	182,728	0.63	2.04	1.55	3.43
West New Brtn	43,886	60,783	88,415	128,117	6.51	4.05	4.92	3.79
North Solomons	71,761	90,382	125,506	-	4.61	3.55	3.92	-
Papua New Guinea	2,150,317	2,435,409	2,978,057	3,520,037	2.49	2.17	2.29	2.15

(1) The 1990 census figures are preliminary and do not include North Solomons Province and the citizen populations are estimates based on the number of non-citizen population for NCD in the 1990 census.

(2) Included with Central Province.

(3) Included with Enga Province

TABLE 9 - KEY INDICES OF FERTILITY AND MORTALITY IN PNG AT DIFFERENT CENSUS PERIODS

GEOGRAPHIC AREAS	1 CRUDE BIRTH RATE (CBR)				2 CRUDE DEATH RATE (CDR)				3 NATURAL INCREASE (NI)				4 TOTAL FERTILITY RATE (TFR)				5 INFANT MORTALITY RATE (IMR)			
	1966	1971	1980	1990	1966	1971	1980	1990	1966	1971	1980	1990	1966	1971	1980	1990	1966	1971	1980	1990
PNG	40.3	-	34.2	34.7	18.1	-	13.2	12.1	22.2	-	21.0	22.6	5.5	5.6	5.4	5.1	135	134	72	52
SECTORS																				
- URBAN	-	-	36.7	-	-	-	7.7	-	-	-	29.0	-	-	5.9	-	-	100	-	-	-
- RURAL	-	-	33.9	-	-	-	14.2	-	-	-	19.7	-	-	5.5	-	-	170	-	-	-
REGIONS																				
SOUTHERN	37.6	-	37.0	34.1	19.4	-	11.5	11.0	18.2	-	25.5	23.1	6.1	6.2	5.7	5.0	-	108	58	47
HIGHLANDS	42.4	-	30.0	28.2	18.6	-	14.6	12.8	23.8	-	15.4	15.4	5.0	5.1	4.8	4.4	-	151	85	56
MOMASE	41.9	-	35.4	37.0	21.2	-	13.8	12.8	20.7	-	28.1	24.2	5.4	5.6	5.6	5.4	-	141	76	58
ISLANDS	43.1	-	40.4	37.9	13.3	-	10.5	9.6	29.8	-	29.9	28.3	6.9	6.8	6.3	5.7	-	81	52	38

NOTE:
a. CBR and CDR are expressed as per 1,000 population
b. Natural increase is the difference between CBR and CDR
c. TFR is expressed as number of children born per woman
d. IMR is expressed as deaths per 1000 live births
e. Figures for 1990 are based on projections by NSO

<u>Sources</u>:

1. Van de Kaa (1971) Demography of PNG indigenous population, 1966 census.
2. Martin Bakker (1986): Monographs on Fertility and Mortality, 1980 census.
3. Social Indicators of PNG - NSO publication (1988)

REFERENCES

1. Van de Kaa D J. The Demography of Papua and New Guinea's Indigenous Population. Australian National University, Canberra, 1971, Page 51, Table 3.8.

2. Above cited, Page 48, Table 3.6.

3. Above cited, Page 48, Table 3.11.

4. Above cited, Page 60, Table 3.12

5. Above cited, Page 68.

6. Rafiq and McDevitt in UN Country Monograph PNG, 1982, Page 63.

7. Bakker M. Monographs on Fertility and Mortality, 1980 census. 1986.

POPULATION TRENDS IN FIJI

H N SHANKAR[1]

TOTAL POPULATION AND ETHNIC DISTRIBUTION

1.1 The population of Fiji consists of two major ethnic groups, the indigenous Melanesian population referred to as Fijians, and the population who are of Indian origin referred to as Indians. According to the 1986 population census, these two ethnic groups comprised 95 percent of the total population of Fiji. Other ethnic groups such as Chinese (0.7%); Europeans (0.6%); Part-Europeans (1.5%); Rotumans (1.2%); Other Pacific Islands (1.2%) and All Others (0.1%) comprised the remaining 5 percent of Fiji's population. Other than the composition of Fijian and Indian populations, the composition of other ethnic groups have not changed significantly over the last decade.

1.2 The latest census conducted in Fiji was on the 31 August 1986 and most of the demographic changes which will be mentioned in this paper will therefore refer to the 1986 Population Census in Fiji. Comparisons with the previous census will also be given. According to the 1986 Population Census, the population of Fiji shows an annual average growth of 1.9 percent. For the period 1977 to 1986, annual growth rates ranged from 1.6 percent to 2.1 percent. The tables below show the estimated mid-year population and annual growth rates and the composition of the Fijian and Indian populations in the period 1977-1986.

YEAR	ESTIMATED MID-YEAR POPULATION (000)	ESTIMATED ANNUAL GROWTH RATE (%)
1977	596	1.9
1978	607	1.8
1979	621	2.0
1980	634	2.1
1981	646	1.9
1982	658	1.8
1983	672	2.1
1984	686	2.1
1985	697	1.6
1986(C)	715	1.9

(C) Census

[1] Government Statistician, Bureau of Statistics, Suva, Fiji.

	FIJIAN			INDIAN		
YEAR	POPULATION (000)	% OF TOTAL	GROWTH RATE	POPULATION (000)	% OF TOTAL	GROWTH RATE
1977	267	44	2.3	301	50	2.0
1978	272	44	1.9	307	50	2.0
1979	279	45	2.5	314	50	2.3
1980	284	44	1.8	321	50	2.2
1981	290	44	2.1	326	50	1.5
1982	297	45	2.4	333	50	2.1
1983	304	45	2.3	339	50	1.8
1984	312	45	2.6	345	50	1.8
1985	319	45	2.2	349	50	1.2
1986(C)	329	46	2.4	349	49	1.7

(C) Census

1.3 The lower growth rates of the Indian component can be attributed to two factors:

(i) The birth rate of the Indian component has declined faster

(ii) The out-migration of the Indian component is higher than the Fijian component

1.4 The population of each ethnic origin at the last two censuses is given below:

	1976 CENSUS		1986 CENSUS	
ETHNIC GROUP	POPULATION	% OF TOTAL	POPULATION	% OF TOTAL
Chinese & Part-Chinese	4,652	0.8	4,784	0.7
Europeans	4,929	0.8	4,196	0.6
Fijians	259,932	44.2	329,305	46.0
Indians	292,896	49.8	348,704	48.7
Part-Europeans	10,276	1.8	10,297	1.5
Rotumans	7,291	1.2	8,652	1.2
Other Pacific Islanders	6,822	1.2	8,627	1.2
All Others	1,270	0.2	810	0.1
TOTAL	588,068	100.0	715,375	100.0

1.5 As a result of declining fertility rates especially amongst the Indian population over the past two decades, and increasing out-migration, a significant shift has occurred in the composition of Fiji's population. At the time of the 1966 Census of Population, Indians comprised 51 percent of the population. However, this share has steadily dropped to 50 percent at the time of the 1976 census and to 49 percent as at the 1986 census. (See Table below).

CENSUS	CHINESE		EUROPEAN		FIJIAN		INDIAN		PART EUROPEAN		ALL OTHERS		TOTAL (a)	ESTIMATED EQUIV. ANNUAL GROWTH RATE
	(000)	(%)	(000)	(%)	(000)	(%)	(000)	(%)	(000)	(%)	(000)	(%)	(000)	(%)
4.4.1881	-	-	3	2	115	90	1	1	1	1	8	6	127	
5.4.1891	-	-	2	2	106	88	7	6	1	1	5	4	121	-0.5
31.3.1901	-	-	2	2	94	78	17	14	2	2	5	4	120	-0.1
2.4.1911	-	-	4	3	87	62	40	29	2	1	7	5	140	+1.5
24.4.1921	1	1	4	2	84	54	61	39	3	2	4	3	157	+1.2
26.4.1936	2	1	4	2	98	50	85	43	5	2	4	2	198	+1.6
2.10.1946	3	1	5	2	118	45	120	46	6	2	8	3	260	+2.7
26.9.1956	4	1	6	2	148	43	169	49	8	2	10	3	345	+2.9
12.9.1966	5	1	7	2	202	42	241	51	10	2	12	3	477	+3.3
13.9.1976	5	1	5	1	260	44	293	50	10	2	15	3	588	+2.1
31.8.1986	5	1	4	1	329	46	349	49	10	1	18	2	715	+2.0

RECENT ESTIMATES OF FIJI'S POPULATION

2.1 The military coups in 1987 saw increased out-migration especially of the Indian population. Two significant changes have been evident as a result of increased out-migration of the Indian population and declining fertility rates. One is the reduction in the overall percent to approximately 1.0 percent. Two, that the Fijian component had overtaken the Indian population 1988.

Estimates for the years 1987 to 1990 are as follows:

ETHNIC GROUP	1987 NO.	1987 %	1988 NO.	1988 %	1989 NO.	1989 %	1990 NO.	1990 %
Fijians	338,882	47.3	344,948	47.9	352,384	48.5	360,102	48.9
Indians	341,787	47.8	340,073	47.3	338,223	46.6	339,784	46.2
Others	34,863	4.9	34,650	4.8	35,638	4.9	36,099	4.9
TOTAL	715,532	100.0	719,671	100.0	726,245	100.0	735,985	100.0

2.2 The Fijians as at the end of 1990 now comprise 48.9 percent of the population; the Indians comprise 46.2 percent of the population and All Other Races comprise the remaining 4.9 percent of the population.

2.3 The number of persons who migrated in the period 1987-1990 were as follows:

	1987	1988	1989	1990
Fijians	351	263	249	307
Indians	4,294	4,808	4,981	5,020
Others	473	425	280	323
TOTAL	5,118	5,496	5,510	5,650

2.4 As will be noted the number of persons who migrated in the period 1983-86 averaged 2,598. In the period 1987-90 the annual average increased to 5,444 which is an increase of 109 percent.

2.5 The number of persons who migrated in the four years prior to 1987 were as follows:

	1983	1984	1985	1986
Fijians	196	179	217	178
Indians	2,152	1,849	2,307	2,362
Others	232	210	252	259
TOTAL	2,580	2,238	2,776	2,799

2.6 It is also to be noted that a significant proportion (26%) of those migrating are in the professional and management category.

FERTILITY AND AGE AT MARRIAGE

3.1 The attitude towards family planning differs between the Fijians and the Indians. Consequently, there has been a marked difference in the fertility history of these two ethnic groups. The Indians on the one hand appear to have taken to smaller size families, whilst the Fijians on the other hand do not appear to have taken to the concept of reduced family sizes. This may be partly explained by the traditional living environment. The major proportion of Fijians still live in rural village-type localities where a larger family does not appear to pose any serious economic problem (subsistence being the major form of livelihood). On the contrary, the Indians mostly live in the urban centres and thus have been exposed to the problems of having large families.

3.2 The total fertility rate (TFR) measures the average number of children borne alive to a woman (or group of women) during the reproductive life span. From rates available since 1977, the fertility for Fijian woman has remained static at around 3.5, while for the Indian woman, it declined from 3.2 in 1981 to 2.8 in 1985. It should however, be noted that these rates have been compiled from the Registrar General's record and may therefore be affected by under-registration. However, the TFR calculated from 1986 Census data by various methodologies also found a faster decline in Indian fertility than the Fijian. Through own children method a rate of 5.6 children for Fijians in 1966 declined to 4.1 in 1986 whereas the Indian decline was from 5.4 to 2.8. The TFR obtained directly from information on live births, gathered in the 1986 Census, gave an estimated 3.9 for Fijians and 2.6 for Indians. For the total population, the TFR from the 1986 Census data was 3.2 children.

<u>TOTAL FERTILITY RATES</u>

YEAR	FIJIANS	INDIANS	TOTAL POPULATION
1977	3.3	3.1	3.2
1978	3.3	3.3	3.3
1979	3.4	3.4	3.4
1980	3.3	3.3	3.4
1981	3.4	3.2	3.3
1982	3.4	3.4	3.5
1983	3.6	3.1	3.3
1984	3.5	2.9	3.2
1985	3.4	2.8	3.1
1986(C)	3.9	2.6	3.2

(C) Census

3.3 Over the period 1970 to 1986 age specific fertility rates (ASFRs) for the Indian population of Fiji have shown declines in all age groups except the 15-19 group. The most significant declines have occurred in the 25 to 34 age group. In the same period ASFR's for Fijians have steadily increased in the 15-19 age group to become the same as the Indian rate, while the 20-24 age group is now above the Indian rate, whereas in 1970 it was below. Significant increases have occurred in age groups 25-29 and 30-34 for the indigenous Fijian population.

AGE SPECIFIC FERTILITY RATES (ASFR)

AGE GROUP	FIJIANS 1970(a)	1976(a)	1985(a)	1986(C)	INDIANS 1970(a)	1976(a)	1985(a)	1986(C)
15-19	39	39	56	62	60	58	61	62
20-24	231	198	208	211	242	255	235	207
25-29	207	200	185	227	215	178	163	162
30-34	142	125	130	171	116	95	70	80
35-39	107	85	78	106	72	46	27	80
40-44	37	31	30	40	25	12	5	10
15-44	132	119	122		134	118	107	

(a) Vital Statistics

(C) 1986 Census

MARRIAGE AGE

4.1 Marriage patterns such as ages of men and women on first marriage, frequency of divorces, and age at widowhood are important determinants of fertility. For demographic purposes, persons living as husband and wife are regarded as married even if they are not legally married.

4.2 The median age at marriage, derived from data on registered marriages, shows very little change for both major ethnic groups during the period 1977-1983. Both Fijian males and females continue to be just over 3 years older at marriage than their Indian counterparts.

MEDIAN AGE AT MARRIAGE

	FIJIANS		INDIANS		ALL COMPONENTS	
YEAR	MALE	FEMALE	MALE	FEMALE	MALE	FEMALE
1977	26.5	23.3	23.1	19.7	24.1	21.4
1978	26.5	23.3	23.2	19.8	24.3	21.4
1979	26.3	23.2	23.1	19.8	24.1	21.4
1980	26.2	23.2	23.2	19.9	24.2	21.5
1981	26.4	23.2	23.2	19.9	24.2	21.5
1982	26.5	23.2	23.3	20.0	24.4	21.6
1983	26.2	23.3	23.2	19.9	24.3	21.5
1984	26.7	23.4	23.5	20.4	24.6	22.0
1985	27.0	23.5	23.6	20.4	24.9	22.0

4.3 The singulate mean age at marriage (SMAM) is a measure of the average age at marriage derived through Census estimates of proportion of males and females who are single in successive age groups. At the time of the Census, all couples who were living together whether legally married or not were considered to be married. As shown below, the Fijian SMAM during the period 1956-1986 Census did not change much, but there is a definite upward trend for Indians indicating increasing age at marriage.

SINGULATE MEAN AGE AT MARRIAGE

	FIJIAN		INDIAN		TOTAL	
CENSUS	MALE	FEMALE	MALE	FEMALE	MALE	FEMALE
1956	25.7	22.3	21.6	18.1	23.8	20.2
1966	26.1	22.4	23.4	20.3	24.6	21.1
1976	26.8	22.1	23.5	21.1	24.5	21.6
1986	26.6	23.4	24.3	21.6	25.3	22.5

FAMILY PLANNING

5.1 Family planning services are available at all government health institutions and private health facilities throughout the country. In addition, contraceptives are subsidised by the government, and are also available at retail chemists and pharmacies.

5.2 Family planning is well integrated into the general health services delivery system. The health nurses from the mother/child health care unit when visiting their nursing districts educate mothers and would be mothers about family planning and the methods available.

5.3 Both the Fiji Fertility Survey (FFS) which was conducted in 1974 and The Knowledge Attitude and Practice (KAP) survey found a high proportion of women who had some knowledge about family planning methods, but a smaller proportion had in fact used a method. The survey found that the proportion of Indian women practicing some form of family planning was 74%, while the corresponding proportion for Fijian women practicing some form of family planning was 55%.

5.4 The Ministry of Health figures also show a difference between Fijian and Indian contraceptive usage. Of the total acceptors in December 1984, Indians made up 68.9%, while Fijians made up only 28.1%. As a proportion of women aged 15-44 years, 33.4% of the Indian women were using one of the methods, while for Fijians, the proportion was 16.3%. The table below shows the acceptor and protection rate for the two major ethnic groups.

FAMILY PLANNING IN FIJI 1978-1984

	FIJIAN			INDIAN		
YEAR	NUMBER	% OF TOTAL ACCEPTORS	% OF WOMEN 15-44 YEARS	NUMBER	% OF TOTAL ACCEPTORS	% OF WOMEN 15-44 YEARS
1978	10,260	28.6	16.1	24,028	66.9	33.8
1979	10,288	28.5	16.1	24,454	67.7	33.9
1980	10,460	28.1	16.7	25,269	68.0	33.9
1981	9,834	27.0	14.8	25,120	69.1	30.9
1982	11,011	27.1	16.0	28,489	70.0	34.3
1983	12,126	29.4	17.3	27,641	67.1	32.7
1984	11,728	28.1	16.3	28,729	68.9	33.4

AGE DISTRIBUTION

6.1 Fiji has a relatively young population, with 38.2 percent of the population below the age of 15 years and 48.5 percent below the age of 28 years at the 1986 Census, compared to 41.1 percent and 53.5 percent at the 1976 Census. These declines can in part be attributed to the declining birth rate over the ten years.

6.2 The median age is often used to describe whether the population is young or old, i.e. ageing. Normally a population is regarded as young if the median age is below 20; it is regarded as intermediate if the median age lies between 20-30 years. From the table below it could be said that Fiji is now experiencing the 'early intermediate' age phase of population maturity.

MEDIAN AGE OF MALES AND FEMALES

	1966		1976		1986	
	MALE	FEMALE	MALE	FEMALE	MALE	FEMALE
Total	16.6	16.5	17.6	17.7	20.5	20.9
Fijian	17.4	18.1	18.5	19.0	20.0	20.5
Indian	15.5	15.0	18.3	18.3	20.8	21.1
European	32.3	29.9	31.8	29.7	33.2	30.9

DEPENDENT POPULATION

7.1 A young population tends to give a high dependency ratio. The dependency ratio represents the ratio of the combined child population and aged population to the population in all the ages between the child and aged groupings. It is the ratio of the number of persons under 15 and over 60 years of age to the population in the 15-59 age group. It is a very crude measure of economic dependency since some persons in dependent age ranges could be producers while in the production age range, some people will be economically dependent, such as housewives.

DEPENDENCY RATIOS FOR 1976 AND 1986

	POPULATION 0-14 YEARS	POPULATION 60+ YEARS	POPULATION 15-59 YEARS	DEPENDENCY RATIO (%)
1976	241,854	24,482	321,732	82.8
1986	273,463	33,032	408,880	75.0

LIFE EXPECTANCY

8.1 Life Tables are in essence a form of combining mortality rates of a population at each age into a consistent statistical model. They are useful not only to measure the age specific level of mortality of a population but also to measure the age specific level of survival of the given population. When a series of life expectancies tables are compared over time, a measure of the changing general health of the population can be obtained. Care must, however, be taken in making such comparisons where the methods of compiling successive tables have changed. In the case of Fiji's Life Expectancy Tables, the 1976 and 1986 tables were compiled using the 'Brass' technique (indirect method) whereas the 1956 and 1966 tables used the direct method.

LIFE EXPECTANCY

	1956 (DM)	1966 (DM)	1976 (BT)	1986 (BT)
Fijian				
Male	62	67	60.7	63.1
Female	65	72	63.9	65.3
Indian				
Male	64	65	59.5	59.6
Female	62	67	62.4	65.1

(DM) Direct Method
(BT) Brass Technique (indirect method)

POPULATION DISTRIBUTION

9.1 The following two tables provide information on the distribution of Fiji's population by province and the distribution of urban and rural population. Some provinces (indicated with an asterik) comprise a group of small islands. These provinces are characterised by having a predominantly Fijian population.

POPULATION DISTRIBUTION BY PROVINCE

	1976			1986		
PROVINCE	TOTAL POPUL-ATION	FIJIAN AS % OF TOTAL	INDIAN AS % OF TOTAL	TOTAL POPUL-ATION	FIJIAN AS % OF TOTAL	INDIAN AS % OF TOTAL
FIJI	588,068	44.2	49.8	715,375	46.0	48.7
Ba	167,095	27.1	69.7	197,633	28.0	69.3
Bua	11,457	65.5	31.4	13,986	69.7	25.9
Cakaudrove	34,251	69.3	16.3	40,433	71.7	15.3
Kadavu*	8,699	98.1	0.1	9,805	98.2	0.5
Lau*	14,452	98.0	1.2	14,203	97.8	1.5
Lomaiviti*	13,568	89.1	4.7	16,066	90.0	4.0
Macuata	57,414	23.3	74.7	74,735	25.2	73.2
Nadroga/ Navosa	45,929	43.6	55.0	54,431	46.5	52.2
Naitasiri	65,111	47.8	47.4	100,227	49.6	44.8
Namosi	3,292	93.3	5.3	4,836	91.8	6.5
Ra	25,523	47.9	50.9	31,285	52.0	47.1
Rewa	87,257	45.7	38.1	97,442	49.1	37.3
Serua	11,263	49.3	45.3	13,356	51.0	43.2
Tailevu	39,952	58.4	39.5	44,249	62.9	35.6
Rotuma*	2,805	1.9	0.2	2,688	2.9	0.8

* Province made up of group of islands

MIGRATION

10.1 In Fiji, internal migration has mostly been from the outer islands and the rural villages and settlements to the urban centres. To avoid concentration in the urban areas, the government has adopted a policy of de-centralising industrial development, and sends government trained teachers to the rural areas to remove the perception that good teachers are available only in the urban areas. When job opportunites are scarce or unavailable in the urban areas, the tendency is to move back to the village or settlement to work on subsistence farms.

10.2 The capital, Suva, which has been the centre of attraction for migrants, has been experiencing a declining growth rate. The annual growth rate of 3.9 percent during the 1966-76 intercensal period declined to 1.8 percent during the 1976-86 period. Similarly, the next largest city, Lautoka, which grew at an annual rate of 3.1 percent during the 1966-76 period, declined to 3.0 percent during the 1976-86 period.

10.3 At the 1986 Census 277,025 or 38.7 percent of the total population were living in urban areas as compared to 218,495 persons or 37.2 percent in 1976. In the 1966 Census, 33.4 percent of the population were living in urban areas. While there was a 1.1% annual increase in this proportion between 1966-1976, the corresponding increase in 1976-1986 was only 0.4 percent.

URBAN RURAL DISTRIBUTION OF POPULATION

	URBAN		RURAL		TOTAL	
ETHNIC ORIGIN	1976	1986	1976	1986	1976	1986
Fijian						
Number	79,314	107,780	180,618	221,525	259,932	329,305
Percent	30.5	32.7	69.5	67.3	100.0	100.0
Indian						
Number	115,632	144,533	177,264	204,171	292,896	348,704
Percent	39.5	41.4	60.5	58.6	100.0	100.0
Others						
Number	23,549	24,712	11,691	12,654	35,240	37,366
Percent	66.8	66.1	33.2	33.9	100.0	100.0
Total						
Number	218,495	277,025	369,573	438,350	588,068	715,375
Percent	37.2	38.7	62.8	61.3	100.0	100.0

POPULATION AND HEALTH SERVICES IN SOLOMON ISLANDS

CHERRY K GALO [1]

1.0 BACKGROUND INFORMATION

1.1 GEOGRAPHY

Solomon Islands, an independent developing nation in the South Pacific, lies between longitude 156E to 170E and from latitude 5S to 12S, covering a land area of 27,750 sq km. There are six main islands and hundreds of little ones.

The country is divided into seven (7) provinces namely:- Western, Malaita, Guadalcanal, Isabel, Central Islands, Makira/Ulawa and Temotu. The Honiara Municipal Authority is regarded as a province.

1.2 DEMOGRAPHY (Annex 1)

The Solomon Islands is predominantly a melanesian country (94%) with pockets of other ethnic groups such as polynesians (3.8%), micronesians (1.4%) and others (0.8%).

According to the 1986 National Census Report, the total population of the country was 285, 176 with 47% of the population under the age of 14 years, and 5% of the population above the age of 60 years, resulting in a very high dependency ratio of 109 dependents for every 100 person aged 15-59.

Compared to other countries of the region, Solomon Islands has one of the highest growth rates of 3.5% with a Total Fertility Rate (TFR) of 6.1 (1986) which is a drop from 7.3 in 1970.

Infant mortality rate is 40 per thousand live births. The life expectancy is 59 years for males and 61 years for females.

If the country continues to grow at 3.5%, the population is expected to double in 20 years.

1 Executive Director, Solomon Islands Planned Parenthood Association

2.0 HEALTH SERVICES AND MANPOWER

2.1 HEALTH SERVICES

Most of the health care services are provided by the Central Government. Much of the top level operative managements of health at central level has been decentralized to the Provincial Governments. The Central Government remains the national policy making body and is responsible for manpower development programmes. All international donor agencies deal directly with the Central Government and not with the Provincial Authorities.

The health referral system is as follows:-

1. National Hospital	: At the national level : (Specialists)	1
2. Provincial Hospitals	: At the Provincial level: (2 church hospitals) (Doctors and nurses)	7
3. Health Centres	: At the area council level: (Senior Nursing Officers and Registered nurses.)	6
4. Clinics	: At the Ward level (RNs and Nurse Aides)	: 138
5. Aid Posts	: At the Ward level (Nurse Aides)	: 69
6. Village Health	: At Village level (Village Health Workers)	: 86

Central Hospital is the national hospital and provides specialized services in surgery, internal medicine, anaesthetics, paediatrics and obstetrics/gynaecology. Divisions provide services in areas of pharmacy, dentistry, laboratory, radiography, and rehabilitation. An eye unit has also been established in the last few years. The Central Hospital also serves as a provincial hospital for Central, Guadalcanal and Honiara Municipal Authority, serving a population of about 110,000.

Provincial hospitals provide general diagnostic and treatment services. All government hospitals are also the headquarters for administration and supervision of provincial health services.

The area health centres are the intermediary link between the rural health clinics and the provincial hospitals. They generally serve a population of approximately 15,000.

Health clinics form the major part of the health facilities and each serve a population of approximately 1,500 - 2,000.

The nurse aide posts generally serve areas of poor access and each cover a population of about 500. The village health workers posts are based in the villages and provide simple care and refer to higher levels. They provide health education to the communities.

2.2 HEALTH MANPOWER (1989)

STAFF	MHMS, MTRI	CENTRAL HOSP	PROVINCIAL HOSP	OUTREACH	TOTAL
Doctors	4	21	17	-	42
Dental	-	11	11	-	22
Nursing	6	98	113	137	354
Admin/Acct	20	-	-	-	20
Pharmacy	-	17	6	-	23
Laboratory	-	19	8	-	27
Physio	-	4	1	-	5
Environ.Health	5	-	28	-	33
Radiography	-	11	4	1	15
Anti Malaria	36	-	-	98	134
Women & Dev.	5	-	3	-	8
Social Dev.	5	-	-	2	7
Suppt Service	-	18	2	-	20
Health Education	4	-	7(+14)	11	22(36)
TOTAL:	**85**	**199**	**200**	**237**	**732**

There is a great shortage of manpower experienced in the country. The Ministry of Health and Medical Services (MHMS) has some short-term, medium term and long-term plans to improve the current situation.

<u>THE BASIC HEALTH ORGANIZATIONAL STRUCTURE</u> (ANNEX 11)

The health services fall into two main areas:

a) Health Improvement covering promotive, preventive, and rehabilitative services;

b) Health Care covering maintenance and development of the health facilities system and staff.

The present organization allocates responsibilities to two under secretaries who advise the Permanent Secretary and Minister on all technical and professional aspects of policies and programmes. They are in turn guided by the heads of divisions and medical officers of all provinces. The Director of Medical Training and Research Institute (MTRI) advises on highly technical and professional matters.

3.0 MAIN CAUSES OF MORBIDITY AND MORTALITY AMONG WOMEN AND CHILDREN:

3.1 MORBIDITY IN CHILDREN:

- Malaria
- Diarrhoea
- Acute respiratory infections
- Conjunctivitis
- Tuberculosis

3.2 MORTALITY IN CHILDREN:

- Infectious/parasitic diseases
- Respiratory system diseases - majority are pneumonia

3.3 MORBIDITY IN MOTHERS:-

- Malaria
- Parasitic diseases
- Pregnancy related problems
- Tuberculosis
- Other chronic chest infections

3.4 MORTALITY IN MOTHERS:-

- Infectious/parasitic diseases
- Pregnancy related problems

Source: Medical Statistics, MHMS, 1988.

Infectious diseases still remain the main causes of morbidity and mortality in mothers and children in the Solomon Islands. Malaria is the biggest public health problem in the country.

4.0 POPULATION GROWTH RELATED PROBLEMS

The population issue and its related problems have been the debate of today in any of the third world nations or so-called developing countries. Solomon Islands is no exception as there have been various problems identified in relation to population growth.

Between 1981 to 1987 it was recorded that the Gross Domestic Product of today in any of the third world nations or so-called developing countries. Solomon Islands is no exception as there have been various problems identified in relation to population growth.

Rapid population growth also has certain impacts on social delivery services such as health services, education and agriculture as well as the labour market.

4.1 HEALTH SERVICES

The main health problems are still infectious diseases, with malaria being the priority disease. Health facilities and trained human-power are virtually static. The increase in both these areas cannot match the fast population growth rate.

Each health facility must therefore serve an ever increasing number of patients as the demand on services increases. With no proportionate increase in health facilities nor trained human-power, the services will deteriorate.

4.2 EDUCATION

An additional attainment assessment by UNESCO in 1987 showed the following estimated percentages above the age of 25 years.

-	Non-formal schooling	55.1%
-	Primary education only	40.0%
-	Secondary education	3.3%
-	Tertiary education	1.6%

In the 1986 census there was a total number of 84,590 primary school age children between the ages of 5 and 14. Unfortunately only 39,563 (47%) were enrolled in primary schools. By the time the 1986 enrollment pass through to secondary school in 1992, there will be only 6,615 (16.7%) places available.

50% of the teachers were not fully trained. The government cannot afford to build more schools, or maintain existing ones.

The 1986 census showed that 53% of primary school age children were not enrolled in schools, and indicated that within the next 20 years 65-70% of all primary school age children will have no primary education. This will further increase the illiteracy rate. If the total fertility rate decreases, a greater proportion of children will have a better chance of attaining some education.

4.3 AGRICULTURE

There has been evidence of population pressure with regard to land and land related issues. Due to population growth the number of customary land disputes have increased, pressures for land for gardening and building has increasingly become a national concern.

As family sizes increase there are more people to feed. In many already densely populated areas, adequate fertile land is scarce and food production per head has decreased, leading to increased malnutrition and ill-health.

With the traditional shifting cultivation, farming gardens are now further into the rainforest. This has resulted in ecological damage such as soil erosion, the destruction of endemic plants and natural habitats. The short fallow period has resulted in increasing areas of infertile land.

4.4 LABOUR FORCE

Together with the high population growth rate and a high total fertility rate there is a fast increase in the total potential labour force. Only a small percentage of this group will obtain employment, and the vast majority will have to engage in other informal economic activities and subsistence food production. According to the 1986 census only 26% of the economically active population are involved in the cash economy.

The total labour force for the next 14 years has already been born and each year an average of 9,643 persons will enter the economically active age bracket. It is extremely unlikely that employment opportunities in all sectors including self-employment will match this average annual increase in the potential labour force.

Unemployment is increasing very dramatically with its related problems both within the rural and urban areas.

The extremely high urban growth rate is resulting in excessive unemployment, alcohol abuse, unlawfulness and discontent.

5.0 POPULATION POLICY FORMULATION

The population issue was discussed directly and indirectly in the Solomons in the early 1980s. Well before 1985 there were attempts within the Ministry of Health to formulate a population policy.

In 1985 a draft of a population policy was formulated by Dr Nathan Kere within the Ministry of Health after a survey throughout the provinces. This draft was presented to the Cabinet in the same year under the leadership of the present Prime Minister, Hon. Solomon Mamaloni, but was not adopted.

Despite the rejection of these initial attempts by the Ministry of Health, another high level workshop was organised in early 1987, jointly by the Ministry of Health and Solomon Islands Planned Parenthood Association. This workshop was attended by high level decision makers such as Permanent Secretaries, Church Leaders, Heads of Non-Government Organizations and International Organizations.

During this workshop a resolution was passed for the formation of a spearhead committee to start work on a detailed policy and programme of action to implement family spacing and welfare services. Having drafted the policy, a questionnaire was finally created for a country-wide survey, and in early 1988 it was carried out. This was targetted at finding people's attitudes towards population issues.

The result of the survey clearly indicated that 75-80% of the repondents recognised population related problems such as customary land disputes, financial difficulties related to education, scarcity of marine resources and shortages of fertile land for gardening purposes. In other words the survey showed that there is a real population problem in the Solomon Islands which needs to be addressed promptly with great concern.

In mid 1988, the first draft of the present population policy was again presented to the same high level decision makers for screening purposes. The screening committee then adopted the draft population policy and recommended it to be tabled in the Cabinet. In November 1988 the first Solomon Islands population policy was adopted in parliament.

5.1 THE POPULATION POLICY OBJECTIVES

a) To foster social and economic development through better interpretation, planning and management of population trends to achieve greater harmony between population and resources.

b) To promote the health of the total population and particularly "Maternal and Child Health".

c) To reduce and maintain the population growth rate to a level that is within the government's capability to support, and at the same time improve the quality of life of all Solomon Islanders through appropriate and relevant awareness education on population issues and family planning.

d) To achieve and maintain a more equitable distribution of the population between rural and urban areas.

5.2 STRATEGIES FOR IMPLEMENTATION

The strategies for a successful implementation of this policy must address the following issues:-

a) The implementation of this policy must go in stages

as follows:-

1. Phase 1

*Educational Awareness Campaign on Population issues	1988 - 1990 intensively, continuing

2. Phase ii - Short Term

   *Increasing Family Planning 1989 - 1990

   Phase ii - Mid-Term

   *Integration of Population issues in all areas of the National Development Plan 1989 - 1995

3. Phase iii

   * Phase ii activities, plus 1995 - 1998

4. Phase iv

   * Review and Forward Planning 1996 - 2000

b) This implementation programme must be completed within a specific TIME FRAME to ensure that the objectives are achieved and the success of the various phases of implementation are properly monitored and evaluated to enable further appropriate action. It is envisaged that within 10 years the total fertility rate will drop to about 4 then to 3 in another decade.

c) Definite funding sources must be identified both internally and outside the country to allow a continuous and full-time involvement with the various phases of the implementation programme.

d) It is absolutely essential that a multi-sectoral approach is adopted in the implementation of this policy, combining efforts from within all government services and non-government organisations, supplemented by relevant and appropriate technical and financial support from certain external funding and agencies with vested interests in population issues and family planning. These funding agencies include UNFPA, SPAFH, IPPF, WHO, AIDAB, SCFA and ILO.

e) It is imperative that the census results in a simplified form be published and widely distributed to the general population.

5.3 IMPLEMENTING PHASES

The population issue has been a major concern to the Ministry of Health since the 1986 census, and there have been a Training of Trainers Workshop and awareness programmes organised by the Health Education Division of the Ministry well before the draft population policy was adopted.

5.3.1 TRAINING OF TRAINERS

The initial Training of Trainers Workshop for family planning workers was scheduled for one week. The programme was jointly conducted by the Health Education Division (MHMS) and Solomon Islands Planned Parenthood Association (SIPPA) and took place from 21st - 25th March 1988. The follow-up Family Planning Training of Trainers Course was conducted for 9 months in 1989 where 19 participants were trained; sixteen local participants, two participants from Fiji and one from Vanuatu. This was based on a training module developed to suit the local situation. The workshops were funded by the South Pacific Alliance for Family Health.

The Training of Trainers Workershops are expected to achieve the following objectives:

a) To teach knowledge and application of new family planning technologies.

b) To enable trainers to relate population issues to fertility control measures.

c) To develop skills in delivering, safe and effective methods for couples desiring to space their children and/or limit family size.

d) To develop skills in communication to effectively deliver population and family planning messages.

The local participants consisted of nurses from the provinces, Honiara, church organizations, School of Nursing, Solomon Islands Planned Parenthood Association and Solomon Islands Plantations Limited. These family planning nurses are actively involved in Population Education and Awareness Campaigns throughout the country, as well as training health workers and supervision Family Planning Programmes in their respective areas of work. The Family Planning Curriculum in the School of Nursing has been strengthened and improved. Each year the MCH/FP Unit of the Ministry of Health and Medical Services conducts a refresher training course for the Family Planning Trainers and also provides assistance/support and supervision.

5.3.2 PROVINCIAL WORKSHOPS

There have been several Population Education Awareness Workshops held in the eight provinces, including Honiara, since 1988. The workshops conducted in 1988 and 1989 were held at provincial level. As from 1990, the workshops are now being conducted at the Area Council level.

Malaita Province		May 16th-20th, 1988
Isabel Province		August 1st-5th, 1988
Central Province		November 7th-11th, 1988
Temotu Province		March 13th-17th, 1989
Makira Ulawa Province		April 3rd-7th, 1989
Guadalcanal Province		July 17th-21st, 1989
Western Province		September 4th-8th, 1989
Honiara Town Council		October 23rd-27th, 1989
Western Province	x2	Area Council Level,1990
Isabel Province	x2	Area Council Level,1990
Malaita Province	x1	" " " ,1990
Central Is. Province	x1	" " " ,1990
Makira Ulawa "	x1	" " " ,1990

1 TO JUNE, 1991

Temotu Province	x1	Area Council Level
Guadalcanal Province	x1	" " "
Central Is. Province	x1	" " "

5.3.3 DRAMATIZED POPULATION EDUCATION PROGRAMMES

The Solomon Islands Development Trust (SIDT) has theatre action groups who dramatize population problems to people in the rural areas. This is an effective means of educating the rural population on this important issue. They also provide educational materials on population issues and distribute this widely throughout the country in the form of comic, strips, magazines (bi-monthly) and calendars.

5.3.4 RADIO PROGRAM

Since 1987 the Planned Parenthood Association of Solomon Islands has been organising radio programmes on population awareness and family planned issues. These programmes are relayed twice a week through the Solomon Islands Broadcasting Corporation.

5.3.5 PRIMARY SCHOOL TEACHERS - AWARENESS WORKSHOPS

Apart from the eight provincial workshops, two other workshops were conducted in 1989 for all primary school teachers in Guadalcanal Province. There is also a population education workshop planned for primary school teachers in 1991, to be funded by UNFPA.

5.3.6 COMMUNITY BASED DISTRIBUTION

Solomon Islands Planned Parenthood Association as promoter of population education awareness has so far trained 100 Community-Based Distributors. These Community-Based Distributors would assist in bringing family planning down to the grass-roots. The Maternal and Child Health/Family Planning Unit of the Ministry of Health and Medical Services is at present planning to investigate the possibility of training women's group leaders to be community distributors of family planning materials as well as motivating and counselling possible family planning clients.

5.3.7 MATERNAL AND CHILD HEALTH/FAMILY PLANNING UNIT

In order to effectively implement the objectives of the population policy, a Maternal and Child Health/Family Planning Unit of the Ministry of Health and Medical Services was established in 1989 and a Senior Population Planner was appointed at the beginning of 1990.

5.3.8 PRIMARY AND SECONDARY CURRICULUM

Population education has been integrated into the primary and secondary schools curricula. Standards 1-6, under Community Studies; Forms 1-4, under Social Studies; Forms 4 and 5 under Science and Home Economics.

6.0 CONSTRAINTS

The major constraints presently affecting the development of population programmes in Solomon Islands are;

a) Lack of adequate finance to develop, administer, implement, monitor and evaluate appropriate programmes.

b) Lack of trained manpower to run the programmes throughout the country especially in the rural areas.

c) Certain traditional socio-cultural beliefs that relate large families to good investment for old age and also financial gains from bride-prices, etc.

d) Lack of awareness by some religious groups of the implications of a rapid population growth rate and its adverse consequences.

f) High illiteracy in the country leading to a low level of educational attainment resulting in:

- Lack of understanding of population issues.
- Lack of awareness of possible problems with large families.

g) The geography of Solomon Islands resulting in:

- A wide diversity of traditions, cultures, customs, and beliefs.
- Increasing problems with transportation and communication.
- Higher rate of possible failure to adequately

implement appropriate planned programmes.

7.0 FUTURE ACTIVITIES AND PROGRAMMES

a) The population awareness programmes particularly at village level will be given priority, and access to family planning services will be strengthened.

b) Women's groups will be trained counsel and motivate clients in order to increase the numbers of users of family planning.

c) The Family, Planning Outreach Programme presently based only in rural health centres and clinics will plan and implement a formal programme that will reach out to the village level. The programme will emphasize the health aspects of family planning, of breast feeding, and responsible parenthood. The programme will be jointly supported and promoted by the Maternal and Child Health Unit and Solomon Islands Planned Parenthood Association, while the supervisory functions will be the responsibility of Provincial Directors of Health Services and Senior Nursing Officers. Maternal and Child Health/Family Planning Unit will also provide support and supervision as required.

d) Work is currently being undertaken by Solomon Islands College of Higher Education to integrate population issues in the teaching trarining programme.

e) On-going methods of family planning including the provision of contraceptive pills, depo-provera injections, loops and condoms will continue to be provided through the health system. Co-operation between Solomon Islands Planned Parenthood Association and "O" Clinic on all family planning related activities would be of paramount importance. he Maternal and Child Health/Family Planning Unit of MHMS will investigate the possibility of introducing another family planning method known as Norplant. Permanent methods, tubal ligation and vasectomy, will continue to be promoted for couples who wish to complete their family.

f) Health education awareness programmes will be conducted in all provinces by the Health Education Division (MHMS). The Statistics Office (MOFEP), Maternal and Child Health Unit (MHMS) and the Health Statistics Office (MHMS) would continue to improve information on maternal health, family planning, data collection and inter-censal studies.

g) A Civil Registration Unit would be established to register all births, deaths, marriages and divorces. The Unit would also monitor and evaluate population trends.

h) The reporting system of the Ministry of Health and Medical Services would be strengthened and improved.

8.0 CONCLUSION

The Solomon Islands will continue to promote population education awareness through the various bodies such as Solomon Islands Planned Parenthood Association, the Maternal and Child Health Unit, the Health Education Division (MHMS), schools (MEHRD), colleges (SICHE), and appropriate non-government organizations.

Refresher workshops are to be continued for those who attended previous Training of Trainers Workshops.

The Solomon Islands Planned Parenthood Association has also planned a Family Life Education Programme for youths, to further involve them in population education awareness.

Rather than using the term family planning which scares some people, SIPPA was reduced its sensitiveness by adopting the term 'HAPI FAMILI'. This does not only aim at the reduction of family size, but also the improvement of basic needs such as proper sanitation, water supply and nutrition.

Finally, but not least, continuous effort will be made to integrate population issues in the Government National Development Plan.

All these on-going activities will be evaluated after the next census in 1996, and finally reviewed for forward planning in the year 2000.

ANNEX 1

DEMOGRAPHIC DATA*

Total Population **	1970:	160 998
	1976:	196 823
	1986:	285 176
Annual rate of increase, 1976 - 86		3.5%
Sex ratio, males per 100 females		108
Age groups, 1986, 0 - 14		47%
15 - 59		48%
60+		5%
	Total:	100%
Life expectancy at birth, 1980 - 84	Males	59.9 years
	Females	61.4 years
Infant mortality, per 1000 live births, 1980 - 84	Males	40 per year
	Females	36 per year
Crude death rate, per 1000 population, 1980-84		10 per year
Crude birth rate, per 1000 population, 1980-84		42 per year
Natural rate of increase, per 1000 population, 1980 - 84		32 per year
Total fertility rate. Number of per woman at child bearing age	1980-84	6.4 children
	1984-86	6.1 children
Singulate mean age at marriage 1986	Males	25.0 years
	Females	21.0 years
Lifetime inter-provincial migrants among population aged 15 and over		22.8%
Inter-provincial migrants since independence among population aged 15 and over		20.0%
Population aged 14 and over working for money	Males	35.2%
	Females	13.0%
Population aged 14 and over working for wages	Males	26.2%
	Females	6.9%
Average Household size **		6.5
Households with no apparent money income **		13.0%
Population aged 10 and over with no education**		39.8%

* Figures are for Solomon Islanders unless indicated with ** in which case all persons or households are involved.

LIMITS TO PAPUA NEW GUINEA'S POPULATION GROWTH - A CRITICAL REVIEW OF THE NATIONAL POPULATION POLICY - PAPUA NEW GUINEA, AND ITS ENVIRONMENTAL IMPLICATIONS

DAVID MOWBRAY[1]

This paper is a brief but critical review of the National Population Policy from an environmental viewpoint. In it I ask questions and make a few suggestions, but I give no answers.

The point is stressed that the environmental implications and possible ecological consequences of a policy which does not directly give clear recognition of the environment as one of the prime components in population planning are clear. Sustainable development for the long term future will be jeopardized.

GENERAL

The sustainability of development and the ensurance of achieving and maintaining a better quality of life are intimately linked to the dynamics of population growth. The issue, however, is not simply one of population size, nor is it one of sufficient resources, nor provision of economic and social benefits, nor of levels of environmental impact....:but rather .....

> Be it that..... A child born in a country where levels of material and energy use are high, and where the technology causes environmental impacts, places a greater burden on the Earth's resources, and the Earth's ecosystem's/biosphere's capacity to tolerate impact, than a child born in a poorer/ developing country.

[1] Senior Lecturer in Biology, and Acting Coordinator Environmental Sciences, Biology Department, University of Papua New Guinea

> Nonetheless, sustainable development can be pursued more easily when the population size is stabilised at a level consistent with the productive capacity of the ecosystem, and its environmental tolerance(1).

Apart from the social and economic consequences of PNG's rapid population growth, there are also profound environmental consequences. There are also biological limitations and ecological constraints to rapid population growth. Necessarily rapid increases in agricultural production, both of crops and livestock, in many areas increase erosion, soil and water deterioration and destruction of wildlife and natural habitats. Pollution by indiscriminant use of pesticides may poison people and domestic and wild animals. In PNG an increasing amount of land is being continually cleared for agriculture either for cash cropping or for subsistence farming, leading to deforestation, erosion, and pollution of coastal areas by increasing sedimentation. Furthermore the demands of increasing population sizes results in the demand for exploitation of our other natural resources to generate necessary income to satisfy peoples needs and aspirations, eg exploitation of forests, fishing and mineral resources. These too result in deterioration of our natural environment due to loss of natural habitats and biodiversity, overfishing and pollution of rivers and coastal areas, such as in Bougainville and Ok Tedi.

The recent gradual redistribution of people from rural to urban areas and from mountains to the coast is making population pressures a primary cause of long-term environmental disturbance. This population movement (together with natural increases) - particularly in the urban areas, is concentrating human wastes and pollution. This adds to the environmental effects of industrial and other developments. Deforestation and erosion problems are getting worse around large urban areas as people seek fuel from timber growing at the periphery of the urban areas(2). Hence rapid urbanisation is leading to many problems of land, water, (and air) pollution apart from those related to provision of clean water and disposal of wastes, faecal or otherwise.

Population density is not currently an impediment to improved standards of living overall in PNG, though large family sizes most certainly limit the fulfilment of individual family's aspirations for a healthy and productive life. Nor is it a primary determinant of environmental deterioration in most parts of the country. But these may not always remain the case.

The fourth goal of the Constitution of Papua New Guinea clearly states:

> **We declare our fourth goal to be for Papua New Guinea's natural resources and environment to be conserved and used for the collective benefit of us all, <u>and be replenished</u> <u>for the benefit of future generations.</u>**

Furthermore the latest restatement of the Government's Development Policies and Strategies states that:

> **Emphasis has been given to responsible development. Development which degrades the environment or leads to a deterioration in the quality of life of the people is not genuine development.**

If we are to achieve this goal due consideration must be given in our National Population Policy to environmental considerations.

We could ask the following questions:

> What is the carrying capacity of PNG (or a province or region of PNG), ie what is the sustainable population size (or maximum number of individuals) that can be supported in our environment indefinitely? Given that we need to conserve and enhance our resource base for future generations - i.e. given due consideration of our land resources, water resources, energy resources, biotic resources, mineral resources, methods of sanitation, and given the types of technologies we choose to utilise these resources, and given the many other interacting social, cultural and economic factors, and peoples' aspirations and needs?
>
> Given the present or expected age compositions and rates of growth, when might these sustainable levels or carrying capacities be reached?

However the point needs to be stressed that:

> consideration of the above also depends upon whether we choose to reorient our technology to pay greater attention to environmental factors, whether we have the political and moral will to ensure a more equitable redistribution of our resources and their benefits amongst the people, and whether we merge environmental and economic factors in our decision making.

It is generally recognised that PNG's population will double to around 7.4 million by the years 2015 - 2025, and given decreasing population growth rates (replacement reproduction?), may stabilise by the late 21st century at around 11 million. With successful implementation of the National Population Policy and rapid acceptance of family planning, coupled with better educational and employment opportunities, better delivery of health services, improved status of women, etc, it may stabilise around 9 million. This is the objective.

But I propose that we also need consider the question:

> **What population size can PNG support? What population size can each region and/or province of PNG support? What are the sustainable population levels?**
>
> **The concept of carrying capacity may be considered too theoretical by many. But the real fact is that if development is to be sustainable we must ensure that the population is sustainable!!**

NATIONAL POPULATION POLICY; CRITICISM

In "Guidelines Towards a National Population Policy for PNG" (3), the issue of environment, or the relationship between environment and population is not listed as a **"key issue"** (p4: 1.12).

However the importance of this relationship is inferred in a number of places in the policy statement:.....but the environment is only mentioned indirectly:

1. On p12: 3.0 mention is made that high population growth (in PNG, est 2.1 - 2.3% with doubling time of 30 - 33 years) **is a deterrent to the attainment of improved standard of life and quality of life of the people, and thus may not be in the best interest of the country..** Examples are given with reference to health, education, employment.

2. Re health - on p12: 3.4 population growth affects health status through resource depletion **and deterioration of the environment caused by population pressure.....**increase pressure on demand for resources on land, water, food,...

3. On p16: 3.23 mention is made that attempts to increase (food) production to maintain subsistence levels and increase cash cropping in the face of increasing population would intensify lands pressures particularly in high density areas, resulting in land disputes **and ecological degradation,** eg Chimbu, the Gazelle Peninsula and Northern Province.

4. On p21: 5.7 point 5. The various research institutions should ..undertake research ...(and) **to define the linkages of population, development and environment.**

The issue of what is the biological/ecological limit to PNG's population size, given social, economic, biological and resource factors is not addressed, nor even mentioned. Also included should be a need to estimate sustainable population sizes for each province, given their own limiting factors and recognizing regional differences...and given the social, economic, cultural, technological, resource-based **and biological/ecological constraints for each.**

I would propose that computer modelling to estimate/guestimate sustainable population sizes may be useful, though the assumptions must be made carefully and the parameters used chosen wisely. Due consideration need be given to all possible factors, and the complex interactions of all.

In Appendix II, the broad role of the Department of Environment and Conservation should be added. A suggested role could be:

1. To promote awareness of the relationship between population size, environment, quality of life, and development at both provincial and national levels.

2. To co-ordinate research to estimate what might be the sustainable level of population/"carrying capacity" for each province/for PNG, given the social, economic, cultural, technological, resource-based **and biological/ecological constraints".**

CONCLUSION

The National Population Policy is a very positive strategy to assist Papua New Guinea on the road to sustainable development. However as the policy evolves I would suggest that consideration need by given to environmental factors. We need to have some idea of what is a sustainable level of population in each of our provinces, in each region and in the country as a whole.

Recognition that our environments have biological limitations and ecological constraints is imperative.

Furthermore we must conserve and enhance our resources base for our children and for those in a thousand years, and beyond.

These are our moral responsibilities and our obligations **to all life** in Papua New Guinea.

REFERENCES

1. World Commission on Environment and Development 1987 Our Common Future. Oxford University Press. pp55-56.

2. Carew-Reid J. 1989. Environment, aid and regionalism in the South Pacific. Pacific Research Monograph No 22. National Centre for Development Studies, The Australian National University. pp25-26.

3. Department of Finance and Planning 1991. Papua New Guinea. An Integrated National Population Policy for Progress and Development. 5th June 1991. pp47.

4. Starke L. 1990. Signs of Hope. Working Towards our Common Future. The Centre for our Common Future. Oxford University Press.

5. Unisearch PNG 1991. Papua New Guinea: An Environmental Situation Report, prepared for the Australian International Development Assistance Bureau, University of Papua New Guinea, February 1991. University of Papua New Guinea. pp53.

6. Unisearch PNG 1991. Papua New Guinea National Report: United Nations Conference on Environment and Development, prepared for the Government of the Independent State of Papua New Guinea, June 1991. University of Papua New Guinea. Draft copy. pp160.

MAPPING AGRICULTURAL SYSTEMS IN PAPUA NEW GUINEA

R. M. BOURKE, R. L. HIDE, B. J. ALLEN, R. GRAU, G. S. HUMPHREYS AND H. C. BROOKFIELD[1]

INTRODUCTION

This is a preliminary description of a project which is mapping subsistence agriculture throughout Papua New Guinea. The mapping is part of the larger Land Management Project based in the Department of Human Geography in the Division of Society and Environment, the Research School of Pacific Studies at the Australian National University. The Land Management Project is concerned with the long-term sustainability of village agricultural systems in Melanesia and Southeast Asia in the context of population growth, rapid social and economic change, and global climatic change and variability. Sustainability in agricultural systems is about change over time, maintenance of soil and plant nutrients, the ability to withstand short environmental shocks or to adapt to longer term changes, while maintaining or increasing production. Essential to the assessment of the sustainability of contemporary agriculture systems is an understanding of how present systems function in relation to their environment, the numbers of people they are supporting, and an estimate of how long they have been in place. The fundamental objective of mapping Papua New Guinean agricultural systems is to provide information that will enable analysis of these elements. The project will also produce much information for more immediate and practical uses.

ORIGINS AND DEVELOPMENT OF THE MAPPING PROJECT

There are few current data with national coverage on subsistence agriculture in Papua New Guinea. Three, national, agricultural censuses were made or attempted between 1947 and 1962 (Allen-Ovenstone and Williams, 1954; Walters, 1963). While the first collected information from a sample of some 300 villages and the last surveyed 100 villages, no original data sheets from any village included in these censuses are currently traceable. National level aggregates of production from the 1961-62 census data are still used thirty years later as the starting point for current estimates. Data at census division level on crops or major food sources assembled in 1966, prior to the first

[1] Department of Human Geography, Research School of Pacific Studies, Australian National University

national population census, provided the basis for two generalised, very smallscale, maps of aspects of subsistence agriculture published in the 1970 Atlas of Papua New Guinea (Lea, 1970; Lea and Ward, 1970). Although the reliability of these data was not great (Lea and Ward, 1970:56), they were later incorporated in a number of other smallscale national maps of aspects of subsistence agriculture (i.e. Brookfield with Hart, 1971; Ford, 1974; Vasey, 1981, 1982). The only new information on food sources with national coverage since the 1960s is that collected by the National Nutrition Survey 1982/83 on selected foods eaten the previous day (IMR, nd).

In 1981, the CSIRO Division of Water and Land Resources and the Papua New Guinea Department of Primary Industry initiated a project to assess the potential of the natural resources of Papua New Guinea for the development of village-based food and cash crop production (McAlpine et al., 1982; Bellamy, 1986). This project created a large database on natural resources, land use and population distribution, known as the Papua New Guinea Resource Information System, or PNGRIS. For village agriculture, PNGRIS includes socio-economic data on cash crops from the 1980 National Population Census, and data on agricultural land use intensity based on interpretation of 1972/73 air photography (Saunders, nd). No data sources with national coverage were available on other components of subsistence agricultural systems. To tap information contained in the large body of micro-level community studies, a partial bibliography linking such sources of subsistence information to the PNGRIS mapping units was prepared (Hide and Cuddy, 1988).

To provide current data with wider coverage missing from the PNGRIS system, R. M. Bourke, who was then Principal Horticulturist with the Papua New Guinea Department of Primary Industry, devised a method, developed from a classification used previously by Brookfield (1962) and Brookfield with Hart (1971), for mapping subsistence agriculture in Papua New Guinea. After recording several characteristics of subsistence agriculture along numerous field transects, Bourke defined the boundaries of those areas with more or less homogeneous features. The map scale chosen was 1:500,000 in order to be compatible with PNGRIS. Between 1980 and 1982 Bourke completed mapping surveys of agriculture in the five highland provinces and West Sepik Province as well as in parts of eight other provinces. This work was deferred from 1983 to 1988 while Bourke undertook postgraduate study at the ANU. In 1990 it was incorporated into the Department of Human Geography's Land Management Project.

The Mapping Project is now partially funded from the Papua New Guinea/Australia Colloquium, through the International Development Program of Australian Universities and Colleges and from the Research School of Pacific Studies at the Australian National University. Although the project is based in the Department of Human Geography at the Australian National University where it involves several members, it is a joint project closely involving staff from the Papua New Guinea National Research Institute and the Geography Department at University of Papua New Guinea (UPNG). Staff of three divisions of the Papua New Guinea Department of Agriculture and Livestock (DAL) are also participating.

In preparation for the first field survey of the renewed mapping project in 1990, the classification and recording systems used by Bourke were revised. Several data categories were expanded and some new ones added. A survey recording form was designed, and a database file system established in dBase IV. The earlier surveys were reviewed and a field programme starting with the highland region planned. To date, two field survey periods have been completed: the five highlands provinces in October-November 1990, and East and West Sepik provinces and part of Madang in June-July 1991. A third survey covering Morobe and the rest of Madang Provinces will be undertaken in October-November 1991.

METHODS: FIELD PROCEDURES AND DATA MANAGEMENT

In summary, the overall approach used in the mapping project involves the following steps: prior to fieldwork literature is reviewed and base maps of agriculturally used land are prepared; a route is planned for field visits so that all major concentrations of rural populations are visited; along these routes food gardens are inspected and villagers interviewed to obtain information on features that cannot be readily observed such as fallow length; landscapes, gardens and other features are photographed; boundaries of agricultural systems are determined; and field survey forms are completed. Between three and six person-weeks are scheduled for fieldwork in each province. After fieldwork, the information is entered into a computerised database, agricultural system boundaries are digitized in a mapping software package, maps of major features are machine plotted, and both data and output are checked.

The field survey method is a form of Rapid Rural Appraisal, and depends heavily on the broad experience of the principal researchers in studying agriculture in many parts of Papua New Guinea. The overall objective of the mapping is to identify agricultural systems in which practices are more or less homogeneous. This is achieved by walking and vehicle traverses, and by aerial surveys, with boundaries between systems identified at a mapping scale of 1:500,000.

To ensure compatibility between data produced by the present project and the PNGRIS database, agricultural systems are mapped only within land classed as used in the CSIRO land use intensity map (Saunders, nd). If major changes in used areas are found during the field surveys, the relevant areas are included. Only minor changes have been recorded to date. Saunders's used-land boundaries are digitized into ARC/INFO, a large map analysis and database package, and base maps are produced and used for agricultural system definition during fieldwork.

The project defines an agricultural system as a set of more or less homogeneous agricultural practices. The variety of crops grown and of techniques used, and the complexities of the resulting combinations, mean that no simple classification is possible. The criteria used to distinguish agricultural systems are:

1. Fallow type (the fallow vegetation which is cleared before cultivation, for example, tall grass, short woody regrowth)

2. Fallow period (the period between cultivations during which the land lies unused)

3. Period of cultivation before fallow

4. Staple food crops

5. Aspects of garden and crop segregation

6. Soil fertility maintenance techniques.
   Agricultural systems in Papua New Guinea include significant variability, some of which cannot be accommodated in the classification system used in this project. For example, if only 5 per cent of garden land follows a forest fallow in a system where the predominant fallow type is short grasses, this is insufficient to effect the classification, though the minor practice is noted. However, if a major difference in fallow type, cropping period, or one of the other distinguishing criteria is used on more than approximately 15 per cent of land cultivated, a sub-system is distinguished. Thus one agricultural system may contain two or three sub-systems in which, for example, the same crops are grown, but in which fallow types, fallow periods and soil tillage techniques may differ.

A range of other information that is not used in distinguishing systems but is nevertheless important in characterizing them, is recorded also. These data include:

1. The main vegetable, fruit, nut and narcotic crops ;

2. Other aspects of soil and water management, for example, soil tillage, placement of pigs in food gardens between crop plantings, use of soil retention barriers, mounding, and irrigation;

3. Other management aspects such as use of fences and planting seasonality;

4. Cash income sources from agricultural production.

Overall, information is recorded on 44 aspects of the agricultural system. Most features are rated for occurrence using a four-class scale: none, minor or insignificant, significant, very significant. A few features are classed descriptively, for example, the cropping period (one crop only before fallow, two crops, 3-5 crops, 6-14 crops, 15+ crops), and the long fallow period (not used, 1-4 years, 5-15 years, >15 years).

For each agricultural system, the following general information is also recorded:

1. Location details (province, district, census division, altitude range, slope);

2. A description of the field surveys, including routes taken and the duration of the survey;

3. A summary of how the system boundaries were defined.

During the survey, the agricultural information is recorded on a 12-page field data entry form. On return from the field, data are entered as text or numerical codes to the database (in dBase IV) which is maintained on IBM type computers. These field observations are supplemented by information from published literature, and the computer record for each agricultural system contains a small bibliography of such items for the area. The system boundaries identified during the survey are digitized into ARC/INFO, and areas are calculated. The procedure for handling post-fieldwork information on agricultural systems and system boundaries is shown schematically in Figure 1.

The Papua New Guinea 1980 National Population Census, in which there was total enumeration of the country's population, is used to establish the rural population resident in the area of each agricultural system. A summary of the data for each census unit is taken from the Village Population File of PNGRIS (Bellamy, 1986), and converted from KMAN format to a dBase IV file which includes an additional field for agricultural system identification. For each province, the map of agricultural system boundaries is overlaid on the Census Unit Maps (Papua New Guinea National Mapping Bureau, updated 1990) and all census units within a system are identified. System codes for each census unit are then entered on the population file, and the total population of each system calculated and transferred to the main database file. Population densities within systems are then calculated in ARC/INFO.

Data from the agricultural systems database are transferred to ARC/INFO and trial maps produced for checking entry errors or field classification and description anomalies. Maps showing any of the data can be produced at provincial, regional or national levels. Further manipulation of data is done either in dBase IV, or in ARC/INFO. New data classes or variables can be produced by combining existing ones (i.e. grouping information on three separate vegetables, pitpit, *Rungia* and *Oenanthe*, to form a crop pattern common in the highlands, or calculating cultivation intensity as the ratio of the cultivation period to the fallow period), and maps showing such new distributions can be plotted quickly.

OUTPUT AND POTENTIAL USES

Output

The project will produce the following:

1. A computerised database containing all the agricultural information recorded. Copies will be available in Papua New Guinea at the Department of Geography, UPNG, at DAL, and other relevant institutions.

2. Hard copies of information in both code and text format directly from the database files. These will be readily available to interested users in Papua New Guinea.

3. A data listing, in the form of a one-page summary sheet for each agricultural system (or subsystem), showing all the information recorded . An example is given in Figure 2.

4. A short text description (two pages) of each agricultural system in plain English. An example is given in Figure 3.

5. A map of each province of Papua New Guinea at a scale of 1:500,000 and of Papua New Guinea at 1:1,000,000, showing agricultural systems.

6. Specific maps of the agricultural features recorded or generated from recorded data. These will normally cover the whole country at 1:1,000,000.

7. A collection of photographs illustrating agricultural techniques for most systems. Documentation for each photograph (date, location. description, agricultural system etc) is held in a data file.

Information for planning and development

Information on agricultural systems is essential for development planning. A number of examples of how the information produced by this project can be applied to development problems follows.

1. Food crops research and extension. Existing information on the significance of staple foods in different parts of Papua New Guinea is poor, particularly in the lowlands and the highland fringes. Most commentators and maps, for example, overestimate the importance of *Colocasia* taro and underestimate that of the relatively recently introduced *Xanthosoma* taro and cassava. Similarly, the literature concentrates on traditional leguminous foods, such as winged bean and lima bean, and understates the significance of peanuts and *Phaseolus* bean. The choice of which crops to select for further research is based presently on outdated information about the numbers of people cultivating crops as staples.

2. **Definition of agro-ecological zones.** The DAL regional Farming System Research teams based at Aiyura, Bubia and Keravat are interested in defining agro-ecological zones for research and extension purposes. The criteria for designating such zones can include types of crops, agricultural techniques, intensity of production, rainfall and altitudinal zone. Information on the first three features is not presently available for Papua New Guinea but this project will provide it.

3. **Intensity of cultivation and the identification of vulnerable agricultural systems.** The intensity of cultivation can be described by the ratio of cultivation period to fallow period. This ratio is a useful indicator of agricultural systems that may be vulnerable to stress, particularly when combined with environmental information from PNGRIS and an estimate of the length of time a system has operated. Information on cropping periods (the number of times that staple crops are planted in major gardens before a long fallow) and long fallow periods is shown for each agricultural system in the Eastern Highlands in Figures 4 and 5 respectively.

4. **Soil fertility maintenance techniques.** Apart from the universally used natural regrowth fallows, a number of other methods are employed to maintain soil fertility in Papua New Guinea. These include: composting; crop rotations, particularly with leguminous food crops; tree planting, particularly of casuarina; the transfer of organic matter from drainage ditches; and soil retention fences (Bourke, 1990). The broad distribution of these techniques in the highlands is shown in Figure 6. Regional and national level maps, such as this one, indicate appropriate locations for more intensive studies of these techniques, and other areas where their introduction might be considered.

5. **Production estimates for the main staple foods.** No reliable up-to-date national production estimates are available for the main staples of Papua New Guinea.

Present estimates are based on 1962 figures updated on the basis of population increases. It should be possible to make more reliable estimates of current production using the agricultural systems database.

Information for a better understanding of how agricultural systems work

A broader understanding of how agricultural systems work in Papua New Guinea and elsewhere will be very important in achieving sustainable food production systems. In Papua New Guinea, the population is expected to double within the next 30 years and food supply will need to increase accordingly if living standards are to be maintained or improved. Food can be imported - at a cost, but in some rural localities where it is no longer possible to simply expand cultivation onto new land will have to increase agricultural production from currently cultivated areas. This is the process known as agricultural intensification. We need to know more about how farmers respond to pressures to innovate and intensify, which techniques can be recommended to farmers in different environments, and which environments are vulnerable to intensified use.

In the highlands, for example, the practice of composting to maintain sweet potato yields is discretely distributed whereas the use of a legume/sweet potato rotation or a planted casuarina fallow is more dispersed (Figure 6). Analysis of the distribution of such techniques in relation to both environmental and socio-cultural factors will help to identify the conditions which may contribute to their introduction and adoption elsewhere in the country. Such analysis also requires data additional to that produced by this project, particularly information on changes over time, estimates of which are sometimes available from published sources, archival records and personal long-term observations.

Short surveys of the kind used in this project cannot gather information on either labour inputs to subsistence agriculture or crop yields, both of which are critical for assessing the sustainability of changing land use practices. That type of data can only be collected, with difficulty, during long and intensive surveys. Nevertheless, observations on possible indices of agricultural stress, such as claimed low crop yields, environmental degradation, out-migration and firewood shortages, are recorded during the field surveys. Such observations can help to define areas of actual and potential agricultural stress, a number of which were identified during the 1990 survey of the highlands provinces. More intensive investigations of environmental degradation, changes in crop yields, population and land use are needed in these locations, and are planned for 1992.

The information generated will also be used to examine existing theories about the evolution of agriculture in Papua New Guinea and elsewhere, and the ability, or otherwise, of people to continually adapt agricultural systems to meet rising demands for production - for both consumption and prestige - without destroying the environmental foundations upon which such systems are based. This is the subject of another paper.

ACKNOWLEDGEMENTS

Financial support for this project is provided by the Australian Government through the International Development Program of the Australian Universities and Colleges, and the Papua New Guinea Government, through the Papua New Guinea National Research Institute; and the Australian National University. The Chief Land Use Officer of the Papua New Guinea Department of Agriculture and Livestock, Mr B. Wayi gave us access to the Papua New Guinea Resource Information System. Mr N. Suvolo of the PNG National Statistical Office provided copies of the 1990 census maps. Mr John McAlpine, Ms Sue Cuddy and other CSIRO staff who worked on the Papua New Guinea Resource Information System have been unfailingly helpful. At the ANU, Ms Anne Cochrane is processing the population data and undertaking many other tasks, Ms Kay Dancey is digitizing maps, and Mr D. Fritsch has designed the software for producing the summary output data as well as giving much advice on dBase use. Mrs Barbara Banks edited the present manuscript.

REFERENCES

Allen-Ovenstone W and Williams E J. Census of native agriculture 1950, Territory of Papua and New Guinea. Report on conduct of census and statistical analysis. Unpublished typescript, Melbourne. 1954

Bellamy J A. (compiler). Papua New Guinea Inventory of Natural Resources, Population Distribution and Land Use Handbook. Natural Resources Series No. 6. Division of Water and Land Resources, CSIRO, Canberra. 1986

Bourke R M. Subsistence food production systems in Papua New Guinea: old changes and new changes. In Pacific Production Systems. Approaches to Economic Prehistory. Yen D E and Mummery J M J (eds). Occasional Papers in Prehistory No 18. Department of Prehistory, RSPacS, Australian National University, Canberra. 1990, pp148-160.

Brookfield H C. Local study and comparative method: an example from Central New Guinea. Annals of the Association of American Geographers. 1962, 52:242-254.

Brookfield H C with Hart D. Melanesia. A Geographical Interpretation of an Island World. Methuen, London. 1971, pp94-124.

Hide R L and Cuddy S M. (Compilers). Annotated and Selected Bibliography of Smallholder Farming Systems in PNG. Part 1 Papua, New Guinea Mainland, New Guinea Islands. Division of Water and Land Resources, CSIRO, Canberra. 1988.

Institute of Medical Research. Papua New Guinea 1982/3 National Nutrition Survey: Provincial tabulations. PNG Institute of Medical Research, Goroka/Nutrition Section, Department of Health, Port Moresby.

Ford E. Crop agriculture. In Papua New Guinea resource atlas. Ford E (ed). Jacaranda Press, Brisbane. 1974, pp16-17.

Lea D A M. Staple crops and main sources of food. In An atlas of Papua and New Guinea. Ward R G and Lea D A M (eds). Department of Geography, University of Papua New Guinea and Collins-Longmans. 1970, pp54-55.

Lea D A M and Ward R G. Crop combinations. In An Atlas of Papua and New Guinea. Ward R G and Lea D A M (eds). Department of Geography, University of Papua New Guinea and Collins-Longmans. 1970, pp56-57.

McAlpine J R, Bleeker P, Freyne D and Keig G. Assessing resource potential for food crop production in Papua New Guinea. In Proceedings of the Second Papua New Guinea Food Crops Conference. Bourke R M and Kesavan V (eds). Departmentof Primary Industry, Port Moresby. 1982, pp325-329.

Saunders J C. Agricultural Land Use of Papua New Guinea. Map to accompany Natural Resources Series Report No. 9. Division of Water and Land Resources, CSIRO, Canberra.

Vasey D. Agricultural systems in Papua New Guinea: adaption to the humid tropics. In A Time to Plant and a Time to Uproot: A History of Agriculture in Papua New Guinea. Denoon D and Snowden C (eds). Institute of Papua New Guinea Studies, Port Moresby. 1981, pp17-31.

Vasey D. Subsistence crop systems. In Papua New Guinea Atlas. A Nation in Transition. King D and Ranck S (eds). Robert Brown and Associates (Australia) and University of Papua New Guinea. 1982, pp50-51.

Walters C L. Survey of Indigenous Agriculture and Ancillary surveys 1961-1962 Technical Document. Bureau of Statistics, Port Moresby. 1963

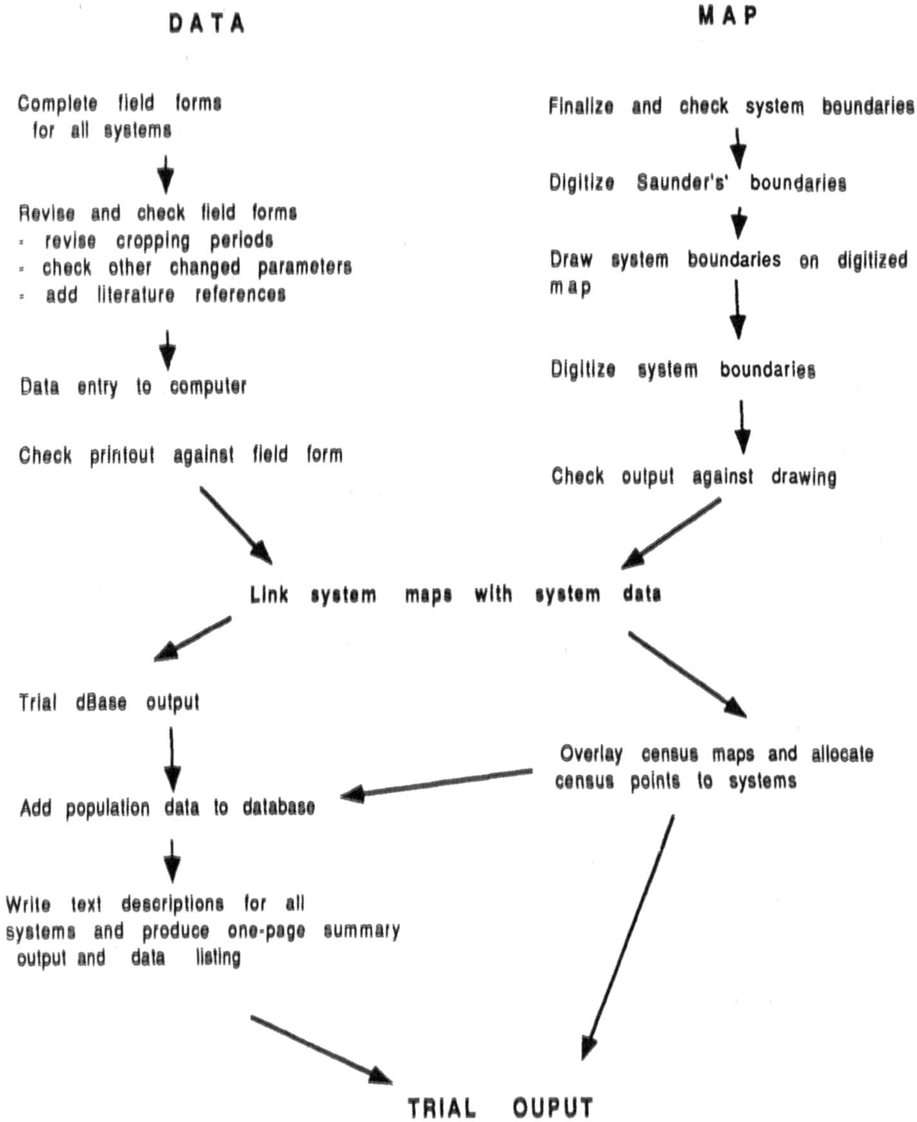

Figure 1. Post-fieldwork data and map preparation methods

PROVINCE 11 Eastern Highlands **AGRICULTURAL SYSTEM No. 1**		
Districts 1 Goroka, 2 Henganofi	**Subsystem No 1 of 1**	**Subsystem Extent** 75-100 %
Area (sq km) 1121	**Population** 57,466	**Population density** 51 persons/sq km

System Summary

Staple is sweet potato, corn and yams are subdominant staples; fallow is short grass. Staple is grown in small mounds on characteristically long drained beds. Typically, fallow period and cultivation period are about the same within an enclosed area. However after several decades of use, some enclosed areas may be abandoned and left to fallow for an unknown number of decades. In other locations, no such abandonment, and crop/fallow cycle continues.

System Crosses Prov. Boundary 12 99

Altitude Range (m) 1200 - 2200 Slope Gentle (2-10 degrees)

CROPS

STAPLES DOMINANT	Sweet Potato
STAPLES SUBDOMINANT	Corn, Yams (D. alata)
OTHER VEGETABLES	Highland pitpit, Oenanthe, Rungia
FRUITS	Banana, Marita pandanus, Sugarcane
NUTS	Karuka (planted)
NARCOTICS	Betel nut (h'land), Betel pepper (h'hland), Tobacco

FALLOW & CROPPING PERIOD

FALLOW TYPE	Short grass
SHORT FALLOW	Very significant
LONG FALLOW PERIOD	1 - 4 years
CROPPING PERIOD	3 - 5 crops

GARDEN SEGREGATION

GARDEN SEGREGATION	None
CROP SEGREGATION	Very significant
CROP SEQUENCES	Significant
MIXED VEGETABLE GARDENS	Significant
HOUSEHOLD GARDENS	Significant

SOIL FERTILITY MAINTENANCE

LEGUME ROTATION	Very significant
PLANTED TREE FALLOW	Minor
COMPOST	None
ANIMAL MANURE	None
ISLAND BED	None
SILT FROM FLOOD	None
INORGANIC FERTILIZER	Minor

CASH EARNING ACTIVITIES

1 Coffee Arabica	Very significant
2 Firewood	Significant
3 Fresh Food	Significant
4 Potato	Significant
5 Cattle	Minor

OTHER AGRONOMIC PRACTICES

Water Management:

DRAINAGE	Very significant
IRRIGATION	None

Soil Management:

PIGS PLACED IN GARDENS	None
BURN FALLOW VEGETATION	Very significant
TILLAGE	Very significant
MECHANIZATION	Minor
DEEP HOLING	None
MULCHING	Minor
SOIL RETENTION BARRIERS	None

Mounding Techniques:

VERY SMALL MOUNDS	Minor
SMALL MOUNDS	Very significant
MOUNDS	None
LARGE MOUNDS	None

Garden Bed Techniques:

BEDS SQUARE	None
BEDS LONG	Very significant

Other Features:

FENCES	Very significant
STAKING	Significant
FALLOW CUT ONTO CROPS	None
SEASONAL MAIN CROPS	None
SEASONAL SEC'DARY CROPS	Significant

References

Howlett, D.R. (1962). A decade of change in the Goroka Valley, New Guinea: land use and development in the 1950s. Ph.D.Thesis, Australian National University.

Bourke, R.M. (1988). Taim hangre: variation in subsistence food supply in the Papua New Guinea Highlands. Ph.D.Thesis, Australian National University.

Bourke, R.M. (1983). Fifty years of agricultural change in a New Guinea Highland village. Unpublished paper, First PNG Food and Nutrition Conference, Goroka.

Figure 2. Example of a one-page summary for a sub-system

Figure 3. Example of a text description of an agricultural system

Province: Eastern Highlands System number: 11-1
File name: Waiehp11.doc

Population: 57,466 **area:** 1121 km2 Population density: 51/km2

Altitudinal range: 1200-2200 m Mean annual rainfall: 1800-2200 mm

Summary description

Short grasses are the most common fallow type with typical fallow periods of about 4-5 years. There are also short fallows (<12 months) between crop plantings. Some gardens are located in short woody regrowth, but the areas are not large enough to warrant a sub-system. The cropping period ranges from 1 to 10 crops with typically 4 crops before fallow. The dominant staple is sweet potato, with corn and yams as subdominant staples. Sweet potato is grown on small mounds on characteristic long drained beds. Food gardens alternate with fallows within fenced enclosures, but these enclosures may be abandoned after several decades and left to fallow for an unknown period. Mixed vegetable gardens are commonly planted. Sweet potato is grown in rotation with peanuts, winged bean and yam. The system is distinguished from EHP 18 where agriculture is less intensive in the short infertile grasslands. Systems to the north (EHP 9) and to the south (EHP 19) are distinguished on the basis of fallow type (tall woody regrowth and cane grass/woody regrowth respectively).

Location, environment and population.

This agricultural system covers the main valleys in the northern part of the province. The Highlands Highway runs through the area and there is good access to the towns of Goroka, Henganofi and Kainantu. The system is used over a wide altitudinal range (1200-2200 m), although gardens are mostly between 1500 and 2000 m. Rainfall is somewhat seasonal, and is more seasonally distributed in the Henganofi area than to the east or west. Various soil types are used, but volcanic ashes are common, particularly on fans where gardens are commonly located. About a quarter of the rural population in the province use the system.

Fallows and cropping period. Short grass is the most common fallow type, but some gardens are cut from short woody regrowth, especially on the eastern side of this system. Tall cane grass is used occasionally. A typical fallow period is 4-5 years.

The cropping period ranges from 1 to 10 crops with typically about 4 crops before fallow. In grassland gardens, sweet potato is generally the first crop after a fallow, and crops of sweet potato are separated by plantings of peanuts or winged bean and short fallows of several months duration. In those gardens cleared from woody regrowth, only one sweet potato crop is usually planted before fallow.

This sequence of crops and both long and short fallows may continue for some decades within an enclosed area. This area is then abandoned and left to fallow for an unknown period while food gardens are moved to another enclosed area.

Major crops.

Sweet potato is the staple crop. Other less important staple foods are corn and yams (**Dioscorea alata** and some **D. bulbifera**). Cassava is important, especially where rainfall is more seasonally distributed, as in the Henganofi area. Commonly grown vegetables include: Highland pitpit, **oenanthe, rungia,** peanuts, winged bean, common bean, pak choi, **Amaranthus** species and cucumber. Significant fruit and nut crops are banana, **marita** pandanus, sugarcane and planted karuka pandanus. Highland betel nut is an important traditional crop in the eastern part of this area. Betel pepper and tobacco are also grown.

Garden and crop segregation.

Separate garden types for different staples are not made, but there is marked spatial segregation of some of the main crops within gardens, especially sweet potato, peanuts, winged bean and yams. Plantings of sweet potato are rotated with those of peanuts, winged bean and yams. Corn and cassava are interplanted within the sweet potato plots. Mixed vegetable gardens as a separate garden type are commonly planted, particularly on flat land near streams and in other drainage depressions. Household gardens are common.

Soil and water management.

Fallow vegetation is generally slashed and then burnt in piles on cleared land. For sweet potato gardens, the soil is generally tilled completely; clods are left on the soil surface; they are then broken again; and the remaining organic matter removed and burnt. The soil is then formed into long beds, typically 2-2.5 wide and 8-12 m long. These are aligned up and down the slope. These neat beds give the agricultural landscape a characteristic appearance. Drains about 20-25 cm deep and wide separate these. Small mounds about 30 cm high are built on the beds for sweet potato. Other crops are not mounded, apart from yams. The soil is not tilled completely in the mixed gardens.

While fallows are the main technique used to maintain soil fertility, rotations of legumes (peanuts or winged bean) and sweet potato are also important. Casuarina trees are occasionally planted in land left to fallow; a little chicken manure and inorganic fertilizer is applied to sweet potato and vegetable crops, but this is not common.

Other agricultural practices. Long timber fences up to 5 km long are widely used to enclose food gardens owned by a number of households. They are made from timber stakes, but occasionally from pig wire.

The following crops are staked: yams (ca 2 m), winged bean (1.5 m when grown for tubers, longer when grown mainly for beans), common bean (ca 2 m), sugarcane (3-6 m).

Sweet potato, peanuts, cassava and sugarcane are not planted seasonally. The following are planted seasonally: mixed gardens (September - December), corn (September - December), winged bean (May - August), cucumber (May - July), yams (May - July). For these crops, the planting season is a little later in locations where the rainfall is more seasonal, that is, in the Benabena Valley and Henganofi area.

Cash earning activities.

Arabica coffee is a very significant source of cash income everywhere. Fresh food, potatoes and firewood are also significant. Fresh food is more important for people living near the Highlands Highway. Food is sold both in local markets (roadside, Goroka, Ukarumpa, Henganofi, Kainantu) and outside the province (Lae, Ramu Sugar, Madang, Port Moresby). Firewood is an important income source for people in the forested areas at higher altitudes (>1800 m). The main foods grown for sale are: sweet potato, peanuts, potato, cabbage, winged bean, cucumber, oenanthe, marita pandanus and karuka pandanus. Some cattle are raised and sold, but to a lesser extent now than in the period mid-1960s to mid-1970s.

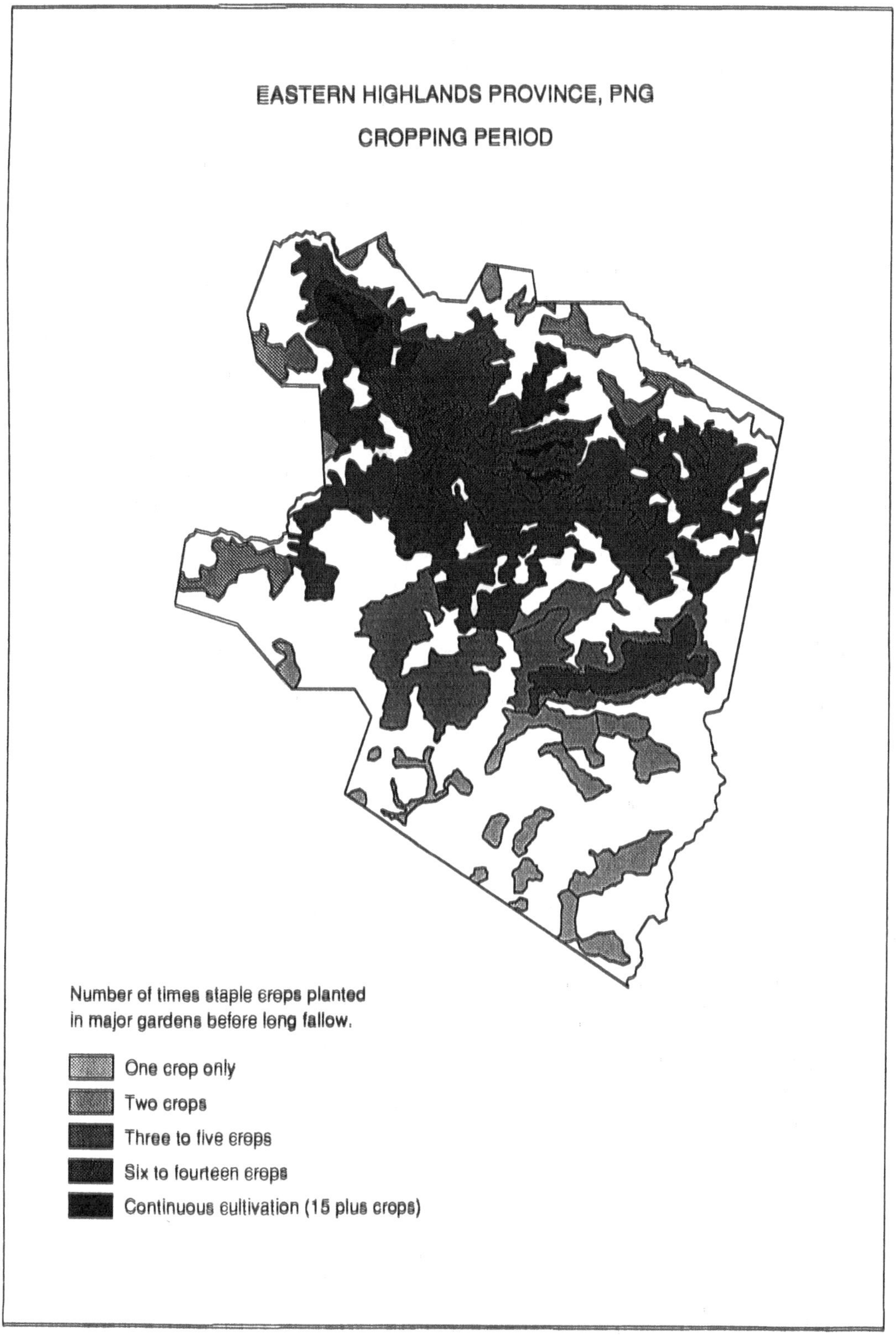

Figure 4. Number of times that staple crops are planted in major gardens before a long fallow in the Eastern Highlands Province

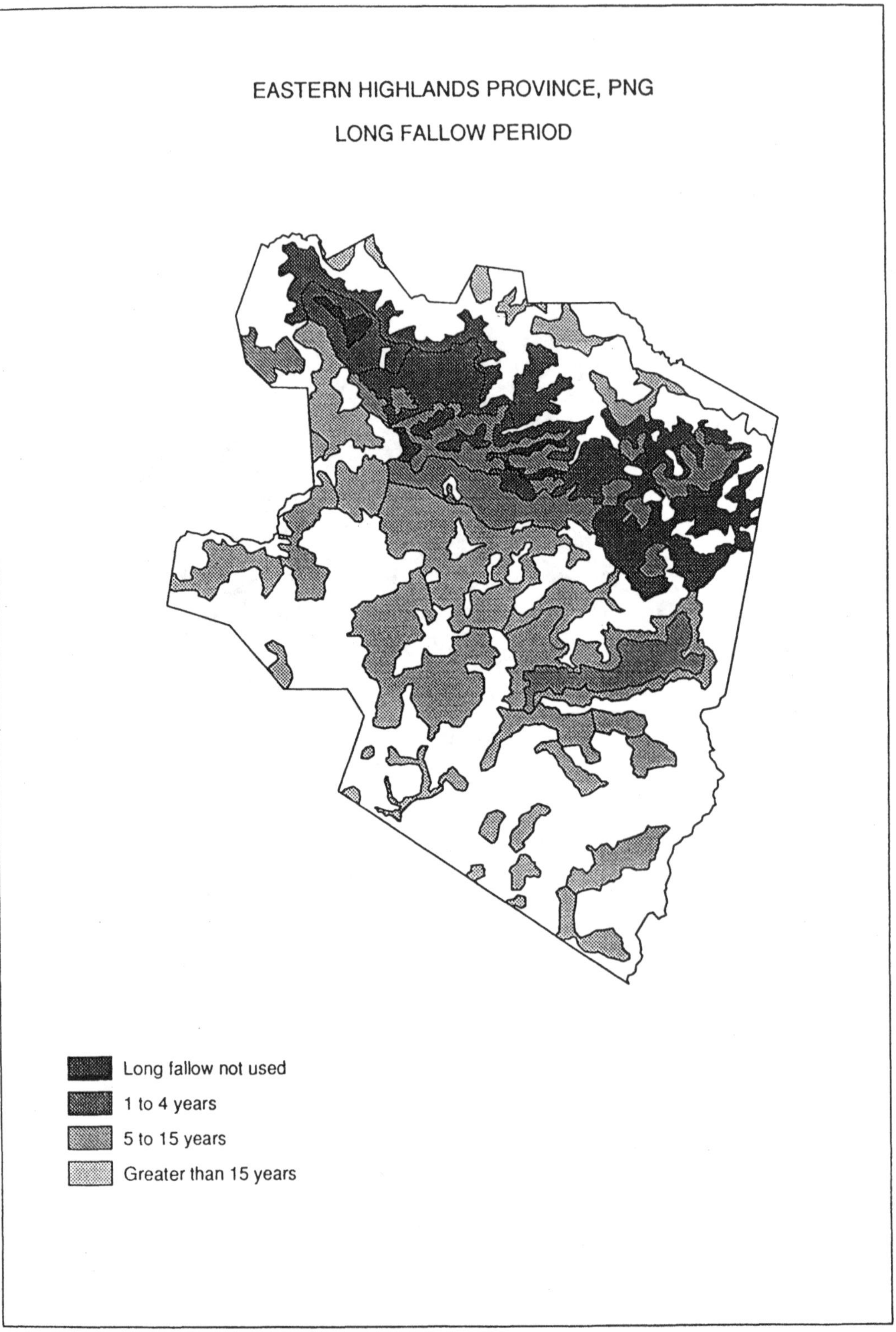

Figure 5. The length of the long fallow period in years in the Eastern Highlands Province

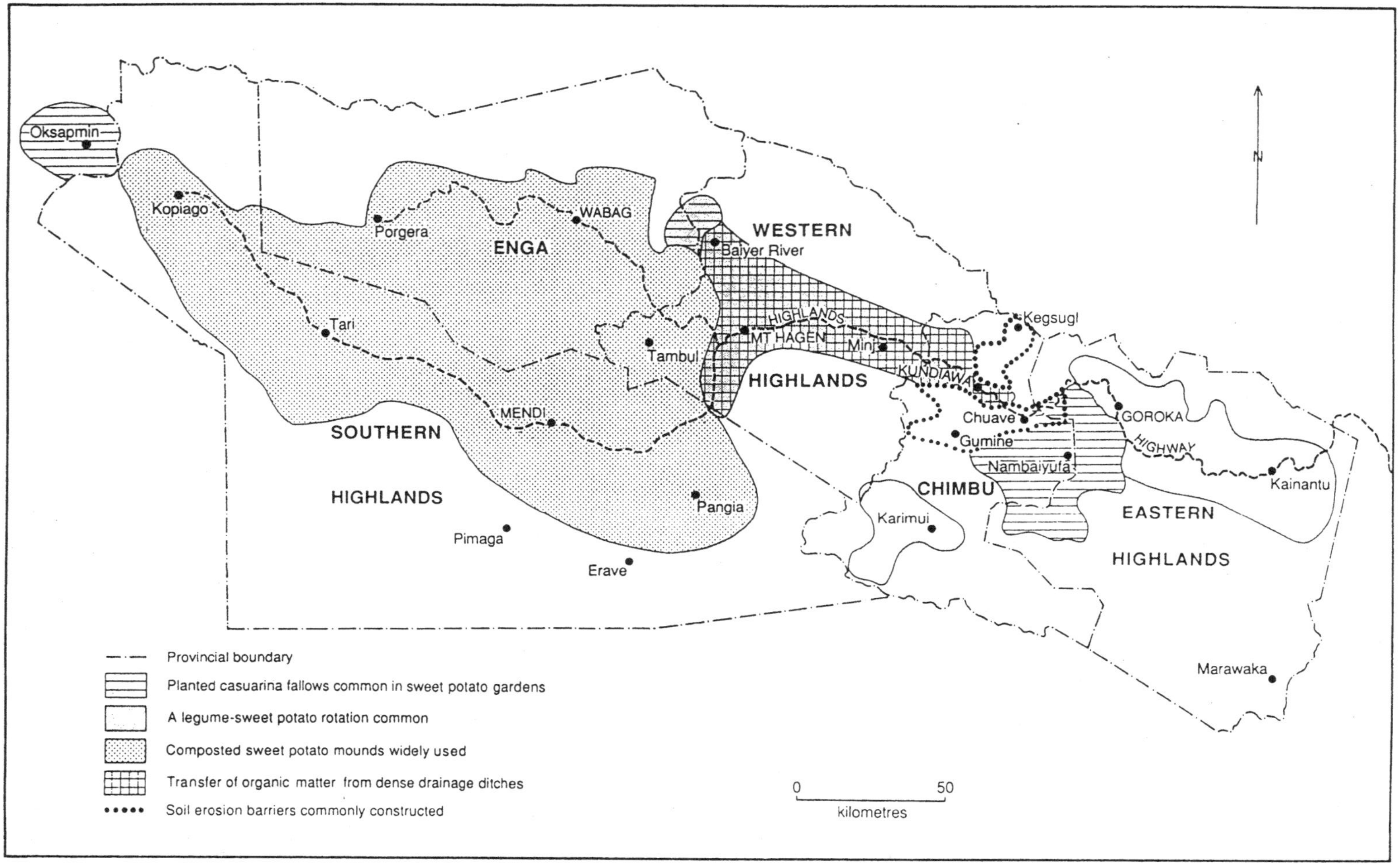

Figure 6. Soil conservation and fertility enhancement techniques used in the Papua New Guinea Highlands

Note: This map is based on surveys done between 1980 and 1982 by R. M. Bourke. Fieldwork in 1990 modified the information slightly and the final format will be different from this map.

Figure 1. Post-fieldwork data and map preparation methods

Figure 2. Example of a one-page summary for a sub-system

Figure 3. Example of a text description of an agricultural system

Figure 4. Number of times that staple crops are planted in major gardens before a long fallow in the Eastern Highlands Province

Figure 5. The length of the long fallow period in years in the Eastern Highlands Province

Figure 6. Soil conservation and fertility enhancement techniques used in the Papua New Guinea highlands

DEVELOPMENT AND ENERGY

D. YEBOAH-AMANKWAH

INTRODUCTION

This year's Waigani Seminar focusses on population, family health and development. Energy has much to do with all of these subjects, particularly, in enabling our plans, whatever they are, to be implemented. Today I wish to concentrate mainly on the subject of development and the influence energy has on its evolution in human societies.

Energy is an underlying enabling factor in all activities, whether human or naturally occurring. From photosynthesis to thunderstorms, from the biological activities in living cells to the gigantic currents of the oceans and the atmosphere, and from the planets to the relentless cosmological transformations in the universe around us, energy, especially in the form of gravitational energy, is the all pervasive factor supplying the force for change. The resulting transformations in the universe, as required by the law of thermodynamics, always leave the total amount of energy in the universe the same, albeit in a more disordered state. These transformations, in fact, provide the only real measure of the continuing steady decline of the universe as it winds down. This steady decline describes the direction of the flow of time from the past to the future - what Stephen Hawkings(1) has aptly described as "the arrow of time". Given the all pervasive properties of energy, it is not at all surprising that our population, our transportation system, our health and medical systems, our agriculture, - indeed, all the developments in a human society - should critically depend upon it.

This dependence of societies on energy is in fact not new, though the subject has not always been perceived in the way it is today. In what follows I shall attempt to show how critically the development of all societies is dependent on the energy that they use. The development process is complex and depends on several factors. Societies that have available supplies of energy may still fail to achieve successful development, but those without adequate supplies of energy have little chance of starting any development at all.

1 Department of Physics
University of Papua New Guinea

ENERGY USE IN THE PAST

Energy has always been essential for the survival and maintenance of all human societies since the dawn of history. Today, no less than in the past, large supplies of energy continue to be needed by man and his society. Wherever and whenever great urban societies have flourished in the past - from ancient Egypt, along the Nile delta, to the Indus river valley of modern Pakistan, and Mesopotamia, along the Euphrates and Tigris rivers - it has been in no small part due to the fact that each society had discovered effective methods for processing more energy. The additional energy supplies usually came from improved agricultural methods to harvest more solar energy, from exploitation of water falls, wind, animal and, frequently, slave power.

The increased available energy went to improvements in transportation; increased food processing, preservation and distribution; shipping, and, quite frequently, increased capacity to wage war. In short, the increase in available energy supplies led directly to increases in the quality of life or development of the society. Such situations inevitably tended to lead to population growth.

ENERGY CONSUMPTION AND DEVELOPMENT

By all accounts, the relation between development and energy is probably much stronger today than it has ever been in all history. This is due to the huge increases in the use of energy in the 20th century. For example, between 1900 and 1970 the world's energy consumption grew ten times, and it is estimated it will grow three more times by the year 2000 (2). The January 1991 Gulf war is the latest example of how far nations will go to neutralize any perceived threat to their future energy supplies. The energy factor appears to be never too far behind in questions of national development and security. National symbols of development such as modern communication networks, efficient transportation systems, elaborate sporting, entertainment and leisure facilities, efficient and mobile military power, etc., are all characterized by one thing: a high rate of energy consumption!

Development is complex and difficult to measure exactly for any society and economists are not in agreement on how it should be done. In the absence of an agreed yardstick, the per capita annual income of societies has frequently been used as a rough measure of development. We shall adopt this practice in our discussion. That there is a close relation between the amount of energy used by a society and its development, as represented by its per capita annual income, has been recognised(3,4,5). A recent study of the relation between the two quantities(6) showed a strong correlation between gross national product per capita, P, and the gross annual energy consumption per capita, E, of nations.

The result of the study which used UN World Statistics for 1979(7) is presented in Figure 1. The regression of E on P yielded eqn 1 and a correlation coefficient of 0.9.

$$P=14.1E^{0.72}$$

Figure 2 is similar to Figure 1 except that the positions of a selected number of countries have been indicated on the plot. Quite clearly energy consumption is strongly related to the per capita income of a nation.

IMPLICATIONS OF THE DEPENDENCE OF DEVELOPMENT ON ENERGY

It is evident from Figure 2 that compared to the per capita energy consumed by persons in the developed countries, the energy consumed by a person in a developing country is small. Fig. 2 shows that the developed countries led by the United States occupy the top of the graph while the developing countries all cluster around the bottom. For example, to point out the great inequality in the use of energy in the world, a United States citizen with an annual income of about 12,000 US Dollars uses a whopping 120,000 Megajoules of energy. The corresponding figures for a Bangladeshi, who lives in a typical developing country, are a mere 140 US Dollars and 1,000 Megajoules respectively. The differences in the figures are staggering and immoral! Indirectly, they point out the sort of energy consumption rates that the developing countries require to develop their societies to levels comparable to those in the developed countries. The message of the figures is simple: third world countries which wish to develop and raise the standard of living of their citizens need to increase their energy generating capacity very significantly in the future!

Already, in the forty years since the last world war, some third world countries such as Korea, Singapore, Taiwan and others, have accepted the challenge, and significant improvements in the standard of living of citizens in those countries has been achieved. Indeed, some of these countries are already on their way to joining the "top league" of developed nations.

To develop at all in the coming years, PNG would need to increase substantially its rate of energy processing. The processing rate should not be measured simply by the amount of petroleum, gas or coal the country sells. Rather it is determined by the industrial, manufacturing and agricultural activities, as well as the general level of economic activity, in the country. For example, PNG may become rich when it exports large amounts of petroleum from the Highlands.

But to develop and improve the quality of life of its citizens in a sustainable way, the energy has to be processed in its economy. In a world-wide race, PNG would need to redouble its effort to win development for its citizens.

DEVELOPMENT PROBLEMS

The problem of development is not simple. The 2,800 million people in the developing world, constituting 66 percent of the world's population, together consumed only 15 percent of the energy processed in the world in 1979. The remaining 85 percent was processed by the industrialized developed 1,300 million people of the world (7). By the year 2,000, it is estimated that on current trends, the share of the total energy going to the third world will have increased to 25 percent. In spite of these anticipated modest gains, development in the third world is not expected to register any significant rise due mainly to the persistently high growth rate of their population. At an annual population growth rate in excess of 2.5 percent in the third world countries compared to less than 0.4 percent in the developed countries, most third world countries are not likely to grow at all! In fact, many of them are headed for decline in their per capita annual income as their populations race ahead of their development effort.

There are other disturbing facts too: the earth's energy resources such as the fossil fuels, on which many developing countries have come to depend for industrial power, are finite, rapidly running out and increasingly expensive to purchase. It is estimated that, in the case of petroleum and natural gas, this resource will be depleted in all but name within the next fifty years. As the fuels become scarcer they will become increasingly more expensive to non-producing countries. Developing countries in this category which have access to only limited foreign exchange are bound to suffer serious disruption of their economies. Even where fossil fuels are available, their polluting effects on the environment are a severe constraint on their use. Destabilising effects such as global warming caused by carbon dioxide and other greenhouse gases released in the burning of the fossil fuels, acid rain and the general environmental degradation resulting from the fossil fuel economy are likely to restrict fossil fuel use in the future.

Even on the most optimistic estimates, energy production, especially the fossil based type, is bound to saturate in the immediate future. The world must quickly learn to develop new and environmentally benign sources of energy such as solar, wind, ocean thermal, hydro- and, certainly, nuclear power. All the rhetoric against it notwithstanding, most major developed countries of the world are increasing their use of nuclear power for electricity generation.

To seriously contemplate the use of these sources in the future, developing countries would need to learn quickly and master effectively the relevant technologies. They need this knowledge to keep their survival options open.

CONCLUSION

In this paper I have argued that the ready availability of energy is an essential pre-condition for ensuring that a country can successfully embark on development. This has always been true, though it needs to be emphasized that energy availability alone will not automatically guarantee development. Any nation that plans to ensure its future development, therefore, must have an effective, efficient and technically balanced programme to build up the rate at which it processes energy. The competitive environment of today's world makes such programmes absolutely necessary for national development.

For third world countries the steady increase in per capita energy consumption is likely to be an uphill task, because of their rapidly increasing population. These increases threaten to absorb all the gains in energy, thereby neutralizing their attempt to increase the per capita energy consumption rate and the accompanying associated development process.

To be effective in supporting development, the energy consumption in a country must not only be efficient, it must also be non-wasteful. For example, in tropical PNG, the architecture and the construction industry should be able to take advantage of the warm environment and avoid the large expensive energy gobbling structures and systems - government and private - which are mostly inoperable in the absence of working air conditioning plants. Strict energy conservation methods must be practiced to reduce energy wastage to a minimum. In this connection, it is difficult to justify the several large multiple-storey office buildings and new hotels that have been constructed in Port Moresby in recent times. Such buildings - mostly windowless glass structures - can not be used when there is no electrical power. Development has nothing to do with "copying architectural practices of the developed temperate countries of the world".

As petroleum runs out in the next fifty years or so, the need to develop new sources of energy has become increasingly urgent. For PNG and many similar developing countries, the obvious alternative sources are solar energy in its various forms, hydropower, wind power and ocean thermal power (Manus Island has the second best site in the Pacific region for this type of power generation)(9). While these sources are environmentally benign, they also make it possibly to save the precious petroleum resource for more essential industries in the chemical and pharmaceutical sectors of the economy. Despite the controversy surrounding nuclear energy, some attention will also need to be given to the use of nuclear power.

All the evidence points to increasing use of nuclear energy by the developed countries to generate electricity, notwithstanding the critical rhetoric against its use.

The short life expectancy of the fossils on which many countries depend for power and the increasing danger to the climate by the greenhouse gasses released by burning fossil fuels pose a serious dilemma to man and his civilization. Nations, especially developing nations, which have little room to manoeuver need to keep their options under constant review if they are not to be overtaken by the imminent depletion of the fossil fuels on which their economies hinge. Petroleum is bound to become expensive as it is depleted in the future so that countries, like PNG, which have deposits on their territory are lucky indeed! Selling the product off in advance for cash to be burned in cars may not be the wisest way of using that resource in the future. Keeping the product for industrial use in the country while concentrating on developing alternative sources of energy may be a far better option for the country's development in the future.

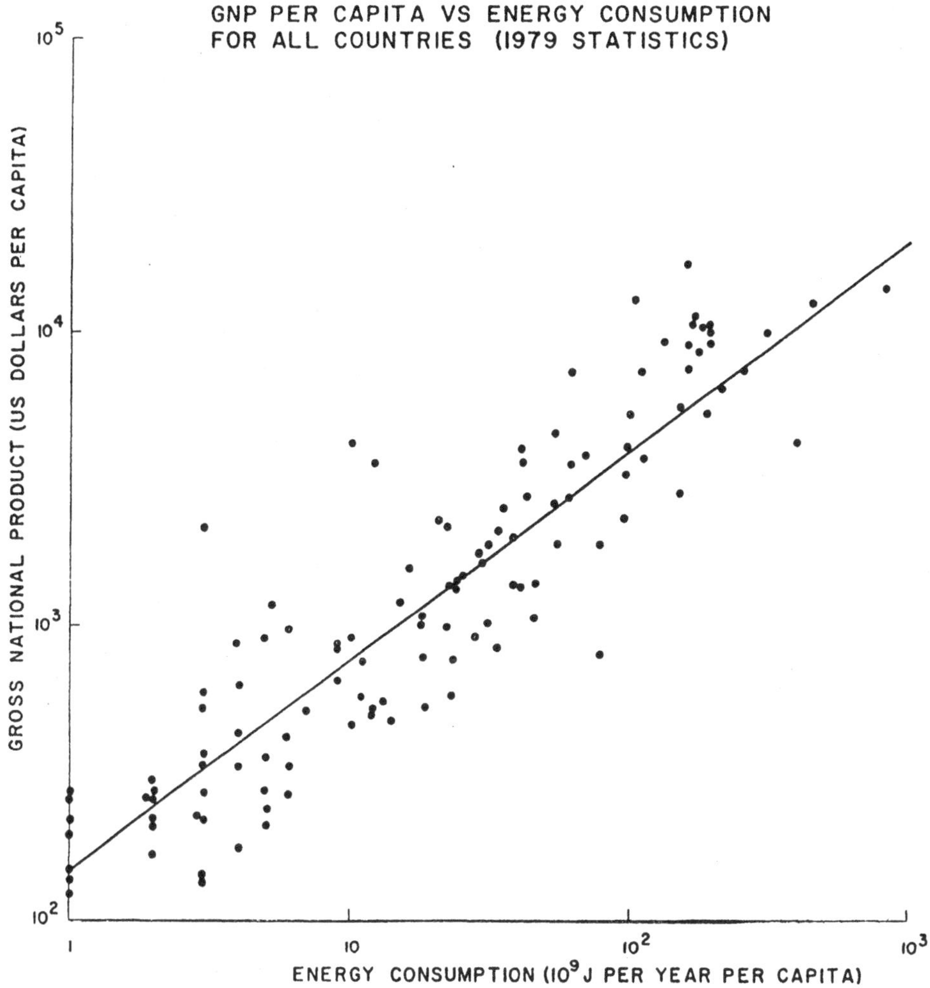

Fig 1. Plot of per capita gross national product (GNP) versus per capita energy consumption for all countries using 1979 UN statistics.

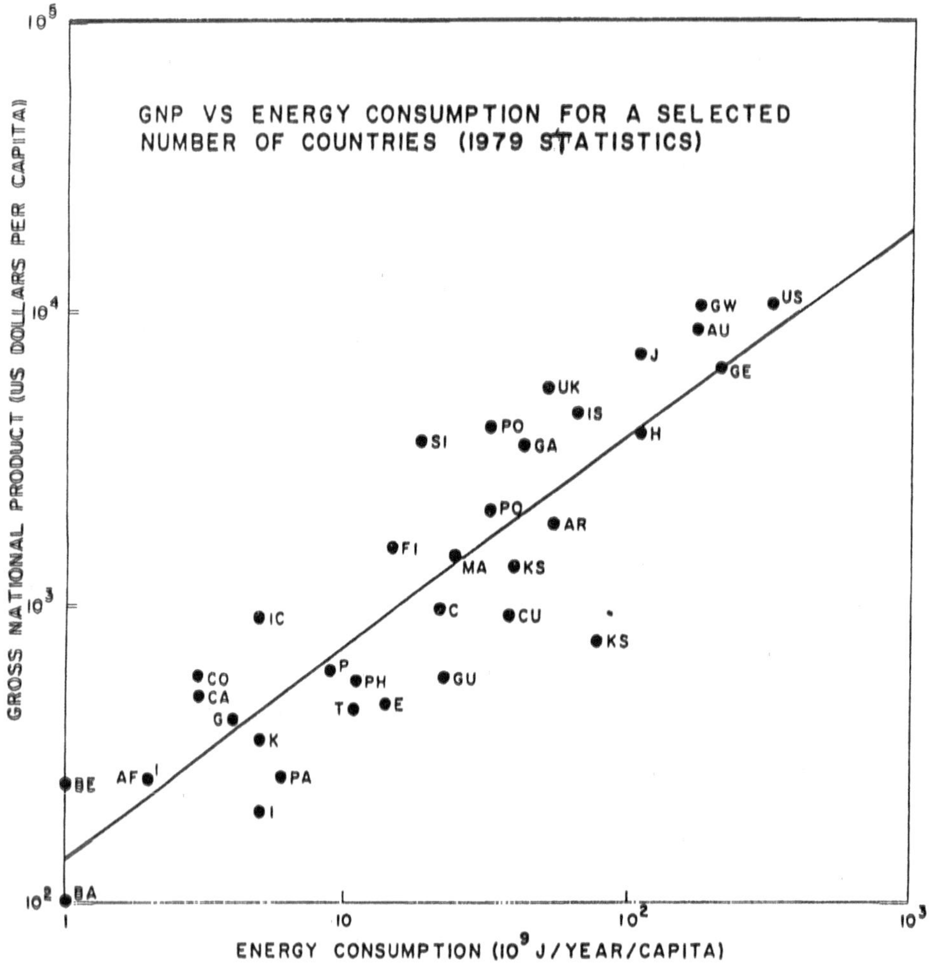

Key

AF	-	Afganistan;	AL	-	Algeria;	Ar	-	Argentina
AV	-	Australia;	B	-	Belgium;	BA	-	Bangladesh
BE	-	Benin;	C	-	Colombia;	CO	-	Congo
CU	-	Cuba;	E	-	Egypt;			
F	-	Fiju;	G	-	Ghana;	GE	-	East Germany
GU	-	Guyana;	GW	-	West Germany;	H	-	Hungary
I	-	India;	IC	-	Ivory Coast;	IS	-	Isreal
J	-	Japan;	K	-	Kenya;	KN	-	North Korea
KS	-	South Korea;	P	-	Pakistan;	PH	-	Phillipines
P	-	PNG:	SI	-	Singapore;	T	-	Tonga
UK	-	U.K:	US	-	U.S			

Fig 2. Plot of per capita gross national product (GNP) versus per capita energy consumption for a selected number of countries. (1979 UN statistics have been used)

REFERENCES

1. Hawkings S. 1990. The arrow of time. 1990 Science Year Book of Science and the Future, page 44. Encyclopaedia Britannica.

2. Sorenson B. 1979: Renewable Energy. Academic Press.

3. Starr C. 1971: Energy and Power. Sci, Amer. vol 225

4. Twidell J. 1979: Energy with harmony in the Third World. Electrical Review International vol 204 No 6

5. McGown L B and Bockris J O. 1980: How to obtain Abundant Clean Energy. Plenun Press.

6. Yeboah-Amankwah D. 1985: Energy: the challenge of the future. University of Papua New Guinea Professorial Lecture.

7. United Nations. 1981. United Nations Year Book of World Statistics.

8. Vaclav S and Knowland W E. 1980: Energy in the Developing World - The Real Energy Crises, page 23. Oxford University Press.

9. Takahashi P K: Renewable Resources for Island Economies. Proceedings of the: Second National Seminar on Renewable Energy for Rural Development, November 1 - 3 1989, Lae, PNG. Edited by F. Welt.

SANITATION AND HEALTH IN URBAN SETTLEMENTS OF PAPUA NEW GUINEA

GILBERT BUKENYA[1]

INTRODUCTION

Approximately one-third of the urban population in Papua New Guinea live in settlements characterised by a lack of potable water, inadequate or no means of disposal of human or animal faeces, no garbage disposal facilities, a high density of insects and rodents, very low standards of both personal and domestic hygiene and intense crowding in rudimentary housing, often with no lighting. In 1974, it was estimated that, on average, 7 people occupied a dwelling in the urban village and 9 people occupied a dwelling in the squatter settlement in the National Capital District. The situation has since worsened. Furthermore, these settlements have a typical physical and social environment that combines a high incidence of domestic and street accidents and extreme poverty with lack of parental supervision, child abandonment, social isolation, insecurity, domestic violence and family break down, drug/stimulant use and cultural conflict.

THE SITUATION: 1988-1990

From studies that have been carried out in urban settlements of Port Moresby, nearly 70% of the inhabitants do not have a proper toilet facility (Table I). The adults defaecate in nearby bushes during the day but it is not clear what happens when one is pressed in the night. Twenty two percent of the settlement inhabitants use pit-latrines, which are often very shallow, smelly and very badly kept, 7% use sanitary pans and, if they have succeeded in paying the collection fees, the pans are emptied by the NCDC services. When they cannot afford payments, which is very common, the mother of the house usually takes charge of the emptying with potentially grave consequences, since it is this same mother who prepares the

[1] Department of Community Medicine
University of Papua New Guinea

food for the family and is likely to contaminate it. This is worsened when there is lack of water for washing the hands, when the mother has poor knowledge regarding hygiene (a very common thing), or simply lacks the time to wash her hands after manipulating faeces because of the burden of work. The very few relatively better-off individuals (1%) use flush toilets with septic tanks or are connected to the sewer system.

Table I: Environmental characteristics of a sample of households living in settlements around Port Moresby

Factor	Number of households using facility No (%)
Type of toilet used by household:	
Bush	543 (69.6)
Pit latrine	174 (22.3)
Bucket	55 (7.0)
Flush	8 (1.0)
Total	**780 (100)**
Type of house:	
Permanent	23 (3.0)
Semi-permanent	94 (12.00)
Temporary	663 (85.0)
Total	**780 (100)**

In most settlements the children as a whole, defaecate indiscriminately in the compounds, and unfortunately this habit is encouraged by mothers because they generally view children's faeces as non-polluting. This implies that baby faeces are not carefully disposed of, care is not taken to wash the hands that handle them, and as a result contamination of food, particularly weaning food, is accentuated.

It must be strongly emphasised that human faeces, especially those of child origin, are among the most contaminating substances with which people can come into contact. They are the principal source of the pathogenic organisms causing many communicable diseases, particularly infections of the intestinal tract. This makes their proper disposal a priority in every community.

Clean water, a requirement of every human being, is often lacking, inadequate, or inaccessible to most people living in urban settlements. The estimate of urban settlement inhabitants connected to the town supply in Port Moresby is about 40% (Table I). As a consequence, water is stored in large quantities for drinking, increasing its chances of contamination. Because the supplies are small, little or no water is used for hygienic purposes, e.g. washing hands after handling faeces, emptying sanitary pans or before handling food. Often lack of hygiene in these poor areas has been blamed on the people themselves, without realising that these people lack the requirements for good hygiene.

A direct link between absence of facilities for the safe disposal of excreta and the incidence of diarrhoea and other faecal-oral diseases such as typhoid has been well established. In the last three years in Port Moresby, virtually all diagnosed cases of typhoid have come from the settlements (Table 2). The most vulnerable age group is that of children below the age of five. It is estimated that in urban settlements, a child born today is 40-50 times more likely to die before the age of five than one born at the same time in a prosperous neighbourhood. A variety of faecal-oral diseases, often exacerbating or precipitating malnutrition, account for a large part of the mortality and morbidity in these children. Although, on average, a Papua New Guinean child suffers one episode of diarrhoea in a year, children from these settlements suffer on average 2.4 episodes of diarrhoea per year (Table 2).

Table 2: The distribution of cases of typhoid, childhood diarrhoea and gonorrhoea in settlement and non-settlement areas of Port Moresby between 1988 and 1990.

Disease	Cases from settlements		Cases from non-settlement areas		Total case in Port Moresby	
	No	(%)	No	(%)	No	(%)
Diarrhoea*.	12583	(70.6)	5243	(29.4)	27826	(100)
Gonorrhoea**:	4289	(75.0)	1430	(25.0)	5719	(100)
Typhoid***:	377	(96.9)	12	(3.1)	389	(100)

* Ratio settlement: non-settlement of 2.4:1

** Ratio settlement: non-settlement of 3.0:1

*** Ratio settlement: non-settlement of 31.4:1
Data from EPINT report

With the emergence of AIDS, sexually transmitted diseases pose a particularly significant public health problem. It has been well demonstrated that those who suffer from other sexually transmitted diseases, especially those causing genital ulcers, are at a high risk of getting AIDS. We found in our survey that for every case of gonorrhoea in more prosperous neighbourhoods, three cases of gonorrhoea will be seen in the settlements (table 2). In addition, although no cases of donovanosis were recorded in the prosperous neighbourhoods, donovanosis was common in the settlements.

DISCUSSION

The situation in the urban settlements is grave, and we may witness extensive epidemics of communicable diseases especially typhoid, the most lethal of all enteric diseases, and AIDS. We may also see more problems related to mental stress such as crime, homicide, and a general breakdown in law and order.

It must be recognised that resources in the past that have been devoted to the social, psychological and physical health needs of the people in these settlements have been very limited. What is worrying is that these people are expected to take responsibility for their own garbage, waste disposal and water while those in middle and upper classes are provided with these services.

The legal status of some of these settlements has also been questioned. This has resulted in the reluctance of local governments to provide basic services, lest they be seen as acknowledging their right to exist. This has been a big draw-back and needs urgent political solution. I would like to propose that services such as water supply, excreta disposal, garbage collection and housing be classified as essential services for human existence, and that they should be available and accessible at a price that can be afforded by the poor sector of the people. It may be stressed that such services protect more than just the people they serve. They also help to minimise the threat to more prosperous rate payers implicit in potential disease foci in their midst. Many of the problems seen in these settlements were major issues a century ago in the industrialised nations, and were associated with high infant deaths and outbreaks of diseases of poor sanitation such as typhoid. The impressive decrease in infant mortality in these nations was due to provision of potable water and sewerage disposal, improved quality of housing, education of mothers, and improved weaning foods.

If this humanitarian concern is acceptable to the authorities, then local governments such as the National Capital District Interim Commission remain the most appropriate level of government from which the cheapest and most effective public action can be initiated to tackle the environmental problem. Furthermore, people in these settlements appear to confide more in these local authorities.

The task of improving this situation is not an easy one but it is not impossible either. Introduction of new technologies must be done with great care and after full consultation with the people they are intended for. The technologies for sanitation, water and housing must be appropriate, affordable, and culturally acceptable. The other activity that must be considered when introducing these new technologies is income-generating technology. This has proved to be an important component of the programme of inner city improvement where such programmes have been carried out.

For these programmes to succeed, a coordinated effort is a pre-requisite, and sustainability with the full participation of the communities concerned must be the pivotal point. Political decisions will have to be made especially about priorities in the allocation of resources for the improvement of housing, water supply and construction of excreta disposal facilities.

Sanitation in these communities is appalling, and has resulted in extensive social, mental and physical ill-health. The distinct possibility exists that, wide spread epidemics, particularly of typhoid will occur in these communities unless something is done. It is thus in our own self-interest, as well as those of the people directly affected, that remedial and preventive measures should be hastened.

ENVIRONMENTAL HAZARDS AND HUMAN HEALTH CONCERNS OF LEAD, MERCURY, CADMIUM AND ARSENIC

K. SINGH[1]

Lead, mercury, cadmium and arsenic cause hazards to human health when people are exposed to elevated levels of these metals. Mercury, cadmium and arsenic are identified often as reaching people via aquatic based food-chains, including fish and shellfish. Lead sources include atmospheric particulates, especially from automobiles and from combustion processes, re-entrainment of lead contaminated dust to children, leaded paints, and foodstuffs contaminated with solder. Lead from water pipes is still a significant problem in some places. Harmful effects of lead were known in the second Century BC in ancient Greece (1).

Over the years, physicians became increasingly familiar with the symptoms of metal poisoning arising in occupational exposed workers and in individuals cases of poisoning. Certain effects only become apparent at particular stages of the exposure scale. In cases of high exposure, clinical signs and symptoms can be observed. At lower exposure levels clinical manifestations may be absent but effects may be observed at the physiological or biochemical level (See Table 1).

[1] Department of Chemistry
University of Papua New Guinea

Table 1: MAJOR METABOLIC FACTORS ASSOCIATED WITH ENVIRONMENTAL EXPOSURE TO LEAD, MERCURY, CADMIUM AND ARSENIC.

Major routes of Entry	**Lead**	**Mercury**	**Cadmium**	**Arsenic**
	Ingestion and Inhalation	Ingestion	Ingestion and Inhalation (tobacco)	Ingestion
Gastrointestinal absorption (%)	~10	~95*	~5**	>80*
Organs of accumulation	Bone, kidney and liver	Brain, liver and kidney	kidney & liver	keratinous tissue
Major routes of excretion	Urine	Faeces	Urine	Urine
Biological half-life	~20 years	~70 days	>10yrs	10 - 30 hours

* Methyl mercury and various arsenic compounds are absorbed efficiently

** Gastrointestional absorption of cadmium is enhanced considerably in individuals with iron deficiency.

Health Effects and Populations Affected

A. LEAD

The major health effects of lead (2) are manifest in <u>three</u> organ systems:

1. **Haematological system**

   Inhibition of ALA-D (aminolevulinic acid dehydratese) and haem synthetase resulting in reduced haem synthesis and causing anaemia.

2. **Nervous System**

   Central nervous system (CNS) impairment at moderate exposure in children, reflected by inattention, cognitive difficulties, fine motor dysfunction and altered EEG patterns. Heavy exposure causes encephalophathy.

3. **Renal System**

Functional impairment of the tubular region characterized by mild aminoaciduria, glucosuria and hyperphosphaturia. Long term heavy exposure may result in irreversible nephropathy.

Children represent the critical group with respect to environmental lead exposure. The particular populations considered to be at most risk are:

i. Pre-school children living in urban areas, particularly in those countries where lead is added to petrol.

ii. Children living in proximity of point sources of lead such as smelters and scrap yards.

iii. Children living in areas with lead plumbing and served by plumbosolvent water.

iv. Children living in housing with high leaded paintwork in poor condition.

B. **MERCURY**

Methylmercury intoxication (3) is characterized by effects on the CNS associated with the sensory, visual and auditory functions and those concerned with coordination.

Early effects are paraesthesia in the tongue, lips and distal extremities. In severe cases, blurred and constricted vision and ataxia may appear.

The developing nervous system of the foetus is more sensitive to methyl mercury than the adult. Prenatal exposure can result in neurotoxic effects in the infant in the absence of effects in the mother. Pregnant women are apparently more sensitive to methylmercury than other adults.

In the last 30 years, there have been several outbreaks of methylmercury intoxication:

<u>From Fish</u>

1. "Minamata disease" took place in Japan in the 1950s and 1960s - this was caused by long term ingestion of contaminated fish.

2. Reported association between several neurological parameters and methylmercury intakes from fish among Canadian Indians.

Other populations with heavy fish consumption have also been identified in the Mediterranean (in Italy), Papua New Guinea, Peru, New Zealand and Seychelles.

From alkyl mercury fungicides

Iraqi epidemic (1971-72) - resulted from consumption of bread prepared from grain dressed with alkylmercury fungicides. Previous outbreaks of this type were: Iraq (1956, 1960), Pakistan (1969), Guatemala (1963-65), Ghana (1967). Clearly the inadvertant ingestion of seed treated with organic mercury as a fungicide is a hazard.

C. CADMIUM

The kidney is the critical organ of intoxication after long-term exposure to cadmium (4).

One of the initial signs of renal dysfunction is an increased urinary excretion of low molecular weight proteins.

Many areas of Japan are contaminated with cadmium, as a result of discharges from numerous non-ferrous mines and smelters. Long-term consumption of rice grown in these areas has resulted in elevated cadmium exposure levels and signs of renal dysfunction in several localities.

A syndrome termed 'itai-itai' characterised by severe renal dysfunction and damage to bone structure has also been identified. The disease predominantly affected elderly women with poor nutritional status.

D. ARSENIC

In the case of arsenic, both inorganic compounds as arsenates (As^{5+}) or as arsenites (As^{3+}), and organic compounds such as arsenobetaine and arsenocholine can give rise to health effects in a large number of organs (5), (Table 2).

TABLE 2: HEALTH EFFECTS ATTRIBUTED TO ARSENIC

Organ affected		Effects
Skin	-	Hyperpigmentation Hyperkeratosis Skin tumours
Lungs	-	Lung cancer
Liver	-	Liver dysfunction
Cardiovascular system	-	Peripheral vascular disturbances leading to gangrene
Nervous system	-	Peripheral neuropathy Hearing defects
Reproductive system	-	Increased frequency of spontaneous abortions

TABLE 3: ESTIMATED THRESHOLD VALUES FOR CHRONIC EXPOSURE TO LEAD, METHYL MERCURY, CADMIUM AND INORGANIC ARSENIC.

Metal	Estimated Threshold	Reported values in the general population background
Lead	15-20 ug/dl Blood lead	10 - 20 ug/dl
Methyl Mercury	20 ug/g (hair) 80 ng/ml (blood)	2 ug/g 10 ng/ml
Cadmium	150 ug/day dietary intake	20 - 70 ug/day
Arsenic (Inorganic Compds)	200 ug/l in drinking water	2 ug/l

REFERENCES

1. Waldron, H A. (1973). Lead Poisoning in the Ancient World. Med. Hist. (London), 17, 391 - 399.

2. Lin-Fu, J. (1980). Lead poisoning and undue lead exposure in children: history and current status. In Needleman, H L. (Ed.), Low Level Lead Exposure: The Clinical Implications of Current Research, pp 5 - 16, Raven Press, New York.

3. WHO. (1976). Environmental Health Criteria 1. Mercury. World Health Organization, Geneva: 131 pages.

4. Bernard, A, Buchet, J P, Roels, H, Masson, P, and Lauwerys, R. (1972). Renal excretion of proteins and enzymes in workers exposed to cadmium. Eur. J. Clin. Invest., 9, 11 - 22.

5. Pershagen, G (1983). The epidemiology of human arsenic exposure. In Fowler, B A (Ed.), Biological and Environmental Effects of Arsenic, pp. 199 - 232, Elsevier/North-Holland Biomedical Press, Amsterdam.

A RETURN TO THE REGIONAL CENTRE

POPULATION POLICY, HUMAN RESOURCE DEVELOPMENT AND URBAN DEVELOPMENT IN PAPUA NEW GUINEA

T S AND S H ILAVE[1]

1. INTRODUCTION

The 19th Waigani Seminar focusses overdue attention on population growth, family health and development issues. The endorsement in 1990, of the new Integrated National Population Policy provides an excellent opportunity to bring to the forefront of development discussions, the required consideration of the human element in development. The need to consider, again, the fact that in addition to other resources that PNG has had the fortune to be endowed with, the further advancement of the country is critically dependant upon the effective use of PNG's human resources and their continued enrichment through education, skills formation, improved health, nutrition and other means. Inadequate attention to human resource development, has immediate and painful short term social consequences such as the increased incidence of crime and the equally undesirable longer term effects of unemployment, destitution and poverty.

This paper, which is part of a larger study(1), discusses Human Resource Development (HRD) issues from the migration and employment perspectives. On the subject of migration, the new population policy recognizes the unbalanced social and economic development between the rural and urban areas as a contributing factor and Paragraphs 1.6 and 1.7 in the Integrated National Population Policy (INPP) brings this out and we quote:

> "...Internal migration, especially rural to urban is a consequence of unbalanced socio-economic development. This is inevitable in an industrializing country. However, urban biased facilities in health, education, employment and labour market and wage structures may influence rural-urban migration. Neither economic efficiency nor social equity can be attained without a balanced and mutually supporting development of the rural and urban sectors.

1 ESCAP/UNDP is sponsoring this study on Small Town development, Migration and Human Resource Development in PNG and five (5) other countries in the Asia Pacific Region

The need for decentralization and expansion of the urban industrial infrastructure is highlighted. Rise in the urban population has always been directly related to urban problems, but concentration of population in one area can make work easier for Government services and industrial development. Urban growth need not be ignored but it should be guided in appropriate ways." **(National Population Policy, 1990: Paragraphs. 1.6 and 1.7; pp 4-5**

The Policy stance we have just indicated, could remain only as such - just rhetoric and tokenism, for additional decades to come, unless action oriented programmes in support of the policy are immediately put in place. Some similar industrial dispersement programmes in other countries have had limited success and part of the reason for this is attributed to imbalances in HRD utilization and availability among different areas.

It seems to us that one of the ways of doing this i.e, guiding urban development in appropriate ways, is perhaps to redefine the concept of Human Resource Development. What is really meant by HRD?

2. HUMAN RESOURCE DEVELOPMENT (HRD) CONCEPT

The Goal of "integral human development" is already established by the National Constitution and a number of Government programmes. In general terms however, it is perhaps not incorrect to say that the issue of HRD has never really been defined in specific enough terms in order to provide a basis from which a plan of action could be formulated and launched. Several implicit tendencies by authorities to address the issue could nevertheless be identified. We go on to discuss the HRD concept below.

Firstly, as an **employment/unemployment** issue; particularly in the light of the concern over a rapidly increasing population and the changing demographic structure of the population which results in a growing youthful labour force, which the formal sector cannot fully absorb. This rapid growth furthermore brings about pressure on the government's public service and budgetary resources in maintaining and expanding education, health, housing, and related infrastructure and other social services. The related issue of internal rural to urban migration, further complicates the concern, since, the spatial distribution of the population becomes unbalanced as human resources in the rural/agriculture sector becomes depleted while simultaneously more pressure is applied for the provision of services in the urban areas.

Secondly, the HRD issue in PNG has also largely been addressed as a narrower **Human Capital** issue, where the greatest need is identified to be that of upgrading human resources to meet economic growth requirements. The Government's progressive localization plan for the labour force since independence has emphasized the need for the country to be self reliant in manpower. Furthermore, its various national Manpower Assessment exercises, as well as the new Training Policy and indeed, all formal education and training programmes are aimed mostly at this skilled manpower development aspect of HRD.

It seems to us that the approach in the INPP goes further and well beyond HRD as just a form of productive capital. A broader concept encompassing both the means and the end of development is implied; the attitude seems to be that the opportunities provided by HRD should facilitate broad-based participation by the people in the development process, with special provisions to enhance the status of the disadvantaged sections of our community including women and youth.

The following are some initial observations on the Manpower and Employment aspects of HRD.

3. POPULATION AND THE LABOUR FORCE

Although, the country is richly blessed with natural resources, the rapid population growth and especially labour force growth in the towns cannot be matched by the employment generating capacity of the economy. In addition, the labour market reflects the dual character of the economy where there is the small stagnant formal wage sector, while a larger proportion of the population is supported by the agriculture sector, which is affected by low productivity and incomes. Non-agricultural employment and income generating activities are basically non-existent. Furthermore, the mining sector is currently an enclave sector which creates very little direct employment.

3.1 Labour Force Structural Characteristics based on the 1980 census

The PNG labour force of 1.54 million represented 74 per cent of the Economically Active Population (EAP) in 1980.

On the relative distribution of the EAP, the 1980 census shows that less than 10 percent of the EAP was in formal sector wage employment, reflecting the small size of the formal sector work force, while over 25 percent were engaged in some kind of money raising activities other than formal wage employment, and over one-quarter entirely within the subsistence sector. A significant two-thirds of the EAP were engaged in activities in and related to agricultural production. The 1980 census data further shows that many of those in small or large scale business and in other sectors of the formal economy were either directly or indirectly engaged in agricultural production.

The distribution of the work force obviously follows the distribution of the population. The share of labour force by the three sectors in 1980 are: urban 9.6 percent, rural non-village 5.4 percent and rural 85 percent.

To calculate the level of unemployment in an economy with a very strong subsistence base proves problematic. Persons who were very actively seeking employment only represent 2.4 percent of the labour force. However if we were to include those who were not openly seeking work, the unemployment rates would be 16.6 percent nationwide, with higher rates of 25 percent for urban areas. The incidence of unemployment by whichever estimates seems to be highest in urban areas.

According to the 1986 National Manpower Assessment document, the PNG formal sector labour force is relatively youthful, inexperienced and has low educational qualifications.

The relatively limited education and experience of the citizen work force is also reflected in the continuing large employment of non-citizens. The chronic shortage of trained Papua New Guineans constitutes a continuing hindrance to self-reliant growth. The progressive localization of the labour force is thus a major government objective. An objective which has since independence become synonymous with HRD.

At the same time the formal sector cannot keep pace with the increase in the labour force let alone reduce the numbers dependent upon subsistence agriculture or upon other informal rural and urban activities. The implication of this is that most efforts to increase the number of job opportunities must concentrate on the informal and rural sectors particularly agriculture, in which the vast majority of the population are involved.

However, in contrast to the urban situation, very little is known about rural labour markets in PNG. Very little is known statistically about trends in the composition of the rural labour force. In the past, the bulk of the rural work force consisted of single men, not normally resident in the province where they were working, living in accommodation provided by the plantation under an agreement system. To what extent this has evolved is not known, particularly the growth in cash-cropping and increasing integration with the market system by those who had been purely subsistence farmers. Today, the rural population retains an alternative to wage employment.

An important observation from the 1966, 1971 and 1980 Censuses is that informal money-raising activities, own-businesses (large or small scale), self-employment including helpers (paid or unpaid), has shown an increasing trend: 1966 - 13.5 percent, 1971 - 22.7 percent, 1980 - 34.6 percent. This implies the possible increase in the number of self-employed 'bisnismen' using unpaid family labour. This trend suggests that opportunities to earn higher incomes in agriculture were being seized by farmers.

Another important observation is that, proportionally, more women are engaged in informal money-raising activities, (farming/fishing for money) than men. This is the only sector in which more women are engaged than men.

In this section, we have seen that most Papua New Guineans live and work in rural village agriculture. While this used to be mainly subsistence, the number engaged in cash cropping appeared to have increased rapidly. In the light of the present formal sector work force scenarios and the enclave nature of the capital-intensive projects of the mining sector, in the long run, these farmers are the vital element in PNG's development.

We now wish to briefly indicate, in the final section of this seminar paper, a couple of policy issues that we think are relevant on the subject of HRD employment generation, population distribution and migration. Basically, that an integrated approach to HRD is a very crucial requirement for the effective utilization of PNG's human resources.

Employment and human resource development issues are now very important topics because of a serious law and order problem arising from increasing youth unemployment, rural-urban population movement, and social dislocation and strain. There is a need to develop both short term and longer term strategies of employment creation, with special attention paid to particular target groups within the rural population as well as within towns.

4. CONCLUSIONS

Two basic conclusions dealing with HRD and Rural Development on the one hand, and HRD and Urban Development on the other, are outlined below

4.1 Human Resource Development and Rural Development

The two main policy considerations in the 1990s would be first the need to integrate rural areas fully and the rural population entirely into the process of socio-economic development, and secondly, to ensure rural transition towards broad-based sustainable economic development with emphasis on employment and income generation. With regard to the integration consideration, commitment to infrastructural investment like the expansion and maintenance of the road and coastal shipping network, and improved marketing and distribution channels to and from remote areas, is needed.

The modernization of the food crop sector is absolutely necessary, especially if improved female working conditions and their overall position in the labour market and the society as a whole is to be targeted. The issues of improving participation rates, as well as increasing productivity of labour and land, are critical in this regard. In addition to infrastructural support, institutional support in the form of extension services, credit and marketing outlets will be necessary.

The key to urban employment must be sought in rural development.

4.2 Human Resource Development and Urban Employment Generation.

Improvement of the absorptive capacity of the labour market in urban areas is necessary as a long term strategy. This involves addressing the issues of expanding and diversifying the urban labour market thus reducing unemployment, but at the same time, ensuring that migration to larger cities like Port Moresby and Lae is not encouraged in the process.
Promoting the development of small scale enterprises, self-employment and selected informal sector activities in smaller towns, as well as the provision of special conditions for access to credit, must be an important component of this strategy.

An ILO employment mission in 1989 listed: skill training with basic managerial training programmes on self-employment, institutional support in the form of advisory services; provision of physical infrastructure, the setting up of small scale estates where entrepreneurs can lease turn key premises; and appropriate fiscal incentives to promote the establishment of enterprises outside the main centres of Port Moresby and Lae.

However, one also needs to look into the level of minimum wages in smaller resource development linked towns, and changes in rules and regulations governing the establishment of smallscale activities in these towns, as preconditions for the start-up of small-scale enterprises.

The population policy reference we quoted at the beginning of this paper, from the new Integrated Population Policy, prepared by the Department of Finance and Planning in December 1990, simply restated an earlier official PNG Government policy declaration, made some 15 years ago, on the attainment of independence in 1975. The official government attitude towards urban development then, was a call for the control and redirection of the patterns and standards of urban development away from Port Moresby and Lae, towards smaller centres. Economic activities were to be encouraged in smaller regional centres; in areas associated with natural resource developments. These centres were to serve as "Growth Centres" for the surrounding rural areas; to provide marketing and other services to rural people as part of the overall strategy to generate rural income earning opportunities (see National Development Strategy 1976: p.35).

Perhaps it is now the time to revert seriously to the concept of these regional centres.

INDUSTRIALISATION AND LAW AND ORDER

P D FRANKLIN[1]

The topic which I have been asked to address is Industrialisation and Law and Order.

Before I move into the major part of my paper, I would like you to understand clearly what the Chamber of Commerce is.

I represent the Lae Chamber of Commerce and Industry which is a part of the PNG Chamber of Commerce and Industry. The PNG Chamber is made up of chambers of commerce in each business centre e.g. Port Moresby, Lae, Mount Hagen etc. We individually and collectively represent approximately 60-70 percent of private enterprise companies and organisations in PNG. Our members are not limited to large overseas companies but also include small nationally owned businesses.

Approximately 80 percent of all private sector employees are employed by our member companies. Therefore the total employment of chamber members is hundreds of thousands.

If one adds dependents, families and wantoks who rely on our employees' income, the number will exceed one million people. Whilst I am talking to you today I would therefore like you to appreciate that the chambers of commerce not only represent the business managers but also those people who rely on our employees to provide an income.

The improvement required to the law and order situation in PNG, coupled with an environment which encourages industrialisation of the nation, are the key areas of concern to our members.

1 President, Lae Chamber of Commerce and Industry

Our companies are only as good as the people we employ and the effect of law and order on our employees has a dramatic effect on the performance of our companies. If our companies do not perform adequately then we will have neither the incentive nor the financial resources to expand. Without expansion of the business base in PNG there will be no industrialisation. We will continue to rely on foreign aid and export income derived principally from foreign owned mining ventures.

Much has been said over the last couple of years about the law and order situation. In 1991, we have had a crime summit in Port Moresby and more recently a Drugs and Crime seminar in Lae. The Prime Minister has also announced certain initiatives aimed at controlling the law and order situation. I believe little would be gained from me presenting any further views on the law and order problems and their possible solutions other than to encourage you to keep applying pressure on the government and its various departments to take action that will improve the situation.

I would prefer now to assume something will be done to arrest the law and order problems in the short term. If we assume this to be true then we have a responsibility to pursue actions which will further promote industrialisation. Obviously an increase in industry will promote employment and the general wealth of the population. In the long term, this will also result in further improvements in the law and order situation.

The government has been looking at various methods of promoting business and took some major initiatives in 1990.

The Lae Chamber of Commerce and Industry with the support of the Morobe Provincial Government and various community groups has developed a concept, which we believe will add significantly to the government's initiatives in this area. I would like to provide you with some background and an outline of our ideas as we believe the concept could be equally successful in other centres.

The basic tenet of PNG policy has been integral development and decentralisation. In recent years this has not been successful, with PNG having <u>negative</u> growth, thus falling behind its trading partners in the Asian Region.

The history of PNG is littered with projects which have failed. Some of these involved the processing of primary products, particularly fish and peanuts, and forestry related projects. In almost every case, once the initial enthusiasm for the projects waned or the aid provided to establish the project had run out, the business failed. In pure manufacturing there have been several attempts which also failed.

Taking into account our expertise in the Morobe area, our proposal for a solution for Lae centres around the concept of an Accelerated Development Zone. At this stage we have developed this concept for the Lae area, since Lae is particularly suitable for this concept for several reasons which I will outline later.

Our concept requires that a broad plan for the industrial development of Lae be prepared. This plan would determine the industries to be encouraged to Lae. These would be the industries which would make the best use of the areas resources, for example, the downstream processing of highlands produce. The concept also requires the fast tracking of relevant infrastructure development for the area, and the approval process, for the identified projects. It also assumes that some hard, quick fix solutions, are applied to curb Lae's law and order problems in the short term.

The administration of the Accelerated Development Zone would need to be placed in the hands of suitably qualified and experienced persons. We have proposed the establishment of a development corporation which would be administered by a two tier structure (Figure 1).

Figure 1: Administration of Accelerated Development Zone

1. **Supervisory Board**

   3 Members from National Government
   2 Lae Chamber of Commerce
   1 Lae City Authority
   1 Morobe Provincial Government

2. **Executive Board**

   2 Members of the Supervisory Board
   3 Executives of the Corporation

Overall, we believe the concept will in itself provide a major incentive for investment. It will reduce the considerable obstacles to new projects and increase the probability of many projects getting started. It will also ensure that only projects which are likely to be successful (and in line with the overall development of the area) get off the ground.

Infrastructure development would also be planned, and correctly sited, built and maintained.

WHY LAE?

We believe Lae is ideally suited to be the prototype for this proposal. Lae has a number of geographic, historical and economic attributes which make it the natural locus of economic activity at the present time. It is more cost effective to concentrate on developing industry in one site rather than spread out among many centres. In particular this is an effective way of reducing set-up costs and the average cost of utilities such as power, communications and water.

Lae also has several problems (population movement, unemployment and law and order) which are considerably worse than other major centres and must be brought under control as soon as possible. Lae has been a magnet for rural migration. This will continue, bringing with it law and order problems and very high unemployment levels. It is only by putting Lae on an economic growth path that will allow proper planning, that these problems will be contained.

Lae has the potential to provide strong industrial and economic linkages both upstream and downstream. Upstream, by creating a viable and consistent market for rural produce, raw materials etc. Lae would also open up new opportunities for service industries, ranging from very low capital to highly technical and capital based industries such as bi-product recovery, engineering and electronics, and the provision of new facilities such as specialised training, private health care etc. Downstream linkages, by providing the volume to support domestic production of products which are currently imported.

Lae's superior shipping services mean that the normal disadvantages of high freight costs, both domestically and internationally, are reduced by using Lae as a base.

Lae has designated a zone at Malahang for an Industrial Development Zone. This would provide a greenfield site for attracting new major industries to Lae and provide a leading edge for the overall policy.

Finally, Lae is the link-point for much of the resources coming into the country and raw materials being exported. This will particularly be the case during the next decade with the expected high level of mineral extraction. It is therefore important that Lae be developed so that as much as possible of the overall development stays on-shore.

In conclusion, I must say we have seen much written in newspapers, discussed on television and argued in Parliament about our law and order problems and our need for industrial development. Unfortunately, we are all good at identifying the problem but particularly inept at physically implementing solutions. The action we seem to take is a band-aid approach which is ineffective in the long term and generally a waste of money. Our proposal will work, it is ready to go, it has been effectively applied in other developing countries, and I ask you to support it wherever or whenever you might hear it discussed.

This is an opportunity that Papua New Guinea cannot afford to miss!

THE IMPACT OF THE MT KARE GOLDRUSH ON THE PEOPLE OF THE TARI DISTRICT

JOHN VAIL[1]

INTRODUCTION

The Mt Kare goldrush commenced in late 1987 following the discovery of gold by a CRA prospecting team in a remote mountain valley in the Enga Province, about thirty kilometres north of Tari (Figure 1). Within a matter of months thousands of people had arrived at Mt Kare, most from Enga and Southern Highlands provinces, but some from much further afield. Conditions on the goldfields were atrocious - prospectors worked in an environment reminiscent of the World War 1 trenches and living conditions were seldom much better. Women worked alongside men, sometimes in separate teams (and it is worth noting that for many women it was their first opportunity to earn a substantial amount of cash). There were many children on the goldfields too and as time went on, whole families moved in from landowning clans, defying the health risks, lack of security, and the high cost of living. Settlements such as Maretana #2, which was occupied mainly by Huli people, were built in swamp or mud. Refuse was scattered haphazardly around the houses, there were no sanitary facilities, and clean water was difficult to obtain. Settlements were based around a makeshift helipad which provided the only means of access (apart from foot), and high transportation costs were the main reason for the exorbitant price of food and other basic necessities on the goldfields. Housing, which was rudimentary, and often grossly overcrowded, was of two main styles - traditional, with timber slab walls and a roof of wild pandanus leaves; and 'modern' (ie plastic-clad and roofed). The latter type of house had the disadvantage that moisture condensed on the ceiling during the night, when the temperature often fell to near freezing point, and dripped down onto the sleepers below.

1 Papua New Guinea Institute of Medical Research, Tari, Southern Highlands Province

EFFECTS OF THE GOLDRUSH ON TARI

The Mt Kare goldrush is said to have been one of the richest anywhere in the world this century, and probably more than 100 million Kina worth of gold was picked up by the prospectors between the end of 1987 and 1990. Its bywords, among the people of Tari at least, were instant riches, sickness, immorality and waste. And the people of Tari were certainly among those who had the greatest involvement in the goldrush: we might estimate their numbers to be about one-third to one-half of all those on the goldfields.

In an attempt to measure the effect the goldrush was having on Tari, in early 1989 we chose a sample of 600 people from three different census units around Tari, for which the Tari Research Unit already had accurate and up-to-date demographic information. The three census units, Kwangiabi, Hangapo and Waralo, were chosen to represent different degrees of involvement with the goldrush, as access to land rights was far from evenly spread within Tari. In fact, only those clans on the northern and eastern fringes of the Tari basin, such as Kwangiabi, claimed direct rights, and people from other areas who joined the goldrush based their claims either on kinship to landowning clans, through marriage, or even through friendship. People in the western half of the Tari basin, such as those at Waralo, were further inhibited from participating in the goldrush by the large scale battles, which, between 1986 and 1988, more or less split the basin in two.

THE GOLDRUSH POPULATION

The various imbalances in the composition of the gold rush population are illustrated, for the Kare Impact Study (KIS) sample, by Figure 2. As well as there being the greatest number of people from Kwangiabi, the census unit closest to the goldfields, males outnumbered females and young people exceeded older people. Neither of these two imbalances are surprising, given, on the one hand, traditional strictures on female movement, and, on the other, the harshness of the environment at Mt Kare. The graph also shows that at the time of our visit in June 1989 nearly 50% of men from Kwangiabi were prospecting, and there were about three times as many men as women on the goldfields.

SOCIOECONOMIC IMPACT OF THE GOLDRUSH

The socioeconomic impact of the goldrush can be measured by a contrast between the three census units in the KIS sample. Figure 3 looks at the sample by occupational group. It compares the foods eaten, possessions and housing of those people who remained in Tari as subsistence farmers, with those who were prospectors at Mt Kare, and those who earned a cash income. Clearly the prospectors are better off than the subsistence group in terms of both diet and possessions, but those in cash employment have the highest overall status. The graph can of course only show the general picture, and some prospectors, who struck it rich, were no doubt very much better off than the average.

Figure 4 utilises data from an earlier Tari Research Unit survey, in 1984, to show how economic status, as measured by the same wealth variables, has changed since the inception of the goldrush. Before the goldrush, Kwangiabi, the census unit designated as 'High' on this graph, was among the worst off in Tari, due to its remoteness and the poor soils in the northern part of the Tari basin. Kwangiabi has the lowest values among the three census units for each of the wealth variables in 1984.

The goldrush has enabled the area, temporarily at least, to catch up and even overtake other areas in Tari, except in respect of housing, which perhaps requires more time to respond to the stimulus of cash income. What is also striking about this graph is the indication of the overall progress Tari has made in the five year period. This growth can be attributed to the construction of the all-weather road linking Tari to the rest of the highlands in 1980, which has allowed the integration of Tari into the regional economy.

THE DEMOGRAPHIC IMPACT

As well as bringing new wealth, the goldrush is also likely to be reflected in changes in demographic variables. For example, we might wonder whether the appalling environment on the goldfields had a deleterious effect on the health of the people who worked there. Diseases such as diarrhoea, dysentery and influenza were common, and there were also a number of typhoid cases, at least two of which resulted in deaths. It is then surprising to find that Kwangiabi reports the least number of deaths per capita of the three census units during the goldrush years. To see whether this result is reflected across Tari district as a whole, we can draw upon the resources of the Research Unit's demographic data base, which covers a population of 30,000 people.

Figure 5 compares the Kare Involvement groups with each other, both before and during the goldrush. It shows that births and deaths varied little from one involvement group to another, though one can note a slight (but not statistically significant) increase in both fertility and mortality during the goldrush within the High Involvement group. Only marriages and transfers have increased rapidly during the goldrush but this effect must be placed in the perspective of longer term demographic trends, as there are quite marked annual fluctuations in the number of marriages in Tari. Having said this, it is fair to comment that the goldrush does seem to have disturbed normal patterns of marriage to some extent, leading for example to earlier marriage among males, and to bride prices being paid in cash, rather than in pigs, in the High Involvement areas. Bride prices also suffered some inflation during the goldrush in these areas. In passing, I can mention that there is supposed to be a spate of post goldrush divorces taking place now, as girls desert husbands whom they thought would support them, only to find that the money has run out!

CONCLUSION

I shall conclude by trying to draw together some of the main effects of the goldrush on Tari. Among its positive effects, we can count the increase in cash income, which allowed people, particularly (and fortuitously) in what had been the most disadvantaged areas, to buy imported foods and items such as mattresses, shoes, clothing and cooking utensils, that contribute to an improvement in living standards.

The women who participated may have experienced the most dramatic rise in their economic status, as many had had little opportunity beforehand to earn a cash income, unlike men, who traditionally travel far and wide in search of employment.

It must be said that these benefits appear to be of a far smaller magnitude than they might have been, given the huge amount of money earned on the goldfields. Although it is difficult to obtain hard data to confirm this, it seems probable that much of the gold wealth was spent either on the sometimes extortionate rates charged for food and helicopter flights at Mr Kare, or was squandered on alcohol and trips to Port Moresby. Little money was set aside for productive purposes. Many of the vehicles that were purchased during the goldrush are now said to have been wrecked or rendered unroadworthy.

As well as the benefits from the goldrush being small, they were also unevenly spread and short-lived. As has been shown, within Tari district participation in the goldrush was concentrated mainly on a few, landowning clans. Prospectors said that the gold seemed to run through their fingers - it was even said that there was a force 'pulling back' the gold as fast as they found it. The belief that the miners could not hold on to their money, and use it productively, was one reason why there have been persistent demands on CRA (now mining the alluvial gold in a joint venture with the landowners) to provide infrastructural developments, including roads, bridges, a high school and a hospital. Few, or none, of these projects seem likely to eventuate in the Tari district, unless the gold mine lasts well beyond its expected three year life (which is probable only if hard rock mining proceeds.)

One must therefore be sceptical about the value of the goldrush in 'development' terms. There were many negative aspects to the goldrush itself, such as large scale intergroup fighting, illness, prostitution, drunkeness and gambling. Unlike planned business activity, the 'pilai laki' nature of a goldrush militates against the sensible use of gains. The wastage was exacerbated by the fact that the authorities were not prepared for the goldrush and provided little assistance or advice to prospectors on how best their earnings should be spent. Had even some of the cash been used to promote sustainable long term development - which in my view, is best served by investment in smallholder farming - then perhaps the goldrush could have been counted as productive. But this opportunity was missed, and as memories of the fabulous wealth of the goldrush days fade, people will have to readjust to a subsistence lifestyle in a deteriorating physical environment and amid a steadily rising population.

ACKNOWLEDGEMENTS

The Kare Impact Study was conducted by the Tari Research Unit and was a team effort. I should like to mention in particular the interviewers Merilyn Lengo, Alia Warago, Bale Pakalu, Mai Teiyabe, Paul Komengi, Hiru Olabe and Stephen Yawari, and reporters Wilson Andane, John Tendeke and Peter Mulungu.

I would also like to thank Paul Lima, Hondale Tagili and members of the Hetapula Association at Maretana, and Ben Probert of CRAE for their assistance and hospitality at Mr Kare.

Bale Pakalu helped with logistics and Dr S Rogers assisted in the planning and preparation of KIS. Don Lewis and Tom Smith, IMR Goroka, provided advice on the statistical analysis of the data. Finally, the study would not have been possible without the cooperation of the Huli people in Tari and at Mt Kare, to whom we are grateful for their patience in answering our questions.

REFERENCES

Jackson, R. Mt Kare Colluvial Gold Project Socio-Economic Impact Study Mt Kare Mining Pty Ltd 1988

Vail, J. The Social and Economic Questionnaire in Tari 1984. Draft Report, Tari Research Unit 1987

Wood, A W. Land for tomorrow. Subsistence Agriculture, Soil Fertility and Ecosystem stability in the New Guinea Highlands. Unpublished PhD thesis, University of Papua New Guinea 1984.

Figure I: Tari Location Map

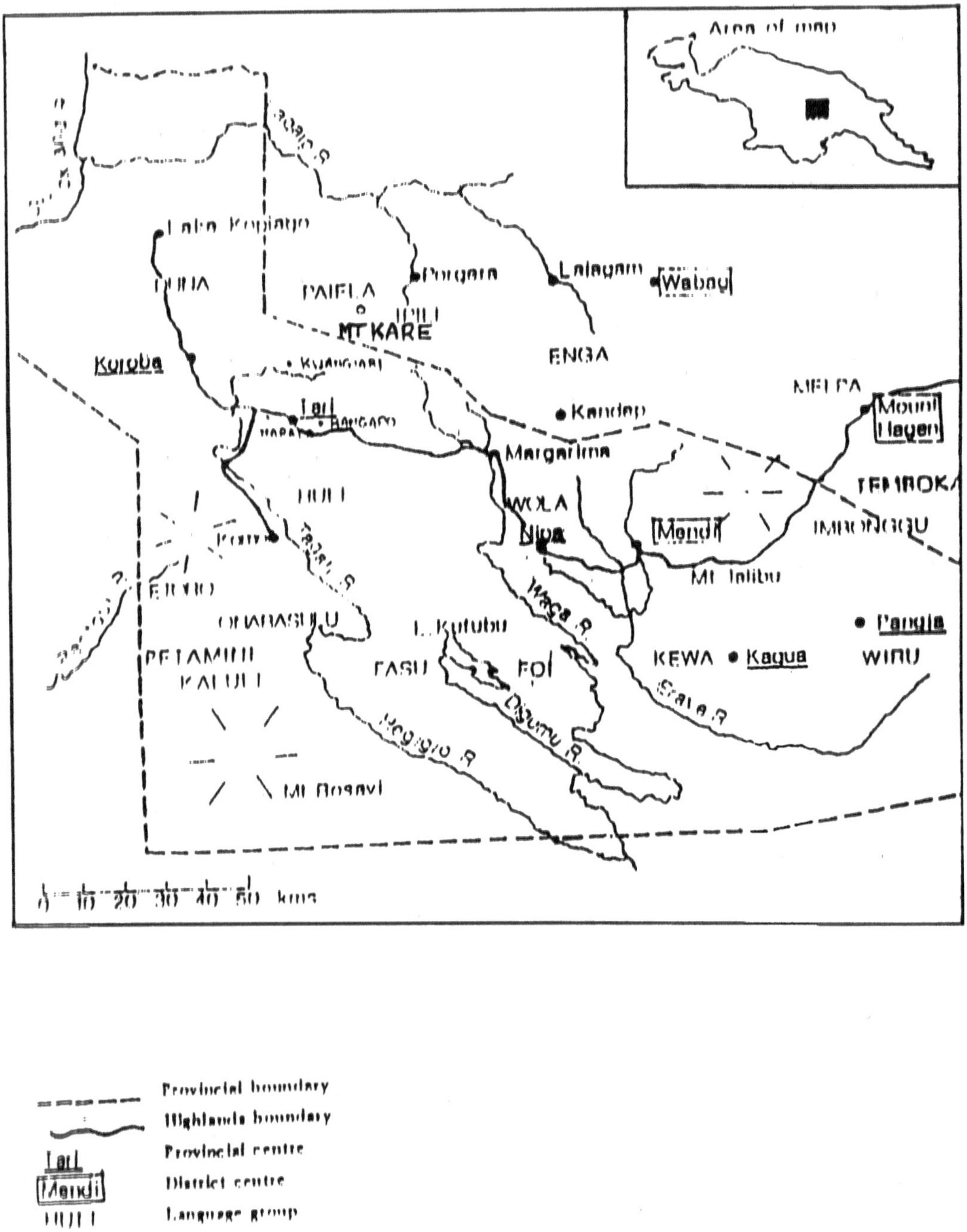

Fig 2

Visitors to Mt Kare

By Age, Sex and Census Unit
From the KIS Sample

Sample Size: Hangapo 107M 93F Kwanglabi 100M 100F Waralo 99M 101F

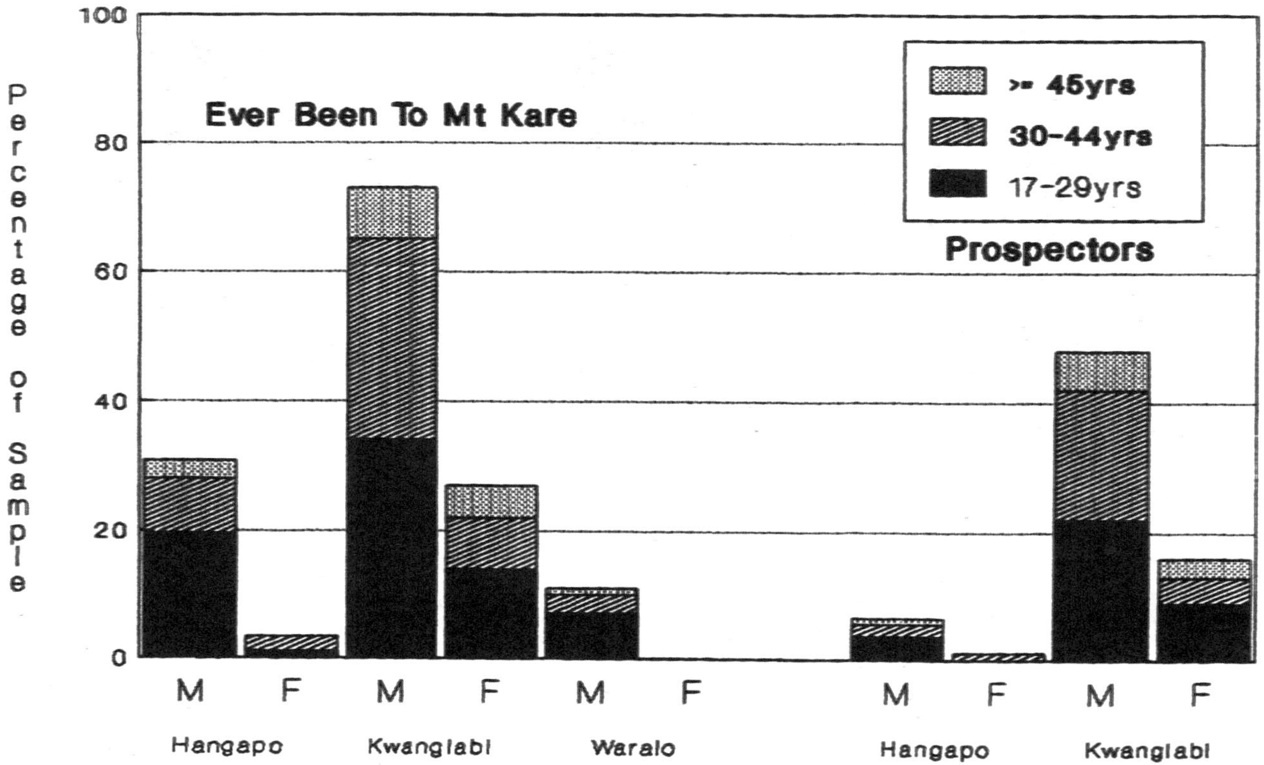

Fig 3 **Indicators of Wealth for KIS Sample**

By Occupational Group

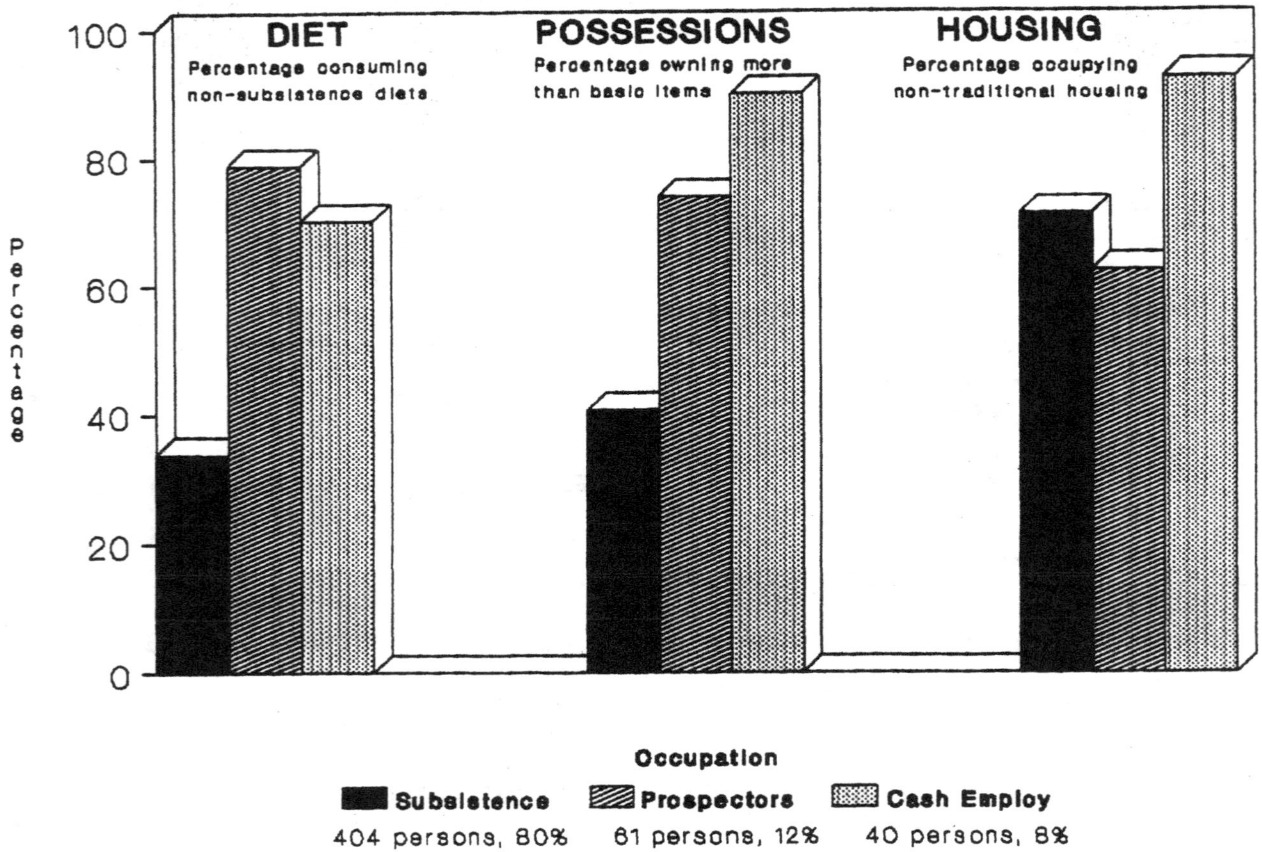

Fig 4 Changes in Economic Status 1984-89

For Census Unit Groups involved in the KIS study

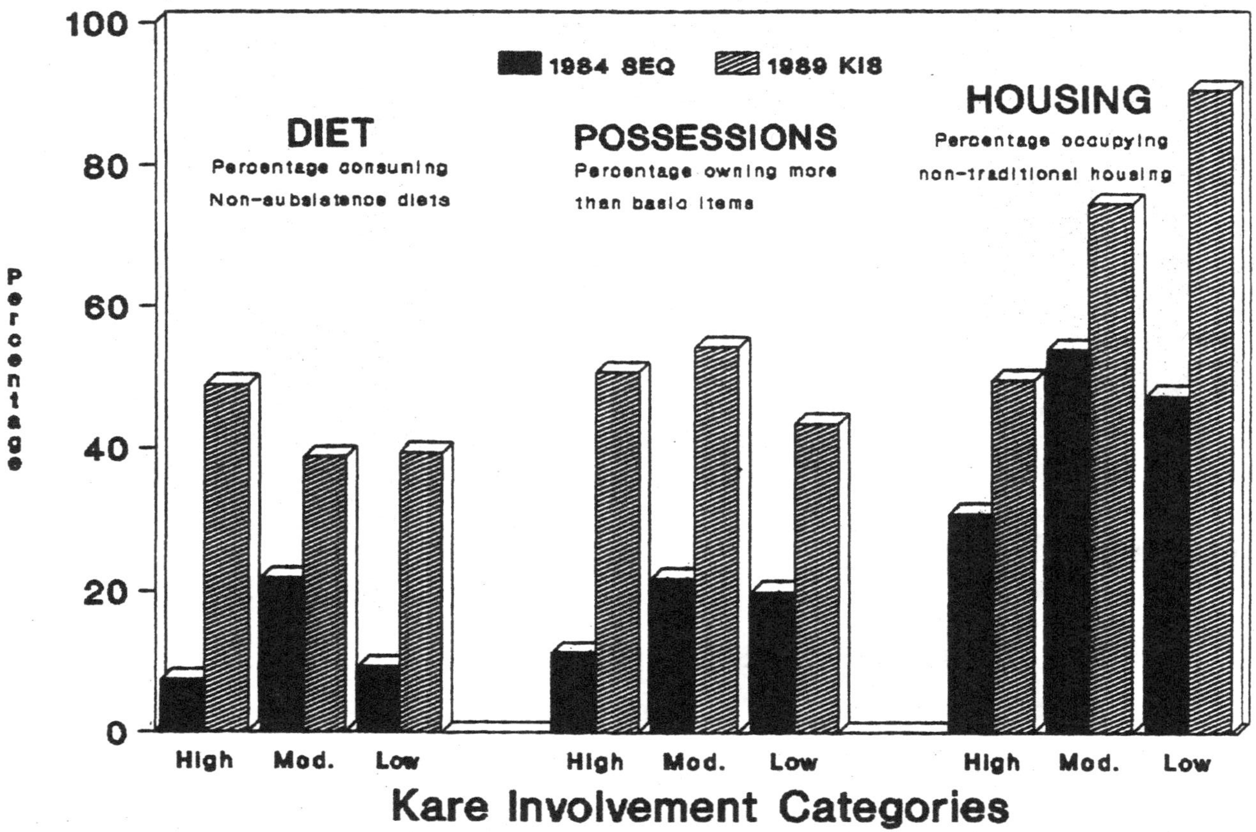

Fig 5

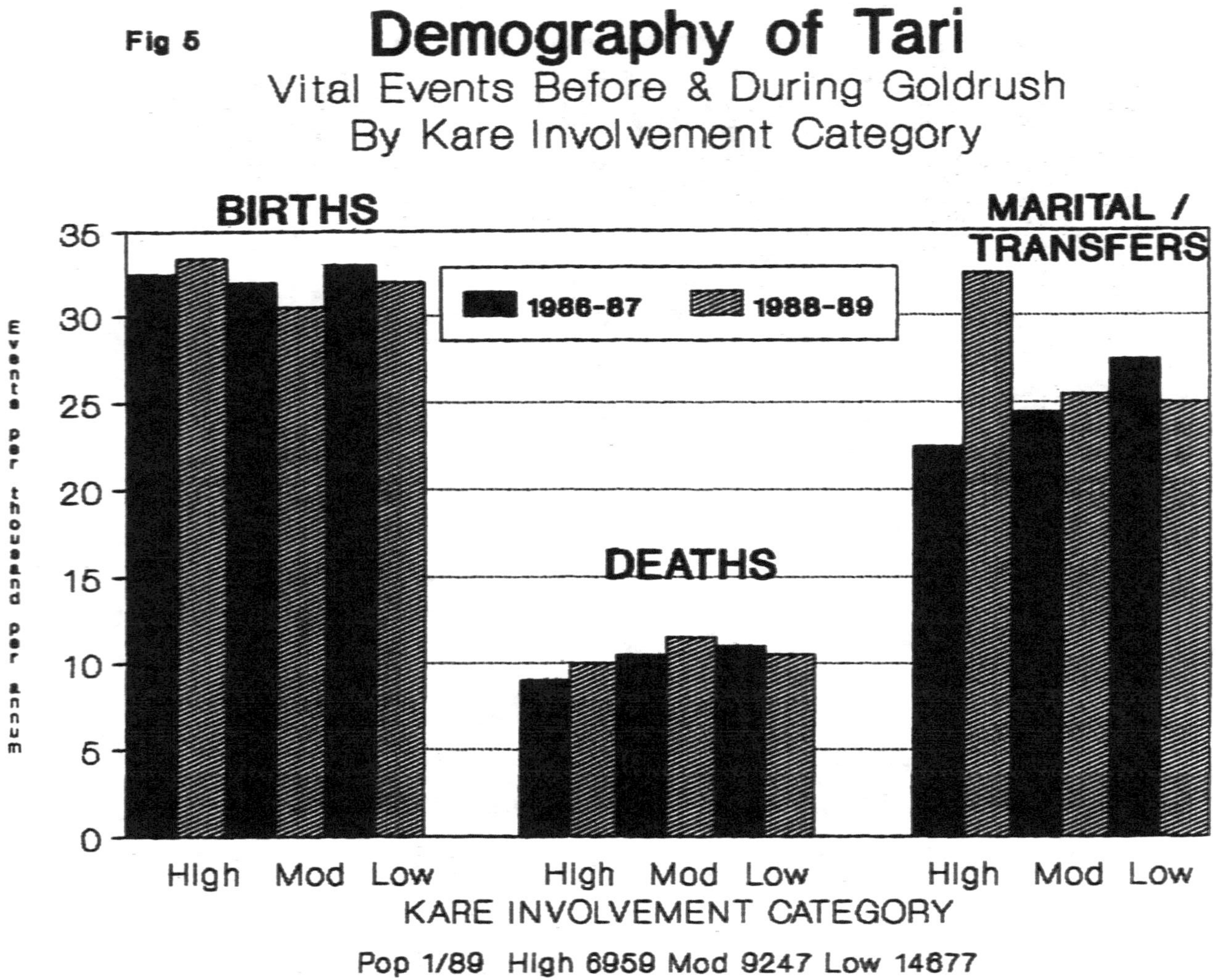
Demography of Tari
Vital Events Before & During Goldrush
By Kare Involvement Category
BIRTHS
DEATHS
MARITAL / TRANSFERS
1986-87
1988-89
Events per thousand per annum
0
5
10
15
20
25
30
35
High Mod Low
High Mod Low
High Mod Low
KARE INVOLVEMENT CATEGORY
Pop 1/89 High 6959 Mod 9247 Low 14677

POPULATION CHANGES AND SOCIO-ECONOMIC DEVELOPMENT

There are four papers in this section. **Asafu-Adjaye's** paper argues that Papua New Guinea can benefit only if the country follows a policy of sustainable development. The policy of sustainable development, according to him, must include issues of health, status of women, population control, human resource development, environment and economic growth. **Helen Hughes** in her paper tells us that the weakness of the Papua New Guinea economy is reflected in the declining standards of health and education, and that this is a reflection not of lack of resources (or resource constraints) but of poor economic management. She also argues that smallness of size is no barrier to growth-ambition; what is needed for economic success is focus on agriculture, outward-orientation and macroeconomic policies in place.

Jennifer Litau deals with the impact of uneven socio-economic development and regional disparities in the distribution of natureal resources on the 1980 inter-provincial migration flows in Papua New Guinea, and the implications of those for contemporary development efforts, policy and planning. According to her, the priorities have ostensibly shifted from urban to rural development. Yet the urban centres continue to draw resources and grow, while rural areas remain neglected. This had resulted in rural decay on the one side, and urban crime, unemployment and squatter settlement on the other.

Jane Thomason first looks at the current state of rural health services and resource requirements for providing health services as indicated by the National Health Plan (1991-95), and then estimates the gap between resource needs and resource availability. Rural health services are important and can be ignored only at great cost to the society.

These four papers make very useful reading.

....

H G MANNUR
Technical Editor
Head, Economics Department
University of Papua New Guinea

POPULATION CHANGES AND DEVELOPMENT

HELEN HUGHES[1]

Until World War II, both population growth and economic growth were slow. Malthusian beliefs of a 'vicious circle' of poverty, in which productivity growth only barely kept ahead of population growth, were widely and sensibly held. Where rapid population growth followed a few years of good harvests, poor seasons soon led to hunger if not war and famine. In Europe (and most other countries) from the Middle Ages to the 18th century, population and economic growth increased slowly from some 0.3 percent to 0.5 percent a year. In the 19th and first half of the 20th centuries, with the application of new technologies, population and economic growth increased to about 1 percent a year (Snooks 1990:36). In developing countries, however, very low rates of population and economic growth, typical of the Middle Ages in Europe, persisted.

The years since World War II have seen a dramatic, unprecedented and unexpected increase in population and economic growth in developing countries.

The application of new technologies to health problems (such as malaria control, vaccination and inoculation and new rehydration techniques) sharply reduced mortality, particularly infant mortality rates, raising the expectation of life and population growth. Fertility rates took time to adjust. Where economic growth was slow, the demographic transition to low fertility rates took time, so that population growth took place at more than 3 percent per annum. Papua New Guinea is one of these countries. Where economic growth, rising educational standards, particularly for women, and social development have been rapid, however, population growth has fallen rapidly even as longevity increased.

THE DEMOGRAPHIC TRANSITION

Population planning has been the key to the delivery of rising living standards. 'Two is enough' has proved to be an effective family planning target in countries as different as HongKong and Indonesia.

Studies of the relationship between population growth and economic development enable conclusions to be drawn about population growth and development (Birdsall 1988).

[1] National Centre for Development Studies, Research School of Pacific Studies, Australian National University

There is a strong relationship between population growth and economic development. Sustained and rapid economic growth not only increases longevity but also encourages fertility to fall so that standards of living rise rapidly.

In neighbouring East Asia, living standards have doubled in every decade since the 1960s. Low rates of economic growth (such as the barely 1 percent a year that occurred in Papua New Guinea since the early 1970s) lead to rapid population growth that undermines development. Instead of deepening investment in terms of capital available per worker, investment has to be widened, so that productivity grows very slowly. Investment in education and health services also has to be widened. This directly affects fertility rates which are highly influenced by attendance at school, particularly for girls, and the opportunity for women to obtain work outside the household.

Low economic growth and high rates of population growth are thus as mutually reinforcing as high rates of economic growth and low population growth.

IS POPULATION GROWTH ALWAYS COSTLY?

Population growth can have a positive effect on the economy. In a rapidly developing, open urban economy in which employment opportunities are running ahead of labour supply, an influx of highly trained and productive immigrants can be very beneficial. This has happened in Europe, notably in the Federal Rupublic of Germany and in Hong Kong. But even in these economies it has been argued that a greater substitution of capital for labour would have been more advantageous to the peoples of the countries concerned.

ECONOMIES OF SCALE

In the past it has been argued that small countries are at a disadvantage in the development process. Large countries apparently have the necessary economies of scale to produce efficiently. But research has shown that this hypothesis does not work in practice. Inward orientation is costly at any population size. No matter how rapidly Papua New Guinea's population grew, and even if its population doubled and trebled, Papua New Guinea would still not be large enough for economic production for the domestic market.

Canned meat, battery chickens, flour and feed, sugar and cement already demonstrate the high costs of production to Papua New Guinea. For mineral-rich countries, in addition, being small means having a small population among which to divide mineral rents.

Some very small countries have been the most rapidly growing economies in the world. They not only include Singapore and HongKong, among Papua New Guinea's neighbours, but also Mauritius and Malta. This relationship is not fortuitous, but arises from the adoption of outward-oriented policies.

ECONOMY-WIDE POLICIES

In the last 45 years, a great deal has been learnt about how to make economies grow. Recent economic research demonstrates that macroeconomic policies not only have more impact on economic growth than microeconomic policies, but that they also affect social variables more deeply.

This means that taxes and how they are spent (fiscal policies), monetary and financial policies (that together with fiscal policy affect the rate of exchange and the rate of inflation) and such economy-wide policies as trade and manpower measures, are the key to growth and development.

Papua New Guinea has succeeded in keeping the rate of exchange fairly stable and inflation relatively low. Such success has been achieved at high cost, overvaluing the exchange rate and hence undermining non-mineral exports and making it very difficult for local producers to compete with imports. Wages have been overvalued in relation to productivity. Recently inflation has been increasing despite the overvaluation of the exchange rate.

Despite ample access to aid funds (at one of the highest per capita inflows of aid in the world) growth has been low because of the inappropriateness of economy-wide policies. The 1990 decline of 4 percent in per capita income worsened a long record of low growth.

The greatest problem is the very low growth of employment and of productive agricultural activities. Out of more than 2 million people in the work force, only some 225,000 work in the formal sector. Rascalism is not a surprising outcome. And without greatly improved law and order, private investment will remain confined to rich mineral prospects, employment will not be created on an adequate scale, agriculture will continue to stagnate and rascalism will be exacerbated.

The weakness of the Papua New Guinea economy is reflected in declining standards of health and education. The lack of resources for health and education in the face of high aid budget contributions reflects poor economic management rather than absolute resource limitations.

The central sectoral problem of Papua New Guinea lies in the stagnation of agriculture. Most Papua New Guineans live in villages, but in the villages there has been almost no improvement in living standards during the last decade. Subsistence gardening is highly developed, but cash agriculture is stagnating, and hence off-farm rural activities are not developing. Present coffee prices are admittedly low, but small holders are not picking coffee because the overvaluation of the kina exaggerates low coffee prices. The reform issues in agriculture are more fundamental than 'band-aid' approaches such as agricultural extension work and the availability of subsidized rural credit. The lack of development of infrastructure makes it impossible to get goods to market economically.

URBAN POLICIES

High costs of living in urban areas are created by the inappropriateness of urban planning. Most of the population are urban fringe dwellers who lack access to drinking water, sanitation and other services. It is estimated that in Port Moresby 70 percent of the population lack such facilities. There has been no attempt to improve urban conditions by 'site and service' and slum improvement approaches. A recent World Bank suggestion on these lines fell on deaf ears. Not only was implementation capacity lacking, but there was no interest in building any but middle income housing for public servants. The lessons of Singapore and Hong Kong, as well as cities such as Kuala Lumpur, which have demonstrated the importance of the supply of appropriate housing for population planning and improving standards of living, go unheeded.

WOMEN IN THE PAPUA NEW GUINEA COMMUNITY

The position of women in Papua New Guinea lags behind that in developing countries at similar levels. Access to education and health is among the lowest in the world. So is access to formal employment.

These factors are reflected in the high fertility and infant mortality rates that lie behind population pressures on Papua New Guinea's economic growth. Prevalent social attitudes to women have not mitigated the traditional role attributed to women in Melanesian society.

POLICIES FOR THE FUTURE

Papua New Guinea is only now overcoming the central myth of the 'Eight Principles' that growth is not essential to development, and that low growth improves the quality of development. Development experience, well documented in research, since the 1950s, has clearly demonstrated that rapid growth is essential to development (Field 1989). Growth rates of 7 percent per annum or more in real terms, are necessary to achieve the social as well as the economic benefits required to improve living standards appreciably.

There is much that the Government of Papua New Guinea can do to strengthen the synergy between economic development and the demographic transition to raise living standards rapidly both by economic and social policies and specifically by implementing population planning measures.

REFERENCES

Birdsall N. Economic approaches to population growth, in: Chenery H. and Srinivasan T. N, eds. Handbook of Development Economics, Elsevier Science Publishers, Amsterdam, 1989; Chapter 12.

Fields GS. Changes in poverty and inequality in developing countries. The World Bank Research Observer, 1989 Vol. 4, No 2: 167-185.

Snooks GD. Economic growth during the last millenium: a quantitative perspective for the British industrial revolution, Working Papers in Economic History No 140, Department of Economic History, Research School of Social Sciences, Australian National University, July, 1990.

SUSTAINABLE DEVELOPMENT: IMPLICATIONS FOR POPULATION, HEALTH AND ENVIRONMENTAL POLICY IN PAPUA NEW GUINEA

JOHN ASAFU-ADJAYE[1]

INTRODUCTION

Papua New Guinea is endowed with rich reserves of natural resources. The natural resource sector, consisting of agriculture, forestry, fishing and mining, accounts for over 40% of Gross Domestic Product (GDP) [Table 1]. Agriculture is the dominant sector, accounting for over 35% of GDP and providing a means of livelihood for about 85% of the population. The PNG economy performed sluggishly during the early eighties, growing at an average rate of 2% per annum in real terms. The world recession and low commodity prices during this period were instrumental in keeping the economy depressed. During the period 1986 to 1988, the average annual growth rate of real GDP was 3.5 (Table 2). There was negative growth of 1.5% and 3.7% in 1989 and 1990, respectively. This decline in economic growth was attributable to the closure of the Bougainville copper mine in May 1989, as well as to the continued decline of agricultural commodity prices. In 1988, the Bougainville mine accounted for about 9% of GDP, while non-mineral production in the North Solomons accounted for a further 8% (Department of Finance and Planning 1991a).

The economy is expected to recover in 1991 with real GDP increasing by 7.8% (Table 2). This optimistic projection is based on the following developments in the mineral sector: the Porgera gold mine will be in its first year of full production by the end of 1991; the Misima gold mine is expected to increase output in 1991; and the Mt. Kare alluvial gold mine is expected to commence production by mid 1991. Meanwhile, construction work (including the laying of an oil pipe line) has begun on the Kutubu oil project, and this is expected to increase growth in the construction, transport and secondary manufacturing sectors. Oil production from the Kutubu project is expected to commence by the end of 1992.

Due to unfavourable commodity prices, minerals have assumed a dominant role in PNG's economic growth. The share of minerals in total GDP rose from 12.4% in 1986 to 15% in 1988, but declined to about 10% in 1989 due to the closure of the Bougainville Copper Limited mine.

[1] Department of Economics, University of Papua New Guinea

Minerals now account for over 60% of total exports (Table 3). Oil exports are expected to reach K640 million by 1995, by which time the share of minerals in total exports would have reached 71%.

In spite of the immense potential, the pace of development in Papua New Guinea has been slow due to a number of socioeconomic, infrastructural and institutional constraints. Some examples of these constraints are, a complex system of land tenure rules, a low level of adult literacy, and social and administrative fragmentation. The problems are compounded by a rugged and mountainous terrain and a wide geographical dispersion of the population. These features make access difficult and hamper efforts to develop domestic markets.

Papua New Guinea now stands on the threshold of a major mining boom, with a unique opportunity to accelerate the rate of development. In this paper, I argue that the only kind of development strategy which will benefit the present as well as future generations of Papua New Guineans is one which is based on the concept of sustainable development (SD).

The remainder of the paper is organised as follows. Section II briefly reviews socio-economic conditions in PNG; section III examines the meaning of SD; section IV discusses the policy implications, and Section V concludes with the summary and recommendations.

SOCIOECONOMIC CONDITIONS

Papua New Guinea has a population of 3.7 million (Table 4). This represents a doubling of the population from the 1960 level of 1.9 million. The population is projected to reach a level of 8.6 million by the year 2025 (UN Population Division, 1989). Although a relatively small country, PNG has a large land area and therefore has a population density of 8 persons per square kilometre, which is among the lowest in the region.

In 1983, PNG had an average per capita gross domestic product (GDP) of K520 (Table 4). Per capita incomes in the National Capital District (NCD) and Bougainville, which account for less than 10% of the total population, were about five times the national average. On the other hand, provinces with per capita incomes of less than K300 comprised 40% of the population, while more than 80% of the population had income levels below the national average.

Analysis of provincial data using indices for socioeconomic conditions reveals disparities for education, health, infant mortality and life expectancy (see Table 4).

Isolated provinces such as the Highlands (except Western Highlands) and the coastal provinces (Gulf, East/West Sepik and Milne Bay), accounting for about half the population, have below average levels of education, health and per capita incomes. In contrast, the Islands provinces, the NCD, Central province and Western province, which have about a quarter of the population, have above average indices of socioeconomic welfare.

It is important to note that even within the so-called "developed" provinces, there are considerable disparities in socioeconomic conditions and access to basic services. In general, the standards of health and education services in the country are below those of neighbouring Asian countries. Nevertheless, considerable progress has been made in the provision of health and basic education services since independence. For example, since 1975, life expectancy has increased from 45 to 54 years, while infant mortality has declined from 130 to 59 deaths/1000 births (UN Population Division 1989). The "less developed" provinces have in the past received preferential treatment in the disbursement of concessional funds for the provision of education and health facilities. However, more needs to be done. As of 1985, only 15% of rural dwellers had access to safe drinking water.

THE MEANING OF SUSTAINABLE DEVELOPMENT

Since the release of the landmark Brundtland Report in 1987 (World Commission on the Environment and Development, WCED, 1987), Sustainable Development has widely been accepted as a desirable goal of development by both developed and developing countries. However, to date, the concept remains a desirable but nebulous objective, which has yet to be defined in meaningful operational terms. The Brundtland Commission defined SD in broad terms as follows:

> **"Sustainable Development is development that meets the needs of the present without compromising the ability of future generations to meet their own needs."**(WCED, 1987, p.2).

Pearce et al. 1989 defined SD as follows:

> **Sustainable development involves a substantially increased emphasis on the value of natural, built and cultural environments.... Sustainable development places emphasis on providing for the needs of the least advantaged in society ("intergenerational equity"), and on fair treatment of future generations ("intragenerational equity").** Pearce et al. 1989, p.2).

Interpretations of SD are many and varied. In a recent survey of the SD literature, the environmental economist John Pezzey counted over 60 different definitions (Pezzey 1989). The Brundtland definition includes two key concepts: (i) the concept of meeting the needs of the poor and disadvantaged; and (ii) the idea of the capacity of the environment to provide for current and future generations given technological and institutional constraints.

In order to operationalize SD, we need to address four crucial areas: (i) economic growth, (ii) equity, (iii) the environment, and (iv) population growth and health.

Economic growth:

While the objective of development is to satisfy human needs and aspirations, it is clear that in a developing country such as PNG, there cannot be economic development without economic growth. Some environmentalists have put the blame for the degradation of the global environment squarely on economic activity associated with the growth process. Calls have been made for such economic activity to be reduced. This point of view is not entirely without merit. After all, unbridled exploitation of natural resources worldwide has imposed huge external costs on the environment. However, less developed countries (LDCs) have few alternatives for promoting growth, other than exploiting their natural resources.

Economic growth is a necessary but not a sufficient condition for sustainable development. According to the Brundtland Report, a minimum GNP growth rate of 3% per annum is required for SD in developing countries as a whole. With specific reference to the developing countries of Asia, a GNP growth rate of 5% per annum is required given the current population growth rates (World Commission on Environment and Development 1987).

Equity:

Rapid economic growth of a country will not necessarily lead to sustainable development if no effort is put into ensuring that the benefits of such growth are equitably distributed not only among the current population (*"intergenerational equity"*) but also future generations (*"intragenerational equity"*). The past patterns of development in PNG have served to exacerbate the disparities between regions, provinces, and among the population. The data in Table 4 portrays inequalities between provinces and regions. There is also inequality among urban and rural dwellers with respect to income (Jackson 1981), access to credit (Gupta 1985), access to basic services, and opportunities for income generation.

The issue of equity in SD also involves safeguarding the rights of women and other disadvantaged groups to equal opportunities, and respecting the rights of traditional land owners in resource development. A transition to SD requires vigorous policies to achieve greater equality between provinces and within the population. There is also an international dimension to SD in that policies are required to achieve equity between the rich and the poor countries.

The environment:

Papua New Guinea's Constitution contains the following important principle on the issue of natural resources and the environment.

> **Papua New Guinea's natural resources and environment must be conserved and used for the collective benefit of us all, and be replenished for the benefit of future generations.**

Thus, PNG's constitution commits the country to a path of sustainable development. The conservation and enhancement of natural resources are required to meet the needs of the growing population. The environmental requirement of SD is that the natural capital stock must be conserved and enhanced. This implies that, for example, land use in agriculture and forestry must be based on the carrying capacity of the land, and annual depletion of topsoil, fish stock, or forest resources shall not exceed the rate of regeneration.

Population growth and health:

The issues of population, health, environment and development are interrelated in complex ways. Economic development can generate resources that can be used to improve living conditions. Improvement in health services reduces the mortality rate and accelerates the rate of population growth. However, a high rate of population growth could deplete resources available for development and compromise the government's ability to provide for the basic needs of the population. Rapid population growth also encourages urban drift, which in turn leads to social and economic tensions. Population growth and lack of options for self-improvement lead to undue pressure on natural resources and the environment.

While population growth and lack of development can put excessive pressure on the environment, it is a fact that inappropriate development also places an undue burden on environmental resources and causes health problems. For example, indiscriminate use of pesticides, which have been widely reported in the Highlands provinces, could adversely affect the health of farmers. Excessive use of fertilizers could lead to high concentration of nitrogen compounds in water and the atmosphere, leading to contamination of groundwater and rivers. Governments in LDCs have carried out development projects regardless of their adverse impacts on health and the environment, due to pressure to meet basic minimum needs.

In the final analysis, the population problem is not simply one of controlling numbers; rather it is a problem of improving the quality of life and providing equal access to self-improvement. Sustainable development requires government to adopt policies which strike the right balance between population size, the country's environmental demands and economic capacity. It is only by following such a strategy that development can truly benefit the present and future generations of Papua New Guineans. I would now like to suggest some policy initiatives.

POLICY SUGGESTIONS

The Status of Women

Research has shown (eg., see Petros-Barvazian 1984, Birdsall 1984) that acceleration of social and economic development will lead to lower population growth. This is due to the fact that fertility rate and family size are inversely correlated to income level. An important aspect of government policy should be to improve the status of women in the society. Such a programme should include improving the literacy rate among women, teaching family planning and resource use, and increasing opportunities for income-generating activities.

Health

A key strategy in this overall plan should be to provide basic health facilities in the rural areas. These should include safe drinking water, sanitation and immunization services. Provision of health care facilities should be complemented by the provision of health education. Some of the negative by-products of increasing development include changes in traditional life-styles and eating habits. Efforts should be made now to avoid chances of increasing cancer, heart disease and HIV infections, the costs of which we can ill-afford.

Human Resource Development

There is an urgent need to promote human resource development since this provides the skills and knowledge required to improve economic performance. Efforts must be made to improve not only educational facilities but also the quality and relevance of the educational process. School curricula must include environmental concepts such as conservation of natural resources and the effects of deforestation. They must emphasise the interaction between population growth, the environment and development.

Population Policy

Papua New Guinea has lacked a clear-cut population policy for several years. Among other things, the lack of government policy to guide the spatial distribution of the population has resulted in settlement patterns (particularly in the urban centres), which are not conducive to sustainable development. Such unplanned settlements limit the capacity of the government to provide clean water and sanitation. They result in increases in disease, and social and law and order problems. In his keynote address to this seminar, The Prime Minister, Hon. Rabbie L. Namaliu, unveiled the long awaited National Population Policy which addresses the issues of health, the status of women, rural development, etc. Thus, there are good prospects for solving the population problem provided the policies are put into effect.

Environmental Policy

The establishment of an Office of the Environment and Conservation (OEC) in 1974, as well as the passage of various environmental protection laws, established a model for other Pacific Island States to emulate. However, since 1982, the effectiveness of PNG's natural resource management programme appears to have been eroded in spite of the impressive administrative structure and legislative support. Budgetary support for OEC work was reduced by 65% to 0.5% of the total expenditure in 1982 (National Planning Office 1981). Spending for environmental protection services has increased from K1.6 million in 1989 to K3.0 million in 1991, which is still a mere 0.2% of total expenditure (Department of Finance and Planning 1991b). Important functions such as environmental education, resource investigations and law enforcement have been curtailed.

The major factors constraining effective environmental management are: lack of adequate guidelines, poor co-ordination between agencies, scarce resources, inadequate staff training and experience, and a lack of local understanding and concern for environmental issues.

From the policy perspective, it is encouraging to note the establishment of the programme, "Environmental Management for Sustainable Development", by the Department of Environment and Conservation. The purpose of the programme is to develop a National Conservation Strategy, to review existing environmental legislation and enact additional legislation, to improve the database on resources, to raise public consciousness of environmental issues, and a host of other objectives.

Integrated Policy Making

A major deficiency in the current public policy making process is lack of integrated decision making. The present approach is to concentrate on individual sectoral plans (eg., health, population, education, etc.), a process which can result in incomplete or contradictory policies. A good example is the proposed National Population Policy which completely ignores environmental factors.

There is an immediate need for a broad-based national policy on sustainable development which strikes a balance between the environment, population and the country's economic resources.

Currently there is no mechanism or public body to integrate long-term plans for sustainable development although a step has been taken in the right direction with the establishment of a Population Unit in the Department of Finance and Planning. There is a need for the creation of a high level advisory council such as the proposed National Advisory Committee on Population Policy. The composition of this council should be broadened to include representatives of the following departments/groups: environment and conservation, forests, agriculture and livestock, fisheries and marine resources, minerals and energy resources, the provinces and private groups.

This advisory body should be responsible for devising strategies for integrating population, health and environmental issues into the core of social and economic development policy making. It should also be responsible for monitoring the social impacts of government policies and development projects, and for co-ordinating the activities of the various development agencies. The body will oversee and monitor the equitable distribution of development benefits, and ensure that there is improved access to essential amenities and basic services. It will identify the most disadvantaged in the society with a view to targeting such segments for development and self-improvement projects.

CONCLUDING REMARKS

Despite abundance of natural resources, development in Papua New Guinea has been slow due to a number of internal and external constraints. The present decade presents prospects for a natural resources boom, which offers the country a unique opportunity to accelerate the pace of development. In this paper, I have argued that it is only by following a policy of sustainable development that present and future generations of Papua New Guineans will truly benefit. A broad-based policy of sustainable development which I have proposed must encompass the issues of health, the status of women, population, human resource development, the environment as well as economic growth.

Government expenditures, as indicated by the 1991 Budget and the 1991 Public Expenditure Programme, are biased in favour of the 'economic' areas (eg., agriculture, minerals and energy), with the 'non-economic' areas (eg., health, education, environmental protection) receiving lower priority. While the 'economic' areas are obviously important for generating resources to pay for development, the 'non-economic' areas also have an important role to play in sustaining development. The two are mutually reinforcing in that expenditure on the so-called 'non-economic' areas leads to an increase in the country's economic and productive activities.

REFERENCES

Birdsall, N. (1984). "Population growth: its magnitudes and implications for development", Finance and Development, Vol 2, No. 3.

Department of Finance and Planning. (1991a.) Economic policies. 1991 Budget Documents, Volume 2, Port Moresby. (1991b). Estimates of revenue and expenditure. Budget Documents, Volume 3, Port Moresby.

Gupta, D. (1985). "Some dimensions of inequality in Papua New Guinea", in P. King, W. Lee and V. Warakai, (eds.) From Rhetoric to Reality, proceedings of the 15th. Waigani Seminar, University of Papua New Guinea Press.

Jackson, D. (1981). The distribution of incomes in Papua New Guinea. National Planning Office, Port Moresby.

National Planning Office (1981). The National Public Expenditure Plan, 1982-1985, National Planning Office, Port Moresby.

National Statistical Office (1991). Citizen Population; Scenario S1 B2 Projections, By Province, 1980 - 2000. National Statistical Office Port Moresby.

Pearce, D.W., A. Markandya and E.B. Barbier (1989). Blueprint for a green economy. London: Earthscan Publications.

Petros-Barvazian, A. (1984). "Family planning: A preventive health measure", World Health, June.

Pezzey, J. (1989). "Definitions of Sustainability," CEED Discussion Paper, No. 9. London: Centre for Economic and Environmental Development.

United Nations Population Division (1989). World population prospects 1988. U.N., New York.

World Bank (1989). Papua New Guinea: Policies and prospects for sustainable growth and broad-based growth. Volume 1, The Main Report.

World Commission on Environment and Development (1987). Our Common Future. New York: Oxford University Press.

Table 1: Gross Domestic Product by Sector, 1985 to 1989 (millions of Kina, constant 1983 prices)

Sector	1985	1986	1987	1988	1989[a]
Agriculture, Forestry, Fishing	699.9	711.5	750.2	777.7	790.9
Mining and Quarrying	274.5	365.8	356.7	367.0	233.9
Manufacturing	242.4	222.3	225.6	236.0	263.4
Electricity and other services	34.4	34.3	36.2	36.4	37.4
Construction	87.8	92.0	87.2	109.4	131.5
Commerce, Transport, Finance	410.0	381.0	417.4	411.2	393.0
Community and Social Services	377.8	379.1	381.4	382.6	404.3
Import Duties	93.4	103.3	117.3	121.8	151.7
Total GDP	2220.3	2289.3	2372.0	2442.1	2406.1

a. Provisional

Source: Department of Finance and Planning (1991a), Table S1.1.

Table 2: Gross Domestic Product (GDP), 1986 - 1991

(Millions of Kina)

	1986	1987	1988	1989	1990	1991
GDP[a] (Current Prices)	2555	2831	3141	3014	3095	3399
	(Growth rates in percentages, year on year)					
GDP[b] (Constant Prices)	4.0	3.6	3.0	-1.5	-3.7	7.8

Sources: a. Department of Finance and Planning, (1991a), Table S1.1.

b. Bank of Papua New Guinea (1991).

Table 3: Export Growth, 1985-95 (selected years)
(Millions of Kina, nominal)

	Actual			Projected	
	1985	1988	1989	1990	1995
Mineral	489.9	861.5	676.1	673.5	1658.4
Gold	318.8	405.1	317.0	366.8	745.5
Copper	164.2	446.9	344.9	389.4	256.6
Silver	6.9	9.5	14.2	17.3	16.1
Oil	-	-	-	-	640.2
Non-mineral	409.6	414.6	375.5	297.8	563.2
Agriculture	330.2	255.2	273.6	193.3	389.0
Forestry	67.3	97.5	93.9	91.0	157.8
Marine	12.1	7.5	8.0	13.5	16.4
Other[a]	46.7	54.4	65.0	79.0	108.4
TOTAL	946.2	1276.1	1116.6	1050.3	2330.0

Sources: 1985, 1988 and 1989: Department of Finance and Planning (1991a), Table S2.3.

1990, 1995: Department of Finance and Planning (1991a), Table S2.7.

a. Includes re-exports and immigrants effects.

Table 4: Socioeconomic Indicators, By Province

Province[a]	Popul-ation ('000) (1990)	Per capita income (Kina) (1983)	Education % Pop. with no schooling (1980)	Health Infant mort. (per 1000) (1980)	Life Expectancy (yrs) (1980)
Nat'l Capital Dist.	158.2	2,116	36	35	56.7
North Solomons	175.9	1,973	50	33	59.6
East New Britain	171.6	770	55	57	52.8
Western	101.1	673	71	83	47.7
New Ireland	171.6	534	59	62	52.7
Central	144.1	528	68	59	51.3
West New Britain	121.5	483	51	60	51.3
Morobe	392.7	473	51	62	50.9
Manus	33.0	416	51	55	51.8
Northern/Oro	99.7	413	61	67	49.2
Madang	274.6	387	80	62	50.7
Western Highlands	323.8	337	89	81	51.9
East Sepik	228.8	320	81	94	49.3
Eastern Highlands	327.1	290	91	55	53.1
Milne Bay	165.4	280	64	50	57.1
Enga	189.0	267	94	91	47.1
Chimbu	191.4	264	93	87	50.2
Southern Highlands	277.0	256	94	116	43.8
West Sepik	138.1	255	84	104	42.1
Gulf	76.7	198	71	71	47.3
Total/Average	3,727.2	520	78	72	49.6

a. Provinces listed in order of per capita income.

Sources: Population - National Statistical Office (1991). Health, education, per capita income, life expectancy - compiled from World Bank (1989), Appendix Tables II.1, II.2

THE IMPLICATIONS OF UNCONTROLLED POPULATION GROWTH FOR THE PROVISION OF RURAL HEALTH SERVICES

JANE THOMASON[1]

INTRODUCTION

The formulation of a national population policy and the consequent prospects of a rational, sustained population programme are encouraging moves which bode well for the long term future of Papua New Guinea. It is not the consequences of <u>this</u> political decision that will largely determine the constraints to provision of health services over the next several years, it is the historical lack of concerted action on population issues and the continuing reluctance of government to recognise the incontrovertible link between population growth and health service requirements. In the medium term, the people of Papua New Guinea will be paying the price for the past sustained high levels of population growth. One likely cost of this will be a decline in provision of health services in terms of coverage, scope or quality.

This paper will focus on the rural health services because they provide health services for the majority of people and because they are the most likely to be adversely affected by a decline in service provision. First, the current state of rural health services will be reviewed, and the resource requirements to provide the level of services indicated by the National Health Plan 1991-1995 will be outlined. Then the gap between these resource requirements and the anticipated available resources will be estimated. Finally, the implications for provision of rural health services will be discussed, including reduction in coverage, reduction in scope of services and reduction in quality of service.

THE CURRENT STATE OF RURAL HEALTH SERVICES

The current National Health Plan (1) outlines a strategy which focuses on improvement of quality and efficiency of existing health services and infrastructure. However, recent reviews of rural health services indicate that the lack of human and material resources is already hampering their effective delivery. Per capita expenditure for health has declined in real terms since 1983.(2) There are also significant inequities in the distribution of health resources between provinces which cannot be justified by the health needs of the population. These disparities are also reflected in the inequitable distribution of staffing between provinces.(3)

[1] Department of Community Medicine,
University of Papua New Guinea

Shortages of skilled human resources have been reported in the rural areas, already. Twenty four percent of health centres and subcentres, the first referral level, have only an orderly or nurse aide on duty in outpatients. This makes the level of initial diagnosis at those facilities equal to an aidpost, except that they would be able to refer more rapidly to a more highly qualified person. Many aidposts are reported to be unstaffed with anecdotal reports indicating that as many as 25% of aidposts may be unstaffed at any one time.

Within provinces, there has been a steady decline in the proportion of non-salary recurrent costs since 1985,(4) which has already adversely affected provision of health worker supervision, health patrols and facility maintenance. While the target for supervisory visits of peripheral health workers is four visits per year, in 1988 staff from only 21 percent of health subcentres and 37 percent of health centres had not made even one visit to their aidposts during 1987. No supervisory visits had been conducted by 42 percent of facilities in the month preceding the study.(5) In the same year, 31 percent of facilities had not received any clinical supervision in the preceding twelve months. Poor supervision has been cited as a major factor in the deterioration of the aidpost system in the country,(6) and a recent study (7) has found that patient examination by aidpost orderlies was inadequate and drug dosages given often incorrect, which is also suggestive of already declining standards in the provision of rural health services.

Another symptom of the recurrent cost problem has been a decline in standards of building maintenance. In 1987 only 33 percent of health centres and subcentres had any expenditure on building maintenance. This represented only 6.4 percent of the recommended level for maintenance expenditure. Further indications of emerging problems in rural health services, which are indicative of inadequate recurrent financing, are poor vaccine stocks, inadequate refrigeration, and declining frequency of maternal and child health clinics, and a consequent concentration of staff on curative care with 60 to 70 percent of staff time spent on curative care and less than 25 percent on the vital area of preventive health.(8) In summary, there is evidence that the system is <u>already</u> failing to respond appropriately to the increasing demands of the population (and the slow economic growth).

RESOURCE REQUIREMENTS TO MEET NATIONAL HEALTH PLAN TARGETS

The National Health Plan 1991-1995 has outlined the objectives for health service provision over the next five years. Although some objectives can be reached within existing resources, as the population continues to grow, inevitably, to reach the increased objectives of the Plan, the resource requirements for health will increase. The main categories of resources for rural health services are human resources, essential drugs, travel and transportation and properly equipped and maintained facilities.

Human Resources

The staffing implications of meeting the targets made explicit in the new five year National Health Plan combined with continuing high levels of population growth are considerable. Currently it is estimated that there are adequate numbers of staff in rural areas to handle current utilisation levels.(8) The National Health Plan 1991-1995 has indicated a desire to improve performance in the area of maternal care so that 60% of all pregnant women make at least three antenatal visits, that 80% deliver their babies under supervision, and that 50% of fertile women utilise family planning services. Assuming that the current rates of curative attendances in rural areas do not change and that the immunisation target of 78% for the third dose of Triple Antigen is also met, the staffing implication of achieving these targets is considerable. Using the Indicators of Staffing Need (ISN), a formula developed for assessing staff requirements for nurses and community health workers in rural health centres and subcentres(9), by 1995, the number of nurses required in rural areas will be 2,797 and community health workers 2,999. The number of staff in rural areas in 1990 was 1,357 and 1,344 respectively. (Figure 1) This will mean an additional requirement of 1,440 nurses and 1,655 community health workers. The cost of such expansion would be in the vicinity of K9.29 million per year.[a]

Aside from the obvious economic implications of the human resource requirements, there are also implications for training (Figure 2). Currently there are approximately 150 nursing graduates and 220 community health worker graduates annually. In five years, 750 nurses and 1,100 community health workers could be trained. Over the forthcoming five years, at present training rates without accounting for attrition from service,[b] only 52% of nursing requirements and 66% of community health worker requirements can be trained.

Essential Drugs

Over the past few years, reports of essential drug shortages[c] are becoming increasingly common. It is easy to see why such shortages have occurred and it is inevitable that they will become more common. The procurement of drugs requires scarce foreign exchange. When the kina was devalued in 1990, by the end of that year, the Division of Pharmaceutical Services was overcommitted by 10%, simply as a result of orders placed prior to devaluation. The devaluation coupled with static appropriations for purchase of drugs over the past five years has made it increasingly difficult for the Pharmaceutical Services Division to

---

a Based on an average salary of K3,000 per annum.

b Attrition from service figures were not available,

c Information on the procurement of pharmaceuticals was obtained by personal communication from the Chief of Pharmaceutical Services of the Department of Health.

maintain levels of procurement. The volume of drugs purchased currently remains at levels similar to that purchased in 1985. Yet as the population has increased and patterns of morbidity and mortality have remained essentially the same, the volume of drugs needed to treat people has increased. Although some savings may be possible through intensifying efforts to reduce wastage and to improve health worker compliance to correct prescribing practice, requirements for expenditure on essential drugs over the next five years will be driven by population growth and the market price of the drugs, and there is no doubt that both of these are rising.

Transport

Transportation and provision of travel allowances for essential extension work are vital to the effective provision of preventive health services. As population increases,the need to both protect and increase allocations for travel and transportation will be important. If insufficient resources are allocated to this, the coverage and frequency of preventive services will decline even further than has been experienced in the past five years.

Maintenance/Building replacement

Because of the already extensive network of health facilities throughout the country, high levels of population growth are unlikely to necessitate significant expansion in infrastructure. The inadequate level of building maintenance in rural areas, however, will necessitate major expenditure in the future. Without preventive maintenance, buildings will reach the end of their useful life more rapidly, and pressure to undertake a sizeable new investment programme to replace the old dilapidated buildings will mount.

Simple estimations can provide an indication of the order of magnitude of this problem. Progressive replacement of all health centres and subcentres over the next 20 years at the rate of 23 per year, would result in an annual cost of approximately K7.7 million[d], compared to the 1989 appropriation for health construction of K3.46 million and 1990 appropriation of K2.56 million[e]. This means more than doubling the current levels of capital investment annually for rural health. If the 2,200 aidposts were also to be replaced, K5.5 million would be required annually making an estimated annual requirement of K13.2 million to achieve replacement of all rural health facilities over a 20 year period. This is approximately four times the current annual capital expenditure.

---

d This assumes that all 469 facilities will be replaced as health centres or sub centres. If any rural hospitals were constructed, the cost would be significantly increased.

e 1989 and 1990 rural health construction figures were supplied by the Projects Section of the Department of Health

RESOURCE EXPECTATIONS

Uncertainty regarding the future growth of the economy of Papua New Guinea makes it difficult to predict the level of resources for the health sector which will be available over the medium term. However, projections based on explicit assumptions are useful in illustrating possible future scenarios. There have been two different sets of projections already made. The first[10], used 1986 as the base year and assumed that population growth would remain in the range of 2.2-2.3% per year and that GDP would rise by 1.3%-1.4% annually (Figure 3).

It assumed that the proportion of GDP for health would be maintained. It was estimated that in 1986, there was a gap of K8.8 million based on shortfalls in operation and maintenance expenditure. By 1995, it was estimated that the gap between the resources required and those available from government will reach the level of K18.4 million.

The second projection[11], assumed that the required level of resources would be the maintenance of 1985 health expenditure in real terms (Figure 4). Projections were done using a "best case scenario" for population growth of 2.3 percent and a "worst case" of 2.7 percent. In the best case scenario: GDP growth is also assumed to be 3.5 percent per annum, which is based on the World Bank medium term projection[12]. In the worst case scenario, GDP growth is assumed to make no change. The proportion of government expenditure on health is assumed to remain the same. The best case scenario projects a shortfall of K8 million in 1995, which would reduce to about K3.4 million by the year 2000. The worst case projects a K24.7 million shortfall in 1995 which would grow to K40 million by the year 2000. The population growth variant plays a key role in determining the differences between the "best" and "worst" scenarios.

Both sets of projections clearly predict that there will be significant shortfalls in expenditure for health services in 1995 ranging between K8 million and K24 million. The simple message is that financial and human resources for health care are becoming scarcer.

IMPLICATIONS

The anticipated gap between requirements and availability of resources will necessarily mean that it will no longer be possible to provide the same level of service as before. The effects on service may be in one or more of the following ways: reduction in scope, reduction in coverage or reduction in quality of service.

Reduction in coverage

Coverage implies the extent to which services are being appropriately utilised by all those who would benefit from them. Inevitably, growing population pressure will mean that coverage will decline. This is likely to compound existing problems with inequity of service provision. Access and political power are related, and the increasing and vocal demands for health services of a growing urban population will inevitably result in an effort to meet their demands. The isolation and relative 'silence' in a political sense of the most remote rural dwellers will tend to mean that services to them will suffer first.

The most likely reductions will be seen in the closure of aidposts and a reduction in preventive services.

Reduction in scope of services

When there are limited resources, it is impossible to do everything at once. One alternative, is to maintain high levels of coverage, but to limit the range and scope of services provided. To do so in any rational way requires the establishment of priorities amongst the range of available health interventions. A debate of such issues has arisen in recent years regarding the inability of governments to respond to the resource requirements of comprehensive primary health care, which has been demonstrated to be costly(13). Proponents have suggested that there are specific medical interventions which could be applied at reasonable cost and which would have a significant impact on infant and child mortality. The measures suggested were immunisation, oral rehydration, breastfeeding and the use of anti-malarials(14). The government could select a deliberate strategy of putting resources into key programmes with identifiable impact on mortality and redirecting resources away from programmes with lower impact such as dental health, mental health, rehabilitation etc.

The National Health Plan outlines the services to be provided at each level of facility. At the lowest service level, the aidpost, the following functions are listed:

1 AIDPOST FUNCTIONS

- outpatient service
- promote family planning
- followup of TB and leprosy patients
- advise community on water, sanitation and nutrition
- promote basic human needs
- assist in MCH clinics and followup after clinic
- refer patients
- report on disease outbreaks

At the health centre, the functions are expanded to include inpatient care, full provision of MCH and family planning services, as well as a range of administrative and managerial functions including, supervision, training and drug distribution.

Plans are articulated in the National Health Plan for a wide variety of activities as listed below.

National Health Technical Plans

- Respiratory Disease Control
- Mosquito Borne Disease Control
- Diseases of Poor Hygiene and Sanitation
- AIDS and other STD
- Hepatitis B Control
- Tuberculosis
- Leprosy
- Yaws
- Diseases of the Eye and Ear
- Nutrition Disorders
- Diabetes Mellitis
- Cardiovascular Disease
- Cancers
- Tobacco Associated Diseases
- Traumatology
- Mental Health
- Oral Disease
- Primary Health Care
- Health Education
- Immunisation
- School Health
- Reproductive Health and Family planning
- Geriatric Health
- Environmental Health
- Support Services

If the selective primary health care approach is followed these health activities could be prioritised on the basis of such factors as, prevalence, mortality, morbidity, feasibility and cost of control and the use of technology.[15] It has also been suggested that in establishing priorities for health expenditure, a distinction should be made between rural primary health services which require planned allocations to promote growth, and hospital services, which tend to grow spontaneously under demand pressures and must have resource limits placed on them to constrain their growth.[16]

It is difficult to make such choices, but to make the choices in a logical and rational way, may be preferable to the alternative. The alternative to a deliberate policy intervention will be that the scope of services will be reduced anyway, but through attrition rather than sound and rational planning. For example, maternal and child health extension work may cease due to lack of staff and transportation, while the curative work of the health facilities continue.

Reduction in quality of service

The impact of health services on the health status of a population depends on: (i) the efficacy of the interventions provided; (ii) the diagnostic accuracy of the health worker; (iii) the compliance of the health worker to correctly provide the intervention or health practice; (iv) the compliance of the patient to correctly use it; and (v) coverage.[17] It has been pointed out already that there is a risk that coverage will be reduced. The diagnostic accuracy of health workers and their compliance to correct intervention and health practice, depend heavily on preservice and inservice training and supervision. The compliance to the correct intervention also depends on the availability of essential drugs. As discussed earlier, the availability of drugs will be increasingly constrained as population pressure increases. The conduct of inservice training and supervision, rely heavily on recurrent funding for travel and transportation. As has already been witnessed, health worker supervision is on the decline. The combination of population demand and sluggish economic growth suggest that there will be little hope of improving these areas in the near future. As a result, it is inevitable that the quality of services provided in the rural areas will decline.

CONCLUSION

This discussion has focused primarily on the implications of population growth, on the provision of health services and health status. Some may correctly argue, that there are other important means of improving health that should be considered. The World Bank, for example, has called the evidence of the significance of the relationship between education and health unequivocal.[18] Other factors have also been linked to improved health status, so the concentration of scarce resources on health services alone may not be the most effective intervention to make changes in people's health status. For example, a number of key areas were found to be important in reducing mortality in Costa Rica, Kerala, in India and Sri Lanka[19], including female autonomy, improved education with equal opportunity for both sexes, adequate nutrition, accessible and efficient health services providing antenatal and postnatal health services, fully trained birth attendants and universal immunisation. On the basis of these findings, it may be that a judicious combination of selected health interventions and channelling of remaining resources into interventions to improve education and the status of women, could be the most successful means of dealing with the resource constraints.

Regardless of how the choices are made, one thing is clear, the combination of high levels of population growth and slow economic growth mean that there <u>are</u> choices to be made. In the medium term at least, there will simply be inadequate public resources to respond to public demand.

Inevitably, either the coverage or the scope of health services will decline, probably either scenario will be accompanied by a deterioration in the quality of those services. These reductions may be carefully planned to minimise their negative effects, or they may be allowed to occur in an ad hoc manner, possibly with the worst effects on the most needy areas.

There is a need for concerted action on the part of the national and provincial governments, the central government agencies and the Department of Health to act to minimise the negative consequences on the provision of health services in a rational and planned way. Clear acknowledgement should be given in the budgetary process to the relationship between population growth and requirements for health services. There is also a need for concerted action to implement the national population policy as a rational and sustained population programme, so that the future provision of health services can be managed within existing resources. Finally, it would be wise to consider a multisectoral approach to the improvement of health, with due consideration to the status of women and education, which elsewhere have been found to be an important complement to the delivery of effective health services in the improvement of health status.

REFERENCES

1. Department of Health, Papua New Guinea National Health Plan 1991-1995, Port Moresby 1991.

2. Thomason J A and Newbrander W C. Health Financing and Budgeting in Thomason J A, Newbrander W C, and Kolehmainen-Aitken R-L (eds) Decentralisation in a Developing Economy: The Experience of Papua New Guinea and its Health Service. Pacific Research Monograph No. 25. ANU Press 1991.

3. Thomason J A, Kolehmainen-Aitken R-L and Newbrander W C. Decentralisation of Health Services in Papua New Guinea: A Critical Review. in Thomason J A, Newbrander WC and Kolehmainen-Aitken R-L. Decentralisation in a Developing Economy: The Experience of Papua New Guinea and its Health Service. Pacific Research Monograph No. 25. ANU Press 1991.

4. Thomason J A and Newbrander W C. A survey of Papua New Guinea's Health Sector Financing and Expenditure. PNG Med J 1991 34: 45-59.

5. Mitchell M D, Thomason J A, Donaldson D, Garner P. 1991 The cost of rural health services in Papua New Guinea. PNG Med J 1991 34:276-284

6. Bouten M. Mission health services. In: Heywood P, Hudson B, Eds. Rural Health Services in Papua New Guinea. Papua New Guinea Department of Health Monograph No 5. Port Moresby:

7. Rogers S et al 1991 Management of potentially serious paediatric illnesses by aidpost orderlies at Tari, Southern Highlands Province. PNG Med J 1991 34:122-8

8. Thomason, J. and Kolehmainen-Aitken, R. Distribution and Performance of Rural Health Workers in Papua New Guinea Soc Sci Med 1991 32(2): 159-165.

9. Kolehmainen-Aitken, R. and Shipp, P. Indicators of Staffing Need: assessing Health Staffing and Equity in Papua New Guinea. Health Policy and Planning 1990 5(2) 167-176

10. Newbrander W C and Thomason J A. Alternatives for financing health services in Papua New Guinea. Health Policy and Planning; 1989 4(2): 131-140.

11. Rosenthal, G. et al. Papua New Guinea Health Sector Financing Study Project. Final Report - Volume I: Health Sector Financing Issues and Options. John Snow Inc. February 1990.

12. The World Bank, Papua New Guinea: Policies and prospects for sustained and broad-based growth. The World Bank, Washington, 1988.

13. Chabot J and Waddington C. Primary Health Care is not cheap: A case study from Guinea Bissau. International Journal of Health Services, 1987 17(3) 387-409.

14. Walsh J A and Warren K S Selective primary health care: An interim strategy for disease control in developing countries. New Engl J Med 1979 301, 18

15. Walsh J A Selectivity within primary health care. Soc Sci Med. Vol 26, 1988 No 9, pp899-902

16. Segall M Health Sector Planning Led by Management of Recurrent Expenditure: An agenda for action-research. International Journal of Health Planning and Management, 1991 Vol.6, 37-75

17. Tugwell P, Bennett K J, Sackett D L and Haynes R B. The measurement iterative loop: a framework for the critical appraisal of need, benefits and costs of health interventions. J Chron Dis. 1986 38, 339

18. Cochrane S H, O'Hara D J and Leslie J. The effects of education on health. World Bank Staff Working Paper, No. 405. 1980 The World Bank, Washington.

19. Caldwell J C Routes to low mortality in poor countries. Popln Devl Rev. 12, 1986 171-220.

Projected Training Potential
for Rural Nurses and CHWs: 1995

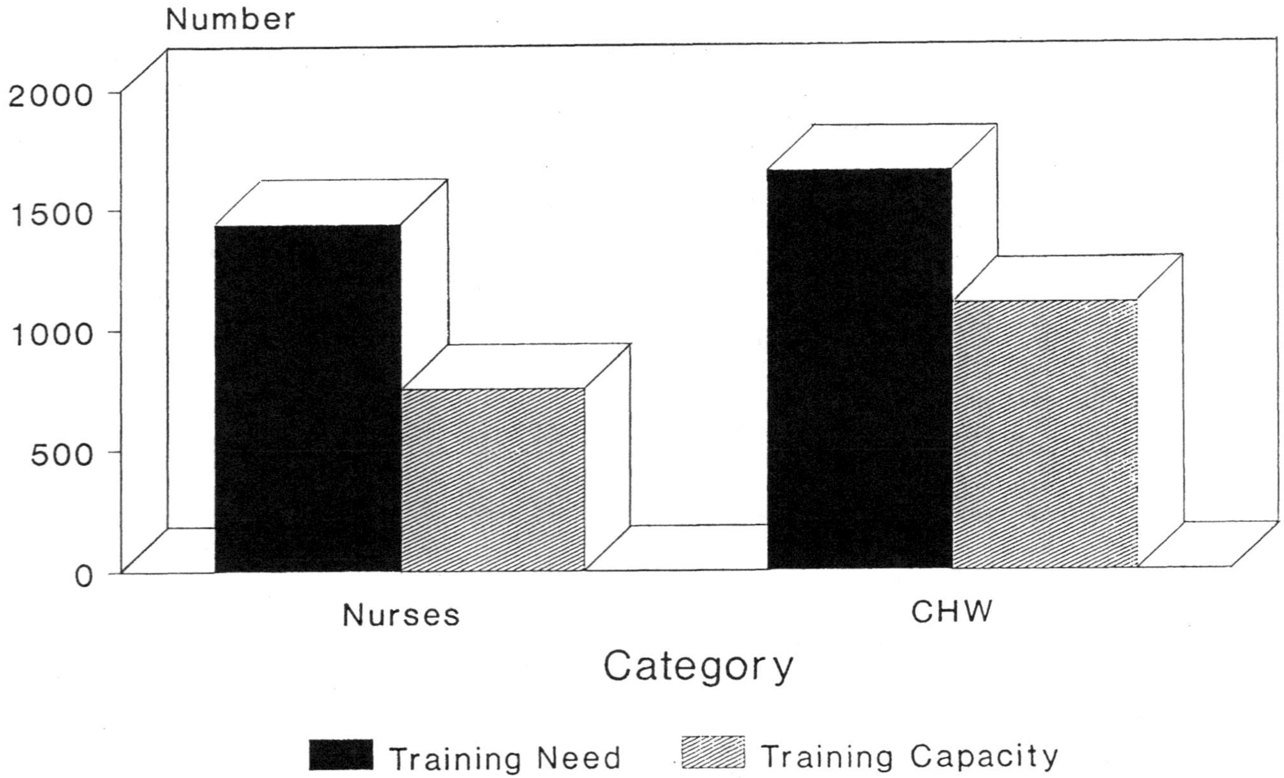

Excluding Aidposts

Rural Health Staff Requirements
Based on Projected Utilisation

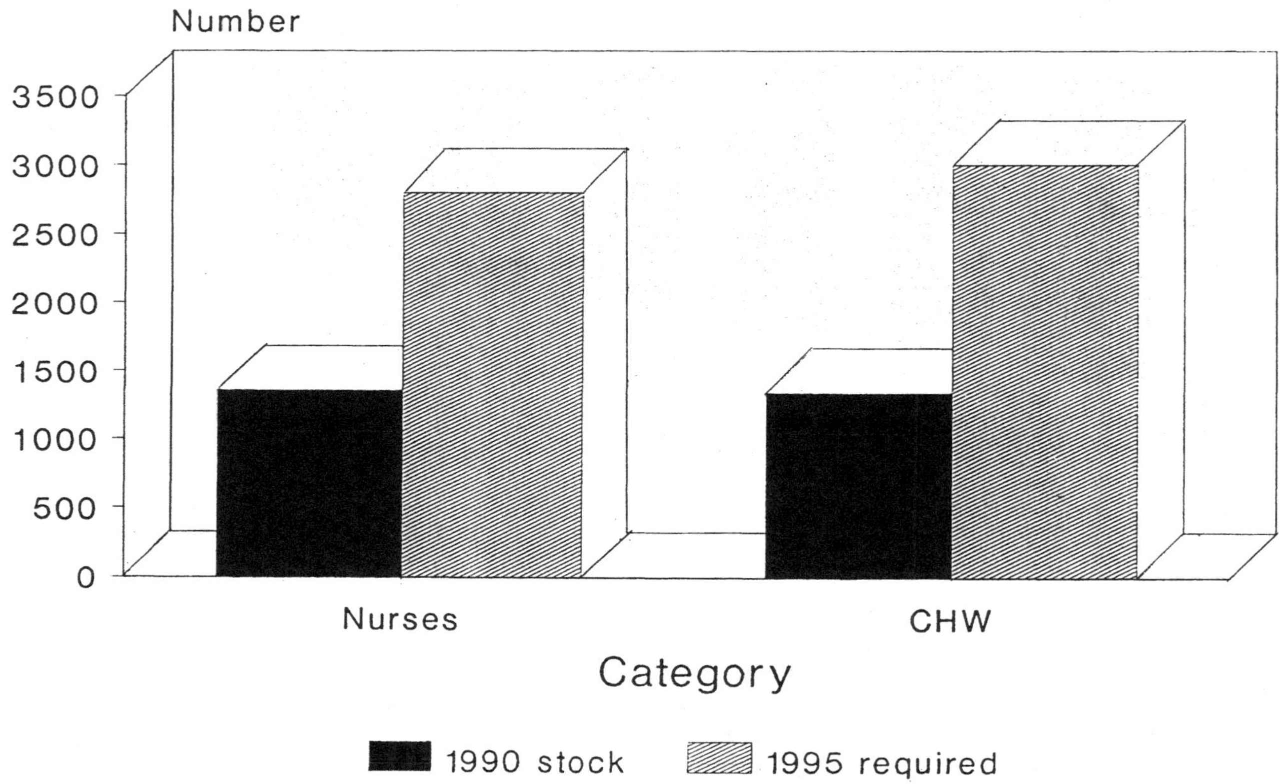

Excluding Aidposts

Projected Shortfall: Health Expenditure
1990-1995

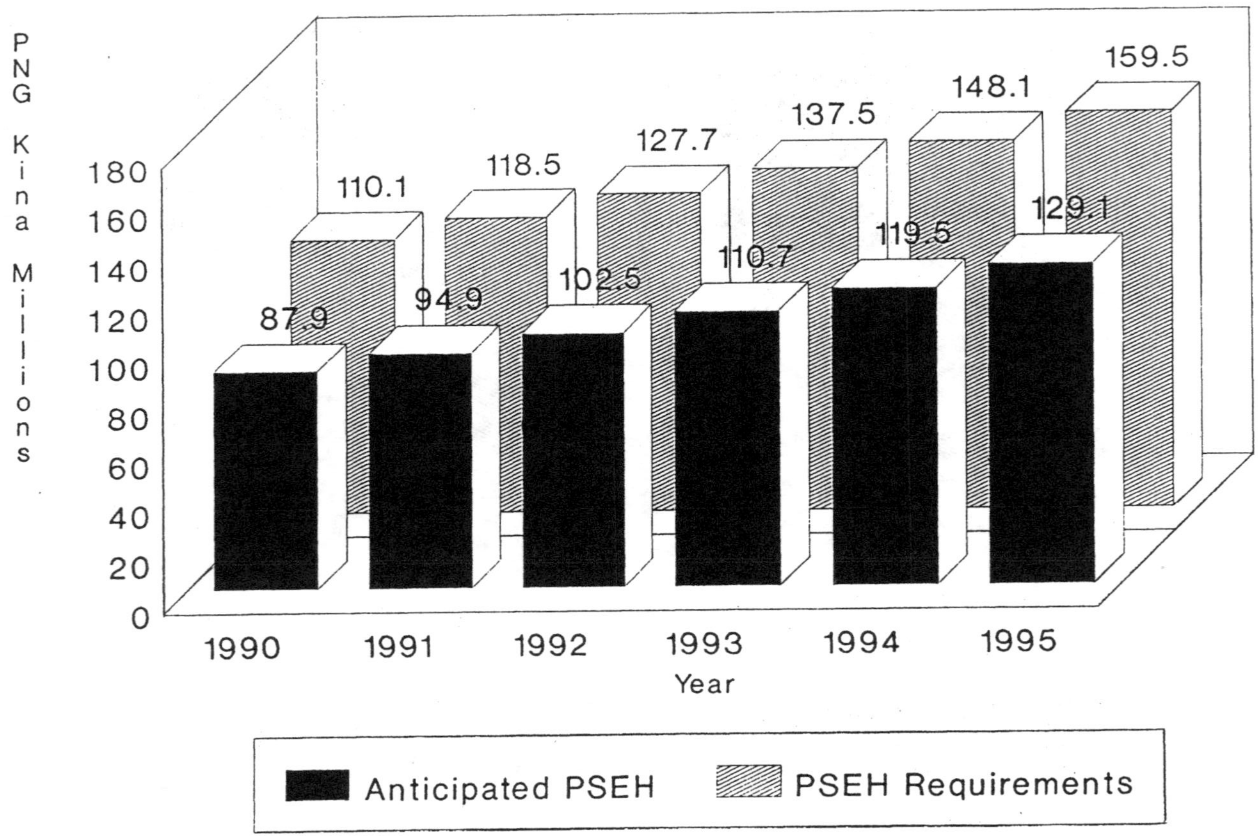

Source: Rosenthal et al

UNEVEN DEVELOPMENT AND MIGRATION IN PAPUA NEW GUINEA: IMPLICATIONS OF 1980 INTERPROVINCIAL FLOWS

JENNIFER LITAU[1]

Introduction

> Structural change or disequilibrium of any sort... may be the single most important progenitor of population movements in Third World settings (Brown and Lawson 1985:3)

An analysis of the causes of population movements must consider causal forces contemporary with movements as influenced by the past, which circumscribe the context within which migration occurs (Riddell 1980). Migration is part of the larger socioeconomic economy. Population movements can, therefore, be understood, by relating them to other socioeconomic changes within the economy. Socioeconomic changes foment migration and are stimulated by it. As migration is part of the larger system, uneven socioeconomic development or regional disparities have an important influence on the magnitudes, patterns and directions of migration.

Migration is defined as the inevitable movement of populations, across regions, in response to imbalances in the unequal distribution of socioeconomic opportunities or regional disparities in the distribution of natural resources. Development is defined as a purpose towards which the state exercises its power, that improves both the present and future lives of its subjects. Uneven development refers to differentials in the distribution of socioeconomic opportunities and natural resources.

Studies concerned with the migration-development relationship generally focus on (a) an historical analysis of migration within the context of social and economic changes or events and (b) the role of individuals in migration. Migration may even be regarded as an inevitable, consequence of macro socioeconomic changes. (Brown and Jones 1985).

Subsequent conclusions therefore pertain to migration processes and patterns which are specific to the locale of study. Generalization about other issues are limited but relevant in practice.

[1] National Research Institute, Papua New Guinea

This paper deals with the impact that uneven socioeconomic development and regional disparities in the distribution of natural resources had on the 1980 interprovincial migration flows in Papua New Guinea (PNG) and the implications for contemporary development efforts, policy and planning.

Background

The relationship between migration and uneven socioeconomic development is generally studied with two main views. The first view called the equilibrium approach advocates that migration must occur in order to correct socioeconomic imbalances which exist. The second view perceives migration as stimulated by broader structural changes which are rooted in specific periods, and this is called the historical-structural approach.

According to the equilibrium approach, migration parallels the imbalances in the socioeconomic structure. Its main focus is on the migration weighing out advantages and costs of the move prior to an actual movement to a destination of 'better' economic opportunities. Inherent in this approach are assumptions that:

(1) no obstacles to migration exist;
(2) migrants are homogeneous in skills and tastes;
(3) migrants have a perfect knowledge regarding employment opportunities; and
(4) they migrate in order to maximize their incomes (Gober-Meyers 1978).

The migration of labour is also seen to involve movement from areas of surplus labour (rural) to labour deficit regions (urban) (Lawson and Brown 1978). Thus, if wage differentials in associated regions were reduced to zero there would be a spatial balance of supply of and demand for labour in the system. In developing countries, labour would be seen to move from rural areas of high labour supply, scarce capital, and few employment opportunities, to mostly urban areas of low labour supply, some capital, and more employment and socioeconomic opportunities.

This view was (and has been) applied with minimal modification to the Third World by Todaro (1970), with expected though limited results. The Todaro model was applied to the ASEAN countries of Indonesia, Philippines, Malaysia and Thailand by Ogawa and Suit (1985), with inconclusive results.

In PNG, the equilibrium approach to development guided the colonial development strategy of the territory. Treadgold (1978) points out that the "colonial (development) objective" was to invest only in economically promising areas such as evolving urban centres, plantations and mines to reap the most revenue. Labour was encouraged to move to these centres. Dahanayake (1982) reiterates that the public policy was directed at promoting spatial equality and resulting economic growth which would lead to a convergence in regional per capita income. The colonial government promoted and perpetuated this development notion through selective investment policies but was minimally concerned with the policy's non-economic impact. Over the years, this development strategy has not only created polarized growth but influenced migrations in favour of destinations with relatively more and better (perceived) opportunities.

The second view is difficult to summarize for two main reasons:

a) because it is found in a variety of theories; and

b) migration can be investigated not separately but as part of the historical analysis of broader socioeconomic or structural changes underway in a society (Wood 1982).

In essence, migration is seen as both a manifestation of, and a response to, the social and spatial arrangements and rearrangements of the national economy, where the State plays a dominant role. Migration must be understood within the context of existing socioeconomic formations imposed both internally and externally, or internally existing but externally reinforced, or externally imposed and subsequently internalized.

This view focuses on classes or class structures rather than people per se. Thus, the positions which people enter and occupy within the socioeconomic system, in terms of their abilities to employ and utilize land, labour and capital to their benefit, determine how economically able they are to survive within this sytem. However, the positions within the socioeconomic environment which people enter and occupy, vary according to their roles, positions and the availability of economic opportunities in a given area. These opportunities, in turn, significantly influence the geographical mobility of labour from one socioeconomic environment to another, such as from the rural to urban centres (Shrestha 1988).

Class structure is seen as an exploitative relationship that assures the unequal appropriation of natural resources and the value which human labour produces. This is based on the principle of capital accumulation and expansion which is realized through the analysis of specific classes and groups and of political and ideological movements within a historical context. Class conflicts in terms of working class rebellion against the employers would lead to a change in the system (Wood 1982).

The principal argument is that capitalist modes of production only partially penetrate an economy, and compete with, and often replace traditional economic systems. This situation subsequently creates a mobile force of 'peasants' many of whom seek jobs in urban areas, under conditions of low wages, weak worker positions relative to employers, and an under-utilization of human resources (Lawson and Brown 1987).

Migration (and social change) is therefore the outcome of conflicts (Woods 1982) or tension resulting from structurally determined "tendencies" and "counter tendencies" or contradictions that are both necessary for, yet destructive of, particular processes and entities (Brown and Lawson 1985: 179). This tension results inevitably from conflicting structural forces which operate within the social and economic system. Structural conflicts reflect variations in the (levels of) distribution of amenities, infrastructure, urbanization, socioeconomic opportunities and government policies. Spatial differentials in structural tension or socioeconomic inequality stimulate migration (Lawson and Brown 1987).

In the Third World, the migration and uneven development relationship was first recognized by Zelinsky (1971) as occurring in stages. Places with different development characteristics in Venezuela were found to generate migration streams which differed in size, explanation and impact (Brown and Kodras 1987). Brown and Lawson (1985) recognized that in Costa Rica, migration flows form a "core-periphery" pattern.

The evidence from the Philippines (Findley, 1987a, 1987b), Lee (1985), and Bilsborrow et al. (1987) also attests this basic relationship between migration and uneven development.

Migration also affects development and underdevelopment through the selectivity of migrants in terms of their age, sex, occupation and capability (Zachariah 1977). Migrants tend to be younger, male, skilled, and relatively more educated in their place of origin but less than the population in their destination (Crowley 1977). They also tend to have a higher level of participation in economic activities (Skeldon 1983). Most of these have been verified in the Third World: Skeldon (1983) for South Asia; Ogawa (1985) for South-East Asia; Riddell (1980) for Africa; Brown and Goetz (1987) for Latin America; and Jones and Richter (1981) for South-East Asia; Ogawa (1985) for South-East Asia and the South Pacific. Specific geographical variations still exist. For instance, Ogawa (1985), Skeldon (1983) and Martine (1975) document short distance, female-dominated migrations mostly for marital and employment reasons for Asia and Colombia, respectively. The impact of education as one of the main promoters of migration is also mixed, as shown by Skeldon (1983) and Zachariah (1977). Such variations amplify the contextual importance of migration and the need for a contextual approach to migration study.

These two views, however, have mutual biases. The equilibrium approach focuses on individual behaviour which the historical - structural approach ignores. Hence, the latter view precludes individual decision making and specifications of costs and benefits which may affect the propensity to migrate. Because of this, the latter approach cannot effectively identify the links between macro-socioeconomic change and population movement because it presumes that individual behaviour can be explained only in terms of the individual location within the economy (Sam 1989).

Despite these criticisms, the historical-structural approach is attractive in practice, relative to the equilibrium approach, in attempting to understand contradictions within the migration setting in the Third World and Papua New Guinea in terms of the migration response to development situation.

UNEVEN DEVELOPMENT AND MIGRATION IN PAPUA NEW GUINEA

Townsend (1985) and Curtain (1981) explicity recognized that the internal and external economic dependence of Papua New Guinea inevitably leads to the role of migration as a survival strategy. Turner (1984) exemplifies that circular migration flows both intensify and foster a high dependency of rural recipients on migrant remittances which is illustrated by King (1980) Morauta (1984), Ross (1984) and Young (1981) as leading to further or repeated migrations. Most other migration studies about Papua New Guinea do not directly relate to the migration-uneven development relationship but are fragmented in foci ranging from descriptive to purely demographic analyses of migration statistics. Ward (1983) first made the call to incorporate into migration studies about Papua New Guinea variables pertaining to the socioeconomic context or institutional factors. Strathern (1985) shares and reiterates this view. In part, this is because other migration processes such as circulation, step and chain migration, urban unemployment and the increasing growth of squatter settlements connected to rural-urban migrations, and why migration does not promote a balance in socioeconomic growth, are inadequately accounted for. However, by delineating these processes within the historical context of socioeconomic change we can begin to understand migration processes in Papua New Guinea much better.

Population mobility has taken place in Papua New Guinea throughout the whole period of human occupation. Such movements included intervillage movements or inter island-coastal trading expeditions of the Hiri and Kula. Movements were relatively permanent for reasons such as changes in tribal and clan boundaries, food or land shortages and disputes, changes in demands for wives, land, security, material goods and trade. Many of these movements were voluntary and more difficult to execute for the individual and family because of the planning and preparations involved. But they were of sufficient magnitude to alter the nature and density of population distribution, and involved the diffusion of agricultural crops and techniques, institutions, artifacts, and behaviour and attitude patterns. Contact with the Europeans and the spread of colonialism generally is understood to have put an end to these old mobility patterns, and brought new ones into play.

The transition from pre-colonial to colonial types of movement first involved the recruitment of local people to work for German planters in East and West New Britain in the 1870s. Next was blackbirding whereby villagers were lured aboard recruiting vessels to go to the sugarcane plantations of Northern Australia, with promises of goods. This practice was permitted to continue throughout the 1880s in East and West New Britain (ENB and WNB) New Ireland (NIP), Bougainville (North Solomons), Milne Bay Islands and Northeastern Papua (See Figure 1). This "laissez faire" era of labour movement ended in 1884 when Papua was formally annexed by Britain and New Guinea by Germany (Turner 1984).

It was during this period that the character of movements changed. Increases occurred in the volume of movements, distances traversed, short-term movements, new movements from the interior to the coast, economically motivated moves, more individual than group migrations, and the settlement of new areas. Transportation greatly facilitated these movements. Greater differences emerged between the new urban and the traditional rural societies which gradually led to disparities between areas.

In Papua, wage labour was quickly institutionalized and regulated, beginning with the Native Labour Ordinance of 1892 which prescribed the terms and conditions of employment. There were two contradictory goals:

(1) survival of village society; and
(2) the continuity of labour supply

Legislation of the labour system in New Guinea evolved more slowly, but the terms and conditions for both colonies were similar. A system of indentured labour was consequently established in Papua New Guinea where the indigenous people moved to government and mission stations, plantations and mines and eventually to urban centres. Gradually, migrants were being drawn to areas of wage-paying job opportunities or alien-sponsored activity.

Between 1920 (when Australia annexed the territories of Papua New Guinea) and the Second World War, indentured or contract labourers were recruited from East Sepik (ESP) and West Sepik, (WSP) Morobe, Madang, Gulf and Milne Bay to work in the plantations of the New Guinea Islands or in the mines of Central, Milne Bay and Morobe. The labourers were brought to the destination of employment at the employer's expense to serve a term, then, as dictated by regulations, repatriated to their areas of origin. Many returned, to repeat migration later, but some remained or moved to the newly evolving towns. The outcome was the well-established settler communities found today in destination provinces.

Indentured labour mobility was formally replaced after the Second-World War by the Agreement Labour System through the Highlands Labour Scheme. The change in name is misleading because it applied only to a change in the recruiting source region; the destination areas and the terms and conditions of employment remained the same. However, in both the contract and agreement systems, movements were temporary and initially circular in nature, as dictated by legislation. Migrants were therefore recruited, brought to plantation destinations; after serving a term ranging from two months to two years, they were repatriated to origin areas.

Return movements by labourers had profound effects on the sending communities; they fostered desires for material goods that could only be obtained through further migrations. Information was also spread about particular employment-source areas which became major recipient destinations of voluntary migrants since the late 1950s. Evolving urban centres of perceived economic opportunities were the main attractions to migrants. These evolved in the most strategic and accessible island or coastal locations, like the colonial towns of Port Moresby, Lae, Rabaul and others currently designated as provincial capitals (Figure 1). The rural non-village sector consisting of plantations, mining enclaves, missions, schools and similar activities not effectively connected with the village nor contained within delineated urban boundaries, was another major attraction as a destination for migrants.

The "colonial objective" was to invest only in economically promising areas in order to reap maximum revenue or benefit. Hence, activities were limited to the urban and rural-non-village sectors of plantations and mines. Such activities mainly involved the domestic production and overseas export of raw materials such as copra, rubber and some minerals. There was little manufacturing and industry but considerable building, service and infrastructure growth in towns, which marked the beginning of polarized socioeconomic growth biased against rural areas. This, in turn, greatly affected mobility and population movements. By the 1960s the Highlands experienced circular migration, mostly to plantations. It was only in the late 1960s that urban-directed movements developed. By 1971, for PNG as a whole, urban centres were very attractive destinations (Skeldon, 1978).

A new dependence on the cash or wage sector, created through the introduction of head tax, school fees, and the desire for consumer goods, 'forced' households to engage in wage-labour migrations which inevitably led to 'voluntary' job searches. Such opportunities were scarce in the villages, and legislation restricted the free movement of people. Yet people migrated from rural-villages to plantations, mines and mission stations, but the largest volume of migration had been from the rural-villages to urban centres (May and Skeldon, 1977). Ward (1977) and Conroy (1977) have identified push factors, or the distressed socioeconomic situation of the villages, as causes.

Since political independence in 1975, the government has initiated many development policies and sectoral strategies as guidelines to its implementation of socioeconomic development. A comprehensive review of these developments was addressed in an IASER sponsored seminar (see IASER: Dahanayake 1982) where the primary goal emphasized was rural development, expansion of commercial agriculture and development of natural resources. This policy, embedded in the multi-export strategy, calls for the development of primary commodities and natural resources. Employment and income opportunities, created by sudden booms in the plantations and mines, "pull" migrants to these related areas. Employers or owners are primarily foreigners. The government, in allowing the development of primary commodities and natural resources, has the intention of promoting employment and the establishment of infrastructure and services. However, inherent within the system are such forces as unfair rates of exchange in terms of money value, environmental destruction and the creation and fostering of high expectations which seem only to be solved by further migrations to these areas.

Current urban centres (Figure 1) had been colonial cities which evolved in the late 1970s in importance and with accompanying population growth. Port Moresby, Lae and Rabaul were the most populous centres until the 1980s when Mt. Hagen, Madang and Arawa caught up. The locations of these places, in terms of access to transportation, communication, trade routes and economic opportunities were important contributing factors.

The 1980s, according to the preliminary results of the 1990 census, show a very high population increase for NCD (Port Moresby) of 56 percent Enga ranks next with a 43 percent increase in its population during the decade. This is followed by West and East New Britain Provinces.

Simbu province has had the lowest population increase of 3 percent and Gulf 6 percent.

Morobe province has recorded the highest population size of 357,000 (1990) from 310,622 (1980). Southern Highlands ranks next with a 1990 population size of 303,000 from 236,052 (1980). Manus then Gulf recorded lowest population sizes in 1990 of 33,000 and 68,000 respectively, a reflection of their positions in 1980 (Times of PNG, 1991).

If as in 1980 where NCD recorded a net inmigration of 56,435 people, then the current increase may be attributed mostly to migration than fertility. This remains to be seen when NSO releases more data. Southern Highlands recorded negative net-inmigration in 1980 so the current positive growth needs to be further examined. Generally, an interesting trend indicated by various provincial population increases is that correlation between socioeconomic and demographic changes during the intercensal period.

In summary, the uneven development in Papua New Guinea, reflects socioeconomic inequalities associated with polarized growth as laid down by the colonial development strategy and reinforced by national government policies. It also includes differentials in the spatial distribution and development of resources, and the resulting awareness by the population. Socioeconomic biases in planning towards urban centres, mining enclaves, plantations, and against other areas. These inequalities are greatly aggravated by the spatial differentiation in the distribution of natural resources, population density, population movements and geographical constraints. As a result of the concentrated colonial development efforts in the agricultural and mining sectors, selected provinces tend to prosper economically over others (Figure 2). Apart from the influence of urban centres, plantations and mines continue to determine the destination of migrations thus resembling migration patterns of the past (Table 1). Such differentials in development were already in existence at the time of political independence in 1975.

Socioeconomic development in Papua New Guinea was, and is, a principal undertaking of the government. Hence, development may be defined as a purpose towards which the state exercises its power, to improve both the present and future lives of its people (Gore 1984). Development regions in Papua New Guinea are classified in terms of homogeneity in geographical, cultural, political and administrative boundaries. However, there is a bias in planning towards administrative regions or provinces, which has been necessitated by decentralization. Much is known about provincial inequality (IASER: De Albuquerque and D'Sa 1986). Within provinces, urban centres dominate in functional, administrative and economic importance. Their importance has been consolidated over the years as evidenced in their population sizes. NSO records show that Port Moresby, Lae and Rabaul were the three largest urban centres in 1980 with populations of 123, 624, 61, 617 and 14, 954 respectively.

Although Papua New Guinea has a long colonial history dating back to 1884, rapid increases in its urban population have occurred only between the late 1960s and 1970s. Rural-urban migration appears to be the most important stream of migration. Other streams such as rural-RNV (Rural-Non Village) and rural-rural areas persist but are less important. According to the 1980 Census, 81.9 percent of the population was resident in rural villages, 5.8 percent in rural-non-villages and 12.3 percent in the urban centres.

Table 1 shows the percentage of migrants from each province who had migrated to rural, rural-non-village, and urban sectors in other provinces by 1980. According to PNG population averages, 54.4 percent of provincial out-migrants had as their destinations urban areas in other provinces, 28.2 percent went to the rural-non-village sectors, while only 12.4 percent migrated to other rural areas. However, Table 1 does not show migration to other sectors within provinces. Within PNG provinces, a population average of 87.2 percent are non-migrants, 3.7 percent are district migrants and 9.1 percent are provincial migrants (Walsh 1985: 49). It can, therefore, be inferred that the rural population, which is in majority is relatively stable. Both district or provincial migrant populations are more likely to participate in multiple moves. The latter groups mainly denote wage labour which is heavily dependent on migration in search of opportunities that seem unavailable in the rural sector. This differential distribution of the population directly reflects the relative attractiveness of each of these respective sectors as potential destinations.

In 1980, these trends had been already consolidated and intensified. Urban migration by most provincial out-migrants dominated the 1980 inter-provincial streams. Migration to RNVs was the next important except for NCD (where retired or retrenched workers were returned to home villages).

Table 1: Outmigration by Birth Province to Sector of Residence, 1971.

Province	Total	RV (%)	RNV (%)	Urban (%)
Western	4,456	18.6	24.8	56.7
Gulf	14,111	3.4	18.7	77.9
Central	9,417	17.8	29.0	53.2
Milne Bay	7,160	8.0	27.1	65.0
Northern	5,834	5.3	31.4	63.3
Southern Highlands	11,916	6.0	77.8	16.2
Western Highlands	9,811	15.2	53.0	31.9
Chimbu	22,531	18.0	51.0	31.0
Eastern Highlands	12,471	7.7	44.4	47.9
East Sepik	18,178	6.0	45.8	48.2
Madang	11,287	13.9	42.4	43.7
Morobe	18,904	14.9	36.1	48.0
West Sepik	7,415	11.0	53.1	35.9
Manus	3,950	13.9	32.2	53.9
New Ireland	4,248	15.8	34.3	49.9
West New Britain	4,882	12.8	43.5	43.7
East New Britain	8,887	19.0	43.2	37.8
Bougainville	2,504	18.0	25.2	56.8
PNG	177,962	12.0	42.1	45.9

Adapted from Ronald Skeldon, Evolving Patterns of Population Movement in Papua New Guinea with Reference to Policy Implications. No. 4, 1978, P.13.

The genesis of uneven development was an outgrowth of the colonial development strategy. Colonial socioeconomic formation or restructuring of the economy manipulated migration through taxes, policies on labour supply and remuneration, and concentration of capital (employers) in some areas to which labour moved. Hence, there was change in the characteristics of migration whereby labour, with different skills, moved to areas such as urban centres, mining enclaves and plantations. These patterns and processes were reinforced by the national development policies after political independence.

Although migration characteristics, patterns and processes established during the colonial period continue to evolve (and perhaps diversify), dominant recipient destinations are still coastal or island provinces, urban centres, and rural-non-village places. In 1971, as Table 1 indicates, in most of the Papuan provinces, but more pronounced for Gulf and Central, major destinations were urban centres (Port Moresby). For New Guinea island provinces, most of North Solomons, Manus and New Ireland out-migrants entered urban centres while for East and West New Britain out-migrants dominant destinations were RNVs, and mostly plantations. East Sepik and Madang out-migrants predominantly entered the urban centres while for West-Sepik and Madang RNVs were major destinations. For the Highlands, 78 percent of out-migrants from Southern Highlands, majority of Western Highlands and Chimbu resided in RNVs or plantations, while most of Eastern Highlands' out-migrants went to urban centres. Essentially, migrations to and probably between rural villages had declined in importance by 1971. Urban centres were becoming more important destinations for out-migrants from provinces with longer histories of contact, and rural non-villages (mostly plantations at that time) were important destinations for out-migrants from provinces with shorter histories of contact.

The early 1980s saw Western and Eastern Highlands Provinces emerging because of the boom in the coffee industry. However, this still resembles established patterns where migration flows in the direction of provincial growth poles, or urban centres, plantation estates, or mining enclaves. This is evident in the migration rates shown in Table 3, where the NCD, Morobe, East New Britain, West New Britain, North Solomons, New Ireland, and Western Highlands have positive net and inmigration rates. Migration to the NCD, Morobe, and East New Britain are dominated by outflows to either urban or rural-non-village sectors in other provinces (Table 2).

Table 2: Provincial Outmigration by Sector Destination, 1980.

Origin Province	Total	Destination of Migrants (%) RV[a]	RNV[a]	U[a]
Western	5,332	12.1	14.2	73.7
Gulf	15,203	7.9	7.7	84.2
Central	22,002	5.3	4.8	89.9
NCD	9,326	34.5	13.6	51.9
Milne Bay	9,676	8.5	17.9	73.6
Northern	7,138	10.6	13.5	75.9
S.Highlands	21,643	7.4	65.2	27.4
Enga	12,021	8.2	45.6	46.2
W.Highlands	7,825	19.1	26.3	54.2
Chimbu	29,684	20.1	36.0	71.6
Morobe	24,456	10.3	30.7	59.0
Madang	15,637	12.8	33.8	53.4
E.Sepik	24,892	10.1	33.7	56.2
W.Sepik	7,486	11.9	41.3	46.8
Manus	5,435	11.6	13.1	75.3
N.Ireland	5,767	15.6	20.5	63.9
E.N.Britain	15,892	17.6	23.9	58.5
W.N.Britain	5,238	16.4	29.5	54.1
N.Solomons	3,423	15.2	19.9	64.9
PNG	269,819	12.4	28.2	54.4

Source: Adapted from A. Crosbie Walsh, <u>Interprovincial Migration in Papua New Guinea.</u> Research Monograph No. 3. Port Moresby: National Statistical Office, 1985, p.47

a R = rural village; RNV = rural-non-village; and U = urban.

Table 3: Provincial Migration Rates, 1980

Province & Region	Born & Resident	Resident[a]	Out	In	Net	OMR[b]	IMR[b]
Western	78,337	76,529	5,332	1,808	-3,524	65	23
Gulf	63,843	61,034	15,503	2,809	-12,695	203	44
Central	116,361	106,408	22,158	9,953	-12,205	173	86
NCD	12,429	46,249	9,745	66,180	56,435	174	589
Milne Bay	127,725	125,085	7,767	2,640	-7,127	72	21
Northern	77,097	70,659	7,232	6,438	-794	93	84
PAPUA	575,792	489,962	69,737	89,828			
% of PNG	19.33	17.98	25.78	33.07			
S.Highlands	23,539	232,044	21,765	3,346	-18,419	82	105
Enga	164,270	162,277	12,044	1,993	-10,051	69	12
W.Highlands	264,129	229,437	7,854	34,686	26,838	33	131
Chimbu	178,013	174,443	29,731	3,570	-26,161	16	20
E.Highlands	274,608	260,836	20,764	13,772	-6,992	74	50
NW EWEW GUINEA HIGHLANDS	1,116,410	1,059,037	92,158	57,367			
%	37.89	31.19	34.07	21.12			
Morobe	305,356	273,422	24,556	31,934	7,378	82	105
Madang	209,650	196,173	15,667	13,483	-3,186	74	64
E.Sepik	220,827	212,858	24,993	7,969	-17,024	105	36
W.Sepik	113,849	110,862	7,528	2,987	-4,541	64	26
NORTHERN	849,682	793,315	72,744	56,373			
%	28.53	29.35	26.89	20.75			
Manus	25,859	23,690	5,449	2,169	-3,280	187	84
N.Ireland	65,657	57,635	5,785	8,022	2,237	91	122
E.N.Britain	130,730	109,567	15,931	21,163	5,232	127	162
W.N.Britain	88,415	68,496	5,250	19,919	14,669	71	225
N.Solomons	125,506	108,726	3,446	16,780	13,334	31	134
N.G.ISLANDS	436,167	368,114	35,861	68,053			
%	14.65	13.62	13.26	25.05			
PNG	2,978,057	2,702,430	270,502	271,627			91

Source: Adapted from A. Crosbie Walsh, Interprovincial Migration in Papua New Guinea. Research Monograph No. 3 PortMoresby: National Statistic Office, 1985, p.43

a. Citizen population only, excluding non-citizens.

b. OMR - Outmigration Rates; and IMR=Immigration Rates.

Methodology

It has been hypothesized that historical and contextual or socioeconomic factors, at both origin and destination provinces significantly influence migration positively and should be explicitly considered in order to understand migration within Papua New Guinea. Additionally, migration streams or flows expect to originate in less developed provinces and flow towards the relatively more developed ones.

The following specific issues will be examined:

(1) Origin push factors associated with social and economic inequalities between provinces play an equally important role in stimulating out migration as destination pull factors do in attracting migrants.

(2) Migration flows are directed at destination provinces either urban in character or endowed with opportunities of income and employment, such as plantations and mines; and these flows tend to reinforce past trends.

(3) A major obstacle to migration is the distance between provinces.

(4) Differentials in the provincial distribution of socioeconomic opportunities associated with wage rates or wage-earning activities significantly influenced the magnitude and direction of flows in favour of higher wage-earning provinces.

(5) Variables closely related to the market or modern economy should play a lesser role in rural settings.

These issues will be evaluated indirectly through employing multiple regression on selected socioeconomic indices adapted or adopted from the Brown-Lawson (1985) migration model which deals with the effect of development on migration, as applied to Costa Rica. The model is based on statistical formulations rooted in economics which account for migration through variables pertaining to wage rates, job opportunities, amenity levels, migration costs and information flows. This conventional modelling is concerned with the search for "universal laws" which apply to migration across geographic locations and time. It generally differs with analyses pertaining to the historical-structural view of migration which guides this study. However, economic growth involves structural changes; therefore, in practice, the use of economic variables and statistical formulations rooted in the equilibrium analyses is justified. Alternatively, employing conventional modelling within a structural analysis is a positive step in bridging the gap between the two different approaches to migration study. Conventional modelling is employed as a method of analysis but the interpretation of the analyses will reflect the contextual "reality".

Model

The Brown-Lawson migration model entails the migration rate-the dependent variable (M_{ij}) which is commonly employed in the empirical estimation of migration in Third World settings and two sub-variables of Om_i and R_{ij}. These dependent variables are defined as:

(1) $M_{ij} = M_{ij}/P_j$

where M_{ij} = number of individuals migrating from province $_i$ to $_j$ in time t to t + 1

P_j = population of province $_i$ at time t

Therefore, M_{ij} is the percentage of the population at risk in province $_i$ at time t, who move to place $_j$ by time t + 1

or

the probability of a person in Province $_i$ moving to Province $_j$ during time t to t + 1. The equation is a composite of (2) the probability of outmigration from $_i$ (Om_i) and (3) finding a new residence anywhere (R_{ij}) defined as,

(2) $Om_i = 1 - (M_{ii}/P_i)$

where M_{ii} = persons remaining in $_i$ from time t to t + 1;

and

(3) $R_{ij} = M_{ij}/M_i$

where M_i is the total outmigration from province $_i$. R_{ij} is the probability that a person from place $_i$ relocates to $_j$ (given that a person moves from place $_i$).

After the Brown-Lawson migration model, Equation (2) reflects the decision to seek a new residence and Equation (3) reflects the decision on where to relocate. Equation (1) embodies both decisions to seek a new residence and where to relocate and represents a joint probability. Estimations of separate models for outmigration and relocation better identify the role of push factors, which estimation of the migration rate itself does not directly bring out.

Three regression analyses using SPSS are performed on the three dependent migration variables: the origin-destination migration rate (M_{ij}), outmigration rate (Om_i) and the probability of relocation (R_{ij}). These migration rates are regressed against independent variables for the Brown-Lawson model. The adapted or adopted independent variables and their operational specifications are:

$DIST_{ij}$ = distance measured in kilometres between provinces $_i$ and $_j$ between provincial capitals.

POP_j	=	destination province $_j$'s residential population in 1980, including both citizens and non-citizens.
$WAGACT_{i\ or\ j}$	=	percentage population in wage-earning activities for both citizens and non-citizens in either province $_{i\ or\ j}$ in 1980.
$PCUJOB_{i\ or\ j}$	=	percentage population in employment by urban-based activities, for either province $_{i\ or\ j}$ in 1980, or the percentage in secondary or tertiary sectors.
$PRES_{i\ or\ j}$	=	population pressure or dependency ratio calculated as a percentage of, too young + old + students, divided by total employed provincial citizen and non-citizen population.
$EDUC_{i\ or\ j}$	=	percentage of adult population (age 15+) of province $_{i\ or\ j}$ in 1980 "not in school" but who have completed one year of school (Grade 1) as a measure of the literacy rate.
$MCHAIN_i$	=	the probability of residing in province $_i$ prior to 1971 and outmigrating by that year. This one is calculated in the same way as the outmigration (Om_i) dependent variable (Equation 2) or provincial outmigration rate (OMR) in 1971 OMR's of province $_i$ are used because they are the latest record to 1980).
POP_i	=	population size of origin province $_i$ in 1980 to represent possible effects of origin province population pressure due to "overpopulation" and its effects on land availability; reasons are non-economic, or availability of amenities.

These independent variables are regressed initially against the migration rate dependent variable (Equation (1)). Then only independent variables pertaining to origin province $_i$ are regressed against the outmigration probability (Equation (2)). Finally, independent variables pertaining to destination province $_j$ are regressed against the relocation probability (Equation (3)). Hence, the interprovincial model, expressed in log-linear form (to denote the multiplicative effects of the independent variables on the dependent variable) is:

$$(4)\quad LnM_{ij} = \alpha_0 + \alpha_1 Ln\ Dist_{ij} + \alpha_2 Ln\ Pop_i + \alpha_3 Ln\ Pop_j + \alpha_4 Ln\ Wagact_j +$$

$$\alpha_5 \text{Ln Pcujob}_j + \alpha_6 \text{Ln Pres}_j + \alpha_7 \text{Ln Educ}_j + \alpha_8 \text{Ln Mchain}_i$$

The outmigration model, in log-linear form is:

$$(5) \quad \text{Ln Om}_j = \alpha_0 + \alpha_1 \text{Ln Pop}_i + \alpha_2 \text{Ln Wagact}_i + \alpha_3 \text{Ln Pcujob}_i + \alpha_4 \text{Ln Pres}_i + \alpha_5 \text{Ln Educ}_i + \alpha_6 \text{Ln Mchain}_i$$

The log-linear relocation probability model is:

$$(6) \quad \text{LnR}_{ij} = \alpha_0 + \alpha_1 \text{Ln Dist}_{ij} + \alpha_2 \text{LnPop}_j + \alpha_3 \text{Ln Wagact}_j + \alpha_4 \text{Ln Pcujob}_j + \alpha_5 \text{Ln Pres}_j + \alpha_6 \text{Ln Educ}_j$$

Interprovincial Migration is expected to vary directly with destination population (Pop_j) size and inversely with intervening distance ($Dist_{ij}$). Pop_j and $Dist_{ij}$ reflect information about wage and employment opportunities between province $_i$ and $_j$ and the extent to which these are communicated between these places. Other interpretations of Pop_j are:

(1) it pertains directly to immigration;
(2) its size also indicates employment opportunities, particularly informal ones, and other amenities. $Dist_{ij}$ also measures indirectly financial costs but its importance should reflect modernity or efficiency of the transportation system; in either case, migration is expected to vary inversely with $Dist_{ij}$.

Expectations about the Wagact $_{i \text{ or } j}$ and $Pcujob_i$ variables assume that migration flows originate from areas of few money-earning job opportunities to areas of more wage and employment opportunities.

Pres $_i$ or $_j$ or a higher percentage of population pressure or level of dependency upon the economic base and its likelihood of providing sufficient support for local residents should relate directly to outmigration flows and inversely to inflows.

Educ $_{i \text{ or } j}$ represents the literacy and human capital component and is expected to vary directly with outmigration and inversely with inmigration. It might also represent indirectly the level and provision of educational services.

Pop_i should represent origin province's push factors arising from population pressures due to land shortages, poor access to or lack of social services. Hence larger origin population sizes should vary directly with outmigration. Alternatively, it may behave like Pop_j.

The strength of $Mchain_i$ represents the strength of interpersonal contact or indirectly it indicates potential access to information flows from media or transportation.

Data

Secondary data obtained from NSO (PNG) of the 1980 Census are used in the analyses. The main data sources are the Provincial Summary Figures (1980) and Interprovincial Migration in Papua New Guinea (Walsh 1983), a research monograph published by NSO. All provincial summaries except West Sepik's are available. The NSO monograph is basically a descriptive study but has valuable information already in tabulated form.

Analyses are conducted using 1980 data within a cross-sectional timeframe. An ideal study would consider and compare both 1980 and 1971 data. This was initially planned but it was later abandoned due to differentials between the way each census was conducted and the use of different definitions, and reclassification of provincial boundaries of central and NCD, and of Western Highlands and Enga Provinces. Subsequent comparisons would be complicated. Also the reliability of 1971 data is questioned.

Furthermore, an ideal test of the effect of uneven development on migration, in the Brown-Lawson model, requires the analyses of migration streams e.g. rural-urban from smallest to largest available scales. For Papua New Guinea, this should have been the test but census data are collected at the provincial level. Hence, though much is known about interprovincial characteristics little is known about intra-provincial characteristics.

Results of Analyses

The first three sets of analyses consisted of the linear model, using untransformed variables which were log-transformed in the second sets of analyses due to evidences of non-normality. Essentially, there is evidence of access in over and under predictions, which did not conform to our expected pattern of variable behaviour. Results greatly improved for all three models. The adjusted r^2 of the "interprovincial" (M_{ij}) flows analysis increased from r^2 = .312 to r^2 = .638 thus accounting for over half the percentage variance in interprovincial migration flows. The adjusted r^2 is used also because of the decrease in the degrees of freedom (df) due to more independent variables. Similarly, the log of Om_i flows increased slightly from adjusted r^2 = .168 to 483. r_{ij} also increased moderately to r^2 =.488, again accounting for almost half of the variation in the inmigration flows (Tables 3, 4 and 5).

Results of the M_{ij} (or interprovincial flow) model of independent variables are reported in Table 3. Considering the log-transformed results only, zero-order correlations (r values), which indicate direct relationships show that the logs of $Wagact_{ij}$, Pop_i and Pop_j encouraged the 1980 interprovincial flows than it was deterred by $Pres_j$, $Pcujob_j$, $Mchain_{ij}$ and $Educ_j$ except $Dist_{ij}$ whose effects exceeded both that of Pop_j and Pop_i. When r, B, and t-values are considered for effects, a slightly different picture emerges. Together, these indicate that $Wagact_j$; (B=.531, t=12.36 and r=.528) is the most significant variable in the M_{ij} model. It suggests that a higher percentage of population engaged in wage-earning activities in province $_j$ relates directly to higher inmigration flows. $Dist_{ij}$ values of B=.431, t=-11.32 and r=.392 indicate that the distance between provinces was an important deterrent to interprovincial migration. $Pres_j$ is of considerable importance (B=.340 and t=6.58) and had the most leverage on the flows (b=4.164) of an inverse relationship. Thus more population pressure in province $_j$ related to lower inflows and lesser pressure corresponded with more inflows. Beta, t and r values for Pop_i and Pop_j (Table 3) suggest that both higher origin and higher destination population sizes relate directly to higher provincial outmigration and inmigration flows; but both variables have a less significant effect. $Mchain_i$, $Educ_j$ and $Pcujob_j$ are also less important, but their relative effects, as indicated by the signs need not be totally discounted.

For the results of the "outmigration" or Om_i flows variables (Table 5), the log of $Wagact_i$ (B=.634, r=621 and t=3.04) also turns out to be the most important variable. Thus, higher percentage of population engaged in wage-earning income in province $_i$ directly influences outmigration from $_i$. This result contradicts the conventional expectation that migration flows originate in province of few money-earning and employment opportunities and flow towards those with more of such opportunities. Its behaviour is consistent, however, with the proposed view, in this study, that structural "pressure" induces migrations. Alien ownership of resources, their means of production, the spatial differentials in location of means of production, economic activities and natural resources imply that labour inevitably also moves to areas in which capital and the means for its production are located. The question whether or not a higher percentage of population in wage-activities should deter migration appears somewhat discounted. In addition, its behaviour could also reflect that even though opportunities exist in province $_i$, outmigration still occurs because there is demand for more services, and that people do actually weigh advantages and costs and decisions about moving.

Table 4: Interprovincial Migration Flows in Papua New Guinea, 1980: All Flows Analyses

a: Untransformed Variables

Independent Variables	r	b	B	t
$Wagact_j$	0.312	63.976***	0.397	7.25
$Dist_{ij}$	-.256	-1.679***	-.307	-5.83
$Mchain_j$	-.146	-9.657***	-.250	-4.01
$Pres_j$	-.068	134.947***	.214	3.11
$Pcujob_j$	-.015	7.312**	.113	2.02
Pop_i	.165	.002**	.102	2.06
$Educ_j$	-.073	79.586	.062	.86

n = 342   Adjusted r^2 = .312   F = 20.307

b: Log-Transformed Variables

Independent Variables	r	b	B	t
$Wagact_j$	0.528	2.509***	0.531	12.36
$Dist_{ij}$	-.392	-0.964***	-.431	-11.32
$Pres_j$	-.136	4.164***	.340	6.58
Pop_j	.292	.765***	.325	5.19
$Mchain_j$	-.180	-.760***	-.263	-5.77
$Educ_j$	-.123	.426***	.244	5.10
Pop_i	.300	.491***	.208	5.86
$Pcujob_j$	-.186	-.125	-.037	-0.87

n = 342   Adjusted r^2 = .638   F = 76.130

Notes

a. West Sepik Province was not included in all the analyses due to unavailable data.

b. r = zero=order correlation. Indicates direct relationships between the independent and dependent variables.
   b = elasticities or the slope of regression.
   B = beta weights. Indicates significance of independent variable's effect on the dependent variable.
   t = t-value. Indicates significance of b values.

c. Significance levels: * = .10, ** = .05, *** = .01.

Tables 5: Provincial Outmigration Flows in Papua New Guinea, 1980: Outmigration Analyses

Independent Variables	r	b	B	t
a: Untransformed Variables				
Pop_i	-0.178	-0.000	-0.390	-1.04
$Pcujob_i$	- .086	.001	.274	1.09
$Mchain_i$	- .090	- .001	- .252	-1.08
$Pres_i$	.079	.008	.178	0.63
$Wagact_i$	.508	.009***	.175	2.92
$Educ_i$	.101	- .000	- .002	-0.01
	n = 19	Adjusted r^2 = .168		F = 1.606
b: Log-Transformed Variables				
$Wagact_i$	0.621	2.058***	0.634	3.04
$Pres_i$	.175	2.131	.253	1.04
$Pcujob_i$	-.577	-.551	-.236	-1.14
$Educ_i$	.367	.249	.208	0.88
$Mchain_i$	.004	-.373	-.179	-0.94
Pop_i	-.200	-.042	-.026	-0.09
	n = 19	Adjusted r^2 = .483	F = 3.801	

Notes:

a. See Notes for Table 3, for explanations for r, b, B, and t.

b. Significance levels are indicated by:
* = .10, ** = .05, *** = .01.

Finally, results of the log of "relocation" variables (Table 6) indicate that the log of $Wagact_j$ has the most important direct positive influence on inter-provincial flows, as indicated by r = .572, B = .501 and t = 10.89. $Wagact_j$ (r value) accounts for over half the percentage of interprovincial flows. $Dist_{ij}$ is next in importance and behaved as a major deterrent to inmigration. Financial or psychic costs and transportation related problems are major obstacles to the probability to relocate, or they hinder inmigration to a province. All other independent variables pertaining to destination province $_j$ turned out to have less significant effects. Elasticities above 1 appear for $Pres_j$ (b=2.447) and $Wagact_j$ (b=2.282) suggesting that together these variables have the greatest leverage on inmigration flows or relocation probability to proince $_j$. Thus more population pressure in province $_j$ relates to a decline in net-inflow.

Residual analyses of M_{ij}, Om_i and r_{ij} yielded 10 important outliers. Standardized residuals tend to indicate an overprediction of inflows and outflows from NCD or towns and underprediction of flows into and between predominantly peripheral provinces. Therefore, results are neither significant nor inconclusive.

Findings

In the Papua New Guinea study, $Wagact_{i \text{ or } j}$ had the most important positive effect on the 1980 interprovincial migrations whereas Brown and Lawson's study on Costa Rica indicated $Pcujob_j$ and Pop_j as having the most positive influence to inter-canton migrations. $Dist_{ij}$ in both studies is an important deterrent to migration. These differences in results are contextually attributed in terms of differences in the history of social and economic penetration and political processes which condition migration processes. The role of $Dist_{ij}$ suggests that in the Third World migration setting, financial or psychic costs and the inefficiency of transportation significantly deter migration between areas.

Socioeconomic inequalities in wage and income earning opportunities and population sizes (indicative of differentials in the distribution of services and employment opportunities) stimulated interprovincial migrations significantly. This finding suggests that past migration trends are consolidated and can be expected to continue in the future.

That higher percentage of urban-based occupations or a larger proportion of secondary and tertiary sector in a province deterred out-migration suggests that they play a key role in attracting inmigration flows. These however were less significant impact upon the inflows.

Overall finding is, in-migration flows were directed at provinces with more employment opportunities, more jobs and amenities, not necessarily urban in character, have lower population pressure, higher literacy rates and lower previous outmigration rates.

Table 6: Provincial Inmigration Flows, 1980: Relocation Analyses

	a: Untransformed Variables			
Independent Variables	r	b	B	t
$Wagact_j$	0.385	0.004***	0.484	9.13
$Dist_{ij}$	-.243	-.001***	-.289	-5.92
$Pres_j$	-.018	.007***	.211	3.52
$Educ_j$	0.620	.011**	.145	2.12
Pop_j	.126	.000	.139	1.74
$Pcujob_j$	-.004	.001**	.119	2.25
n = 432		Adjusted r^2 = .248		F = 19.719

	b: Log-Transformed Variables			
Independent Variables	r	b	B	t
$Wagact_j$	0.572	2.282	0.501	10.89
Pop_j	.327	0.942***	.426	6.74
$Dist_{ij}$	-.277	-.696***	-.323	-7.88
$Educ_j$	-.037	.349***	.208	3.94
$Pres_j$	-.152	2.447***	.207	4.04
$Pcujob_j$	-.192	-.357***	-.109	-2.38
n = 342		Adjusted r^2 =.488		F = 55.218

Notes:

a. See Notes for Table 3, for explanations of r, b, B, and t.

b. Significance levels are indicated by:
* = .10, ** = .05, *** = .01.

These flows originated in provinces with relatively more wage-earning activities, higher population pressure, lower literacy levels, and higher previous outmigration rate or higher incidence of chain-migration. It is unexpected and irrational that there would be out-migration from provinces also with relatively more income-earning opportunities. The finding suggests that out-migrations from provinces occur for non-economic reasons. Greater dependence by people upon the wage sector means that (change in) forces dictating wage and employment opportunities strongly influence the tendency to outmigrate from a province. Alternatively, outmigration from provinces of relatively better employment opportunities imply that people are seeking or demand better non-economic services.

"Chain-effects" or family links seem partly responsible for the behaviour of $Wagact_i$. That is, people outmigrated to join relatives, friends, or wantoks. Chain-migration encouraged interprovincial flows but varied with outmigration flows suggesting that provinces with higher previous OMR are likely to experience further future outflows. The strength of interpersonal contacts or wantoks is demonstrated here. It also implies disparities in information flow caused by uneven development in communication or transportation networks.

The findings support the deterrent effect of distance between provinces $Dist_{ij}$. $Wagact_j$ reinforcing past trends, over the push effects of low literacy ($Educ_i$), population pressure ($pres_i$) and $Mchain_i$. The hypothesis that push factors compare equally to pull factors is not supported. Contradictory findings in regard to the roles of $Wagact_i$ in outmigration and $Pcujob_j$ in relocation to a province have stressed the importance of an explicit consideration of the socio economic context in understanding migration processes in Papua New Guinea.

Critique of Conventional Modelling

Conventional modelling has served basically as a method of analysis permitting the explicit analysis of socioeconomic variables affecting migration processes in Papua New Guinea, which are not otherwise permitted by the historical - structural approach that guides this study. Conventional models have been shown to describe market economy variables relatively better than social variables in terms of (1) contradictory findings regarding $Wagact_i$; and (2) overprediction of inflows to relatively larger market economy provinces of NCD, Western Highlands, and East New Britain, and subsequent underprediction of flows from and to the peripheral provinces of Western, Enga and Manus.

This does injustice to the social variable drawing major criticisms from the historical-structural approach within which both social and economic processes have equally significant effects on migration processes and patterns in Papua New Guinea. Other essential elements of this approach such as historical, political, and social processes, the qualitative effects of labour migrations on the peripheral provinces, and how this affects labour production, supply and remuneration, cannot be accounted for statistically. Similarly, continuous migrations to economically prosperous provinces which affects capital and labour conditions, cannot be simply reduced to a few statistical equations. Integrating conventional modelling into a structurally based migration study is a positive step towards bridging the gap between the two different approaches. Further work could be done to improve the use of conventional modelling to understand the structural effects or migration processes and patterns, like the "development paradigm" of migration by Brown and Sanders (1981).

Socio-Economic and Political Implications for Policy and Planning

1. Since the interprovincial migration flows of 1980 resemble the past trends, where policy strongly influences the directions of movements, it is likely that these types of flows will continue into the future. The Constitution encourages and protects the right to freedom of movement. Socioeconomic inequalities cannot be totally eradicated. However, government policy or action could redirect, stop or encourage further movements, conditioned by the socioeconomic context. In essence, public policy can reverse patterns already established. Creating employment opportunities and providing basic services in rural areas would hold people back or attract in-migrants.

2. The urban and the RNV components of provinces continue to develop over and above the levels for the rest of Papua New Guinea. This would make these sectors or provinces more attractive destinations, leading to unequal population growth and distribution. Relatively higher population growths in these provinces means pressure on existing levels of services for health, housing and education; the need for an increase in quantity and levels of provision of amenities and job opportunities; social pressure on wantoks; increase in rate of unemployment; a rise in crime levels and squatter settlements. It also means a lag in providing for adequate needed services. A positive implication of this is more potential voters and better representation by elected representatives. However, unless there is an increase in the rate of provision of these services, more unemployment related problems will result. There is a need to 'balance' migration and economic investments, or to promote integrated urban and rural development. The population policy is committed in this direction and must be supported.

3. The influence of the extended family or wantok system, seen through the effects of chain-migrations will continue to directly affect migrant types, their places of destination, their activity, household sizes and levels of food consumption, housing, health and education services. Longitudinal studies of this

phenomenon are required because of its implications on the population distribution and their levels of consumption of services.

4. The distance cost, and the efficiency of transportation or communication networks will continue to act as a major deterrents to interprovincial migrations. Where these distance-associated effects are minimal, we could expect higher degree of mobility. Plans drawn in terms of providing employment and social services need to take this into account, in NCD and other larger urban centres.

5. Provinces with higher wage-earning opportunities will continue to attract in-migrants; but population pressure, education level and urban-based opportunities in prospective destinations will tend to reduce the probabilities of inmigration to a province. The effects of these factors can be regulated by government action or public policy.

Conclusion

Government planning, policy making and implementation of social, economic, and infrastructural growth in provinces have historically affected migration processes and patterns and vice versa. Contemporary government actions reinforce migration and uneven development patterns and processes established during the colonial period. Although, priorities have shifted over time from urban development to agriculatural/rural development, the urban centres continue to absorb resources and grow, while rural areas remain neglected. Even though the importance of plantations fluctuates, resettlement schemes, mining enclaves or the RNV sector continue to grow and attract migrants. The urban and RNV sectors develop over and above the levels of the rest of the country, which makes these sectors, or provinces where they are located more attractive destinations. In the light of the growing urban-related problems of crime, unemployment and squatter settlements, and 'rural-decay' in some provinces, the planners and implementers have a vital part to play.

LIST OF ABBREVIATIONS

ASEAN	Association of South-East Asian Nations
ENB	East New Britain Province
ESP	East Sepik Province
NCD	National Capital District
NIP	New Ireland Province
NSO	National Statistical Office
OMR	Out Migration Rates
PNG	Papua New Guinea
RNV	Rural Non-Villages
SHP	Southern Highlands Province
SPSS	Statistical Packages For Social Sciences
EHP	Eastern Highlands Province
WNB	West New Britain Province
WSP	West Sepik Province

REFERENCES

Bilsborrow R E, McDevitt T M, Kassoudji S. and Fuller R., The impact of origin community characteristics Demography 1987; 24: 191-210.

Brown L A and Goetz A R. Development-related contextual effects and individual attributes in Third World migration processes: a Venezuelan example, Demography 1987; 24: 497-516.

Brown L A and Jones J P. Spatial variation in migration processes and development: a Costa Rican example of conventional modelling augmented by the expansion method, Demography 1985; 22: 327-352.

Brown L A and Kodras J E. Migration, human resource transfers, and development contexts: a logit analysis of Venezuelan data, Geographical Analysis 1987; 19: 243-263.

Brown L A and Lawson V A. Migration in the Third World setting, uneven development, and conventional modelling: a case study of Costa Rica, 1985; 75: 29-47.

Brown L A and Sanders R L. Toward a development paradigm of migration, with reference to the Third World settings, in G F Dejong and R W Gardner, ed., Migration Decision-making: Multidisciplinary Approaches to Micro-level studies in Developed and Developing Countries, Pergamon Press, 1981; pp. 49-69.

Crowley R. Population distribution: perspectives and policies, in A A Brown and E Neuberger, ed., Internal Migration: An Interdisciplinary Perspective. New York: Academic Press, 1977; pp.255-276.

Conroy J. Population distribution: perspectives and policies, in A A Brown and E Neuberger, ed., Internal Migration: An Interdisciplinary Perspective. New York: Academic Press, 1977; pp.255-276.

Conroy J. Urbanization in Papua New Guinea: a development constraint, in R J May, ed., Change and movement. Canberra: Australian National University 1977; pp. 59-70.

Curtain R L. Migration in Papua New Guinea: the role of the peasant household in a strategy of survival, in ed., G W Johns and H V Richter, Population Mobility and Development: Southeast Asia and the Pacific. Canberra: The Australian National University, 1981; pp. 187-204.

Dahanayake P ed. Post-independence Economic Development of Papua New Guinea. 1982; Monograph 19. Waigani: IASER.

Davis K. The effect of out-migration on regions of origin, in ed., A A Brown and E Neuberger, Internal Migration: a Comparative Perspective, New York: Academic Press. 1977; pp. 147-166.

De Albuquerque K and D'Sa E. Spatial Inequalities in Papua New Guinea: a District Level Analysis, 1986. Discussion Paper No. 49, Waigani: IASER.

Findley S E. Rural Development and Migration: a Study of Family Choices in the Philippines. 1987 Colorado: Westview Press.

__________, An interactive contextual model of migration in Ilocos Norte, the Philippines. 1987 Demography 24: 163-190.

Gober-Meyers P. Employment, migration and growth in post-industrial market economies, Progress in Human Geography 1978; 2: 207-229.

Gore C. Regions in Question. 1984 London: Methuen.

Harris J R and Todaro M P. Migration, unemployment and development: a two-sector analysis, American Economic Review 1970; 13:126-142.

King D. Small towns in Papua New Guinea: in-migration and out-migration: case studies of Losuia and Kwikila, working paper. 1980

Lawson V A and Brown L A. Structural tension, migration, and development: a case study of Venezuela, 1987 Professional Geographer 39:179-188.

Lee S H. Why People Intend to Move: Individual and Community-level Factors of Out-migration in the Philippines. 1985 Colorado: Westview Press.

Martine G. Volume, characteristics and consequences of internal migration in Colombia, Demography 1975; 12:193-208.

May R J and Skeldon R. Internal migration in Papua New Guinea: an introduction to its description and analysis, in R J May ed., Change and Movement, The Australian National University, pp. 1-26. 1977

Morauta L. Left Behind in the village. Monograph 25. 1984 Boroko: IASER.

Ogawa N and Suits D E. An application of the Harris-Todaro model to selected ASEAN countries, in Urbanization and migration in ASEAN development, ed. P M Hauser and D B Suits and N Ogawa, 1985; pp 131-146. Tokyo: National Institute for Research Advancement.

Provincial Summary Figures. Port Moresby: National Statistical Office. 1980

Riddel J B. African migration and regional disparities, in R N Thomas and J M Hunter, Internal Migration Systems in the Developing World: with Special Reference to Latin America. 1980; pp.120-50. Massachusetts: Schenkman Publishing Co.

____________ Beyond the description of spatial pattern: the process of proletarianization as a factor in population migration in West Africa, Progress in Human Geography 1981; 5: 370-392.

Ross A C. Migrants from Fifty Villages. Monograph 25, 1984 Waigani: IASER

Sam J. Uneven Development and Migration in the Third World: 1980 Provincial Migration Flows in Papua New Guinea, Unpublished Thesis. 1989

Shrestha N R. A structural perspective on labour migration in underdeveloped countries, Progress in Human Geography 12: 179-206.

Skeldon R. Migration in South Asia: an Overview. Bangkok: ESCAP. 1983

Strathern M. The disconcerting tie: attitudes of Hagen migrants towards home, in M Chapman and R Prothero, Circulation in Population Movements: Concepts and Substance from the Melanesian Case. London: Routledge, 1985; pp. 360-376.

Times of PNG, April 11, 1991:3.

Todaro M P. A model of labor migration and urban unemployment in less developed countries, American Economic Review 1969; 59:138-148.

________, Internal Migration in Developing Countries. Geneva:ILO. 1976

Townsend D. Articulation, dissolution and migration: the partial intergration of Hube area, Papua New Guinea, Tijdschrift voor Economise en Sociale Geografie 1980; 71:285-294.

Treadgold M. Regional inequality in Papua New Guinea: some evidence, Pacific Viewpoint 1978; 19:129-148.

Turner A. Labour Mobility and Rural Development: the Use of Remittances in Ayuan and Aioa; Oro Province, Papua New Guinea, Masters Thesis (Unpublished). 1984

Young E. Processes influencing the evaluation of migration, from rural communities in Chimbu and New Ireland provinces, Typescript. 1977

Walsh C A. Inter-Provincial Migration in Papua New Guinea. Research Monograph No. 3. Port Moresby: National Statistical Office. 1985

Ward R G. Internal migration and urbanization in Papua New Guinea, in R J May, ed., Change and Movement. Canberra: The Australian National University, 1977; pp. 27-51.

Wood C H. Equilibrium, and historical-structural perspectives on migration, International Migration Review 1982; 16:229-316.

Zachariah K C. Measurement of internal migration from census data, in A A Brown and E Neuberger, ed., Internal Migration: a Comparative Disciplinary View. New York: Academic Press, 1977; pp.121-134.

Zelinsky W. The hypothesis of mobility transition, Geographical Review 1971; 61:219-249.

Papers presented at and arising from the 19th Waigani Seminars, University of Papua New Guinea, 16 - 22 June 1991

Population, Family Health and Development

Volume 2

These Volumes are dedicated

to our Patron

the late Ms Margaret Nakikus

TABLE OF CONTENTS

FAMILY PLANNING, FAMILY HEALTH, HEALTH AND DEVELOPMENT

ACKNOWLEDGEMENTS

We gratefully acknowledge the financial assistance of our donors, The Australian High Commission, The World Bank, SPAFH with funding from USAID, IPPF, UNICEF, UNFPA, Air Niugini, the Bank of Papua New Guinea, the Post and Telecommunication Corporation, Ramu Sugar, and the Summer Institute of Linguistics.

Thanks are due to the hardworking 19th Waigani Seminar Organising Committee, our Patron Mrs Margaret Nakikus, Treasurer John Vince, Deputy Chairman N.G. Patil, and Committee Members Homolpi Warom, Arai Pula, Beatrice Avalos, John Shadlow and Eleina Butuna. Many thanks also to our technical editors H.G. Mannur, Beatrice Avalos, John Shadlow and Lance Hill, and to Aoare Lomai.

Our Special thanks go to Philomena Boden for the enormous amount of work she has put into word processing this entire publication. Her dedication and skill have been invaluable in the production of these volumes.

Tukutau Taufa
Caroline Bass

EDUCATION FOR ALL

In 1990 the developing nations of the world gathered in Jomtien, Thailand to discuss progress towards the achievement of the right of education for all, or more precisely the degree to which this right had become a reality for most people in the world of the late twentieth century. A gloomy consideration of statistics and a record of failures in many areas, led to the commitment of governments and of donor agencies to support much more drastic steps towards improvement of educational provisions.

Papua New Guinea became a signatory of the Declaration which indicated adherence, among others, to the following goals:

> Universal access to, and completion of, primary education (or whatever higher level of education is consideration as 'basic') by the year 2000.
>
> Education programmes for women and girls ... designed to promote equal opportunities in all aspects of their lives.
>
> ....equal access to education to every category of disabled persons as an integral part of the education system.
>
> Strong intellectual and scientific environment for basic education. This implies improving higher education and developing scientific research. Close contact with contemporary technological and scientific knowledge should be possible at every level of education.
>
> Reduction of the adult illiteracy rate ... to, say, one half its 1990 level by the year 2000, with sufficient emphasis on female literacy to significantly reduce the current disparity between male and female illiteracy rates.

Papers in this section address some of the issues highlighted by Jomtien and therefore represent a contribution to policy discussions in Papua New Guinea in the light of its commitment to the Jomtien Declaration.

James Quarshie examines the socio-economic context from the perspective of demographic variables and the kind of planning that will be needed if decisive steps towards Education for all in Papua New Guinea are to be taken. **Sheldon Weeks** notes the slowness with which historically Papua New Guinea has moved towards universal primary education and points to low cost and straight-forward alternatives for achieving the goal. **Maba Lohia**, vehemently reminds us that disabled children are as much a part of the population with a right to education as are normal children who profit from the regular system. He indicates that Education for All policies must contemplate a much stronger investment in and action in favour of the young disabled people who possibly constitute at least 5 percent of the population of Papua New Guinea. The status of technical and vocational education in Papua New Guinea was the object of an extensive investigation and report achieved with technical assistance from GTZ (Germany). **Rainier Janisch** examines the implications of the findings of the study and the way vocational/technical education should go if viable alternatives are to be offered to sixth and tenth grade leavers in Papua New Guinea. Finally, from a more specialised perspective **Timothy Curtin** discusses critically the economic theories that undermine the concept of extending educational opportunities for as long as a person is able to pursue these, showing how the average length of education correlates with economic growth in developing nations.

....

BEATRICE AVALOS
Technical Editor
Education Department
University of Papua New Guinea

DEMOGRAPHIC TRENDS IN PAPUA NEW GUINEA AND THEIR IMPLICATIONS FOR EDUCATIONAL POLICY AND PLANNING

JAMES D QUARSHIE[1]

INTRODUCTION

I deem it important to comment on the relevance of demographic trends to educational policy and planning in Papua New Guinea at this seminar for a number of reasons. First, I have strong interest in educational policy and planning; and come from a third world country where I have been exposed to demographic and educational issues similar, in many respects, to those of Papua New Guinea. Thus the seminar presents me with an opportunity to exchange ideas with you on this topic. Finally, I have known an educational jurisdiction in an advanced country which expanded educational facilities to meet rising school age population only to find years later that it had permanently constructed school facilities without students. Hopefully, by sharing ideas on topics such as this, countries like Papua New Guinea and other third world countries with limited resources can avoid that kind of situation.

Psacharopoulos and Woodhall (1985) stressed the need for analysis of demographic trends for its relevance to school enrollments. From such analysis could be developed appropriate educational policies and strategies for dealing with emerging characteristics of the society. Such policies have implications for educational planners working on areas of funding, facilities, teacher supply, curriculum, and others.

It is the purpose of this paper to examine demographic trends of Papua New Guinea vis-a-vis community and provincial high school enrollment trends and patterns with the view to suggesting educational policies that could be pursued in terms of access, facilities, teacher supply, curriculum, and funding to meet the pronounced goals of education for Papua New Guinea. The planning implications of such policies shall also be discussed.

In the analysis which follows, it is assumed that the Government of Papua New Guinea subscribes to the U.N. declaration that everyone has a right to education as described in Omari and others (1983:9, 10). Hence social demand is the major factor in planning, at least, basic education.

[1] Professional Studies Department, Goroka Teachers' College, University of Papua New Guinea

ANALYTICAL FRAMEWORK

The framework for analysis of the implications of demographic trends for educational policy and planning is adapted from Kotler and Murphy's (1981) strategic planning process model and Dunn's (1981) types of policy-relevant information. Strategic planning 'involves the ongoing analysis of the institutional environment to ascertain what long term changes are occurring which may provide opportunities with relation to emerging educational needs or demands' (Young, 1981:1). Young further emphasized that by this analysis the institution might also be able to influence the changes rather than always responding to such changes. Thus this planning strategy promotes 'strategic fit' between the organization and its changing environment (Kotler and Murphy, 1981). Dunn identified five types of policy relevant information, one of which was 'policy alternative' which he described as a 'potentially available course of action that may contribute to the attainment of values and the resolution of a policy problem' (Dunn, 1981:60). The adapted framework which is shown diagrammatically in figure 1 below consists of five main components as follows:

1. External environmental scanning for demographic trends.

2. Internal environmental analysis of the resources of the system, namely, funding, school facilities, and teachers, as well as enrollment trends and patterns of the system.

3. Pronounced educational goals.

4. Policy Issues on access, facilities, teachers, curriculum and funding.

5. Policy alternatives and planning implications on access, facilities, teachers, curriculum and funding.

Fig. 1 An Adapted Strategic Planning Process

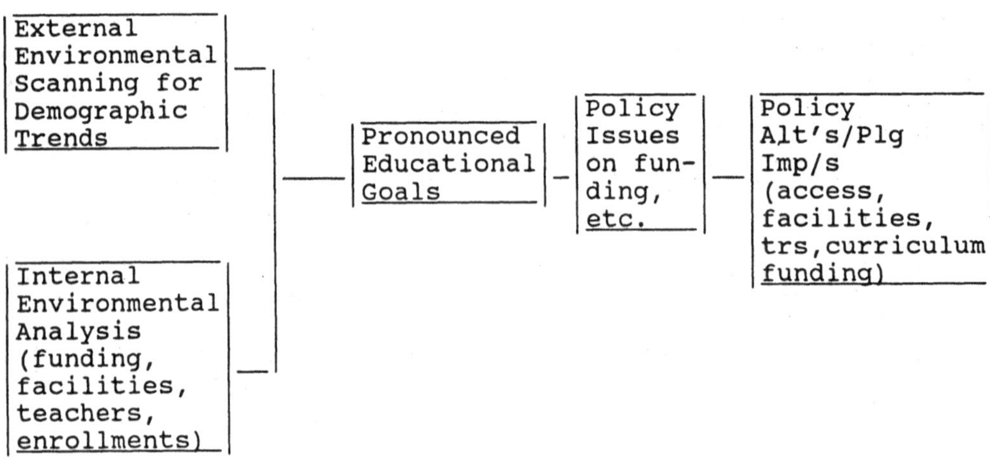

EXTERNAL ENVIRONMENTAL SCANNING FOR DEMOGRAPHIC TRENDS

What is the nature of demography of Papua New Guinea as a whole and the provinces? What demographic trends likely to influence education in the country are evident? Unless otherwise stated, census and growth rate data reported in this paper are from the 1990 National Population Census: Preliminary Figures Census Division Populations (1991) and the 1980 National Population Census, Final Figures: National Summary (1988).

The citizen population of Papua New Guinea in 1966, 1971, 1980 was 2,150,313, 2,435,409 and 2,978,057 respectively. The preliminary figures of the 1990 population census show a total population of 3,529,538 including the relatively small non-citizen population. These show growth rates of 13.3% from 1966 to 1971, 22.3% from 1971 to 1980, and 18.5% from 1980 to 1990.

In 1966, 1971, and 1980, the relevant school population aged 5 to 19 consisted of 740,363; 868,650; and 1,124,592 respectively (1980 National Population Census Final Figures, United Nation, 1982). These give growth rates of 17.3% from 1966 to 1971, and 29.5% from 1971 to 1980. The breakdown of the 1990 population into age cohorts was not available at the time of preparing this paper. But the 1966, 1971, and 1980 data confirm that the growth rates in the 5-19 years age group have been greater than the growth rates in the whole population. These also confirm a disproportionally young population (Walsh, 1985; Agyei, 1988). The 1980 census indicated 43% of population under 15 years (Brogan, 1985).

Other demographic indicators of interest to education which have been identified for Papua New Guinea are;

1. Uneven distribution of the population with highest densities in the National Capital District, Western, Chimbu and Eastern Highlands provinces and lowest densities in Western, Gulf, and West Sepik provinces (Walsh, 1985).

2. The population is overwhelmingly rural with over 80% of the population found in rural villages (Walsh, 1985). The preliminary figures of the 1990 National Population Census, however, indicate that the population growth rate between 1980 and 1990 has been much faster in urban areas than in rural areas.

3. Rural village populations, ... are overwhelmingly non-migrant (Walsh, 1985).

4. The greatest proportion of the young people (0-14 years) reside in rural villages (Walsh, 1985).

5. Urban centers have an attraction to migrants (Skeldon, 1978).

6. Migration up to the 1960s was largely to Morobe, the Islands, and Central provinces (including the National Capital District) but substantial portion of recent migrants has destinations that include the Eastern Highlands, Western Highlands, North Solomons (probably until the Bougainville crisis), West New Britain and the Northern Provinces (Walsh, 1985).

What does the future hold in terms of demographic indicators of relevance to education? Scenario B in population projections suggested by experts in the field, namely, Brogan (1985), Bakker (1985), and Bakker (1984, cited by Brogan, 1985); and reckoned by Albuquerque and Tauge (1987) as most likely to occur assumes gradual decline in mortality, continuing slow decline in fertility (Brogan, 1985). This scenario gives population projections with high youth population. As determined by Brogan (1985) under the above assumptions relating to mortality and fertility, there would be approximately 40% and 38% of population under 15 years by the years 2000 and 2015, respectively.

Comparing the 2000 and 2015 under 15 years projections of 40% and 38%, respectively, with the 43% of 1980, it could be said that there would be only a small decline in the proportion of the school age children in the population. But in absolute terms, the number of under 15 year old people will actually increase as evidenced in the table 1 below:

TABLE 1 - Under 15 year Olds in the PNG Citizen Population, 1980, 2000 and 2015

Year	**Citizen Population**	**Under 15 Years Old Population**	
		Percentage	**Number**
1980	2,978,050	43	1,280,562
2000	4,706,370	40	1,882,548
2015	6,628,490	38	2,518,826

Source: Derived from Brian Brogan Population and Economic Development in Papua New Guinea 1980-2015 (1985:20)

INTERNAL ENVIRONMENTAL ANALYSIS

In this section, we shall briefly look at the resources of the system, namely funding, facilities, and teachers for providing educational services, as well as the enrollment trends and patterns at the community school and the provincial high school levels.

Funding

Although education agencies and parents contribute in some ways to the financing of education, the costs of education in PNG (are) largely borne by the State (Department of Education, 1985b:1). Table 2 below shows the percentage of PNG national government budget devoted to education (for recurrent and capital expenditure) in selected years as reported by the World Bank (1986a:49), the PNG Department of Education (1985b:1), and Education Plan 1976-80 (p.112):

TABLE 2 - Percentage of PNG Government Budget Devoted to Education, 1965-1985

Year	% of Budget Devoted to Education
1965	14.4
1970	13.2
1975	17.0
1980	14.2
1985	15.0

If we compare the 1.8% increase in the proportion of the government budget devoted to education between 1970 and 1985 to Papua New Guinea's real growth rate of 1.4% in the GNP between 1973 and 1985 (World Bank, 1986b:8), then it could be said that education receives a fair share of the government budget.

The above figures, however, show a slow growth in terms of the proportion of government budget devoted to education from 1965 to 1985, as compared to the growth of the relevant school age population for the same period. Furthermore the contribution of 14.2% of the government budget to public education in 1980 (the most recent year for which there was comparative data) was small relative to educational contributions of many developing nations, and even some advanced countries such as Japan, Australia, and New Zealand, in the same year. In that year, a World Bank (1986a:49-50--see Appendix table 1) report indicates that as many as 35 out of 68 developing nations in Africa, Asia, South America, and South Asia, East Asia, and Pacific spent more than 14.2% of their government budget on public education. Some of these nations, including two in South Asia, East Asia, and the Pacific region spent over 20% of their budget on education in 1980. The contributions in these 68 countries ranged from 5.0% in one country (Pakistan) to 36.6% in another country (Comoros), with an average of 15.7% (World Bank, 1986a:49, 50), showing that Papua New Guinea's contribution of 14.2% was below the average.

It appears from the above data that it might be desirable for the government to increase its spending on education substantially more than the 0.8% from 1980 to 1985; as well as to seek other sources of educational funds. This seems inevitable from the international perspective, and from the rate of growth of the school age population.

Facilities

Although there are many types of facilities that go to promote education, schools are the most basic and most expensive facilities for education in Papua New Guinea as in other parts of the world. Appendix Table 2 contains the growth of community schools in PNG over the five-year period, 1985-1990. The table shows that in many provinces, there has been good progress in the provision of community schools. In five provinces, namely, Western, Eastern Highlands, Western Highlands, Madang, and West Sepik, and the District of Kiunga Lake Murray, there was a 20% or more growth in community schools from 1985 to 1990.

However, two provinces, namely, the Southern Highlands and Chimbu fell far below the national average in the growth of community schools. Chimbu had a growth rate of 4% over the five-year period, while in Southern Highlands there was a 2% fall, that is, a negative growth.

At the provincial high school level, the number of schools in the provinces in 1990 ranged from three in Western and Manus to 10 in Morobe. Kiunga also had two high schools. Comparing the 1990 number of high schools in the provinces (see Appendix table 3) against their 13-16 year old population in 1980 (1980 National Population Census Final Figures: Provincial Summary--All Provinces, 1985--except West Sepik), and assuming a desirable provision of 1 high school for every 1000 of the relevant age group (13-16 years), it was found that the Province of Manus with a 13-16 year old population of 2954 and three high schools was the province most well served. Seven provinces which were found to be most in need of high schools were: Eastern Highlands, Morobe, Western Highlands, East Sepik, Madang, Enga, and Southern Highlands. On the basis of their 13-16 year old populations, each of these provinces in 1990 would need at least ten more provincial high schools, a rather expensive and financially unrealistic venture. But the analysis points out to the need for a minimal provision of some additional schools in these provinces. Albuquerque and Tauge (1987) have also argued that by 1995, there would be need for an additional 36 to 152 new schools though they also see the latter figure as unrealistic given financial and other constraints.

In addition to Manus, four other provinces which were relatively well endowed with high schools on the basis of their 13-16 year old populations were the National Capital District, New Ireland, Gulf and Central. Each of these provinces, by the standard used would be in need of two or three more schools. High schools needs were not estimated for the North Solomons and Kiunga because of lack of data. The use of the 1990 census data for the 13-16 populations (not available at the time of writing) rather than the 1980 census data would provide a more up to date estimate of high school requirements of the provinces.

Teachers

Education statistics (Department of Education, 1990) indicate that in 1990, there were 12,514 community school teachers all of whom were Nationals. Out of this total number of teachers, 3,958 (approximately 32%) were females. At the provincial high school level, there was a total of 2,138 teachers consisting of approximately 85% Nationals and 15% Non-Papua New Guineans. 687 (32%) of the total teaching force in the provincial high schools were female. One would expect the community schools to have a much higher proportion of female teachers than the high schools. Given the size of the female population in the country, and the need for female role models that would also encourage more female enrolment in the schools, it would be desirable that attempts be made to increase the proportion of female teachers at both the community and the provincial high school levels.

The 15% expatriate teachers in Provincial high schools in 1990 is a reduction from the rate of 40% in 1975 (PNG Education Gazette, September, 1985). Although this may be seen as an achievement, the existence of 15% of expatriate teachers in the provincial high schools is an indication that perhaps more National teachers need to be produced. Any attempt to expand educational facilities to meet increased demand would also call for more teachers at both the community and high school levels.

School Enrolment Trends and Patterns

Enrolments at the community school level have been growing at a very fast rate since 1975. For example, between 1975 and 1984, enrolments in community schools increased by about 45%, this rate of increase being faster than the rate of increase in the population (PNG Education Gazette, September, 1985:22). By 1990, the community school enrolments had reached 402,948 from 351,171 in 1985 (Department of Education, 1990, 1985a).

There are, however, a number of issues surrounding this growth. First, this growth in community school enrolment has not been uniform across all the provinces. As evident in Appendix Table 4, even though some of the highest increases in the enrolment rates between 1974 and 1983 were recorded in the Highlands provinces, the lowest enrolment rates in community schools in 1983 (50%, 53%, 54%, 56% and 58%) were found in Southern Highlands, Enga, Western Highlands, Eastern Highlands, Madang, and Chimbu provinces, in that order.

Secondly, the enrolment rates are substantially different between boys and girls. As evident in Appendix Table 5, even though from 1976 to 1983 the enrolment rates for girls went up in all provinces, particularly in Enga, Southern Highlands, Western Highlands, Chimbu, and Eastern Highlands, the enrolment rates for girls in 1983 were 10% or more below those of boys in 10 provinces, and 5% or more below those of boys in all but two provinces (North Solomons and NCD). Girls enrolment in community schools in 1983 as a proportion of all 7-12 year old girls was lowest in six provinces, namely, Enga (with the lowest), followed by Southern Highlands, Madang, Western Highlands, Eastern Highlands, and Chimbu.

As evident in Appendix Table 6, from 1985 to 1990, seven provinces which had in most of the six years fallen below the national level in terms of female enrolment relative to students enrolled in community schools included four of the provinces with lowest enrolment rates for girls in 1983. These were Enga, Madang, Eastern Highlands, and Chimbu. The other three provinces which fell below the national level in terms of female enrolments in most years were Gulf, Morobe, and West Sepik, plus the Kiunga Lake Murray District.

Finally, it must be noted also that enrolment rates (i.e enrolment as a percentage of 7-12 year olds) could be inflated because of a number of reasons including the existence of over-age and under-age students enrolled in the community schools, hence decline in enrolment rates in some provinces between 1974 and 1983 might be due to decline in the under-age or over-age enrolments (Albuquerque and Tauge, 1987; Institute of Applied Social and Economic Research, 1979).

Enrolment projections to the year 1995 by Albuquerque and Tauge (1987) and the less than 15 years population projection to the year 2015 by Brogan (1985) and Bakker (cited by Brogan, 1985) suggest a pattern of steady growth in community school enrolments to the years 2000 and 2015. Under three different sets of assumptions, Albuquerque and Tauge's (1987) projections of community school enrolments show a continuing growth.

In fact, the 'no change' and 'Medium Variant A' assumptions have both failed since the 1990 enrolments of over 400,000 (Department of Education, 1990) have already surpassed the 1995 projections of 319,000 and 364,000 under these two scenarios. Given the 1990 community school enrolment of over 400,000 it is likely that the enrolments into the 1990s will be well over 500,000. This, together with the projected under 15 years population of 2,518,826 by the year 2015, confirms a strong pattern of consistent growth in community school enrolments well into the 21 Century.

While community school enrolments are growing and will continue to grow in the years ahead, concerns are being raised about a number of issues. First, there is the concern whether community school leavers at the age of 13 can effectively work or be useful in their communities (Department of Education, 1985, Institute of Applied Social and Economic Research, 1979,Memorial, 1974). Hence ...most parents don't appreciate their spending on children who only leave the primary school (Memorial, 1974:17).

The second relates to questions about the need of education for girls in some areas (Education Plan, 1976-80, Memorial, 1974.) Third is the fear that large scale movement of people (across the country) can result in schools being poorly sited (Education Plan, 1976). Fourth, there is a fear of oversupply of teachers following the period of expansion (Education Plan, 1976-80).

At the provincial high school level, enrolments between 1975 and 1984 nearly doubled (PNG Education Gazette, September 1985). From 1984 to 1990 there has been a consistent growth in enrolment from 44,420 (Wari, 1990) to 52,555 (Department of Education, 1990). Albuquerque and Tauge's (1987) projection in also suggests continuing growth in high school enrolments to the year 1995 under three different sets of assumptions.

Given the fact that the percentage of 13-16 year olds enrolled in high schools has been 14.3%, 14.5%, 15.0%, and 15.5% for the years 1984, 1986, 1988, and 1989 (Wari, 1990) respectively the 'no change' in enrolment rate assumption is not valid. Evidence (Wari, 1990) shows that enrolment in high schools increased between 1984 and 1988 by over 2% more than was anticipated under the Education III Project. This suggests that we could expect higher enrolment growth. This, together with the projected high youth population by the year 2015, suggests that it is reasonable to assume a pattern of consistent growth in high school enrolment as well. Just as for community schools, some provinces are better served than others with high schools as pointed out above under facilities. Similarly, some provinces lag behind in female enrolments (Wari, 1990:2). A concern has been expressed about the possibility of expanding High School enrolments faster than the number of jobs... (Albuquerque and Tauge, 1987:14; Education Plan, 1976-80:36; Wari, 1990:4). Additionally, the issue of funds for financing expansion in both the community and the high school levels has been expressed in various quarters, including Albuquerque and Tauge (1987), and Department of Education (1985b).

Educational Goals

The goals of education consistent with Papua New Guinea's Eight Aims and the National Goals and Directive Principles (see Department of Education, 1983:99-101; A Philosopy of Education for Papua New Guinea--Matane Report, 1986) are contained in several documents of the Government in the form of aims or policies on education.

From the Educational Developments in PNG 1978-84 (Department of Education, 1985b:3), PNG Education Gazette (September, 1985), Report of Study on Universalization of Primary Education (Department of Education, 1983), and Papua New Guinea Education Plan 1976-1980, the following are goals of education:

1. To provide a relevant education, which will equip children with skills that can be used in their everyday living through a relevant school curriculum.

2. To ensure equal access to education in all provinces.

3. To increase enrolments at all levels of the educational system.

4. To increase the proportion of females in schools.

5. To achieve 82% and 92% primary school enrolment by the years 1980 and 1985, respectively, and Universal Primary Education (UPE) early next century.

6. To maintain good standards in education provided for the children of the country.

7. To reduce the number of expatriate staff at the various levels of the educational system.

Some of these goals have been modified over the years. For example, in a statement at the Goroka Teachers' College in March this year (1991), the Minister of Education indicated that UPE by 2000 would be unattainable.

These goals incorporate principles of equity, efficiency, and quality all of which are necessary in a democratic society such as Papua New Guinea. Comparing these goals to the outcome of our analysis of the demographic trends and internal environment, what policy issues emerge?

Policy Issues

A number of important questions regarding educational planning can be raised from our analysis to this point. For example, at what rate should enrolment at various levels increase to attain specific enrolment objectives in the future? Where should specific schools be located? How many schools and teachers shall be needed in the years ahead? The first two are technical questions not dealt with in this paper. The third question has been well dealt with by Albuquerque and Tauge (1987). Readers interested in these technical questions may see Albuquerque and Tauge (1987) and Chesswas (1969).

Rather than look at these technical issues, the paper will present options or alternatives with regard to the following policy questions, and their implications for educational planning in terms of what kinds of planning activities would be needed to implement those policies:

1. Access: How can enrolments be improved generally, and particularly in underprivileged areas and of girls?

2. Facilities: What types of facilities can be used to accommodate increased enrolments?

3. Teachers: How can teacher supply be increased without creating the problems of oversupply beyond the period of expansion alluded to elsewhere in the paper?

4. Curriculum and programs: What can be done to ensure that graduates of the school system are found useful by the community without also creating unemployment, particularly among provincial high school graduates?

5. Funding: What sources of funds are available to support any expansion at both the community and provincial high school levels?

Policy Alternatives and Planning Implications

The policy alternatives and their implications for planning will be presented in line with the five broad areas identified above and in the analytical framework, namely, access, facilities, teachers, curriculum and programs, and funding. Most of the policy alternatives presented below are based on ideas from the literature including the Education Plan, 1976-80 (PNG Department of Education 1983), Institute of Applied Social and Economic Research (1979), World Bank Education (2nd Quarter, 1987; July 1986; Fall 1986), World Bank 1986a) Circa (1980) and Chesswas (1969); from practices that have been found feasible and successful elsewhere, and from discussions with colleagues.

Access

Alternative 1. Allow voluntary demand for education with government providing the facilities where demand is strong. Educational planning activities would consist of monitoring the system to determine where demand is greatest and planning for the necessary facilities.

This alternative has the effect of education flourishing in areas where education has at this point been most supported. The other areas would tend to wait until they realize the importance of education before fully making use of the opportunities. These areas would thus always tend to fall behind the other areas where education has traditionally been well supported, because schools have existed there for a longer period of time. This alternative is not consistent with the Government's equality goals.

Alternative 2. Government should deliberately stimulate demand for education by adopting policies that promote interest in education. Such policies could include:

a. Beginning with the current underprivileged areas, basic education (to be defined below) to be fee-free, and the fee-free education gradually phased-in to all other provinces.

b. Reward parents who send their children to school at the exact age of school entry, namely, seven yeares. Such reward could be a school uniform for the child, or a government education coupon with a good value redeemable for school materials.

c. In provinces with low female participation rates, provide financial reward to parents who send their daughters to school.

Planning concerns would include identifying population centres, determining catchment areas for schools in all areas, and estimating the size of educational facilities to be needed. Other major planning activities would consist of determining the cost of fee-free policy and other incentive programs, and where coupons would have to be redeemed. The problem with this alternative is that it could become very expensive.

Facilities

Alternative 1. Build additional facilities to accommodate increasing enrolments. Major planning activities would include determining locations of facilities and when they would be ready; and planning for enrolments to coincide with the completion dates. This alternative is not only expensive but takes time and hence slows down the educational development process.

Alternative 2. Better utilisation of existing school facilities by having two streams of students with two sets of required number of teachers using the same facilities on shift basis (Chesswas, 1969), say one from 7.00 am to 12.00 noon and the other from 12.30 pm to 5.30 pm.

Secondly, additional community resources such as church buildings and community centres could be utilised for educational purposes during the school hours in the course of the week when many of such facilities are idle.

Additionally, the current migratory trends in the country, the reported fast rate of growth of the urban sector relative to the rural sector (1990 National Population Census Preliminary Figures, 1991) and the current state of the economy with strong potential for industrial activities in many parts of the country, suggest that the population movements in the country is in a state of flux and very volatile with possibility of new movements at any point in time. Hence instead of putting up permanent new buildings, any new additional school facilities that have to be constructed could be of a pre-fabricated nature so that they could be easily dismantled and reconstructed in another location if need be. Construction of new facilities should involve community labor contribution, an idea which has been suggested in the Education Plan (1976-1980:27) but which may have to be sold to local community people.

Planning activities would include identifying additional community facilities, allocating students to various facilities for the shift system, identifying proper pre-fabricated materials for the construction of additional new facilities needed, and planning for the locations of new facilities.

This alternative has the advantage of ensuring a good pace in educational development. But the shift system may have disadvantages such as tiredness among the afternoon stream of students following playing in the early part of the day, and reducing the contact hours.

Teachers

Alternative 1. Expand community school and high school teacher training facilities and intake to meet the demand for more teachers. A major planning activity would consist of determining the number and nature of teacher training facilities and annual intake to ensure that targets are met. Additionally, the number and sources of temporary expatriate teachers to be needed until a regular flow of graduates from the teacher training institutions begins would have to be determined.

This alternative has the advantage of ensuring that relatively good quality teachers are available but it also has some limitations. For example, it could be very costly and restrict the pace of educational development since expanding teacher training facilities would be expensive and preparation of teachers takes time. There is also the danger of having teachers on hand at the end of the expansionary program, a problem that has been alluded to.

Alternative 2. Tap teaching resources from existing environment through any or a combination of any of the following programs:

a. Attract teachers who have left the system back into teaching by offering appropriate incentives (World Bank Education News Vol. 2, No. 1, 1987).

b. Use high school and university graduates as untrained teachers (Chesswas, 1969) for designated classes, after a short (6-8 week) intensive teacher training prior to taking up appointment. For example high school graduates after the intensive course can teach Grades 2 and 5. The proposed national service scheme could be used to recruit such untrained teachers.

c. Re-institute the 2-year teacher training programs to run concurrently with the 3-year programs until sufficient numbers of teachers are available by which time the 2-year program would be phased out.

d. Upgrade community school teachers through in-service programs to become high school teachers, and in their places engage some untrained teachers as suggested in 'b' above.

e. Allow local communities to select some teacher trainees so that upon graduation these persons would be required to go back to the communities to teach. This would save the Government from having to build houses for such teachers.

Planning activities would include identifying and estimating trained teachers outside the school system, planning for short intensive courses for untrained teachers planning the development of teacher training programs at a relatively slow pace to produce needed teachers, and determining appropriate programs for phasing out untrained teachers as qualified teachers become available. This alternative would be likely to provide sufficient numbers of teachers for educational expansion.

The disadvantage of this alternative is that relatively poor quality teachers would handle selected classes. But as the World Bank Education News (Vol. 1, No. 3, 1986) correctly pointed out, in a period of low enrolment rates and with need for improving equity and accessibility, priority must be on quantitative expansion.

Curriculum and Programs

Alternative 1. Maintain the existing 6-year community school followed by the 4-year provincial high school. No radical planning changes would be required, except the production of more curriculum materials to meet demand from increased enrolments. The limitation of this alternative is that many of the problems relating to usefulness of community and high school graduates could still be with us.

Many aspects of suggested alternatives 2 and 3 below have been expressed in the National Education Strategy (Institute of Applied Social and Economic Research, 1979:25-27).

Alternative 2. Introduce 3-year day Senior Community Schools to be attached to the existing Community Schools and any new Community Schools which together with the Community Schools would provide a 9-year (rather than the current 6-year) Basic Education. The present grade 6 would thus become a transitional stage for all pupils, rather than a terminal stage. With the shift system proposed under "facilities" above, existing Community Schools, if not used for a second Community School stream, could be used as Senior Community Schools as well.

Programmes at the Senior Community Schools would, in the main, consist of cultural studies (traditional customs, festivals, drumming and dancing, etc. to reinforce and develop appreciation among the pupils for their roots) and vocational studies with emphasis on vocations available in the local communities such as fishing, farming, crafts, and new programs such as dress making and tailoring, shoe making, poultry, and watch repairing.

Given research findings (Agyei, 1988:72, 104) that more educated women in Papua New Guinea tend to have fewer children, and that relative to other sources, schools provide less exposure to students on birth control, parenting should be incorporated as a required course or as a unit of a required course in the new Basic Education program. By this, we might be able to influence the demographic trends instead of always responding to them, as pointed out under the analytical framework.

This 3-year Senior Community School programme could render education for both girls and boys more useful. As well, it could ensure that pupils leave school at a more mature age able to participate effectively in community development; hence the proposal here is for three years of Community School rather than two as suggested in the National Education Strategy. And like the Continuation Education programme in Ghana the last two years of a 9-10 year Basic Education, would help pupils who are finishing their formal education to make the important decision to settle in productive occupational activities in the rural areas (Anim and Kwansa, 1978:10).

The recently poposed changes to the Papua New Guinea education system (Education Sector Report, 1991) in which the community school will end with grade 8; and selection to high school (which will have two rather than the present 4-year program) will be placed at the end of grade 8. Since in the current Provincial High School, "...the two years covered by grades 7 and 8 should instigate a positive change in attitude of pupils towards agriculture and manual work and life in a rural setting, and would prepare....young men and women for active participation in aspects of rural development..."(Institute of Applied and Economic Research, 1979:35), and since a Senior Community School would appear to do this better than the current Provincial High School, the Education Sector recommendation seems appropriate. Incorporating two years of the present high school programme into this practically oriented Senior Community School would also make it better respected than the "Skulonka", a proposal similar to the Senior Community School which failed because of it being perceived as a second class institution. For the reason of maturity stated above it would be better that students who do not proceed to provincial high school at the end of grade 8 spend an additional year at the Senior Community School.

Among the major planning activities under this alternative are identification and selection of teachers who could include local artisans, provision of facilities such as extra classrooms for certain courses, eg. workshop oriented courses, equipment and materials, and the development of programmes and instructional materials.

This alternative has the advantage of being seen as a more community oriented venture. As well, as argued by many people, it could keep pupils in their environment at a time when we want to create in their minds a positive image of that environment rather than have them removed to remote boarding institutions as is the case under the present provincial high school system.

Alternative 3. Instead of having Senior Community Schools, the present provincial high school could become a Community High School admitting all pupils from Community Schools with the first three years being considered as part of Basic Education and providing the same program suggested for the Senior Community Schools. As much as possible the Community High Schools should be day schools.

Planning activities under this alternative would include determining locations of new schools (to become Community High Schools), in addition to the other planning activities under alternative 2. The disadvantage of this alternative is that because of the historical perception of the provincial high school, even if they become Community High Schools, their program may not be seen as a community venture and it may be more expensive to initiate.

Funding

Alternative 1. Continue to tap the traditional sources of funds, including all those identified in the Education Plan 1976-1980 (pp. 110-115) such as from the normal percentage of the national budget, church agencies, school fees, Australia, New Zealand, the World Bank, and the Commonwealth Secretariat.

Planning activities under this alternative would include determining how much would be derived from each of these sources and deciding on the allocation of these funds to the various educational projects. The problem with this alternative is that it may not yield sufficient funds.

Alternative 2. This alternative which would be consistent with the goal of promoting accessibility would consist of the following programmes towards raising appropriate amounts of revenue for educational projects:

a. Beginning with currently underprivileged provinces, abolish fees and gradually phase this in all other provinces at the Basic Education level suggested above, except in the case of boarding, that is, if boarding becomes necessary.

b. Beyond the Basic Education level, impose user fees with the level of fees charged increasing, the higher the grade level.

c. All boarding facilities at all levels of the educational system should be self supporting, since day students fully pay for their boarding at home or with wantoks.

d. The Government of Papua New Guinea should increase its contribution to education more in line with other third world countries.

e. Funding from other sources under alternative 1 be pursued.

f. All profit making organisations be required to pay annual Education Tax on the basis of the principles of benefits received from education and ability to pay, an alternative source of educational funding that has also been proposed elsewhere (Circa, 1980). This will also streamline the efforts being made by some organisations to help education.

Planning activities under this alternative would include those under alternative 1 as well as determining the level of funding to be derived from the new sources.

NOTE OF CAUTION AND CONCLUDING REMARKS

Education should not be seen as a panacea for the ills of society. For educational programmes to be most effective, they should be reinforced with appropriate and relevant social programmes. For example, loans need to be ensured if young schools leavers from the Basic Education programme are to be able to start off in productive ventures in the rural areas. There will also be the need for the provision of basic social amenities such as health clinics and good drinking water in the rural areas, if these youngsters are to stay in the rural areas. At the same time, the reward system in the employment sector should recognise the importance of the skills developed in the Senior Community Schools by offering better remunerations to people with such skills.

If education is to be seen as relevant by the people of Papua New Guinea, it has to be seen to contribute effectively to community development. It is my belief that proposals in this paper could contribute to making education relevant to the people of Papua New Guinea.

REFERENCES

Albuquerque, Klaus de and Mariget Tauge (1987)
Social Implications of Population Growth in Papua New Guinea, 1980-1995. Port Moresby: Institute of Applied Social and Economic Research (IASER).

Agyei, William K A (1988)
Fertility and Family Planning in the Third World: A Case Study of Papua New Guinea. London Croom Helm.

Anim, N.O. and K. Bassa Kwansa (1978)
The Continuation Education System in Ghana. A Paper presented at the International Institute for Education Planning, Paris. Institute for Educational Planning and Administration, University of Cape Coast, Cape Coast, Ghana.

Bakker, M L (1985)
Population Projections for the Citizen Population of Papua New Guinea for the period 1980-2015. Port Moresby: National Statistical Office.

Brogan, Brian (1985)
Population and Economic Development in Papua New Guinea 1980-2015. Port Moresby: Institute of National Affairs.

Chesswas, J D (1969)
Methodologies of Educational Planning for Developing Countries (1 Text). Unesco: International Institute for Educational Planning.

Department of Education Gazette, PNG (September, 1985)
Port Moresby: PNG Department of Education.

Department of Education (1990, 1989, 1988, 1987, 1986, 1985a)
Education Staffing and Enrollment Statistics National Education System. Port Moresby: Management Planning Unit, PNG Department of Education.

Department of Education (1985b)
Educational Developments in Papua New Guinea 1978-84.
Port Moresby: PNG Department of Education (A Report Prepared for the 5th Regional Conference of Ministers of Education and those Responsible for Economic Planning of Member States in Asia and the Pacific).

Department of Education (1983)
Report of Study on Universalization of Primary Education.
Port Moresby: PNG Department of Education.

Dunn, William N. (1981)
Public Policy Analysis: An Introduction. Englewood Cliffs: Prentice-Hall.

Education Plan Papua New Guinea, 1976-1980.
Education Sector Report

Institute of Applied Social and Economic Research (1979)
National Education Strategy: Papua New Guinea Education Plan Review and Proposals. Boroko, PNG: Institute of Applied Social and Economic Research.

Kotler, Philip and Patrick E. Murphy (1981)
"Strategic Planning for Higher Education" The Journal of Higher Education, Vol. 52, No. 5 (Sept/Oct)

Memorandum from the Faculty of Education, University of Cape Coast, Ghana to the Adade Commission on Education (Circa 1980)

Memorial, Anasain (1974)
"Parents and Children Talk About Education" in J.P. Powell and Michael Wilson (ed.) Education and Rural Development in the Highlands of Papua New Guinea. Port Moresby: The University of Papua New Guinea.

Ministerial Committee Report (1986)
A Philosophy of Education for Papua New Guinea.

Omari, I M, A S Mbise, S T Mahenge, G A Malekela, and M P Besha (1983) Universal Primary Education in Tanzania. Ottawa, Canada: International Development Research Center (IDRC).

Papua New Guinea 1980 National Population Census Final Figures: National Summary (1988). Port Moresby: National Statistical Office.

Papua New Guinea 1980 National Population Census Final Figures: National Summary. (All Provinces except West Sepik) (1985). Port Moresby: National Statistical Office.

Papua New Guinea 1990 National Population Census Preliminary Figures Census Division Populations (1991) Port Moresby: National Statistical Office.

Psacharopoulos, G. and M. Woodhall (1985)
Education and Development. Washington, D.C: The World Bank.

Skeldon, Ronald (1978)
Evolving Patterns of Population Movement in Papua New Guinea with Reference to Policy Implications. Boroko, PNG: Institute of Applied Social and Economic Research.

United Nations (1982)
Population of Papua New Guinea ESCAP/SPC Country Monograph Series No. 7.2. New York: United Nations.

Walsh, A. Crosbie (1985)
Inter-Provincial Migration in Papua New Guinea Research Monograph No. 3 Port Moresby: National Statistical Office.

Wari, Pala (1990)
"Education 111 Project Indicators, 1984-1989." Port Moresby: Research and Evaluation Unit, Ministry of Education, Department of Education.

World Bank Education News Vol. 2, No. 1 (2nd Quarter 1987); Vol. 1, No. 3 (Fall, 1986); Vol. 1, No. 2, (July, 1986).

World Bank (1986a)
Financing Education in Developing Countries: An Exploration of Policy Options. Washington, D.C: The World Bank.

World Bank (1986 b)
The World Bank Atlas 1987. Washington, D C: The World Bank.

Young Stanley (1981)
"Some Dimensions of Strategic Planning for Higher Education" Planning for Higher Education, 9:4 (Summer) 1-7.

ACKNOWLEDGEMENT: The author is grateful to Mr Tony Wrightson and Sr Theresa Flaherty both of the Department of Professional Studies, Goroka Teachers' College, University of Papua New Guinea for reading the first draft of this paper and providing him with suggestions and insightful comments.

Appendix Table 1

Share of Public Educational Expenditure in the Public Budget, 1980

REGION AND COUNTRY	%	REGION AND COUNTRY	%
Africa			
Burkina Faso	19.8	Nepal	8.3
Botswana	11.7	Pakistan	5.0
Burundi	17.5	Papua New Guinea	14.2
Cameroon	20.3	Philippines	10.3
Central African Republic	19.9	Singapore	7.3
Comoros	36.6	Solomon Islands	10.6
Congo, P.R. of	23.6	Sri Lanka	8.8
Cote d'Ivoire	29.8	Thailand	20.6
Djibouti	11.5	**Latin America and Carribean**	
Ethiopia	9.3	Argentina	15.1
Kenya	18.1	Bahamas	22.9
Gambia	9.7	Barbados	19.6
Liberia	24.3	Bolivia	25.3
Malawi	12.9	Chile	11.9
Mali	30.5	Colombia	14.3
Mauritius	11.6	Costa Rica	22.2
Niger	22.9	Dominican Republic	16.0
Nigeria	16.2	Ecuador	33.3
Rwanda	21.6	El Salvador	17.1
Seychelles	14.4	Guatemala	16.6
Somalia	8.7	Guyana	14.0
Sudan	9.1	Haiti	10.7
Swaziland	14.1	Honduras	15.0
Tanzania	10.7	Jamaica	13.1
Togo	19.4	Mexico	16.7
Uganda	11.3	Nicaragua	10.4
Zambia	7.6	Panama	19.0
Zimbabwe	13.7	Paraguay	12.4
S.Asia, E.Asia and Pacific		Peru	15.2
Bangladesh	8.2	St. Christopher & Nevis	10.2
Burma	12.2	St. Lucia	16.8
India	10.0	Suriname	25.0
Indonesia	8.9	Trinidad & Tobago	9.5
Korea, Rep. of	23.7	Uruguay	10.0
Malaysia	16.4	Venezuela	14.7

Source: World Bank Financing Education in Developing Countries An Exploration of Policy Options. Washington, D.C. The World Bank (1986a:49-50).

Appendix Table 2

Growth of Community Schools in Papua New Guinea by Province, 1985-1990

PROVINCE		S C H O O L S		
		1985	**1990**	**% Increase,1985-90**
1.	Western	55	71	29
2.	Gulf	71	79	11
3.	NCD	33	36	9
4.	Central	150	176	17
5.	Milne Bay	150	161	7
6.	Oro	82	91	11
7.	Southern Highlands	143	140	2
8.	Eastern Highlands	153	188	23
9.	Chimbu	98	102	4
10.	Western Highlands	115	138	20
11.	Enga	84	94	12
12.	Morobe	218	252	16
13.	Madang	138	167	21
14.	West Sepik	116	139	20
15.	East Sepik	192	208	8
16.	Manus	52	60	15
17.	New Ireland	98	103	5
18.	East New Britain	119	129	8
19.	West New Britain	109	125	15
20.	North Solomons	142	--	--
21.	KLMD	40	51	28
	Total	**2358**	**2510**	6

Note: The Department of Education considers Kiunga Lake, Murray as a separate entity from Western Province because of the Copper Project (Department of Education, 1985a, table 7).

Source: Department of Education <u>Education Staffing and Enrolment Statistics National Education System</u>. Port Moresby: Management Planning Unit, PNG Department of Education (1985 and 1990). (Percentage increase in number of schools derived by author).

Appendix Table 3

Growth of Provincial High Schools and Enrolment by Province, 1985-1990

PROVINCE	SCHOOLS AND ENROLMENTS			
	1985		1990	
	No. of Schs.	Enrol.	No. of Schs.	Enrol
1. Western	2	1043	3	974
2. Gulf	3	964	4	1305
3. NCD	6	2964	7	4294
4. Central	8	3011	8	3200
5. Milne Bay	5	2250	5	2261
6. Oro (Northern)	2	1065	4	1422
7. Southern Highlands	8	2982	9	3354
8. Eastern Highlands	6	2784	8	3770
9. Chimbu	6	2784	7	3040
10. Western Highlands	8	2730	8	3424
11. Enga	5	1711	5	2153
12. Morobe	9	3766	10	5012
13. Madang	5	2915	7	3384
14. West Sepik	6	1671	6	1841
15. East Sepik	8	2900	8	3190
16. Manus	3	977	3	1203
17. New Ireland	5	1989	5	2057
18. East New Britain	8	3953	8	3981
19. West New Britain	4	1639	4	1997
20. North Solomons	5	2207	-	-
21. KLMD	1	512	2	693
Total:	**113**	**46317**	**121**	**52555**

Note: The Department of Education considers Kiunga Lake, Murray as a separate entity from Western Province because of the Copper Project (Department of Education, 1985a, table 7).

Source: Department of Education <u>Education Staffing and Enrollment Statistics National Education System</u>. Port Moresby: Management Planning Unit, PNG Department of Education (1985 and 1990).

Appendix Table 4

Community School (Gr. 1-6) Enrolment as Percentage of Population 7-12 Years by Province, 1974 and 1983

PROVINCE		1974	1983
		% OF 7-12	% OF 7-12
1.	Western	68	69
2.	Gulf	63	67
3.	NCD	62	77
4.	Central	76	77
5.	Milne Bay	76	70
6.	Oro (Northern)	63	66
7.	Southern Highlands	43	50
8.	Eastern Highlands	32	54
9.	Chimbu	53	58
10.	Western Highlands	45	54
11.	Enga	30	53
12.	Morobe	53	59
13.	Madang	57	56
14.	East Sepik	57	67
15.	West Sepik	51	70
16.	Manus	65	102
17.	New Ireland	81	79
18.	East New Britain	103	85
19.	West New Britain	78	81
20.	North Solomons	79	72
	PNG (All Provinces)	56	63

Sources: 1. Papua New Guinea Education Plan 1976-1980 p.9

2. PNG Department of Education Report of Study on Universalization of Primary Education (Port Moresby) 1983: 82

Appendix Table 5

Community School (Gr. 1-6) Enrolment as Percentage of Population 7-12 years by Province and Sex, 1976 and 1983

PROVINCE	ENROLMENTS AS % OF POPULATION 7-12			
	1976		1983	
	Boys	Girls	Boys	Girls
1. Western	72.8	47.3	74.4	63.9
2. Gulf	71.4	48.1	76.0	58.0
3. Central	79.0	55.3	80.2	72.7
4. NCD	62.1	57.2	78.4	76.1
5. Milne Bay	85.3	67.2	72.5	66.8
6. Oro (Northern)	62.4	45.0	70.5	60.4
7. Southern Highlands	67.0	24.4	54.2	45.1
8. Enga	56.9	18.2	63.8	41.2
9. Western Highlands	64.5	32.4	58.6	49.2
10. Chimbu	64.9	30.0	65.6	49.9
11. Eastern Highlands	54.6	26.5	58.3	49.5
12. Morobe	65.1	37.4	65.9	51.1
13. Madang	71.1	41.2	64.0	46.7
14. East Sepik	74.7	47.8	76.0	57.1
15. West Sepik	75.5	41.7	84.9	53.3
16. Manus	65.9	55.8	105.1	99.3
17. New Ireland	87.2	71.9	82.5	75.4
18. East New Britain	110.8	108.8	90.1	80.2
19. West New Britain	106.6	91.4	85.9	74.5
20. North Solomons	74.6	71.2	73.3	70.7
Total	**70.9**	**44.5**	**69.3**	**57.0**

Sources: 1. United Nations and South Pacific Commission Population of Papua New Guinea: Country Monograph Series No. 7.2 (New York and Noumea, New Caledonia) 1982: 259.

2. PNG Department of Education Report of Study on Universalization of Primary Education (Port Moresby) 1983:83.

Appendix Table 6

Percentage of PNG Student Enrolment as Girls in Community Schools (Gr 1-6) By Province, 1985-90

PROVINCE	PERCENTAGE OF ENROLMENT AS GIRLS					
	1985	**1986**	**1987**	**1988**	**1989**	**1990**
1. Western	47	47	46	47	47	47
2. Gulf	41	41	42	41	41	42
3. NCD	47	47	48	47	47	47
4. Central	45	44	45	45	45	45
5. Milne Bay	47	47	47	47	47	48
6. Oro (Northern)	44	44	46	45	45	45
7. Southern Highlands	45	43	44	45	45	45
8. Eastern Highlands	43	44	43	43	43	43
9. Chimbu	42	41	42	41	42	45
10. Western Highlands	45	45	46	45	45	45
11. Enga	40	40	40	40	40	40
12. Morobe	42	42	42	43	43	44
13. Madang	41	41	41	42	42	43
14. West Sepik	39	39	40	40	40	41
15. East Sepik	44	45	45	46	46	46
16. Manus	46	48	47	48	49	48
17. New Ireland	48	47	47	47	46	47
18. East New Britain	47	47	47	47	47	46
19. West New Britain	45	45	44	45	45	44
20. North Solomons	48	48	48	48	49	--
21. KLMD	38	40	41	43	43	44
Total:	**44**	**44**	**44**	**44**	**44**	**44**

Note: The Department of Education considers Kiunga Lake, Murray as a separate entity from Western Province because of the Copper Project (Department of Education, 1985a, table 7).

Source: Derived from Education Staffing and Enrollment Statistics National Education System, 1985, 1986, 1987, 1988, 1989 and 1990. Port Moresby: PNG Department of Education, Management Planning Unit.

STRATEGIES TO ACHIEVE UNIVERSAL EDUCATION

SHELDON G WEEKS[1]

HISTORICAL PERSPECTIVE

Papua New Guinea is a long way from achieving universal primary education, yet alone universal education for all from preschool through Grade 12. To develop appropriate strategies to achieve universal education one must begin with a consideration of past efforts to promote universal primary education and evaluate what has gone wrong. At this moment a number of the papers for the Waigani Seminar on related issues are not available to me. These include Tim Curtin's on economic implications of expansion, and James Quarshie's on the implication of demographic trends for educational planning. Whether the actual growth rate is 2.03 or 2.2 or 2.4 percent per annum, and the implications of differing growth rates, is not my immediate concern - I want instead to explore strategies that might be used to help achieve universal education.

1. <u>Events through 1950s</u>

The first time universal primary education was announced as official government policy was during the period when Paul Hasluk was administrator (Hasluk 1976). A plan was set in 1958 that was to achieve UPE by 1975. By 1970 only one third of the target of 750,000 pupils had been reached. Universal primary education was an ideal which never was attained because it was only rhetoric - the steps required to translate universal primary education into reality were never taken: increasing the budget for primary education, expanding the flow of trained teachers, establishing the district (now province) and Local Government Council capacity to plan and execute the development of new schools, and the creation of a system which captured the commitment of children and parents so that they would stay in school instead of dropping out (Smith 1987).

2. 1960s to Independence

While lip-service to universal primary education was made during this period, the reality was that resources were directed to expand secondary and tertiary education. There was a proliferation of post-secondary institutions (with Grade 8 and then Grade 10 entrance requirements) till at independence there were approximately 67 tertiary institutions compared to 78 high schools (Weeks 1977, NDOE

[1] **Division of Educational Research**
National Research Institute

1985). The institutions where teachers were trained were rationalized from a variety of small church agency run colleges to the present core of nine (ten with the SDA college at Sonoma) of which only two were run by the government - Madang and Port Moresby Teachers' College. The nine community teachers' colleges reached a combined enrolment of 1,957 in 1980.

3. Failure to Achieve UPE Since Independence

The budget allocated to education has risen steadily up to 1983 and since 1988. Though planners and policy makers have talked about universal primary education, their priority has been the expansion of secondary and tertiary education, and their focus has been on quality over quantity. This orientation was encouraged by the review of education that took place in 1980 (Kenehe 1981).

The National Department of Education has released a number of surveys supporting universal primary education (Neuendorf 1983, Yoeman 1987). But looking backwards over the fifteen years since Independence it is possible to conclude that the government has never been serious about universal primary education. The resources to establish universal primary education have never been made available, the number of community teachers' colleges has declined by one (Port Moresby In-service College was established instead) and the number of trainees has gone down continuously to an intake in 1991 of around 600 students following the introduction of the three year course.

Dropping out from community school has never been confronted. Yet it remains the Achilles heel of the education process, with the proportion dropping out rising steadily from year to year (Bray 1984b, Tawaiyole and Gibson 1989). Between these and other studies there is no shortage of recommendations to deal with dropping out.

STRATEGIES FOR THE FUTURE

To be able to achieve universal education in the next nine years (by the year 2001), the approaches of the past and those currently being taken will have to be abandoned. New strategies will have to be developed if even universal primary education from Grades 1 to 6 is ever to be achieved. A complete mobilization of human and other resources is required if universal education from preschool to Grade 12 is to become a reality.

1. Resolve Contradictions Inherent in Management and Administration

Policies to support the development of universal education must be established and given the full support of both national and provincial governments.

Universal Education for All

The time may have come to introduce an education system that allows those students who want to progress from one level to the next to move on. One reason the high rates of dropping out are experienced, the non-enrolment, and the withdrawal of community support occurs, is because children, and their parents, perceive that they have no future in the present system where two-thirds are eliminated at Grade 6 and again at Grade 10. What people want is universal education for all.

Preschool through Grade 12

A new structure for the education system is required that will capture the imagination and support of the people. There is wide spread frustration over the present education system which produces a nation of 'pushouts' and 'failures' by having space for only one third of the students to go on after Grade 6 and 30 percent after Grade 10.

The present proposals coming from the National Department of Education's Education Sector Study for a new structure (3-6-2-2) or North Solomons Interim Education Authority for slightly different structure (1-7-5) are to be welcomed (Momis 1991).

Multigrade teaching

It is essential that all teachers learn how to teach small ability groups, to reach those who are under-achieving and encourage those who are bright. The community teachers' colleges programme must be reformed to allow for and support these changes.

Every School an Intake Every Year

Level II schools with biennial, triennial and staggered intakes (one, two or three teachers) are the weak link in the chain. Children are told to wait until they are older, to come back again in one, two or even three or four years. Many do not come back at all. Every school should enrol students every year, but the goal of one teacher for 35 pupils can still be striven for if teachers are trained and prepared to teach two or three or more classes under one roof (ability group teaching).

Relevant Education through Integrated Teaching

When education is universal the range of ability of the students increases, particularly at lower and upper secondary schools, because there is minimal or no selection. To be able to educate a diverse group of students a new syllabus is required. One possible approach is that which was pioneered by SSCEP and continued by the Curriculum Extension Office - the development of Integrated Teaching Projects, community extension and outstations. Curriculum extension was designed to provide an education that would benefit both those students who were going to return home and those who would continue on to further studies. All students studied the same material and streaming was not required.

The approaches developed through Secondary Schools Community Extension Project and the Community Schools Agricultural Project were endorsed by the Matane Report in 1986 and became official national policy in 1987. All schools are meant to use Integrated Teaching Units (primary) and Integrated Teaching Projects (secondary). A Curriculum Extension Office was created to help develop such materials, provide advice, circulate a newsletter and bulletins, run in-service training and in general promote integrated teaching. It was abolished at the start of 1990.

2. Overcome Failures in Educational Planning

In order to overcome the dual phenomenon of non-enrolment and dropping out, to gain the full support of the community for formal education, a number of radical changes are required that must take place at the same time.

Priority to Teacher Training

The development and expansion of the nation's teachers' colleges has not been given the support it requires. The number of graduates from the community teachers' colleges remains grossly inadequate, and will decline even further following the introduction of the three year course. To achieve universal primary education we require not 600 teachers a year, but at least twice that many.

As universal secondary education evolves, the need for more high school teachers will increase dramatically. Goroka Teachers' College must be expanded to take in more students and steps taken to develop a second secondary teachers' college in the islands region. This emergency teacher training college could be in North Solomons Province.

If the demand for more primary and secondary teachers is not met, and expansion of schooling occurs without increasing the capacity of the community and secondary teachers' colleges, the consequence will be a dramatic increase in the number of untrained teachers in primary schools, and the rapid promotion of community school teachers into secondary school teachers.

Priority to Preschools

We believe that if Tokples preschools were to spread throughout the country the resulting rise in the level of understanding of schooling through increased comprehension (if one learns to read and write in one's own language first, than one learns better in English later) might go a long way to decrease absenteeism, dropping out, and negative attitudes to education.

Priority to Continuing Education

If the examination at the end of Grade 6 can be eliminated, and the proposed Grade 8 examination avoided; we will have gone a long way towards creating an education system which is accessible to the majority of children. The 'pushout' phenomenon at Grade 6 and Grade 8 will no longer exist if universal education is provided. A priority must be given to expanding the education system so that the majority of children who want to go from primary to secondary schools are able to do so.

When a community has its 'own' schools, both primary and secondary institutions, enrolments rise, dropping out decreases, and general support for schooling improves (Weeks 1987).

Alternative approaches to formal secondary education need to be fully utilized until the transition to universal education can be achieved. CODE is our largest high school (with over 20,000 students). In Manus, high school education for all was to be achieved, at first, through the establishment of CODE study centres on remote islands. Community Secondary education, if re-established, would have tremendous potential to absorb youth. There is also capacity for more vocational centres. Such approaches are ultimately more sound than squandering K50 million on a 'National Guard' employing 5,000 Ghurkas from Nepal.

3. Establish a Commitment to Universal Education

Financial resources must be released to support the expansion of preschool and primary and secondary schooling. More schooling costs more, but if people are mobilized to support education, not all the costs have to be borne from the centre. Many of the projections as to expansion and possible costs are based on old models and old assumptions. Even preschools can become expensive if those at the centre attempt to provide all the materials-if instead each school is helped to have paper and a silk screen printing outfit, then they can begin to produce their own materials.

4. Devise Ways to Remove Bottlenecks

The major bottleneck that exists is fear of lowering standards, fear of diluting an elite system, fear of the high costs of a mass education system, and fear of the consequences of an overproduction of educated people.

Standards

The question of 'Standards' are often raised as a smoke screen to oppose educational development and expansion. What is forgotten is that expansion, by definition, means lower mean scores (and therefore lower standards)! If I open a university with one student, the best in the country, as soon as I enrol the next student, second best, I have lowered my standards.

Diluting an Elite System

The time has come to abolish national high schools. The government has not been able to build a new national high school since Passam in 1979. Instead of more, narrow, elite institutions we should spread the benefits across the whole system.

Reducing Costs while Raising Quality

By the year 2001, if we were to expand secondary schooling rapidly to meet demand, we would have not 130 high schools as in 1990, but approximately 780 high schools. This sounds impossible because each small boarding high school (2-2-2-2) now costs K2.8 million. To build a new national high school is now estimated to cost K16 million. Instead of 16 new national high schools for K256 million if we were to spread this amount across 650 new high schools it would provide around K400,000 each. If each community worked to build their own community high school this amount would go a long way to providing the required facilities. Day high schools will be cheaper and they do not require the extensive reticulated water systems with flush toilets present in current boarding high schools.

Improved plans for low cost teachers' houses and classrooms have already been implemented in some provinces compared to those of National Works (the costs is K3,000 a classroom instead of K42,000 and K2,000 a teachers' house instead of K27,000). These plans must be adapted more widely. They represent costs for cement, roofing and hardware when the community builds the structures using approved provincial plans. High schools could also use such plans and could probably cost K500,000 to K1 million instead of K2.8 million (libraries, laboratories, technical divisions and facilities will still be costly). New high schools will be cheaper because more and more of them will be day schools (saving on the cost of boarding facilities).

The major cost of any rapid expansion of the education system is teachers' salaries. The average cost per-teacher is at least K7,000 (including leave fares and other benefits). In 1990 there were 12,500 community school teachers and 2,400 secondary school teachers. By 2001 the education system will require at least 20,000 community school teachers and 10,000 high school teachers - or twice as many teachers as in 1990. This doubling of the salary bill at first may seem to be prohibitive, but if only a proportion of the benefits from the new resource development projects (gold, gas, oil, timber) are channelled into education, even more should be immediately affordable, or at least beginning in 1992.

The Merits of Overproduction

'Does expanding the secondary education system make good economic sense for a developing country?' Tanzania has been compared to Kenya and called a 'natural experiment' (Knight and Sabot 1990). It is 'natural' because both countries share a similar size, colonial heritage, resources, and patterns of economic development - they differ in one notable aspect, the proportion of the age group in secondary school is only 4 percent in Tanzania compared to 19 percent in Kenya. This is because Tanzania for 25 years had an extremely restricted post-primary system compared to Kenya's 'no-holds barred' approach to secondary schooling. Knight and Sabot found that secondary education develops cognitive skills that are related to increases in the productivity of workers, that an investment in secondary schooling yields a higher rate of return, and that expansion contributes significantly to economic growth. This is in sharp contrast to the general received truth that 'fragile' Third World states expand education to their own peril (Fuller 1991).

CONCLUSION

UPE is attainable. We can adapt strategies now to demonstrate our commitment and resolve to achieve universal primary education. Educational developments in a few provinces (Manus and New Ireland Provinces, and National Capital District) demonstrate that UPE can be achieved in the next decade. But are people really committed to universal primary education?

REFERENCES

Bacchus, M K (1984) A Review of Educational 'Needs' at the Secondary Level in Papua New Guinea. Report 48, Educational Research Unit, Waigani, University of Papua New Guinea.

Brammall J and May R J (1975) Education in Melanesia. Canberra. Australian National University.

Bray, M (1984a) Educational Planning in a Decentralized System: The Papua New Guinean Experience. Waigani, University of Papua New Guinea Press and Sydney, Sydney University Press.

Bray, M (1984b) Dropping Out from Community Schools: the Extent, the Causes and Possible Remedies. Report No. 49, Educational Research Unit, Waigani, University of Papua New Guinea.

Conroy, J D (1976) Education, Employment and Migration in Papua New Guinea. Canberra, Australian National University.

Fuller, Bruce (1991) Growing-Up Modern: The Western State Builds Third-World Schools. London, Routledge.

Gibson, Margaret (1990) 'Equity for the Nation's Smallest Schools', Papua New Guinea Journal of Education. 26(1) forthcoming.

Gibson, Margaret and Weeks, Sheldon (1990) Improving Education in the Western Province. Research Report 66, Division of Educational Research, National Research Institute, Waigani.

Hanson J, Agard J and Smith P. eds. (1978) Underway on a Five Year Plan. Proceedings of the Fourth Extraordinary Faculty Meeting of the Faculty of Education, Waigani, University of Papua New Guinea.

Hasluck, Paul (1976) A Time for Building: Australian Administration in Papua New Guinea, 1951-1963. Melbourne, Melbourne University Press.

Kenehe, Simon Chairman (1981) In Search of Standards, Gordons, Hebamo Press.

Knight J B and Sabot R H (1990) Education, Productivity and Inequality: The East African Natural Experiment. Oxford, Oxford University Press.

Matane, Sir Paulias (1986) A Philosophy of Education for Papua
New Guinea. Ministerial Commitee Report, Waigani, National Department of Education.

Momis, Fr John (1991) 'Education in North Solomons Province' Times of Papua New Guinea, 6 May, two pages.

National Department of Education (1985) Growth of Education Since Independence: 1975 - 1985. Waigani, NDOE.

Neuendorf, Alwyn (1983) Universalization of Primary Education. Bangkok, Unesco, Apeid.

Rogers, Cyril (1979) A National Education Strategy. IASER Monograph 9, Waigani, Institute of Applied Social and Economic Research.

Smith, Geoffrey (1975) Education in Papua New Guinea. Melbourne, Melbourne University Press.

Smith, Peter (1987) Education and Colonial Control in Papua New Guinea: A Documentary History. Melbourne, Longman Cheshire.

Tawaiyole, Pani and Gibson, Margaret (1989) Survey of Enrolments and Wastage in Papua New Guinea Schools, 1971 - 1988. Paper presented for the Apeid-NIER Planning Workshop, Tokyo, Japan 28 June - 11 July.

Thomas, E Barrington (1976) Papua New Guinea Education, Melbourne, Oxford University Press.

Yoeman, Lyn (1985) Universal Primary Education: Factors Affecting the Enrolment and Retention of Girls in Papua New Guinea Community Schools. Evualation Unit. Waigani, National Department of Education (Published by Apeid, Unesco, Bangkok 1987).

Weeks, S G (1977) The Social Background of Tertiary Students in Papua New Guinea. ERU Report No. 22, Waigani, University of Papua New Guinea. 191 pp.

Weeks, S G (1987) Education and Change in Pangia, Southern Highlands Province. ERU Report No. 56, Waigani University of Papua New Guinea, 121 pp.

Weeks, S G (1989a) 'What is the Practical Option', in Piniau, S.ed. High School Education for All in Manus (report of the Seminar, Lorengau, July 11-13, 1988). Rabaul, Hanns Seidel Foundation, 181-188.

Weeks S G (1989b) 'Manus Builds a Third High School at Bundrahei', in Piniau, S.ed. High School Education for All in Manus (report of the Seminar, Lorengau, July 11-13, 1988). Rabaul, Hanns Seidel Foundation, 101-104.

Wormald, E and Crossley, A (1988) Women and Education in Papua New Guinea. Waigani, University of Papua New Guinea Press.

EDUCATION FOR ALL: RIGHTS OF THE DISABLED

MABA LOHIA[1]

What is Education?

Is education a right, a need or a privilege?

In theory, most people including academics and politicians would agree that education is a right of every person, and that education or learning begins at home and does not end until the person dies. If education is a right, then a responsible government is obligated to provide for it at all costs.

In Papua New Guinea, however, not enough money is allocated to education and as a result education has become the privilege of a minority group instead of a RIGHT BELONGING TO ALL.

What is Special Education?

For those who do not quite fit into the regular education system, special education is also a right. Governments have the responsibility to provide for it just as much as they do for the regular system.

Unfortunately, because of limited funds allocated to education in Papua New Guinea, the tendency is to give priority to the brightest normal children who it is assumed will give the most back to the society or nation. However, it is equally important that disabled children be given the opportunity of education and training to their maximum potential to enable them to participate and contribute in their way to the society to which they belong and not become a burden to their government.

1 Port Moresby Special Education Centre

Regular Education Compared to Special Education.

The diagram below shows the different paths that normal and disabled children have for achieving the same goal of becoming an educated person. For a normal child the path towards the goal is shorter than for a special child who will have different aims set according to the level of his or her disability and functional capacities. A longer time is expected to become fully educated and more stepping stones have to be set along the way.

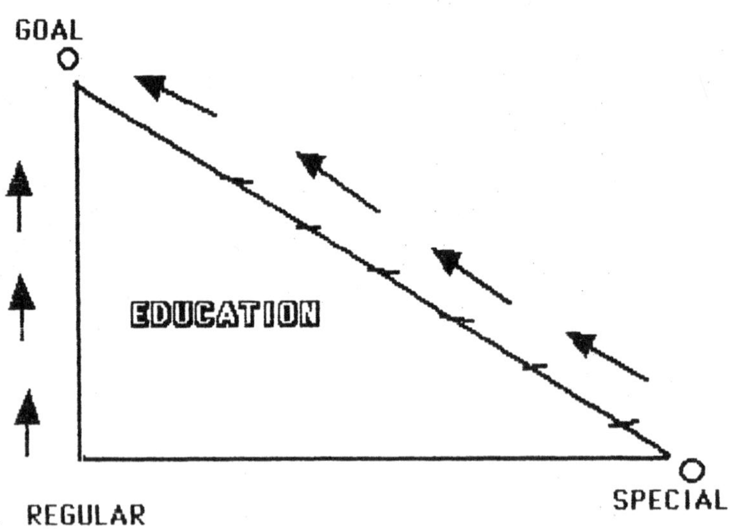

Goals may be different - and some achievements may appear smaller, but they are no less important. For a severely handicapped child to achieve independence is similar to a normal student being successful in his degree programme at the university. It also brings pride, satisfaction and freedom to the family of that child who can then turn to its other responsibilities of bringing up a good and happy family.

If every teacher in the country were to receive one disabled child in his or her classroom, the government policy of education for all could be easily achieved within the next ten years without further social unrest and without injustice to the disabled portion of the population.

Policy in Papua New Guinea

A draft plan or policy on integration and rehabilitation written by the National Board for the Disabled Persons is now before the National Executive Council for consideration. The plan calls for integration and provision of rehabilitation services for the disabled within the government infrastructure.

It is recognised that integration of disabled persons in the village community takes place extremely well thanks to the support of the extended family system. This system of caring for the disabled has also to be encouraged by the government through the support of technical and manpower assistance.

In an increasingly urbanised society such as Port Moresby, however, many people do not have the type of support that the village or extended family provide. There is need therefore for special education units to be attached to the regular education system to cater for such situations. These units can serve as resource centres staffed by rehabilitation specialists (teachers, occupational, speech, physiotherapists, psychologists etc.) to monitor special education programmes and to provide backup services throughout the country.

Statistics

There are no true figures about numbers of disabled people in the country as yet. However, if the United Nations assumption is correct that ten percent of the world population suffers from some form of impairment then in Papua New Guinea we might be looking to at least 50 percent of that figure, at a disabled population of around 200,000 persons.

A pilot survey carried out in 1978 in some parts of the Central Province By Griew and Cohedy from the Community Medicine Department at the University of Papua New Guinea, revealed that 2.5 percent of the population suffer from impairments such as deafness, blindness and lameness. This was quite a disturbing revelation for Papua New Guinea.

Unless the Government is prepared to introduce some form of preventive measures the problems associated with disabled people are likely to increase dramatically in the next decade due to:

a) Improved medical facilities that allow a disabled child who would otherwise have died to remain alive;

b) Parents who have children when there is risk of a genetically transmittable disorder;

c) Lack of awareness about risks of taking medication during pregnancy;

d) Increased family size which involves risks for mothers who do not plan their families properly;

e) Hazards resulting from industrialisation and modernisation such as:

   - industrial accidents
   - pollution
   - environmental hazards
   - traffic accidents, etc.

Causes of Disability

There are many causes of disability; some known and others yet to be identified. The most commonly known causes are the following:

- meningitis
- rubella
- malnutrition
- premature births
- traffic accidents
- hereditary factors
- taking of pills by mothers resulting in impairments such as deafness, blindness, paralysis, mental retardation, social disorders etc.

The Future.

If the government of Papua New Guinea is concerned with checking rapid population growth, it should also begin to think about reducing the rate of growth of the disabled population.

Disability prevention programmes need to be run alongside the existing Health Department Health Services such as community nursing, immunisation and family planning programmes.

In addition to the above measures, there is urgent need to have the National Department of Education include and fully recognise special education programmes, by:

a) Affiliating the few existing private special education centres to the National Education System, and using these centres to develop or design curriculum material for implementation in the community teachers colleges.

b) Incorporating advanced and specialised training programmes at degree level within the Medical Faculty of the University of Papua New Guinea.

VOCATIONAL/TECHNICAL EDUCATION AND LABOUR MARKET CONDITIONS IN PAPUA NEW GUINEA

RAINER JANISCH[1]

INTRODUCTION

There are narrow interrelationships between the educational system and the sectors of work and vocational life. The representation of these interrelationships is one of the tasks of research on the vocational and labour market and of the research in the economics of education.

The goal of research carried out in the above fields is to provide those people who are active in the field of educational planning with information on the problem areas listed below:

- Determination of the significance of human capital for development and foreseeable specialisation requirements of the state's economy;
- Representation for the purpose of planning of the existing linkages between the education sector and the remaining sectors of the economy;
- Making conscious and transparent the significance of the educational system as a mechanism for equitable distribution of opportunities to young people.

Based on the above theoretical guidelines and on terms of reference set by the governments of Papua New Guinea and the Federal Republic of Germany a study was undertaken to examine, on the one hand, the interdependence between the general and vocational education systems and, on the other, between the educational system and the economic sector of Papua New Guinea (GTZ 1991).

This paper examines some of the findings of the above study and discusses these in three sections:

- The first section deals with the qualitative and quantitative aspects of the state of development of education and the urban economy sectors and looks at the consequences, which in our opinion, result from this development;
- the second part discusses the different explanatory approaches found in theory and their significance in relation to the situation in Papua New Guinea;

[1] University of Hanover

- the third part considers possible macrosystems of vocational education, explains their effects and refers these to the Papua New Guinea system; this part is followed by a brief conclusion.

Qualitative and Quantitative Aspects of the Development of the Educational System, the Labour Market and Employment in Papua New Guinea.

1. Labour Market and Employment

Compared to other developing countries the availability of statistical data on the labour market situation and on the employment structure and development (formal sector wage employment) is extremely limited; even basic data are not available -or, if available, are not up to date.

The central problem of the Papua New Guinea labour market situation is that of an annual growth of the labour force by approximately 50,000 and small sized labour market (at present of only about 250,000) coupled with relative stagnation of growth in the eighties. The economically growing sectors of the mining and mineral oil industry have a low employment intensity, while employment in small and medium-sized labour intensive enterprises in the trades and industrial sector and the non-formal sector play a negligible role in Papua New Guinea's economic structure. The consequence of this situation is a high unemployment rate concentrated in the agglomeration centres where to a degree it has contributed to a rise in criminal activities.

Manpower planning as worked out in 1982 and 1986 for Papua New Guinea (a new review has been initiated by the Department of Finance and Planning) will, for methodical reasons and poor availability of data, be limited to the employment situation in the formal sectors. The National Manpower Assessment Plan 1982-1992 (1986) was based on an estimated total employment of 194,174 in 1984, only 9 percent of whom were in the industrial sector, and attempted to give an estimate of the specialists required in individual professions and the needs in training courses using the traditional 'manpower requirements approach'. Although the methods and results of this kind of manpower planning have been massively criticised, the estimates that were made in the plan had consequences for the Pre-employment Technical Training (PETT) courses in the Technical Colleges.

Survey of Employers and Employees

In order to gain some idea about the significance of qualifications earned in vocational training centres and technical colleges in relation to the formal economic sector, a survey of employers was carried out in the Lae region. One hundred and thirty three companies were questioned; 36 of these were in the industrial sector. The companies employed a total of 8,345 persons of which 2,791 could be included in the professional categories covered by the training offered in vocational centres and technical colleges. Of the group of 2,791 a random sample of 405 employees were chosen as subjects for a tracer study. Of these, 138 persons had attended courses in vocational centres while the rest had completed their education in a technical college.

Asked about their expectations in relation to employment opportunities in the next five years, the companies indicated that there would be an astonishing rise in demand (+41 percent). In relation to the professional categories relevant to the study, the companies indicated that they had at present some 807 vacancies, and when these were related to the number of staff presently occupied it could be predicted that the current demand would last at least for the next one to two years. In terms of the type of vacancies available the employers indicated the need for skilled technicians at certificate level as opposed to PETT types of qualifications, and for skills such as carpentry, joinery, cabinet making and plumbing which are peculiar to the particular labour market requirements of Lae. In terms of recruitment practices, the companies questioned indicated that if they were unable to recruit technicians qualified at the certificate level then they preferred to get unqualified persons and train them on-the-job. Only a small percentage would recruit PETT graduates with apprenticeship or PETT graduates and train them on-the-job. The skills considered to be in short supply by these employers were those at the higher technician certificate level as well as persons with electrical and electronics skills.

The interviews to employees with vocational training and with technical college education provided additional information of interest. The general level of formal education was high among them. Eighty one percent of those questioned had attended provincial high schools and 64 percent had completed grade 10, even though for vocational school only grade six is required. Over a third of those interviewed had financed their education with private funds (38.4 percent); another group of equal size had received public scholarships (38.1 percent) and 15 percent had been funded by employers. Most of those who had attended vocational centres (82.7 percent) had funded their own education.

Asked about how they found employment after conclusion of their education, only a minority had done so through the intervention of the National Employment Service (6.7 percent). the rule was rather to find a job as a result of own initiative. Comparison between the activities performed in their employment with those for which they had been trained showed conformity in professions such as 'fitting and machining', 'electrical' or 'motor mechanics'. It was not the case however in the case of more specialist qualifications acquired through certificates from technical colleges and vocational centres. While jobs with a predominantly theoretical content are preferentially filled with graduates from technical colleges, those with a predominantly practical component are filled with persons who attended vocational training centres.

Finally, the comparison between the wage structure of the two groups of employees, from training colleges and from vocational centres, showed a marked difference. The income of former vocational training centre students ranged from 110 Kina per fortnight (metal fabrication/welding) to 141 kina per fortnight (carpentry/joinery); while the average wage of a former technical college student ranged from 170 kina per fortnight (motor mechanics, carpentry/joinery) to 241 kina per fortnight (printing). Professions with higher and predominantly theoretical qualification requirements are paid higher salaries. Thus a major influence on salary allocation for comparable types of occupations is the higher education grade of technical college students. What is noticeable in this respect is that the stated average income exceeds by a small amount the renumeration to be paid to apprentices as fixed by the Apprenticeship Board.

Results obtained from this survey of companies and employees in the Lae region, which represents the industrial agglomeration centre of the country, indicate that the labour market lacks manpower with vocational skills and qualifications. However, in interpreting these results, it should be kept in mind that many of those who attend vocational centre and PETT courses have difficulty in getting their first employment in the formal employment sector.

2. Transition from General to Vocational Education.

Transition and drop-out (push-out) rates from one level of education to another represents one of the most important problems affecting education and the planning of training in Papua New Guinea. There is a drop-out rate of approximately 30 percent among the community school age group, and this figure needs to take account of the fact that only 70 percent of this age group are actually enrolled in community schools.

The minimal requirements for entry to vocational training centres is grade six. A comparison between the number of pupils leaving community schools with the entrance capacity of vocational centres shows a disparity: only 15 percent of 6th grade leavers are accepted by these centres. The situation is similar for the transition from lower secondary school (grade 10) to continuing schools among which are the technical colleges. Thus only 34 percent of grade 10 leavers are able to continue their education in upper secondary or other continuing institutions. Of these, only 24 percent will be able to enter PETT courses which constitute the first stage of the formal vocational education system. The entrance capacity to these courses has decreased steadily in the decade from 1980 to 1990 by almost 50 percent and there has been a simultaneous decline in the figures continuing on to the second stage of the vocational education system which is the apprenticeship.

If results of the survey alluded to earlier are compared to the situation of school leavers and their chances of further education, the following is noted:

- companies state that they have important requirements for skilled, qualified employees;
- technical colleges have diminished their training activities;
- more than an insignificant proportion of young people who have gone through the vocational education system do not find employment in the modern sector of the economy.

Therefore, there does seem to be a qualitative discrepancy between the vocational education system and the labour and employment system. The qualifications strategies and considerations of both systems seem to be located at different points. Offer of qualifications and demand for qualifications are not harmonically related.

The reasons for this qualitative discrepancy shall be elucidated in the second and third parts of this papers.

MANPOWER PLANNING PHILOSOPHIES AND ECONOMIC GROWTH

The process of economic growth and structural change, the development of industry and the modernisation of agriculture, the introduction of new production technologies and the establishment of a modern institutional framework conducive to change -all require the concomitant development of the human resource potential of a country as a factor in its growth and modernisation. Human resource development foremost depends on the knowledge, competencies, orientations and values imparted by education and training.

For the task of planning the growth and structure of education systems as part of an overall development strategy, three 'philosophies' and technical approaches can be distinguished:

- the 'manpower requirements approach' to educational planning sees the development of the educational system as dependent on the qualification needs of the system of employment and tries to translate these needs - via technical coefficients and relationships - into outputs of the educational system (number of graduates at various levels and fields of specialisation) that must be produced to guarantee a structurally balanced labour market development;
- the 'rate of return approach' which is of a more economic nature, perceives education as investment in human capital earning a rate of return that is determined by the education-specific wage differentials that can be derived from the actual wage

structure of the labour market. The logic of this planning approach accordingly is that if the rate of return for a specific type of qualification is relatively high it must be particularly scarce and production therefore should be expanded; on the other hand, if qualification is in oversupply it earns low rates of return and the number of graduates in such fields should be reduced;

- the third approach starts from the presumption that the education sector develops and expands in a relatively autonomous way and that the demand for education is a relevant point from which to start in educational planning. The problem of linkages with the sector of production and employment then becomes a question of the 'absorptive capacity' of the economy for the supply of qualifications of different levels and types, and educational planning should try to gear output levels and structure to that absorptive capacity.

Insofar as all these planning approaches are quantitatively oriented and take the structure of the educational system as given, in some important respects they are obviously deficient. What also matters for educational planning but also for the relationship between education and the economy are issues of organisationa and curricula content, i.e. the qualitative aspects of schools and their programmes, of narrowly or broadly defined concepts of occupational competence, of relevance of university studies etc. Thus existing deficiencies of the educational system and the planning of organisational and curricula reforms to overcome such qualitative problems may be more important than the quantative imbalances and the need for expansion. Analysis of these deficiences and recommendations for reform have to start from qualitative studies of the educational process, the functioning of the labour market, the recruitment policies of firms, the career development of graduates, etc.

Whatever approach is adopted to tackle the problem of steering vocational training and technical education in Papua New Guinea towards the labour market and employment, it will run into the difficulty of extreme scarcity of statistical data. Most commonly in the context of planning a manpower analysis in Papua New Guinea the needed data is simply not available. There is also the question, of course, of whether this planning approach is at all relevant to the particular subsector of the educational system we are considering here.

Vocational training and technical education are understood to mean training given in vocational centres and in technical colleges in Papua New Guinea. Most vocational centres are located in rural areas and their training is oriented towards improvement of living conditions, traditional agriculture and the needs of small rural workshops, the handicraft sector and possibilities of self-employment in the more or less informal economic activities of rural areas. A manpower planning approach, besides the lack of data, is not suited to this sector of small-scale, informal activities. More relevant would be the concept of the 'absorptive capacity' of a particular rural area for specific qualifications. This would lead more or less to individual programmes for each vocational training centre geared towards the actual situation and possible development of economic activity in the small-scale informal sector.

The technical colleges, on the other hand, are mainly engaged in the system of apprenticeship training in that their programme of extension courses complement the practical apprenticeship training in established firms. The PETT courses at technical colleges serve as the basis for apprenticeship training and their course content should be oriented (as was originally designed) towards broader occupational fields rather than particular ones. The increase or decrease of the particular trade for which apprentices are being trained at present depends on the decision of individual firms and their judgment about future manpower requirements. The programme of extension courses at the technical colleges therefore mainly reflect the development and the occupational structure of apprenticeship training decided by individual firms. These firms do not require and would not observe an economy-wisde manpower approach to planning. It could be useful in this respect to provide better incentives for firms to carry out apprenticeship training and to advise and guide them in their training decisions, but in fact the role of the technical colleges' subsector here is a reactive and passive one.

MACROSYSTEMS OF TECHNICAL AND VOCATIONAL EDUCATION

The macrosystems of vocational education depend on the regulatory means determined by political institutions. The following are the essential regulatory means of a vocational education system:

- regulation of responsibilities and functions (role of the state, of the private economy, or other supporters);
- regulation of the financing of education;
- classification of educational institutions within the overall education system;
- regulation of the certification system linked to professional fields;
- regulation of initial and further training of teachers, as linked with salary scale;
- regulation of entrance requirements for vocational and technical courses;
- regulation of responsibilities and procedures for curriculum development.

Below is a classification of models according to the role exercised by the state in relation to vocational and technical education. It relates to the functions, influence and intervention possibilities of the state including its role in applying regulatory means.

1. Types of Formal Vocational and Technical Education.

In analysing the numerous national systems of technical and vocational education, it is possible to distinguish the following three basic models:

Market Model

The government plays a minor or no role at all in the vocational qualification process

Bureaucratic Model

The government is the sole authority responsible for the planning, organisation and control of technical and vocational education

Government-Controlled Market Model (Dual-System)

The government provides a more or less tight framework for technical and vocational education in private enterprises or other private institutions.

Model 1

The government plays a minor role or no role at all in vocational training. This is the liberal model. It is better, however, to term it a market economy or market model. Most countries using this model have well developed educational systems with 10 to 12 years of compulsory schooling which is rather strongly influenced by the government. All young people in these countries attend a secondary school, and the number of secondary graduates going on to college and universities is high.

Technical and vocational education to a great extent, however, is not under government influence. It is directly related to productive work and to the labour market. Its development and organisation is left to the citizens' initiative and to the commitment of enterprises, local authorities and other training providers who, without reference to government regulations, offer and organise vocational education and training geared to practical work situations.

Usually there are also state school programmes for marginal and problem groups that provide vocational qualification; however, here the historically evolved traditional structures still dominate. Enterprises remain the major training providers. Above all, the big enterprises usually achieve an outstanding position in the market owing to their economic superiority, as is the case for example in Japan.

The following are the main mechanisms responsible for the functioning of the market-oriented system of technical and vocational education:

- The market model determines the quantitative relations between qualification requirements and vocational education. Vocational qualifications are provided according to demand. Demand is determined by customers, that is, enterprises.

- The type of qualification (qualitative aspects) is determined exclusively by what the enterprises desire. Inter-company qualification transfer depends on the market, but usually is not very strong.

- The market mechanism of vocational qualifications functions best when potential customers provide their own training and thus control results.

- Training is financed by the customers, that is, governed by the principle of cost minimisation. Usually it is more related to productive rather than pedagogical principles (on-the-job-training).

- The providers of vocational training select the trainees irrespective of higher order social values (e.g. equal opportunities). Trainees, in principle, have the same legal status as regular workers.

Model 2

In this model, the government is the sole authority responsible for the planning, organisation and control of technical and vocational education.

For logical reasons, this model should be termed bureaucratic; however, in view of its predominantly institutional form it may be called the school model.

School-based systems of technical and vocational education to a great extent are similar in structure and origin. Their special feature is a graded vocational school system closely linked to the general education system and, in developed countries, it is always located at the upper secondary level.

Access to the different training courses which provide qualifications at clearly defined levels is determined by the applicant's completion of lower secondary education. This link between school education and the technical-vocational institutions is also evident from the direct connection existing between school leaving qualifications and vocational qualifications (often included in wage agreements) which may even result in double qualifications (e.g. university entrance and skilled worker qualification).

School-based systems of technical and vocational education in principle constitute hierarchical elite systems and are found mostly in countries with a centralised administration. Owing to their elitist character, they usually carry an educational monopoly in the field of technical and vocational education which virtually precludes the development of competing forms of training, e.g. 'dual' systems. Private enterprise does not play a role in such systems of technical and vocational education, except perhaps as provider of places for students who are required to spend practical work periods in industry. The stronger the government's claim to the sole responsibility for technical and vocational education, the more closed is the bureaucratic system of planning, organisation and control. This does not preclude in some cases cooperation by enterprises indirectly with the technical-vocational system.

Below are some of the important characteristics of the system as described:

- The quantitative relations between qualification requirements and technical-vocational education are determined by public planning authorities. Demand-oriented planning is most efficient when it refers to a limited number of established basic occupations.

- The type of vocational qualifications (qualitative aspect) is not primarily determined by practical work situations, but usually also take account of individual and social requirements. The more the vocational schools are related to general education including its performance and selection criteria, the more their technical qualification is influenced by the system-related problems of general schools.

- The planning, organisation and control of the process of technical and vocational education are determined to a great extent by the bureaucracy; the implementation of the related universal principles tends to guarantee that the provision of systematic training is strongly influenced by teaching theory.

- School-based technical and vocational education is financed from public funds. Since such funds, by definition, are limited there usually are no national training models aimed at providing vocational qualification for the entire age group.

- School models function best for occupations and occupational fields that do not involve much training of psychomotor skills, e.g. commercial occupations.

Model 3

In this model the government provides a more or less tight framework for technical and vocational education which is carried out in private enterprises or other private training institutions.

The system could be called a government-controlled market model; however, it is precisely what we call a dual system.

Such systems are commonly called dual because the two places of learning, enterprise and government-supported schools cooperate with the common aim of providing trainees with vocational qualifications. However, the dual structure may vary.

Government controlled market models are characterised by a strong dividing line between the system of technical and vocational education and the general public school system. This is demonstrated above all by the existence of a more or less detailed specific technical and vocational legislation which cannot be categorised as school legislation. The legal responsibility for technical and vocational education under such sytems lies therefore as a rule with the ministries of finance or labour.

What is essential about the functioning of this model is neither the location of training nor a specific enterprise structure, but the existence of a training sector which is designed according to the private enterprise (i.e. free market) rules and which can be modified by government rules.

The dual system can be defined as a system involving two places of learning only with regard to its institutional form. With regard to its function, the dual character depends on the integration of two different sets of regulations governing technical and vocational education. This integration is most closely reflected in the legislation on technical and vocational education which, in a target-oriented approach, combines the private market oriented law system with the public law of government.

The functional criteria derived from this model are the following:

- The quantitative relations between qualification requirements and technical-vocational education depends on the market (which provides the training opportunities); however, the enterprises offering training accept government-issued rules.

- The type of vocational qualifications (qualitative aspects) is determined primarily by practical work situations in the enterprise. The definition of qualification goals involves not only the enterprise but also the government and other interest groups (e.g. trade unions, professional associations).

- The enterprises are training providers. However, vocational training processes have to be organised according to government rules and are subject to direct or indirect government control.

- The costs of training are, in principle, borne by the enterprises. Dual training models are, however, characterised by the application of regularised financing models (e.g. fund financing) and/or co-financing by the government to a greater or lesser extent.

- In dual systems of technical and vocational education, the extent to which vocational training is designed systematically and governed by pedagogical principles can be modified according to the demand. The most important instrument in that respect is the modification of financial incentives.

2. The Situation of Technical and Vocational Education in Papua New Guinea.

A uniform vocational education system defined by legal regulations does not exist in Papua New Guinea. Rather what exists are two different systems, a formal one where the educational institutions are the technical colleges and the enterprises, and a non-formal vocational system organised in absolute independence from the formal one, without any common structural elements. Persons who attend the non-formal vocational system have no possibility of changing to the formal one in conformity with their obtained certificates.

The formal educational system is characterised by a horizontal basic structure consisting of elements of basic vocational training (PETT courses), dual skilled worker training (Apprenticeship Training) and a technician/master training (Certificate Course). The structure of this system conforms with manpower requirements of the modern urban employment system.

The curriculum for both technical colleges and enterprise training institutions is determined by competent boards (Apprenticeship Board, Technical Education Committee). Due to lack of specifications for the professional fields and lack of regulations for the conduct of examinations, but also due to missing regulations on competencies and responsibilities, the required co-ordination is not performed adequately.

Although the basic structure of formal technical institutions conforms with the requirements of the employment system for qualified manpower, it contains considerable social injustice documented by the lack of career development potential and lack of acceptance by the Papua New Guinea educational system of the persons who have been trained in the technical system. There is no vertical career development potential; technical education in Papua New Guinea constitutes an educational deadlock. This is particularly true of those who attend the non-formal vocational training system.

The non-formal vocational training system (vocational training centres) is oriented to rural requirements. Most of the male persons who pass through this system try, however, to find employment in the modern sector although their qualifications for the most part do not cover urban employment requirements.

The responsibility regulations and regulations of the responsible supporting bodies of both systems are particularly problematic. A clear responsibility is found only in the field of basic vocational education. In all remaining areas there are complex regulations which can relate to national, regional or public/private levels. Furthermore, responsibilities in the public administrations are not clearly defined and lead to a permanent information and communication gap.

Financing of vocational education is heterogeneous. In the formal system, there are two supporters: the state and the private sector. In the non-formal sector there are state, private and other sponsors, but they are not able to provide sufficiently for the required needs but they are not able to provide sufficiently for the required needs of the institutions. The centres therefore are forced to resort to alternative funding sources (e.g. selling products and services). Vocational centres which are not able to make use of such resources find themselves in deplorable conditions.

Comparative Evaluation.

On the basis of this brief description of technical and vocational education in Papua New Guinea, the following can be stated of its relation to the above discussed three models. Vocational education in Papua New Guinea contains elements of all three basic models. The non-formal vocational training of vocational centres is predominantly characterised by the criteria of the market model. According to this system, the State plays only a marginal role. The type of vocational qualification depends on the presumed usefulness it has in the region in which the institution is located; transferability of qualifications to other regions is low. Funding of the relevant educational activities is predominantly private and subject to cost minimisation. It is a type of education which is partly linked to production and less of a pedagogical type.

In the formal technical system, the PETT courses offered in technical colleges are organised according to the bureaucratic model. State planning acts between the qualitative relations of the market needs and technical education. The type of qualification obtained is not oriented towards professional usefulness in a particular region at a particular point in time. It is essentially determined by the performance and selection principles of the general educational system. It is almost exclusively funded by government.

Contrary to these systems, there are dual training structures represented in the Apprenticeship Training and Certificate Course, the models of which have been described earlier.

The educational institutions in the non-formal system are the vocational training centres. Due to lack of data and the absence of clearly regulated formal responsibilities, individual vocational training centres cannot be compared to each other. There is no exchange comparability of the vocational centre qualifications in the labour market.

The effects of this model heterogeneity in the vocational education system is largely known and has been documented elsewhere:

Papua New Guinea's vocational and technical education system does not offer enough labour market relevant qualifications for those persons attending the system. From the point of view of educational achievement, it is a political deadlock. the employers of vocational qualifications (companies, enterprises, public institutions) are forced to satisfy their needs by taking other measures (training on-the-job, foreign experts, in-house training).

CONCLUSION

A 'qualitative improvement' strategy for the vocational-technical system is needed in order to realise a connection between education and the labour and professional sector of Papua New Guinea.

Such a strategy could be achieved through the establishment of an institution responsible for eliminating the heterogeneity in the system, as detailed above, and of defining clear responsibilities, structural conditions and generally valid regulatory means for the technical vocational sector.

REFERENCES

Sector Study: Technical and Vocational Education in Papua New Guinea. Interim Report on the Project of Technical Cooperation in the Field of Vocational Training. Parts I, and II and III. Cologne. 1992 GTZ MBH.

THE ECONOMICS OF EDUCATION - WILL PAPUA NEW GUINEA BE READY FOR THE 21ST CENTURY

TIMOTHY CURTIN[1]

The Royal Economic Society and the Economic Journal recently celebrated their centenary by inviting their most distinguished contributors to set out predictions for the future of economics in the next century. William Baumo(1) was one of the few out of 22 to give more than a passing glance to the economics of growth and development, and called for a return to Adam Smith's concern 200 years ago to seek out the causes of the wealth of nations.

Baumol comments:

> The pertinent theory still has a long way to go (and) recent events in eastern Europe, Latin America - (and, he could have added, Africa, the Indian sub-continent, and the South Pacific) - have demonstrated dramatically the threat of political turmoil ... that failure to achieve viable growth rates entails.

And he concluded:

> attention to this subject will .. require more intensive use of standard analytic techniques ... and examination of topics such as the economics of education which have largely escaped the attention of mainstream economists...(We need to) understand more fully just what education contributes to (economic) growth, what types of education are critical for the purpose, and what allocation of expenditure can be most effective in facilitating growth. In several countries, notably the United States, the growing proportion in the labour force of groups with inferior education constitutes a threat not only to themselves but also to the remainder of society.

The recent history of Papua New Guinea demonstrates the force of Baumol's prediction - in the last analysis the Bougainville crisis could even be said to represent as much a revolt by the least educated inhabitants of that Province against the rest, as a secessionist movement.

[1] Department of Finance and Planning

I have myself attempted to respond to Baumol's call for a newer economics but one hopes his remarks will encourage many more of the economics profession to build on the understanding that education is - as Denison [2] was the first to demonstrate - the single most important determinant of the processes of economic growth and development.

It is not before time: the modern theory of economic growth has been for far too long locked into intensely mathematical but ultimately sterile formulations which, as a direct result of the requirements of elegant mathematical constructions, abstracted from any participation by human beings other than as automatons.

Thus the standard growth model - that of Harrod and Domar - consists (in the form described by Stern, 1991)[3] of no more than a pair of tautologous (i.e. true in all states of the world) equilibrium conditions: given that Investment results in K', where K' is the stock of Capital (K) <u>after</u> the investment, and that by definition Investment must be equal to savings (S), the proportion of income which is saved must be equal <u>ex post</u> to the contribution of Capital to Income:

$$I = S$$

$$K'/K = s/u \qquad \text{......(1)}$$

where $s = S/y$ and $u = K/Y$

and $rY = Y'/Y = s/v$ ......(2)

where v is the incremental capital output ratio (ICOR),

$$\text{i.e. } v = K'/Y$$

Now since in equilibrium $s = u = v$, s/u must be equal to unity, and no further growth is possible:

for if $K'/K = 1$

then $K' = K$

which means of course no growth in the capital stock K, and therefore no growth in national income Y.

Stern (3) comments that this simple theory has been and remains very influential - depressing might have been a better word, or dismal. Yet although all it consists of is accounting relationships between the ratio of saving to the national income, and the proportion of national income which is accounted for by investment, the model was indeed influential in countries like India which strove hard to raise the savings ratio and the ICOR, but which for all their efforts ended up with growth rates not significantly different from zero.

Although in later developments a partial way out of the cul de sac which this theory led to came with recognition that people do matter, but even then the growth theorists were only able to conclude that the growth of the economy was in the long run restricted, in the absence of technical progress, to the rate of growth of the population and the labour force. But the resulting forcus on technical progress ... which came to be seen as the main factor was viewed as being exogenously determined, that is, independently and arbitrarily determined by factors outside the system (Stern, p.125).

This extraordinary belief, which implied that investment contributed nothing to technical progress, was modified when some authors allowed for increases in labour productivity - but such increases were restricted only to those obtainable from learning by doing, Arrow, (4). Thus the mainstream of economic growth theory ended by concluding either that stagnation (in the sense that growth could not in the long run exceed the rate of growth of the labour force) was inevitable, or that growth at rates faster than the growth of population was impossible in the absence of technical progress, a subject about which the growth theorists and their models had nothing to say, except that like the growth of the population it could not be affected by policy.

This fatalistic approach has latterly begun to be modified, notably by Schultz (5) who has stressed the importance of understanding that technical progress must be treated as an endogenous or integral part of the system, and that there are no exogenous factors which could explain technical progress, which is instead the outcome of the process of human capital formation. But there is as yet no indication that the theorists have found a way to incorporate human capital formation into their models.

Part of the problem has been that almost all human capital theorists took a fatal wrong turning, led by Blaug (6) whose misinterpretations of the fundamental tenets of investment analysis led them to the conclusion that for the great majority primary schooling was all that was required to equip them for employment in a modern industrial economy - but properly treated, the theory of human capital formation does have a great deal to offer to growth theory. In fact it provides the missing ingredient without which most economies would indeed be doomed to stagnation.

This interpretation is supported by the earliest econometric studies of the determinants of the process of economic growth. Denison in particular had found that when all the obvious causal factors had been accounted for, like the growth of the labour force and the rate of investment, there remained a substantial residual, of no less than 66% of the observed growth of the national income of the United States; and he suggested that this residual should be identified with the contribution of human capital formation to economic growth (1962).

But by what in retrospect may seem a perversion of economic analysis, Mark Blaug quickly reinterpreted Denison's residual, which accounted for 66% of national income growth, to suggest that only 66% of the additional earnings observed to be associated with further education could be attributed to such education, with the balance to be ascribed to such factors as innate ability or IQ, the social and educational status of one's parents, the type of school attended, and so on. This alpha coefficient as Blaug called it - sleight of hand would have been a better term - formed a major part of Blaug's case against investment in higher education, for cost-benefit analysis implied that if only 66% of an individual's additional earnings arising from education was due to education, the resulting rate of return on investment in providing that education would be "sub-economic" (Blaug, 1965).

One possible source of the confusion between the Denison and Blaug coefficients - a confusion which Denison shared equally with Blaug - lies in a fundamental misunderstanding of the analogy on which the concept of human capital formation is based. If people are the raw material of human capital just as iron and steel are the raw materials of physical capital such as machinery, then of course the initial quality of the input - whether people or steel - does have a bearing on the final outcome or rate of return to be expected from the processes of education or manufacturing specific lots of people or steel.

But what Blaug and all subsequent writers have all had difficulty in accepting is the statistical evidence such as that cited in Becker (7) showing that for people of <u>equal</u> abilities, there is a close relationship between the amounts of education they respectively receive and their lifetime earnings - just as steel of consistent quality produces uniform output.

Secondly, Denison's econometrics were based on extending the concept of the production function, in which a firm's output is determined by the quantities of inputs - labour and capital - to the whole economy. Blaug may initially have had in mind an analogy between such a production function and that for an individual, whose income could be considered to be determined by a set of inputs, of which his education is only one. Such an analysis would be instructive, since those other inputs - such as the equipment available for individual employees - are all themselves owned and produced by other people, who in turn have had varying amounts of education.

Blaug is far from being the only economist who seemingly never came to terms with the formulations of the national accounts, since the national income is of course no more than the aggregate of all the personal incomes of the members of the nation, and all complementary physical inputs (raw materials - iron and steel - and machinery) are treated as intermediate goods, while the value of all final goods is exactly equal to the aggregate of personal incomes. But this may explain why he turned instead to a series of sociological explanations for the differentials in earnings associated with successive furthering of education, amongst them the so-called screening hypothesis which alleges that education per se has no value to employers, except as a means of screening the more suitable of potential employees out of the total labour force (for a defence of this view see Maglen, (8) and for a critique, see Curtin, (9).

My own assessment of the rather remarkable amount of evidence that is available to chart the impact of education - or lack of it - on economic growth in Papua New Guinea is that Denison was right: education is the single most important determinant. This can be illustrated by the data on the growth of education and employment in Papua New Guinea.

Table 1 disproves the conventional view that whatever the private benefits of further/higher education may be, the tendency for the marginal social rate of return to be lower at the tertiary than the primary level of education indicates that priority should be accorded to primary education alone...anything which tends to increase enrolments at the primary level and to decrease them at the secondary and tertiary is a step in the right direction (Blaug, 1976, p.279).

The Table shows first, that when cumulative social net present values are considered, they are maximised when the educational cycle is completed for each individual, despite the apparent decline in the social rate of return as education proceeds.

The data in Table 1 also show that when all incremental taxation is taken into account, as it NEVER has been before, the resulting public rate of return indicates that further education yields a fully financial and economic rate of return to government (the unpublished paper by Bowman, Millot and Shiefelbein, (10) is a partial exception, but considers only taxation of those with higher education).

Tables 2 and 3 constitute further refutations of the conventional view established by Blaug (11) that the present value of the national income will be maximised if educational resources are concentrated on provision of primary education and diverted from secondary and tertiary. The historical record for the growth of education and employment in PNG shows that the contribution of the relatively small numbers of the post-primary educated employees to national income has been growing much more rapidly than that of the vastly larger numbers of primary leavers, most of whom are permanently unemployed. Moreover the data suggest that GNP growth per capita in Papua New Guinea has been constrained more by the slow growth of further education than by any shortage of primary school leavers.

Table 4 shows how what matters for economic growth is the average years of education obtained by each member of the labour force - the measure here is correlation of the rates of growth of exports in 16 developing countries with the rates of expansion of primary, secondary, and tertiary schooling and of the average years of schooling of new entrants to the labour force. The coefficients imply that horizontal growth of primary and secondary schooling alone (i.e. more at each level) is of less importance than vertical growth, in the sense of the average years of schooling obtained by the new entrants to the labour force every year.

Table 5 refutes the screening hypothesis. Clearly the belief by Arrow (1962) and Blaug (1965) in learning by doing is not supported by regression analysis of the relative earnings of the labour force at the Ok Tedi copper mine, where length of service makes a much smaller contribution than level of education and training to the explanation of relative earnings.

CONCLUSION

Standard methods for appraising investment in education based on assessing private and social rates of return which ignore the associated net present values, and fail to account for all incremental taxation, have produced misleading assessments of the relative ordering of priorities to be accorded to investment in human capital formation.

In particular, Blaug's advocacy of maximisation of rates of return by concentrating resources on rates of return does not maximise net present values of the national income.

Blaug's social rates of return do not correspond to the government's public rate of return arising from its own benefits (in the form of ALL incremental taxation associated with provision of further education); the public rates of return on primary and tertiary education are the inverse of the social.

Moreover all statistical analysis by the human capital theorists, including those who have written on the economics of education in Papua New Guinea such as Gannicott (12) and McGavin (13) has exaggerated private rates of return by taking into account only income taxes and ignoring incremental indirect taxation payable by the more educated members of society.

Thus complete calculations of private and public rates of return and net present values do not confirm standard policy prescriptions of exclusive incremental indirect taxation payable by the more educated members of society.

Thus complete calculations of private and public rates of return and net present values do not confirm standard policy prescriptions of exclusive priority to investment in primary schooling before secondary and tertiary.

THE POLICY CONCLUSION IS THAT EDUCATION SHOULD BE PROVIDED FOR ALL TO THE LIMITS OF THEIR ABILITIES.

When that is being done Papua New Guinea will be able to look forward to the 21st century with confidence.

REFERENCES

1 Baumol W J (1991). Towards a Newer Economics: the Future Lies Ahead, Economic Journal, January, P.7

2 Denison E F (1967). Why Growth Rates Differ. Washington: Brookings Centre for Economic Development

3 Stern N (1991). The Determinants of Growth, Economic Journal, January, P.124

4 Arrow K J (1962). The economic implications of learning by doing, Review of Economic Studies

5 Schultz T W (1990). Restoring Economic Equilibrium: Human Capital in the Modernising Economy. Oxford: Blackwell

6 Blaug M (1965). The Rate of Return on Investment in Education in Great Britain, Manchester School, September.

7 Becker G S (1983). Human Capital. 2nd edition, Chicago: University of Chicago Press.

8 Maglen L (1990). Challenging the Human Capital Orthodoxy, Economic Record, December.

9 Curtin T (1991). The Economics of Public Investment in Education in Papua New Guinea. Faculty of Education, Occasional Paper No. 1, UPNG.

10 Bowman M J, Millot B, Schiefelbein E (1986). The Political Economy of Public Support for Higher Education, World Bank, Discussion Paper (unpublished), Washington

11 Blaug M, Layard R, Woodhall M (1969). The Causes of Graduate Unemployment in India. London: Allen Lane.

12 Gannicott K (1989). The Evaluation of Human Capital in Papua New Guinea, Papua New Guinea Journal of Education.

13 McGavin P A (1991). Policy Evaluation of Investment in Education: a Papua New Guinea study, Economics of Education Review.

TABLE 1 **PUBLIC INVESTMENT IN EDUCATION IN PAPUA NEW GUINEA RATES OF RETURN AND TOTAL AND MARGINAL NET PRESENT VALUES**

(PNG Kina = US$1.05 in 1991) (Discount rate 5%)	PRIVATE	PUBLIC (Kina)	SOCIAL
1.NO SCHOOLING			
NPV - to age 45	18742	3153	21895
- to age 64	22885	3850	26735
2.PRIMARY GRADE 6 (Increase over No Schooling)			
NPV - to age 45	2312	108	2419
- to age 64	3969	771	4741
IRR (%) (to age 45)	27.7	5.4	10.5
IRR (%) (to age 64)	27.7	6.9	11.4
3.SECONDARY GRADE 10 (Increase over Grade 6)			
NPV - to age 45	8180	3641	11821
- to age 64	12915	8994	21909
IRR (%) (to age 45)	28.9	12.4	18.6
4.SECONDARY GRADE 12 (Increase over Grade 10)			
NPV - to age 45	7246	5067	12313
- to age 64	11161	13770	24931
IRR (%) (to age 45)	Inf.	13.8	27.5
5.DEGREE (Increase over Grade 12)			
NPV - to age 45	3726	2486	6212
- to age 64	12406	25131	37536
IRR (%) (to age 45)	8.7	6.0	6.8
IRR (%) (to age 64)	10.8	9.3	9.7
6.POST-PRIMARY (Cumulative Increase from Grade 6 to Degree)			
NPV - to age 45	19152	11193	30345
- to age 64	28496	49768	78264
IRR (%) (to age 45)	20.8	8.2	11.4
7.COMPLETE CYCLE (Grade 1-Degree over No Schooling)			
NPV - (to age 64)	40360	48666	89027
IRR (%)(to age 64)	21.8	10.6	12.9

TABLE 2 - AGGREGATE NET PRESENT VALUE OF THE LABOUR FORCE IN PAPUA NEW GUINEA

	NPVs PER CAP KINA	1979 NUMBERS	TOTAL NPV K MN	1982 NUMBERS	TOTAL NPV K MN	1988 NUMBERS	TOTAL NPV K MN	GROWTH RATES PERSONS 1979-1988
1. HIGHEST SCHOOLING OF								(% p.a.)
LABOUR FORCE AGED 18+		1341786		1440732		1661051		.0240000
PRIMARY G1-G5		383892		417846		509567		.0319670
PRIMARY G6		85226		125758		233875		.1186968
SECONDARY G7-G9		74649		92297		138937		.0714628
SECONDARY G10		6359		9860		26549		.1720932
GRADES 11-12		155448		22090		45264		.1268747
TERTIARY		1987		4063		8900		.1812850
TOTAL EDUCATED (G1+)		5675614		671914		963092		.0605161
TOTAL UNEDUCATED		774225		768818		697959		-.011456
2. EMPLOYED IN FORMAL SECTOR								
(i) CITIZEN EMPLOYEES								
NO SCHOOLING	26735	57600,65	1539,953	56548	1511,811	57850	1546,620	.0004801
PRIMARY G1-G5	29105,5	31493,35	916,6297	32974	959,7248	34851	1014,356	.0113197
PRIMARY G6	31476	28341.46	892.0757	27645	870.1540	37532	1181.357	.0316996
SECONDARY G7-G9	42668.5	31406.09	1340.051	32549	1388.817	41553	1773.004	.0315964
SECONDARY G10	53385	42555.82	2271.842	43125	2302.228	79232	4229.800	.0715033
SECONDARY G11-12	78317	6202.985	485.7992	7582	593.7995	10158	795.5441	.0563330
DEGREES	115853	2395.138	277.4839	2575	298.3215	6907	800.1967	.1248809
Total national Employees		199996		202998		268083		
- excluding self-employed	115853	319	36.95711	1488	172.3893	1993	230.8950	.2257812
(ii) EXPATRIATES	149861	13418	2010.835	13964	2092.659	16917	2535.199	.0260812
3. UNEMPLOYED/INFORMAL SECTOR								
NO SCHOOLING	26735	716624.4	19158.95	712270	19042.54	640109	17113.31	-.012468
PRIMARY G1-G5	26735	352398.6	9421.378	384872	10289.55	474716	12691.53	.0336601
PRIMARY G6	26735	56884.54	1520.808	98113	2623.051	196343	5249.230	.1475725
SECONDARY G7-G9	26735	5930.094	158.5411	22083	590.3890	26701	713.8512	.1819724
SECIBDARY G10	26735	616	16.46876	367	9.811745	683	18.26001	
SECONDARY G11-12	26735	500	13.3675	510	13,63485	1106	29.56891	.0922183
TERTIARY	26735	-408.138	-10.9116	1488	39,78168	1993	53.28286	
		1132545						
TOTAL UNEMPLOYED/ INFORMAL S	26735	1141790	30525.76	1219703	32608.76	1341651	35869.04	.0180842

	1979 PERSONS	1979 NPVs	1982 PERSONS	1982 NPVs	1988 PERSONS	1988 NPVs	GROWTH RATES 1979- PERSONS	GROWTH RATES 1979- NPVs
EDUCATED NATIONAL EMPLOYEES	142395.4	6183.881	146450	6413.045	210233	9794.258	.0442406	.0524223
TOTAL NATIONAL EMPLOYMENT	199996	7723.835	202998	7924.856	268083	11340.88	.0330912	.0436019
-Post Primary	82560.03	4375.176	85831	4583.166	137850	7598.545	.0586135	.0632545
-Primary	59834.81	1808.705	57427	1829.879	72383	2195.713	.0213791	.0217777
TOTAL UNEMPLOYED/ INFORMAL	1141790	30278.60	1237734	32608.76	1392968	35869.04	.0223391	.0190042
TOTAL LABOUR FORCE	1341786	38002.44	1440732	40533.62	1661051	47209.92	.0240000	.0243989

TABLE 3 EDUCATION, EMPLOYMENT, AND NATIONAL INCOME 1973-1991

	1973/74	1979	1982	1984	1986	1989	1991	
DISTRIBUTION OF EMPLOYEES BY EDUCATION LEVEL (%)								
NONE TO G5)	.645	.4454700	.4541170	.4498666	.0755245	.0208333	.0208333	
PRIMARY G6)	.186	.1417073	.1384715	.1352480	.1636364	.0708333	.2769195	
SECONDARY G7-G10	.1582	.3698095	.3602145	.3647950	.5608392	.3083333	.5337079	
TERTIARY G11-BA	.01	.0430132	.0471971	.0500904	.2	.6	.1685393	
	.9992	1	1	1	1	1	1	
TOTAL SAMPLE	9349	132936	202960	198818	715	240	712	
ALLOCATION OF EMPLOYEES BY HIGHEST ATTAINED SCHOOLING								
TOTAL	150000	200000	216018	214722.2	226416.0	257090.0	246952.0	
NONE TO G5	96750	89094.00	98097.44	96596.33	17099.95	5356.042	5144.833	
PRIMARY G6	27900	28341.46	29912.33	29040.75	37049.89	18210.54	68385.81	
SECONDARY G7-G10	23730	73961.91	77812.82	78329.58	126982.9	79269.42	131800.2	
TERTIARY G11-BA	1500	8602.636	10195.41	10755.52	45283.20	154254.0	41621.12	
NET PRESENT VALUE OF EMPLOYEES' EARNINGS AT 1988 AVERAGE EARNINGS-BY-SCHOOLING LEVELS								GROWTH '73-'79
NONE TO G5	2586.611	2381.928	2622.635	2582.503	457.1671	143.1938	137.5471	
PRIMARY G6	878.1804	892.0757	941.5204	914.0868	1166.182	573.1950	2152.512	.0541530
SECONDARY G7-G10	1186.5	3698.095	3890.641	3916.479	6349.147	3963.471	6590.011	.1061170
TERTIARY G11-BA	150	860.2636	1019.541	1075.552	4528.320	15425.40	4162.112	.2158932
TOTAL	4801.292	7832.363	8474.338	8488.620	12500.82	20105.26	13042.18	.0605446

SOURCES

Garnaut, Wright, and Curtain 1977;

McGavin and Ross, 1988; McGavin 1990 (INA); Ok Tedi Mining Ltd. (April 1991 Payroll)

Curtin, UPNG Faculty of Education Occasional paper No. 1, 1991.

National Statistics Office, Tax Incidence Studies, 1986, 1988

TABLE 4 CORRELATION OF EXPANSION OF EDUCATION WITH GROWTH OF FERTILIZER USE AND EXPORTS

COUNTRY	PRIMARY	SECONDARY --1965-1986--	TERTIARY	AVERAGE SCHOOLING	FERTILIZER (kg/ha)	EXPORTS (1966-1986)
EGYPT	.0229545	.0779871	.884545	.023176	.0571621	.1069438
PAPUA NEW GUINEA	.0400436	.0880992	.1543597	.0238185	.1113321	.0855592
ZAMBIA	.0585233	.1559227	.2743827	.0352422	.0451622	-.000138
PAKISTAN	.0481972	.0507213	.0599854	.0180044	.1173704	.1073087
GHANA	.0087102	.1317062	.1521051	.0156374	.0413236	.0602226
KENYA	.0604343	.1321161	.280563	.0324811	.0498072	.081158
BANGLADESH	.0346422	.0542177	.0952903	.0143047	.0952347	.0907727
INDIA	.0639531	.038136	.0611902	.029863	.1084158	.1061884
MALAWI	.0464525	.0776955	.2371301	.0191426	.059447	.0836347
ETHIOPIA	.1036611	.1317073	.1227937	.0851804	.1914964	.0728494
INDONESIA	.039951	.1019711	.1058076	.0291744	.1329504	.1667139
PHILIPPINES	.0285947	.061724	.0741106	.0153178	.0248415	.0912248
THAILAND	.0361296	.0571937	.1260831	.0197299	.0905077	.1363846
CAMEROON	.0420855	.0992278	.2694384	.0247796	.0506883	.1418991
NIGERIA	.0575257	.119529	.1743802	.0440527	.2720557	.1115844
MAURITIUS	.007874	.0861437	-.027681	.0103792	.0075787	.1194639

REGRESSIONS

INDEPENDENT VARIABLES	DEPENDENT VARIABLE (EXPORT GROWTH) COEFFICIENTS AND STANDARD ERRORS			
	1. SCHOOLING ONLY		2. SCHOOLING & FERTILISERS	
AVERAGE ANNUAL GROWTH OF				
1.PRIMARY ENROLMENTS	-1.72	1.57	-1.79	1.35
2.SECONDARY ENROLMENTS	-1.67	0.69	-1.93	0.61
3.TERTIARY ENROLMENTS	0.25	0.23	0.26	0.20
4.SCHOOLING PER HEAD	2.37	2.24	3.77	2.04
5.FERTILISER USAGE	-	-	-0.44	0.20
R SQUARED	0.48	0.65		
STANDARD ERROR OF y est.	0.045	0.039		
CONSTANT	0.19	0.22		

NOTES: 1. Average annual growth of enrolments derived by applying age-enrolment ratios to population structure.

2. Schooling per head - for new entrants to the labour force (age 15).

SOURCE: Development Reports, World Bank (annual)

TABLE 5 DISTRIBUTION OF EARNINGS OF OK TEDI LABOUR FORCE 1991

1. STAFF:	TERTIARY	OTHER	ALL STAFF	2.AWARD	3. TOTAL	%	ALL PNG	
KINA P.A							1988	%
0.2600				52	52	3.128761	55935	27.53249
2601-5199		5	5	492	497	29.90373	80336	39.54322
5200-6239	13	90	103	455	558	33.57401	22709	11.17789
6240-7280		0	152	152	152	9.145608	17813	8.76966
7281-8319	23	135	158	1	159	9.566787	6393	3.146781
8320-10140	18	-78	96		96	5.776173	8025	3.950089
10141-12220	26	70	96		96	5.776173	5020	2.470959
12221-15080	13	2	34		34	2.045728	4479	2.204666
15081-20280	8	6	14		14	.8423586	1563	.7693444
20281-30160	3	1	4		4	.2406739	614	.3022248
30161-40040							121	.0595590
40041+							152	.0748179
TOTALS	104	406	510	1152	1662	100	203160	100

NOTE: The Labour force is divided into "Award" and "Staff". "Tertiary" includes Graduates, Diplomas, and unfinished undergraduate courses.

Two award workers with tertiary qualifications are included in the Staff data here.

SOURCE: OTML Payroll print-out of 2nd April 1991
Table A5 (for national data).

REGRESSION RESULTS

DEPENDENT VARIABLE (Y): WEEKLY GROSS EARNINGS

INDEPENDENT VARIABLES: X1. QUALIFICATIONS (YEARS)
X2. AGE
X3. LENGTH OF SERVICE AT OTML

	Y	X1	X2	X3	R^2
TOTAL LABOUR FORCE (1,662)					
- Coefficients		16.78	1.97	1.47	0.54
- Standard Error	36.0	0.4	0.1	0.29	
- Constant: -96,4857					

EXAMPLE: Predicted earnings (Y) of graduate (16 years of) education) aged 30 on staff at OTML for 5 years:

(16 x 16.78 + (30 x 1.97) + (5 x 1.47) - 96.4857 = 238
(Actual earnings of only graduate at OTML aged 30: K230)

THE CHILD AND MELANESIAN VALUES

ENNIO MANTOVANI[1]

INTRODUCTION

From 2.6 percent in 1970 the 1990 Census for Papua New Guinea gives a 2.1 percent increase of the population over the last 10 years. The question is, how to slow down this birth rate further during the next decade?

It is my thesis that the child, above everything else, is a key value representing identity, meaning, and especially security for people. As a consequence the less identity, meaning, and security in life the greater the psychological need for more children; and the more identity, meaning and security, the lesser the urge to have many children.

If this is true, the best way to solve the birthrate issue is to provide people with the means which will enable them to claim identity, meaning, and economic security and wellbeing. However, because we deal with felt values, promises will never suffice: it is only the experience of security and wellbeing that will lessen the emotional fear which is expressed in the need for many children.

This paper presupposes and supports the concern for family planning. Its purpose is to show the way which has proven successful so far in lowering the birth rate in Papua New Guinea.

I propose to base my argument on the research results and the data from the Melanesian Institute on Marriage and Family Life in Melanesia. Secondly, I shall analyse the results within the Melanesian value system. Thirdly, I shall highlight those elements from the analysis which seem relevant for the future. Finally, I shall end with some conclusions.

THE DATA

The preferred number of children

The question is: how do Melanesians look at the issue of family size today?

1 The Melanesian Institute

Anthropological Survey

Recently the Melanesian Institute conducted anthropological research on Marriage and Family Life in Melanesia particularly in Papua New Guinea and the Solomon Islands. There were 1325 people interviewed of whom 385 were from the Highlands, 392 from the Coastal mainland and 539 from the Islands. The research was carried out almost exclusively in the rural areas of those three regions where the linguistic groups are living. In some cases, such as the Tolais and Simbus, the research covered the urban areas as well so as to assess the cultural change.

In each of the 31 linguistic groups we interviewed at least 40 people: twenty men and twenty women. These interviewees were selected in equal number from four age groups: the group of those men and women who were preparing for marriage, of those parents with the first child, of those fathers and mothers whose first child was in high school (or of that age) and of those whose first born was married.

When asked how many children the couple should have, nearly 50 percent opted for a four to seven child family. This means practically every second person in the rural area opts for a four to seven child family. There are nearly three times as many people opting for the four to seven child family than for the two to three child. The one child family was hardly considered: only 0.2 percent of the females chose it. The eight plus child family did not go beyond a 3.8 percent. A sizeable 21 percent were of the opinion that it would be up to the couple to decide the size of their family.

This statistic seems to show that the difference between the males and females is minimal: we are dealing with a common value. This evidence does not support the motion that the women <u>always</u> want fewer children but the husband forces them to have more. The following tables testifies to this point.

Table 1: Preferred number of children, by Sex

No. of children	% average	females	males
0-1	0.6	0.3	0.8
2-3	17.7	17.2	18.3
4-7	45.7	44.8	46.7
8-9	3.2	2.7	3.8
10+	3.5	1.2	5.8
(Up to couple	22.0	28.7	15.3)
(As many as possible	3.9	2.2	5.7)

If we try to correlate the age of the respondents with the size of the family for which they opted the following picture emerges:

Table 2: Preferred number of Children, by age

Size	Unmar	Young	Mature	Old
0-1	0.5	1.0	0.9	0
2-3	26.9	20.7	15.0	9.4
4-7	47.8	52.4	49.5	35.2
8-9	2.1	2.1	3.8	7.5
10 +	4.9	2.7	8.2	7.5
up to couple	10.4	13.1	15.5	23.8

The correlation between age of respondent and ideal number of children seems to show some difference of expectations. The older group are the stronger on the seven plus child family. The older the group, the more freedom they give to the couple to decide the size of the family they want. The unmarried group however, are the strongest on the two to three child family, although a good 47 percent opt for the four to seven child family. There seems to be a downwards trend: the number of children one expects gets smaller the younger the couple. The people who are not married yet have the lowest expectation. Can we learn anything for the future? This question poses the question whether urbanisation trends will bring any further change.

Sociological Survey

In the Melanesian Institute's sociological survey concerning Marriage and Family Life, 887 households were interviewed in Port Moresby, Lae, Arawa/Kieta/Panguna, Goroka and Wewak. The towns were subdivided into three types of residential area: high cost, squatter settlement and urban village. In each household only one person was interviewed. Of the people interviewed, 444 were females and 443 males.

The results are shown in Table 3 regarding the ideal number of children:

Table 3: Preferred number of children by urban dwellers

No of children	average	females	males
1	1.9	2.7	1.1
2	9.0	10.8	7.2
3	15.8	17.3	14.2
4	35.6	34.7	36.6
5	14.7	15.1	14.2
6	10.3	10.1	10.4
7	3.9	2.7	5.2
8	2.0	1.4	2.7
9	0.9	1.1	0.7
10	1.1	0.5	1.8

What is apparent is that 67 percent of the males and 66 percent of the females opt for a family of 3 to 5 children with four being the favourite choice. One out of three urban dwellers opts for a family with four children. In towns there is also a broad agreement between females and males on the number of children they would like to have. These figures are more accurate than those in the Point Issue 17 and in Catalyst, 1989, No. 2. They have been arrived at by rechecking all the data. While slightly different, they confirm the reports in Point and Catalyst.

There seems to be a downwards trend when compared with the results from the rural research. If we add the percentage of those who opted for two and three children we come to an average of 24.8 against the 17.8 of the rural area. The four to seven children group, with its average of 60.6 percent, is higher than in the rural area which has only 47.7 percent average; however, the more than six children families are not in favour anymore. What are some of the variables which might have influenced this downward trend? Beside age we shall test employment, education, and church affiliation in that order.

Employment

A high percentage of the people interviewed had a job and some economic security. To the question of employment we received the following answers: 20 percent of females said they were 'self employed' and 80 percent of males responded 'self employed'. In the case of spouse employment 88.5 percent of male respondents claimed that their spouses work for cash wages while only 10.6 percent of female interviewees pointed out that their spouses are employed.

A correlation between the job holders and number of children shows the following results.

Table 4: Preferred number of children by employment status

No. Children	1-4	5-10	other
Males employed	61.3	32.4	6.3
Males unemployed	48.8	46.5	4.8
Females employed	69.0	28.3	3.0
Females unemployed	64.5	32.2	3.3
Husband employed	66.7	30.2	3.1
Husband unemployed	57.4	36.2	6.4

Employment provides economic security which seems to have an impact. The women whose husbands are employed show the same tendency. This is a fact to keep in mind when working towards population control.

Education

The correlation between education and desired number of children gives the following results:

Table 5: Preferred number of children according to educational status

No. children	1 to 4	5 to 9	other
Primary	58.7	34.7	6.6
University	77.3	19.3	3.4

Age

In addition Table 6 shows a correlation between age and desired number of children:

Table 6: Preferred number of children according to age

No. children		1 to 4	5 to 9	other
Age	0- 30	73.7	21.4	4.9
	31-45	58.0	36.4	5.6
	45 +	43.0	46.6	10.4

There is no doubt regarding a correlation between age and number of desired children: the younger the respondent the lower the number of desired children.

Church Affiliation

Table 7: Preferred number of children according to church affiliation

No. children	1 to 4	5 to 9	other
Anglicans	64.6	25.0	10.4
Catholics	60.1	34.0	5.9
Lutherans	60.8	32.4	6.8
United Church	58.2	36.9	4.9
SDA	62.9	34.2	2.9

This evidence seems to show that church affiliation is not important in deciding the ideal size of the family. This may be due to the fact that church affiliation includes too many other factors like education, employment, and age.

The purpose of marriage

Another way to ascertain attitudes towards children in Melanesia was to ask about the main reasons for marrying. According to the responses there is no question that the child is the main reason for marrying. The anthropological interviews gave the following data.

Table 8: Reasons for Marriage

Reasons	average	females	males
Offspring	90.9	92.5	89.7
Coop btw families	81.4	82.1	80.8
Bonding groups	72.9	70.9	74.5
Old age insurance	78.6	74.6	81.8
Companionship	75.6	71.0	79.2
Sex	73.6	71.0	75.5
Labour	73.4	75.1	72.0
Status	70.1	61.3	77.0

If we correlate the attitudes to the age of respondents we obtain the following picture as given in Table 9.

Table 9: Reasons for Marriage according to age

	unmar	young	mature	old
Offspring	89.7	92.2	90.5	91.4
Coop btw families	79.2	79.7	85.0	82.1
Bonding groups	69.2	72.0	75.8	75.6
Old age insurance	76.9	75.8	80.4	81.8
Companionship	75.7	73.2	77.0	77.0
Sex	71.3	74.1	75.0	73.6
Labour	69.4	73.2	75.8	75.3
Status	64.9	68.1	73.8	74.6

It seems that age does not change the basic attitudes. Will urbanisation change them? In Table 10 the following picture emerges from the urban survey.

Table 10: Reasons for Marriage according to habitation

Reason	average	females	males	H/C	L/C	St1	U/V
Offspring	68.1	68.2	67.9	70.0	61.1	75.6	66.1
To be a family	39.5	36.9	42.0	45.0	38.8	35.0	40.4
For love	35.5	40.3	30.7	42.6	34.4	33.4	40.4
Get partner	30.3	30.0	30.7	39.7	31.7	25.8	21.3
Mutual help	21.8	22.3	21.2	16.1	24.3	25.8	16.9
Continue "line"	6.9	4.5	9.3	6.7	8.4	3.9	9.5
Strength. clan	6.2	4.7	7.7	3.9	5.7	7.1	8.8
Sex	6.2	5.6	6.8	3.4	4.7	11.1	4.4

What is top priority in marriage in the rural area is still top priority in the urban situation. This is borne out by a correlation between age, education, and reasons for marriage in Table 11 and 12.

Table 11: Reasons for Marriage according to age

Age	Chld	Fam	love	partner	help	continue line	strength clan	sex
- 30	66.9	37.7	36.5	29.9	20.7	6.4	4.0	5.5
31-45	68.5	40.3	33.7	30.1	23.5	6.8	7.5	6.8
45 +	68.6	41.8	40.6	32.5	18.6	8.2	3.7	6.7

Education

It seems that higher education lowers the priority of the child. Among the same group the role of love and companionship gains considerably, but not so the family. It is the personal element gaining over the structural and the social aspect of the family life as obvious in Table 12.

Table 12: Importance of children in marriage according to educational status

Primary	68.9	46.1	30.2	28.5	24.0	4.0	6.1	4.8
Tertiary	58.2	32.8	42.5	38.8	18.6	8.2	3.7	6.7

To further test the role played by the child in the family, in the anthropological interviews we asked whether a marriage without a child is considered a marriage at all. The answer was shown in Table 13.

Table 13: Importance of children in marriage

Answer	average	females	males
No	53.6	50.9	55.6
Yes	41.8	45.0	39.4
Blank	4.6	5.0	4.1

To come to the issue from another angle we asked what people would do if there was no child in marriage and the answer was apparent in as follows:

Table 14: Action taken in childless marriage

Answer	average	females	males
Get another spouse	47.00	48.7	45.7
Adopt	42.3	36.5	46.7
Divorce	34.9	30.7	38.3
Go without	4.4	5.5	3.5
Tradit. medicine	3.5	5.8	1.8

Once again this data supports the evidence in Table 7 that church affliation has very little influence on the choice of the ideal family size. For practising Christians these are very strong statements speaking for the high value of the child. These answers are even more relevant because the people interviewed knew that the interviewers were working for a church institution. A century of Christian teaching could not sway the majority of the people interviewed. For the sake of the child they were willing, at least so they said, to put themselves outside the church. The child is too important a value. Anybody trying to touch the issue of children should be aware of this fact. Any policy aiming at reducing the number of children will have to face this deep appreciation for the child.

ANALYSIS OF THE DATA

The next question would be to try to explain why the child acquired such a high value in the life of Papua New Guinea? The data refers to attitudes, expectations and preferences regarding the family size, and not about actual family size. The data present the ideal of the people. By presenting the ideal, these data give us the chance to analyse the underlying values.

A few facts emerge from the data: firstly, there is a great appreciation for the child; secondly, there is a move away from the five plus child family towards a smaller family; thirdly, the one to four child family seems to be the ideal for the majority of the people; fourthly, the younger the respondent the smaller the ideal number of children; fifthly, the higher the education the lower the number of children they wish to have; and lastly, those with a job prefer smaller families.

How can we explain these facts? One important way is by understanding and interpreting them from within the Melanesian value system. In this section I shall touch on only two aspects of the rich symbolism of the child in relation to the community on the one hand and its relation to the parents as members of that community on the other.

<u>The child was value</u>

<u>The Child and the community</u>

I argued for the centrality of the community in the traditional value system.

Whichever form the community might have taken concretely in the various parts of PNG there was and often there still is a group of people linked together by ties of blood and affinity which was very important for the survival of the individual. This community answered all the human needs of the individual; the physical, the emotional, the social, and the spiritual needs. The data in this paper confirms my impression which appears also to be true in the Solomon Islands. Over the millennia the community was experienced as the only way to true and lasting well-being in Melanesia.

However, experience taught that the community was able to provide the service to all the individuals only as long as it was strong and was kept that way. A weak community meant a weakening of the security and identity of the individuals of that community. To care for and serve the community meant to care in the best way for one's own well-being.

The key aspect of this service to and care for the community was the child, the new blood which kept the community young and strong. The child over the millennia became the symbol of one's service to the community and of the guarantee of the security the community would provide.

This millennial experience has been internalised into what we call basic values. It is in the subconscious, motivating people, causing actions and reactions, moods and attitudes. Reason cannot argue away these attitudes and moods. Only a new and lasting experience might weaken and change them. Often the socio-economic aspects of a culture might change but the underlying values continue and lag behind the general evolution. As a matter of fact, according to our research on Melanesian family life, the one value which hardly changed is the child. That is to say, in the value system in Melanesia the child appear to be the only 'constant' factor throughout the ages.

In summary the child is the symbol, the visible guarantee of security and the best hope for future well-being of both the community and the individual.

The child and the parents

Looking at the child from the point of view of the parents as members of the community the child assumes a different value. A person takes his or her identity and value from and in relation to the community. 'The big man', the important woman are those who are experienced as very helpful to the community. The "rubbish" person is the one who does not contribute much or even harms the community.

The most basic contribution to the community and the vehicle for self-worth and identity is marriage and procreation of offspring. The child is the basic contribution to the community: the child renews the community, strengthens it. The more healthy children there are, the better the service by the individual to the community, the greater the sense of self-worth by the visible sign of success, accomplishment, of worth and dignity for a person. Several children enhanced and enriched this sense of worth.

The child, the data and priority of the child in marriage

These considerations help us understand the figures we obtained from our research.

A person without a child can feel worthless and endangered. Worthless because he or she fails the community, and endangered because the community will not be strong enough to help him or her. A marriage without a child is difficult to reconcile with the need for keeping the community young and strong.

Given the experience of infant mortality one needs to procreate a significant number of children to fulfil one's responsibility to the community and to experience security and self-worth.

The young opt for smaller families

We noticed that the young tend to lower the size of the ideal family. This is understandable for two reasons. On the one hand the young never experienced the total dependence on the community and therefore the loyalty to and the expectations from the community. The young generation feels less loyal to the community and expects little in return from the community. The child as the future of the community is not as important as it was for the older generation.

The younger generation has also experienced medical care and has never been required to face the high rate of infant mortality of their parents and grand parents. Therefore they will be concerned to have enough children, but not as many as their elders. The shift might be small and the data confirm it.

Better educated people opt for smaller families

We further noticed that tertiary education seems to lower the need for big families. Tertiary education is supposed to open the mind of the student to new horizons, to new possibilities of self-actualisation based on different kinds of service to the community, to a wider community. The child is still important, but there are other elements on which the identity and self-worth of the person can be built. Education of this type lowers the ned for many children.

Successful tertiary education, and the big high-cost house, are a mark of somebody who has 'made it'. The future is not based on what the children will give but on what the parents have achieved. The child will still remain important, but not as important as for the man who depends very strongly on the support of the community and so on his children.

Those with a job wish for smaller families

As was already stated, the child is symbol and guarantee of security. If there is extra security coming from outside the community, through employment, the need for many children is not felt so strongly anymore and so the expectations are for a smaller family.

Before we conclude this paper we make several observations. Firstly, the child as value is based on the experience generated by a certain socio-economic system where the community was the only feasible way to well-being based on village subsistance gardening. People felt obliged to bear many children. Once the socio-economic situation changes the security, identity, and self-worth comes from other sources such as cash earning, and there will be less need for many children.

Secondly, an emphasis is placed on the element of real life experience. It is not the talking, it is not the promising, it is not the dreaming of a new socio-economic situation, but the actual experience of it. More than experience of the situation itself, it is the experience of its continuation and of its stability. People must experience the new situation, must experience its reliability, must experience the failure of any other system. The third observation is the time factor. To create a common and shared attitude one needs a period of continuous experiences. Nothing can fully replace the time factor.

THE FUTURE

What can we learn for the future?

Looking at the figures and the analysis of the data, we can learn something which is very important for population control.

<u>One must find alternatives to the security offered by the Community</u>

A new socio-economic experience caused by cultural change helped the young and the employed people to lower their need for big families. The reasons seem to lie in the community which lost some of its relevance because people experienced alternatives to the security offered by the community. As a consequence the psychological need to support the community with many children is not that strong anymore. If this trend continues the birth rate will drop further. However, the downward trend depends on the future experience of security and well-being by the people of Papua New Guinea.

At this point in time the whole issue of social security comes in when the child is not regarded as an absolute value: it stands in relation to the experience of security and well-being. It is unwise for population control policies to overlook these facts. Social and economic security is the best method to bring the birth rate under control.

<u>One must provide education</u>

A further help in lowering the need for big families seems to come from higher education. The analysis has shown that success depends on the identity, the sense of self-worth, the purpose in life this type of education has generated, and the economic security it provides. As a consequence, any education, whether formal or informal, which provides people with these values will, everything else being equal, probably succeed in bringing down the birth rate by lowering the need for many children.

This consideration brings us to the thorny issue of education in Papua New Guinea. The high dropout rate, which robs young people of dignity and self-respect, and the growing number of unemployed young people who feel worthless, renders no good basis for population control. One does not need to be a prophet to predict that if the present situation of a high rate of drop-outs continues, and youth unemployment grows, and if economic security continues to deteriorate, population control policy is ignoring the real issues affecting the birth rate. In a word, unless the human needs which are met by the child are satisfied in other ways, any policy of lowering the birth rate will meet with resistance and will face failure.

The link between birth rate and poverty

We do not agree with the idea that the high birth rate and the ensuing overpopulation are a cause of poverty. A few observations supported by Table 15 might clarify this issue. It is true that overpopulation and scarcity of natural resources, including scarcity of arable land, can cause or aggravate existing poverty. However, we cannot talk about overpopulation in Papua New Guinea as the statistics below show.

Table 15: Density of Population per square Km.

Bangladesh	699
Korea, Rep.	422
Netherlands	356
Japan	326
Belgium	325
Germany West	246
India	233
Italy	190
China	112
Indonesia	88
PNG	8

This table puts the figures from the 1990 Census into perspective. This does not mean that we should relax and forget about the family planning programme, but only that we should not introduce panic legislation into Papua New Guinea.

All of us who have worked the land in this country know that by using better agricultural techniques it can yield much more. The land and subsistence can support and maintain a bigger population if land reforms are introduced and agricultural methods are improved.

A further look at the statistics on the density of population per square kilometer shows that one can have high density and wellbeing as in Korea, Netherlands, Japan etc. and low density and hunger. PNG is not poor by any stretch of the imagination and one cannot talk as yet of hunger.

We fear that the number of children can be taken as an excuse for covering up failures in development strategies.

PNG is not poor because of lack of resources, or because it has too many children, but because with all the resources it exports, it gives work to the Japanese, Koreans, and Europeans instead of developing local industries where its own youth can find employment and a sense of self-worth.

The real danger today, if we take seriously the results of the research, is not the failure of the family planning programme as such but the process of pauperisation because of a lack of real rural and industrial development, and the lack of proper education.

If we do not use our human resources to develop our natural resources to give social and economic security to all the people, we will see an increase in the birth rate in spite of all the family planning programmes. As the research shows, it is the insecurity that causes the need for many children.

CONCLUSIONS

This paper concentrates mainly on the child as a symbol of values for the parents. The data show that the ideal family, of which the majority of Papua New Guineans dream, is the four child family. However, there are clear "natural" downward trends. I say natural to contrast them with the trends which might be introduced artificially by modern family planning. From Government documents it appears that there is a drop from 2.6 percent growth in 1970 to the present 2.1 percent. The 3 percent who use family planning are too small to cause such a considerable decline in population growth. It would be unwise to look for new methods when the old ones are proven very effective.

The factors that supports the decline in population growth are the alternative security offered by better health care and by development, employment opportunities and better education.

This is explained by the fact that the child over the generations has become the symbol of identity, of human worth, and of social and economic security. The child is more than a biological reality that can be medically prevented. It is the symbol of key human values which cry for satisfaction. One cannot stop people having as many children as they think they need without first satisfying the needs for which the child stands.

The best population control is to invest heavily in the rural sector to give increased pride and identity to the rural population which is nearly 90 percent of the total population. The Government must support the kind of education which seeks to give a sense of worth and identity. It must set all its resources to giving economic security to every sector of its population. This is the only safe and sure method of population control.

Once people are freed from their insecurity, family planning programmes can help, but they cannot initiate the decision to have smaller families.

CONCERN AND CARE FOR THE MELANESIAN FAMILY

FRANK DIMI [1]

INTRODUCTION

The theme of the seminar titled, "Population, Family Health and Development" touches on a number of issues relating to the building up of good family living. My programmes in the province are mainly centred around families, and I would like to share some of my views on this topic. I discuss marriage and family, family and society, parents and children, responsible parenthood and rights and duties of individuals within a family, as I agree with John Bowring who once said, **"A HAPPY FAMILY IS BUT AN EARLIER HEAVEN".**

MARRIAGE AND FAMILY

The family, as I see it, is the basic unit of a society, and the strenth and solidarity of a society is highly dependent on how this basic unit performs its functions. I am confident in saying that some social problems among our children today can be traced back to failure of parents/families to perform their functions that include responsibilities and obligations.

In the Melanesian context, marriage is not something for the couple only. The big family or the relatives or clan members of the couple really take part in this marriage, because they feel that they are part of the couple. The newly formed family will feel that they can get a good name or prestige, status and pride within the community. This is borne out, in some societies, through the collective contribution towards the payment of brideprice.

Thus, the Melanesian marriage means the coming together of two groups to form a new relationship, and to strengthen the already established or existing one through the occasion. The couple plays an essential role for the two groups to come together. In addition married life unites husband and wife in a very close and intimate partnership.

[1] Family Service C M Wirui, Wewak

This partnership of life and love has been established by the Creator. Married life is rooted in the contract made between husband and wife. This is a permanent contract made by both partners - freely, willingly and personally. Even in the eyes of society, this is a lasting relationship providing security for the spouse, the children and society.

Furthermore, the family, which is founded and given life by love, is a community of persons: of husband and wife, of parents and children and of relatives. Its first task is to live with fidelity the reality of Communion in a constant effort to develop an authentic community of persons. The inner principle of that task, its permanent power and its final goal is LOVE: without love the family is not a community of persons and, in the same way, without love the family cannot live, grow and perfect itself as a community of persons.

All persons have the right to free choice in their state of life, and thus to marry and establish a family, or to remain single. Also every man and every woman, having reached marriage age and having the necessary capacity, has the right to marry and establish a family without any discrimination whatsoever. Legal restrictions to the exercise of this right, whether they be of a permanent or of a temporary nature, can be introduced only when they are required by grave and objective demands of the institution of marriage itself and its social and public significance: they must respect in all cases the dignity and the fundamental rights of the individual.

Today, the human family is living in a modern age. There are great changes in our society and in the world at large. For example, modern technology, medicine, education, economic development to name but a few, have a great influence on the way of life and functions of the family in our society. The social life has changed very much. Indeed, we can say that there is a true social and cultural transformation taking place all over the world as well as in Papua New Guinea. This social and cultural change taking place in society is also effecting the family and life style of our people. This leads to confusion to many families of not knowing how to cope with the drastic changes. When this happens, the family members often become victims in such processes.

To be more aware, the couple needs suitable instruction and guidance on dignity, responsibilities and practical points to maintain the moral values of their family life in accordance with these changes. Couples should have the need and the obligation to be fully and correctly informed, and the right to be educated, to make reasonable decisions.

RESPONSIBLE PARENTHOOD

Responsible parenthood includes care of mother, father, children that are born and future children, as well as the needs and potentials of the country and the world. Thus, conjugal love requires in husband and wife an awareness of their mission of "responsible parenthood" which today is rightly much insisted upon, and which also must be correctly understood.

With regard to biological processes, responsible parenthood means the knowledge and respect of the functions that the human intellect discovers in the power of giving life - thus biological laws are a part of the human person. Responsible parenthood above all, implies a profound relationship to the moral order established by God, of which a good conscience is the faithful interpreter. The responsible exercise of parenthood implies, therefore, that husband and wife recognise fully their own duties towards their creator, towards themselves, towards the family and towards the society in a correct hierarchy of values.

THE CHILDREN

Children are indeed the greatest gift of marriage and are a blessing to the parents. Very special concern and care for the child, even from the first moment of conception and then throughout the years of infancy and youth, requires a very special relationship. The parents become the sole responsible persons for the total growth and development of the child. Even though a child is sick, suffering from pain or is handicapped, special concern and care is still given by the parents. That special concern and care which it receives from parents is LOVE. The most fundamental element that every child should receive from parents is this LOVE. In return the children will compensate their parents by making them special and holy in their own special ways. From their parents children receive, as well as life, an inheritance of values, duties, aspirations and support.

SUPPORTIVE POINTS

Some supportive points on Human Rights and Dignity include that the Catholic Church openly and strongly defends the rights of the family against any abuse by society and the State. I mention a few of these family rights. They include the right to exist and progress as a family; that is to say, the right of every human being, even if he or she is poor, to found a family and to have adequate means to support it; the right to exercise its responsibility for the transmission of life and the upbringing of children, and the right to the intimacy of conjugal and family life.

Secondly, as pointed out earlier spouses have the inalienable right to start a family and to decide on the spacing and the number of children to be born, taking into full consideration their duties towards themselves. Moreover, the family has a right to assistance by society in the bearing and rearing of children. Even those married couples who have a large family should not be subjected to discrimination.

Thirdly, the Catholic Church agrees with the population policy that any activities which attempt in any way to limit the freedom of couples in deciding about their children constitutes a grave offence against human dignity and justice.

Fourthly, with regard to the children's education it must be said that since parents have conferred life on their children, they have a most solemn obligation to educate their offspring in conformity with their moral and religious convictions, taking into account the cultural traditions of the family which favour the good and the dignity of the child. Parents take on the task as educators to help their children live a fully human life.

Finally, no country or society can look to the future other than through its children.

LIFE & DEATH: FACTS & FIGURES, MYTHS & FANTASIES

SIRUS NARAQI[1]

The medical profession deals with the preservation of health and protection of human life, and often witnesses the death of many individuals. It is natural, therefore, that medical doctors ponder upon issues related to life and death, and that they raise questions about facts and figures as well as myths and fantasies associated with these subjects.

Table 1 compares certain information about the general state of health and related issues in high and low income countries.

TABLE 1: GENERAL INFORMATION ON HEALTH IN THE WORLD

	HIGH INCOME COUNTRIES	LOW INCOME COUNTRIES
HEALTH SPENDING	$277/CAPITA	$2.6/CAPITA
FOOD SUPPLY	134%	94%
WATER SUPPLY	100%	29%
INFANT MORTALITY	11/1000	130/1000
CHILD MORTALITY	1/1000	22/1000
LIFE EXPECTANCY	74 YEARS	48 YEARS

Tables 2, 3 and 4 demonstrate general information about health status in Papua New Guinea. It is evident that the major causes of hospitalization and death are preventable or treatable diseases and that infectious diseases dominate the medical scene.

TABLE 2: PAPUA NEW GUINEA - GENERAL INFORMATION ON HEALTH

LIFE EXPECTANCY	49.5 YEARS
INFANT MORTALITY	72/1000 LIVE BIRTH
RATIO OF MEDICAL PRACTITIONERS	1/10,000
HEALTH SPENDING/PER CAPITA	US$20
POPULATION:	3.5×10^6
HEALTH BUDGET:	50×10^6
NUMBER OF DOCTORS:	300

[1] Professor and Head, Division of Medicine
Clinical Sciences Department, Port Moresby General Hospital

TABLE 3: PAPUA NEW GUINEA MAJOR TREATABLE/PREVENTABLE CAUSES OF HOSPITALIZATION

DISEASES	1972	1982
TUBERCULOSIS	18.2	1.3
LEPROSY	15.7	6.3
PNEUMONIA	6.8	13.8
MALARIA	2.4	11.3
TOTAL	43.1%	32.7%

TABLE 4: PAPUA NEW GUINEA - MAJOR CAUSES OF DEATH

	1972	1982
TREATABLE/PREVENTABLE		
PNEUMONIA	18.1%	22%
MALARIA	4.9%	9%
MENINGITIS	4.3%	6.5%
TUBERCULOSIS	4.1%	4.8%
NON-TREATABLE		
ALL CANCERS	5.1%	2.1%
HEART DISEASES	3.8%	4.9%

The following questions are raised as examples of the difficulties facing clinicians and medical administrators during the course of performing their duties. Manpower and financial resources are used generously at hospitals to save the lives of young and old. However, what is saved at hospitals one by one, are lost at wars thousands by thousands. How long should one continue to save lives in the hospitals and lose them at wars?

The following question raises moral and ethical questions as well as problematic and contradictory actions taken concerning allocation of resources. Firstly, let us consider items of interest in the World:

- Kill one person, you are a murderer,
  Kill one million, you are a Hero!

- Millions are spent to save life in Hospitals,
  Millions are spent to take life at Wars!

- Many die of starvation,
  Many die of overeating!

- Many are hungry,
  Many destroy their extra food!

Secondly, in the developing countries, it costs about US $150,000 to train a specialist medical doctor and about US$15,000 to train a rural health worker. Both are vital elements of health care. Rural health workers treat village people especially ordinary folks and children, and specialist doctors care for people of the cities including the elites and the elderly. Should we train one specialist medical doctor to save the lives of the elderly and elites, or ten rural health workers to save the lives of children and commoners? In Papua New Guinea it takes a long time to train medical manpower for Health Care. The training periods range between a few months to train a village health worker and twelve years to produce a specialist:

VILLAGE HEALTH WORKER	(FEW MONTHS OF TRAINING)
AIDPOST ORDERLY	(2 YEARS OF TRAINING)
HEALTH EXTENSION OFFICER	(3 YEARS OF TRAINING)
GENERAL PRACTITIONER	(7 YEARS OF TRAINING)
SPECIALIST	(12 YEARS OF TRAINING)

In Papua New Guinea, the largest nation of the Pacific Islands, the infant mortality rate has dropped significantly. However, the average life span is still less than 50 years. This indicates that many die young. Should one continue to concentrate on saving the lives of the children and leave the adults, so that the children will be raised as orphans? Table 5 reveals some interesting answers for this question.

TABLE 5: CAUSES OF DEATH AT PORT MORESBY GENERAL HOSPITAL

	Early	**Late**	**Total***
Preventable	2	5	7
Treatable	7	28	35
Untreatable	8	23	31
Undetermined	18	29	47
	35	85	120

Source: Papua New Guinea Medical Journal 1989 32:171-176,

* Note that the total is out of 1242 admissions in six months in the Medical Wards.

Thirdly, in most developing countries malaria is the major illness affecting all strata of the society. A patient suffering from malaria may be treated at a cost of US$1.00. On the other hand, myocardial infarction affects a small number of highly placed government workers and professionals. A patient with myocardial infarction needs to be treated in coronary care units and to have bypass/angioplasty at a later date in another country at a total cost of US$10,000. Should one concentrate on treating a case of myocardial infarction, to allow a small elite segment of the society to provide professional services, or on treating 10,000 cases of malaria from various strata of the society? Tables 6 & 7 provides some of the expenditure between treating illnesses in the rural and urban areas.

TABLE 6: CHLOROQUINE RESISTANT FALCIPARUM MALARIA ESTIMATED COST OF TREATMENT

MEDICATIONS		COST
CHLOROQUINE	(150mg BASE) 10 TABLETS	9 TOEA
QUININE	(300mg BASE) 18 TABLETS	85 TOEA
FANSIDAR	(500mg) 3 TABLETS	13 TOEA
	TOTAL:	K1.07

TABLE 7: MANAGEMENT OF ACUTE MYOCARDIAL INFARCTION ESTIMATED COST

TRAVEL TO AUSTRALIA	(2 PEOPLE)	K2000
HOSPITALIZATION	(2 WEEKS)	K4500
SURGERY/ANGIOPLASTY		K1500
MISCELLANEOUS		K2000
	TOTAL	K10,000

Fourthly, war and disease are the two long-time enemies of man; both compete to bring tragedy to human societies. In the final years of the 20th century, war, a symptom of immaturity in mankind, is still claiming the lives of people in large numbers. Health problems such as infectious diseases and cancer are also abundant. In peace time in most parts of the world, infectious diseases, most of which are preventable or treatable, continue to be the major cause of death. Man's coming of age signals the possibility of elimination of war from the face of the planet and the establishment of a lasting peace. Is the world going to move from disease to health with a comprehensive global approach? Table 8 presents the prevalence of common infections throughout the world.

TABLE 8: PREVALENCE OF COMMON INFECTIONS (WORLD WIDE)

Disease	Number
MALARIA	$270X10^6$
SCHISTOSOMIASIS	$200X10^6$
LYMPHATIC FILARIASIS	$90X10^6$
CHAGAS DISEASE	$18X10^6$
ONCHOCERCIASIS	$17X10^6$
LEISHMANIASIS	$12X10^6$
LEPROSY	$12X10^6$

In conclusion I suggest that mankind is in desperate need of a new approach to health care, and other problems which the world is facing. This new approach should have a proper balance, a global vision and a universal scope.

REFERENCES

Naraqi, S. Hospitals and Battle fields: A different point of view on International Peace: Address given to the Annual Meeting of the Medical Society of Papua New Guinea Sept 5, 1985, Port Moresby, Papua New Guinea.

Naraqi, S. The Role of Internal Medicine in Health Care and Training in Papua New Guinea. Australia and New Zealand Journal Medical 16: 301-303,1986.

Naraqi, S. Barefoot Doctors and Specialists: Planning of Post-Graduate Medical Training and Health Care Delivery in Papua New Guinea. Papua New Guinea Medical Journal 30: 219-227, 1987.

Naraqi, S and Gena, M. Mortality in the Medical Wards of a University Teaching Hospital in Papua New Guinea. A Study of 1242 Admissions: Papua New Guinea Medical Journal 32: 171-176, 1989.

Severe and Complicated Malaria Vol. 84: Supp. 2 1990 pp1-65. W.H.O Division of Control of Tropical Diseases.

Kevau, I H. Clinical Documentation of Twenty cases of Acute Myocardial Infarction in Papua New Guineans. Papua New Guinea Medical Journal 33: 275-280, 1990.

HEALTHY MEN, HEALTHY FAMILIES: THE NEED FOR PERSONAL GROWTH

HELGI EYFORD [1]

INTRODUCTION

This presentation is not the result of research because there is no research or even systematic work being done in the area of men's development here in Papua New Guinea. This presentation, as the title suggests, is a statement of need, a statement of interest, that I hope will attract others to work with me in this uncharted field.

I was intrigued and encouraged when I saw the posters advertising this conference. Most development thinking and most government programmes still separate development activities into distinct disciplines: economics, health, population, agriculture, etc.

Yet, the lives and insights of community people that I have talked with on my travels throughout central province Papua New Guinea and in rural communities elsewhere in the world make it very clear to me that development is an integrated affair. Certainly, the social traditions surrounding family size, economic activity and health are very much related. In real life people's health is a serious economic concern and having a job is an important health matter.

This conference seems to be part of a relatively recent trend to integrate rather disparate fields in an effort to improve real lives. And it was this integration, implied in the theme, that first attracted me to participate in this conference.

The picture on the poster and on the cover of this publication caught my attention. The image, that I guess is supposed to represent the family, is a women and child.

That's nice, but unless I am mistaken, I think there is someone missing. That baby did not grow on a tree or fall from the sky. Somewhere, sometime, a man was involved. Now I understand the artists decision. My mental image of a family also includes a mother and child and may be a house. My colleagues at the University of Papua New Guinea and my friends in the village would probably picture a larger group than just two - their families rarely shrink below nine or ten on any given day. But that would make a rather crowded graphic

[1] Education Department, University of Papua New Guinea

Why is it that we do not always think of men as an integral part of domestic life? Indeed the only picture of a family including a man that I have seen drawn on a poster in this country is the one on family violence which shows the man beating the women and the child crying.

This is not a very good advertising strategy by the way. Don't show pictures of what you are against. The image will stay in people's minds and condition their behaviour. Plato figured this out over 2,000 years ago and advised educators to take great pains to control the music, pictures and images that students experience:

> we must issue...orders to all artists and prevent them portraying bad character, ill-discipline, meanness, or ugliness in painting, sculpture, architecture, or any work of art, and if they are unable to comply they must be forbidden to practise their art... For rhythm and harmony penetrate deeply into the mind and have a most powerful effect on it. Plato (1)

Robert Browning, the poet, re-asserted this concept very convincingly some 100 years ago stating that we become what we behold. He advised educators to "do the thing that shall breed the thought", implying that our lived example is more important than our words. The message is confirmed in the modern parody of ineffective parents shouting "do as I say not as I do."

The point is if we all think men are so bad and talk about them as such brutes and portray them as such animals, then they will be nasty brutish and short tempered.

THE NEED FOR VISION

What we need is a vision, an image of what it is to be a man. The popular vision, whether here or in North America, is not a very good one. I am often bothered when some feminist crusader calls agression and brutality a male characteristic. It is not male, it is dysfunctional. A healthy man is neither aggressive nor brutal.

It is not normal for men to beat their wives, regularly drink themselves silly, or fly into a purple rage when frustrated. It is not normal for men to father many children with many women and not support them. It is not normal because it is an identity built on the oppression of another and it is behaviour which does not sustain a society. A healthy personality is one that can live in a constructive relationship with another.

And I will not accept that it is part of traditional culture in Papua New Guinea to beat your wife or to be an emotional cripple. No healthy personality in any culture can be built on the diminishing of another. No healthy family or community can rely on men who fly into a violent rage when someone bumps into their car. To argue that such dysfunctional behaviour is simply a part of PNG culture is either racist, because it demeans a culture that has sustained life for thousands of years, or it is an excuse not to deal with personal growth issues.

We need a vision of healthy men that can inspire and condition modern men in Papua New Guinea. But where do we get it? I think it must largely be recreated, it is not sitting on a shelf in a department store in New York and it is not buried in the comfortable past. We have to create a new vision of healthy manhood that is culturally appropriate as well as appropriate to the needs of the age in which we live.

The place to start is in stories. Our traditional stories and myths are important windows into our psychological nature. Traditional folklore and mythology are extremely important expressions of basic human verities. Joseph Campbell argues that while science and experiment have made it impossible to interpret myths literally, the attempt to live without myth is disastrous. Myths represent facts of the mind,

> telling us in picture language of powers of the psyche to be recognized and integrated in our lives, powers that have been common to the human spirit forever, and which represent that wisdom of the species by which man has weathered the milleniums. Thus they have not been, and can never be, displaced by the findings of science, which relate rather to the outside world than to the depth that we enter in sleep. Through a dialogue conducted with these inward forces through our dreams and through a study of myths, we can learn to know and come to terms with the greater horizon or our own deeper and wiser, inward self. And analogously, the society that cherishes and keeps its myths alive will be nourished from the soundest, richest strata of the human spirit. Cambell (2)

Campbell spent much of a distinguished career documenting the astonishing similarities between myths of, for example, China, India, Yucatan, the Bible, and the North American Indian. Indeed, one of his major contributions was his description of the Monomyth, an archetypal story which is found in almost all myth systems. From this he concluded that many of the themes, emotions, fears, described in myths are universal and vary only in their particular expression depending on the society.

Robert Johnson, a Jungian psychologist, describes the importance of myth:

> Mythology was sacred to primitive people; it was as though their myths contained their very souls. Their lives were cradled within their mythology, and the death of their mythology, as happened with the American Indians, meant the destruction of their lives and spirits.
>
> Myths stand in relationship to mankind in general as a dream does to the individual. A dream shows the individual an important psychological truth about himself. A myth shows an important psychological truth that applies to mankind as a whole. A person who understands a dream understands himself better; a person who grasps the inner meaning of a myth is in touch with the universal spiritual questions life asks us all. Johnson (3)

So it is recommended that we look to the myths of Papua New Guinea to find the images and rhythms that should guide our lives. This will be a challenging endeavour for a country with so many different cultures and so many different stories. But everyone does not have to read the same stories anymore than they have to live the same lives. There is an incredibly rich and varied storehouse of stories and myths in this country that can be used to develop the national ethos of this country.

THE NEED FOR CEREMONY

Another thing we lose in the mad rush to mimic western industrialised countries is our sense of ceremony and ritual. Ritual and ceremony are key elements in the value training of any human. Ceremonies and ritual are designed to re-connect us with fundamental rhythms, actions, positions, and ideas. Campbell argues that the function of ritual is to give form to human life at the deepest level:

> In ancient times every social organization was ritually structured and the sense of depth was rendered through the maintenance of a religious tone. Today, religious tone is reserved for the exceptional, very special, sacred occasions. Yet ritual survives in the patterns of secular life - in the decorum of courts and the regulations of military life, but also in the manner of people sitting down to table together (ibid).

In Papua New Guinea we have the advantage of being relatively close to the initiation rites and practices of our ancestors. From these ceremonies we can learn much about what it is expected of us as men. I do not mean we have to start doing initiation ceremonies in exactly the way our ancestors did. But we can learn from these ceremonies and perhaps construct our modern ones.

I was a witness to an interesting attempt to recreate an initiation ceremony in a modern town in Canada. The parents were non-Natives who had been working in Native communities for over 10 years and had come to appreciate the role of ceremony in Native life. So on their son's fifteenth birthday they asked a Native elder to conduct a ceremony.

The father invited four men of different ages whom he felt represented positive masculine qualities. The mother invited four women of different ages whom she thought represented good feminine qualities in their lives.

These role models were seated in the inner circle, the men on the west side and the women on the east. The rest of the guests looked on from outside the circle. After the elder burned some sweetgrass and chanted some prayers, each of the role model adults stood up and presented the boy with a gift that symbolized their wish and advice for the boy. After all eight had had their say, the mother and father had something to say. They reminded the boy of his birth and childhood and talked about the challenges before him. Then the young man stood up and addressed the circle. Then the elder summed up what was now expected of the young man and gave him an eagle feather and some coloured cloth. After this, in a more light hearted manner, the rest of the assembled guests gave their gifts and wishes to the young man.

It was both a profoundly moving experience as well as a community building one. But most important it was clear for all there what was expected of the young person as a man. Also the young man expressed his personal vision and acceptance of his manhood. This, to me, symbolized a successful effort to restore ceremony in modern life, drawing from the past, combining it in the present and building a vision for the future.

One important thing we can do for the health of the family and the health of women is to develop a vision of what a healthy man is in reference to myths, stories and rituals.

A NEEDED INSIGHT

Something we learn from mythology is that men are different from women. Stories and legends from around the world, from every culture attest to this. My own personal experience has largely corroborated this radical statement that psychologically men must go through different struggles than women. The young man must leave his mother, strike out on his own. Myths from around the world tell of young men going out on adventures to find something or other. They must leave home and family and endure some hardships before they attain their goal and return home.

I referred earlier to Robert Johnson's, book about male psychology that I highly recommend. He uses a well known myth of Parcifal, a young knight in the court of King Arthur, as a metaphor to explain a man's journey to discover himself. Along with Jung, Johnson argues that every man has a feminine side, which Jung called the anima, and every woman has a masculine side, called the animus. If we don't develop both sides of our nature we become unbalanced and unable to realize our potential.

Myths and legends from around the world are replete with stories of active wandering men in search of completeness and understanding, that is, their feminine side. Men, both here in Papua New Guinea and around the world, seem to be in a desperate search to discover this feminine part of themselves. Unless we can facilitate this search for the feminine then the active, wandering element will be distorted into violence and irresponsibility.

Stories and rituals with similar themes can be found in Papua New Guinea. To come of age a boy must be taken from his mother, endure serious pain, maybe have a vision, learn some special knowledge, and thereby prove himself, before he can come back to his village and take up his place as a man. Tension has been created when boys who have not gone through the traditional initiation ceremonies come back to the village. This conflict arises because they have been initiated in the western system by their school experiences.

I had a revealing conversation with a long time teacher up in the highlands. She said that the boys traditionally would go out on a hunt or prove themselves in warfare. Recently they transferred this test of manhood to doing well at school and getting a job. But now they come to school and jobs are not readily available. They must find other, alternative, means to prove themselves, and some of these alternatives are not so healthy. She felt that many of the rascals were simply acting out an age old desire to do the difficult and daring thing as had been accomplished by their parents in the traditional cultures.

THE NEED FOR HEALING

Reading myths and inventing rituals alone will not be enough. Men are hurting, men are afraid, men feel powerless, and unless we deal with these feelings and fears, the more constructive vision cannot take root. I realize it sounds strange to some people to describe men as afraid and powerless but Warren Farrell, in his book Why Men are the Way They Are (4), argues just this. He says that men feel powerless in the face of the roles society expects of them. To attack them as chauvinist aggressors is not helpful in understanding the feelings of men and only furthers their clinging to outmoded or dysfunctional behaviour patterns.

When attacked as primitive chauvinists in the fight for women's rights, men respond in the only way they are allowed, either with phsical outburts or with intellectual games. The point we must recognize is that men feel as powerless as women in a system which alienates both. Men are only the nominal oppressors, the real oppressor is the dysfunctional relationships in our society. And both men and women are responsible by association with this dysfunctional system of relationships.

It is not enough to criticise and blame men. We must ask ourselves why men are such jerks. Why do they beat the only people in the world who love them. Why are gangs of young men wondering around Moresby doing nasty things. We have to ask these questions, develop reasonable hypotheses, and start working with men.

Anne Wilson Schaef (5) argues that our society is caught in an unbalanced and inhuman pattern of behaviours, it is a unhealthy society that behaves like an addict, a drug addict or alcoholic. It is this pattern of behaviour which is the oppressor, not the male or female victims.

Schaef argues that modern industrial society rewards certain inhuman behaviour such as aggression, materialism, dishonesty, compulsive work. She originally called it the white male system because white men were at the top, but she came to realize that men are as alienated in this system as women. Both are addicted to perverse and inhuman behaviours.

Schaef defines addictions as anything that takes control of us and talks about substance addictions and process addictions. We all know about substance addictions; alcohol, cocaine, tobacco, and my personal favourite, coffee, and what they can do to an individual. But we don't often think of being addicted to processes; ways of interacting, ways of behaving. Process addictions include accumulating money, gambling, sex, work, religion, worry.

A classic process addiction is control. Many men are addicted to being in control, and will lie, cheat, steal and physically intimidate people to maintain the feeling of being in control. You can recognize an addiction by what people will do to satisfy it. An addiction to control is often evident in male or female first-borns who are left to look after the family while the parents are doing something else. The first born builds a sense of identity as manager and controller and only feels good when managing. This will last a lifetime without treatment.

Men are particularly susceptible to this addiction because they are taught that a real man exerts his will on those around him. If such a man is challenged effectively by outside forces such as a boss, a stronger neighbour, etc.; he will often run home and bash up his wife to rekindle the feeling of mastery and control he may have lost.

The road to healing for Schaef lies in first admitting the addiction. If we can admit we are functioning with unhealthy expectations of one another, we can begin to explore how we got this way and how we might change.

If men in this country, and elsewhere for that matter, can recognise that they are behaving in ways that are not in their best interests, that are not getting them what they truly want, i.e. love, security, completeness, then they can begin to change. After naming the addiction, we can build our vision in reference to myths and through talking with one another, through sharing. Then comes mutual support as we try to build new personalities. All of these stages can be facilitated in groups, non-threatening, supportive groups of men.

Men usually don't deal with their feelings. This is not by choice but by conditioning. I have heard male interaction described as watching something together, as for example a rugby game, other people, as contrasted to women who watch each other. But this habit can be overcome if you create a safe environment for men to share. You will be surprised what men can and will talk about given the right conditions.

A PARTIAL HISTORY OF THE ADDICTION

We have to ask ourselves why men in PNG have lost the vision of healthy manhood and why these men are feeling confused and afraid.

The process by which men in PNG traditionally discovered their sense of purpose and pride has been undermined and confused with colonization. Traditional practices were scorned and sometimes outlawed. In their stead, white religion and education and wage employment were offered. The result for most is confused role model development in the changing society.

Over 100 years of colonization and rapid modernization have fatally undermined the traditional role of men. Before the coming of whites men in many PNG cultural groups were unquestionably capable. They provided the meat, security and religious direction for the community. Then the white man comes along with vastly more wealth, power, and magic.

What happens to the value of men in the colonized society? The men are humiliated and made theoretically redundant. This has happened in all colonized societies. It is evident in Africa, in India, in North America among the indigenous people. There have been even some interesting studies done about afro-american males and the subculture that has arisen to compensate for the loss of traditional masculinity. The common phenomenon is serious psychological trauma for the men followed by dysfunctional, often violent behaviour.

Papua New Guinean men had a very interesting adaptive technique - cargo cults. Cargo cults were, among other things, mechanisms to explain these white men who had such amazing wealth and such superior weapons. It was a way of explaining why they were so superior to indigenous men in all the areas that counted. At first the whites were often greeted as returning dead. Then they were seen as thieves intercepting the goods sent down by ancestors for Papua New Guineans. Some of the beliefs and practices of cargo cults are pretty bizarre but if you see them as attempts to preserve male pride, male identity, then their passion and logic can be appreciated.

Don't underestimate the need to preserve male pride, or female pride for that matter. A person who does not feel appreciated or respected will either seek desperately to earn it, possibly through deviant behaviour, or he will internalize it, believe, accept it. This is really dangerous because a person who really believes he is second rate, that he is no good, will not do good. At the root of most of the alcohol and sexual abuse that is epidemic in Native communities in Canada is a self-loathing internalized from the wider society's contempt for Native culture.

CONCLUSION

Most efforts to address the problems of family health tend to deal with women. They are after all the ones who are suffering as a result of the status quo. In fact one entire day of this Seminar was devoted to discussions of women's health. The government of Papua New Guinea has a Department of Home Affairs and Youth which has a special women's Division. I think all of this attention is good and needed.

I want to suggest, however, that men are part of the problem and they will have to be part of the solution. If you really want to change family health in this country, it is not enough to work only with women. You must deal with men. I suggest we need a Division of men within Home and Youth Affairs.

Family health is much more than the aggregate health of individual members. A family is more than the sum of its members. The family is a set of relationships that transcends and conditions each individual. The health of the family is primarily the health of the relationships between the members. As such, we must help our men folk deal with their hurts and confusion before we can have healthy families in Papua New Guinea.

A primary and urgent need in this country, I suggest, is the need to forge a new style of being men that is based on traditional, life sustaining values, but which has applicability and meaning in the modern world.

How do we achieve this new synthesis of being male? The first steps might include the following:

- men must be helped to understand the nature of their oppressor. This can be achieved with discussion or encounter groups where men can share their feelings and frustrations. This is possible even with so-called callous and tough men.

- Secondly, we must encourage our parents and grandparents to read myths and stories to recite legends and participate in rituals. We need to expose ourselves to the best of our own culture and other cultures.

- Thirdly, we train boys in our schools to be emotionally competent. Boys need to learn how to handle frustration and anger in constructive ways if they are to grow up to be useful members of society.

I suggest those three steps are what men can do. Women must also strive to understand a new maleness. If they continue to respond in the old ways to men who are trying to change, then nothing will change in the end. Women are as much a part of the current problems in our families as are men. We all must work together to create more constructive modern role models.

Unless we take these initiatives and others that will allow men the opportunity for personal growth, which has been denied them in this changing modern world, then our hopes for development and family health will necessarily be frustrated.

REFERENCES

1. Plato, The Republic, trans. H.D.P. Lee (London: Penguin Books, 1963) line 402, p.142

2. Joseph Campbell, Hero with a Thousand Faces (Princeton: Princeton University Press, 1973) p.13

3. Robert A. Johnson, He: Understanding Masculine Psychology (New York, Harper and Row: 1977) pp.1-2

4. Warren Farrel, Why Men Are the Way They Are (New York: Berkley Publishers, 1988)

5. Anne Wilson Schaef, When Society Becomes an Addict (San Francisco: Harper & Row, 1987)

NATIONAL STRATEGY MEETING ON THE HEALTH OF WOMEN IN PAPUA NEW GUINEA

KEYNOTE ADDRESS BY MARGARET NAKIKUS
Patron to the 19th Waigani Seminar

I will not dwell on the current health status of the women in this country. Many of us here today already know and are aware of how poor it is. You have been invited to participate in this important meeting because you do know and because each and everyone of you is in a position to do something about it.

Let me remind you of a few key facts about the situation of our women.

Women make up 47% of the population of this country.

45% of the women are in the child bearing years of 15-44.

On average, woman in this country will bear 5.4 children.

Each of these women stand a lifetime chance of 1 in 26 of dying during one of these pregnancies.

A woman's access to family planning is limited and less than 3% of women are using modern means of family planning.

The current situation is unacceptable and for the benefit of the women and of the country as a whole this problem must be addressed now.

Some would say that this is an overstatement of the situation. I have good reason to say the situation is critical. Even though we have seen some major improvement in some health indicators in the country, for instance, the infant and child mortality rates have been decreasing, we cannot say the same for the indicators that measure the health of women. In fact there are some indications that the situation is worsening.

One of the difficulties in assessing the problem is that it is often hidden because of the current poor reporting of illness and death in this country. The maternal mortality rate is estimated to be from 7 - 18 per 1,000 live births in Papua New Guinea. This is a very high rate by world standards. However, in a village only one mother may die during childbirth every 2-3 years.

It therefore may not appear to be a major problem. It is estimated that only one in ten deaths that occur during childbirth are reported. It therefore may not appear to be a major problem.

The diagnosis of sexually transmitted disease is difficult. Only the very ill women present for treatment and many suffer the consequences of the disease in silence. It therefore does not appear to be a major problem.

For many of you here today this meeting is a part of a process that you began earlier this year. We want to thank you for your input and for the ideas and the information you supplied, to bring us to this point in time. For those of you who have only recently become a part of this process, I would like to give you some brief background information on what has happened up until today.

In August 1990 the Papua New Guinea Institute of Medical Research in co-operation with UNICEF released a monograph that summarised the current state of the Health of the Women of Papua New Guinea. As you are aware the monograph did not paint a very positive picture.

As a follow-up to the release of the monograph the National Department of Health and the National Department of Youth and Home Affairs in conjunction with UNICEF and the Papua New Guinea Institute of Medical Research identified a group of individuals to form a National Steering Committee on women's health.

The job of this committee was to decide what steps should be taken next to ensure that action was taken to improve the health of women in Papua New Guinea.

The committee recognised that improving women's health will not be a health issue alone and that participants in such a meeting must represent both government departments and non-government agencies. The committee also recognised that the task was large and to address it in a one day meeting would not be possible.

Two things were done to address these concerns.

Firstly, a wide range of government and non-government agencies were invited to participate in the meeting.

Secondly, invited participants were asked to do some preliminary work prior to today's meeting.

In March of this year a questionnaire was circulated. Respondents were asked to identify what they felt were the most important factors affecting women's health. They were also asked to identify the areas in which efforts should be made by Government and Non-government sectors to improve the current status of women's health. The information from this questionnaire was put into a working document which was circulated to all participants earlier this month and it will be the focus of our discussions today.

The appendices of the document contain the verbatim responses to the questionnaire. I am sure many of you will recognise your input. This information was then summarised outlining the key factors affecting women's health which are listed on page 4 of this document.

The social/cultural situation in Papua New Guinea affects the lives and health of all women today. Adverse living conditions, lack of basic services such as water and sanitation, place a strain on the lives of all people. In addition to this, women are also affected by an extremely high rate of violence, while experiencing a reduction in the traditional support from families and friends. The society in general is one that favours males, whether that is in the power given to them to make decisions, or to the basics of who receives food first at meal times.

The low social status of women in Papua New Guinea is a key factor which affects their health status. The heavy physical workload carried by the women of this country was identified as a major factor. Furthermore low self-esteem was seen as interfering with their ability to deal with general development issues and limiting their involvement at all levels of development.

There is no question that education affects the health status of any population. There may be some debate as to why that is so, but not to the fact that better educated women have different attitudes to health and health care.

In Papua New Guinea lack of education is a problem for everyone, and especially for women. More women than men are illiterate. Fewer women than men are given the opportunity to attend school, especially school beyond the Grade 6 level. Formal education is important in the long term improvement of women's health, but another educational aspect which could be amenable to change in the short term is that related to sound health practice. It was identified that there a general lack of knowledge of health and health issues such as hygiene, treatment of disease and disease prevention. Health problems such as poor nutrition and malaria are important to all but can have a more dramatic impact on a woman who is frequently pregnant or who is breast feeding.

It was felt that there is generally poor recognition of illness and a lack of action to seek medical help. In addition, cultural taboos often do not allow women to follow professional medical advice given to them.

The role of Health Care Services was seen as a key factor. However, many of you felt that at present the health services are not fulfilling the role expected of them in regard to the health of women. The lack of services, access, appropriateness, the inability to use existing services and the quality of the services delivered were frequently mentioned.

The lack of economic opportunity for women and general lack of emphasis on women's issues were also identified as factors responsible for women's poor health.

It is clear from the responses to the questionnaire that respondents accept the fact that the current poor health status of women in this country is not a health issue alone, but is affected by a number of factors.

The next job was then to summarise what areas the respondents felt we should concentrate our efforts on to help correct the current situation. You can see from the listing on page 5 of the document that these have been summarised for today's discussions. It is not a comprehensive list. Other criteria was used to identify areas that could be addressed in the short and medium term.

In the social/cultural area there was no question that the status of women in the country needed to be improved. There was also a strong feeling that a reduction in the present workload of women was necessary if we are to see an improvement in their health status.

With regard to education, many indicated that there was an urgent need to increase literacy rates and to increase the amount of health related knowledge. It was emphasised by many that this education was needed by both men and women.

Health Services are of course essential. It was felt that there needed to be improved access to services. This was especially true for all rural areas. In conjunction with this is also the appropriateness of services provided, and the training of community, health workers, nurses and health officers to deal with women patients.

There were then two issues that were grouped under the title of generic or global issues. These included the need to improve the co-ordination and integration of activities within the country. Such coordination/integration would prevent duplication of activities and allow for more effective use of existing resources to improve the health status of our women.

The other key issue that was raised in this area was the need to establish a programme to assist women to manage the social changes that are affecting their ability to deal with the day to day activities of their lives, especially the decreasing level of support from family, friends and other traditional sources of support.

The topics were worded so that discussions could focus on questions such as:

If this is what we think we should have - for instance "increased literacy rates" - what are the current facilitating factors. What opportunities can be found in the present situation to facilitate improvements?

Secondly, what is stopping change from happening - what are the barriers to achieving change?

What strategies shall we develop to take advantage of existing opportunities and resources as well as to circumvent the barriers that may prevent the long term improvement in women's health? And finally how do we get these strategies put into action?

These questions must provide the basis of our work today.

In your information material you were given summary sheets to help you begin to formulate your ideas on each of these topics.

Today, each of the eight topics will be discussed by one group. Each group has been assigned a facilitator who will help the group to focus on their discussion topic. The groups will then report the results of their discussion to the plenary session. These results will be summarised and at the end of the day we will have identified key strategies to achieving each of our objectives and will have identified lead Departments or Agencies that will be responsible for overseeing the development of action plans.

This is not an easy task. We have in the room today both policy makers and policy implementers. We hope that the balance of these two groups will result in the presentation of workable strategies that both groups believe in and will act on to implement.

In summary, I must reiterate that the current situation related to the health of women in this country is at a critical point. There are indications that the situation is worsening and we have the opportunity today to design strategies and action plans to reverse that trend.

I urge you to take this task seriously, as your discussions today will have an important impact on the future of the women of Papua New Guinea. I wish you well in your discussions and I look forward to the recommendations and actions that result from this meeting today.

PROCEEDINGS OF THE NATIONAL STRATEGY MEETING ON THE HEALTH OF WOMEN IN PAPUA NEW GUINEA

RUMONA DICKSON[1]

STEERING COMMITTEE MEMBERS

Ms. Marjorie Andrew
Ms. Rumona Dickson
Dr. Naomi Martin
Ms. Margaret Misso
Ms. Margaret Nakikus
Mr. Enoch Posanai
Ms. Marie Powell
Ms. Jane Thomason

SUPPORTING DEPARTMENTS AND ORGANISATIONS

Commission for High Education

National Department of Health

National Department of Youth and Home Affairs

Papua New Guinea Institute of Medical Research

UNICEF

University of Papua New Guinea

Waigani Seminar Organising Committee

1 Scientific Officer, Papua New Guinea Institute of Medical Research, Madang

BACKGROUND

The National Strategy Meeting on the Health of Women in Papua New Guinea was held on June 18, 1991. It was held in conjunction with the 19th Waigani Seminar in Port Moresby and was funded by UNICEF. The work began four years earlier with the production by the Papua New Guinea Institute of Medical Research(PNGIMR), UNICEF and CUSO of the monograph, "The Health of Women in Papua New Guinea" by Joy Gillett. The purpose of the monograph was to bring together current information on the health of women in the country. The monograph was released in August 1990 and more than 5000 copies were distributed throughout the country.

Following the release of the monograph the National Departments of Health and Youth and Home Affairs, UNICEF and the PNGIMR identified key individuals to form a national steering committee. The objectives of this committee were to identify a way to bring the issue of the poor status of women's health to the attention of decision makers in the country and to identify strategies to address the main women's health issues.

As a first step this committee organised the National Strategy Meeting on the Health of Women in Papua New Guinea. The planning and preparation for this meeting began in early 1990.

The committee compiled a list of possible participants from both the government and non-government sectors. These individuals were contacted by the steering committee members and the purpose of the meeting was explained. Participants were asked to complete a questionnaire to identify what they felt were the five most important factors affecting women's health and the areas in which government and non-government agencies should be concentrating their efforts to improve women's health.

The responses were summarised and this summary was used as the discussion paper for the June 18 meeting. Discussions were carried out in pre-assigned groups that ranged in size from 8-15. Group discussion was led by an assigned facilitator and utilised a nominal group process.

The advance work done by participants allowed discussions during the one day meeting to focus attention on the identified areas of concern. Discussions during the meeting concentrated briefly on identifying factors that are facilitating the improvement of women's health and the barriers that impede this improvement. Next discussions focused on the identification of strategies to utilise the facilitating factors and to overcome the identified barriers. The groups then identified specific projects which totally or partially fit within these strategies. Group reporters presented the findings of their group to the meeting as a whole.

This paper summarises the advance work done for this meeting as well as the responses to the questionnaires and the results of the group discussions held during the one-day meeting.

STAGE 1: THE QUESTIONNAIRE

The questionnaire was mailed to 85 previously contactindividuals. A total of 49 were completed and returned. The questions and the summarised responses are listed below.

Question 1: List the 5 most important factors that you believe affect the health of women in Papua New Guinea.

Responses to this question were summarised into six categories. There has been no attempt to put this list in priority order.

1. STATUS OF WOMEN

- Heavy workload
- Low self esteem
- Lack of equal opportunity
- Limited input into family or community decisions
- Traditional attitude to women and their role

2. SOCIAL/CULTURAL

- Violence against women
- Adverse living conditions
- Decrease in traditional support to families
- Preference for men in the society
- Food taboos

3. EDUCATION

- General illiteracy
- Lack of educational opportunities for girls and women
- Lack of education and knowledge related to health and health issues: eg: personal hygiene, disease prevention, treatment of disease

4. HEALTH PROBLEMS

- Problems related to the role of being mothers, including frequent pregnancies
- Limited use of family planning and child spacing
- Poor nutrition
- Infectious diseases, e.g. malaria, pneumonia, diarrhoea
- Poor recognition of illness and lack of action to seek medical treatment
- Cultural taboos that forbid seeking care and/or following medical advice

5. HEALTH SERVICES

- Inadequate health care services, including availability, access and often poor quality of services delivered
- Inadequate availability of family planning

6. ECONOMIC/POLITICAL

- Lack of economic opportunities for women in the country
- Lack of emphasis on women's issues
- Unemployment (in general, and also particularly for women)

The list clearly illustrated that respondents felt that the poor state of women's health is not a health issue alone. The health of women in the country is affected by a number of factors and therefore, any strategies to improve this situation will require a multi-sectoral approach.

Question 2: In what 5 areas do you believe we should be concentrating our efforts to improve the health of women in Papua New Guinea?

The identification of a wide variety of factors affecting women's health led to the identification of a wide variety of areas in which efforts should be concentrated to improve women's health. These were summarised into four areas.

1. EDUCATION

- Increased literacy rates
- Increased health related knowledge

2. SOCIAL/CULTURAL

- Improved status of women
- Decreased workload for women

3. HEALTH SERVICES

- Improved access to services
- Improved appropriateness of services

4. GENERAL ISSUES

- Improved coordination/integration of activities
- Improving women's management of social change

These areas formed the basis for the discussions during meeting.

STAGE 2: WORKING DOCUMENT

The information from the questionnaire was returned to the participants in the form of a working document for them to review prior to the meeting.

STAGE 3: NATIONAL STRATEGY MEETING

1. PARTICIPANTS

Participants in both the questionnaire and the meeting portions of the process represented a broad spectrum of government and non-government agencies and departments. Participants included policy makers, program planners and program implementers. There was representation from both national and provincial levels. A list of meeting participants is included in Appendix A.

National government departments that participated included the Departments of the Prime Minister's Office, Health, Home Affairs and Youth,Education, Finance and Planning and the National Waterboard. Provincial government representatives came from Milne Bay, Oro, West New Britain, Western Highlands, Manus, Madang, Southern Highlands, East Sepik, Morobe,Central, West Sepik and NCD. Non-government groups included the National Council of Women, Project Concern, the Child Survival Support Project, the University of Papua New Guinea, the Melanesian Council of Churches, The Melanesian Institute, the PNG Nursing Association, the Church Medical Council, the Institute of Medical Research and the National Research Institute. Aid donors including UNICEF, WHO, USAID, World Vision Australia and Save the Children Fund were also represented at the meeting.

2. DISCUSSION GROUPS

Participants had been requested in advance to identify the discussion topic area in which they preferred to participate on the day of the meeting. These preferences were considered during the pre-assignment of the discussion groups.

For the purpose of the discussion groups, the following definitions were used:

Facilitating factors: Anything that assists in the achievement of the goal.

Examples of facilitating factors could be existing projects or any available resources (material, financial or human) that could be used to achieve the goal.

Barriers: Anything that impedes the achievement of the goal.

Strategies: Any method or combination of methods used to make better use of facilitating factors and current resources to overcome the barriers and achieve the goal.

Project ideas: Any projects that incorporate the strategies to reach the goal.

3. GROUP FACILITATORS

Steering committee members identified key individuals that they felt would fill the role of group facilitators. These individuals represented a broad spectrum of experience and a number of government departments and non-government agencies (Appendix B).

Facilitators were individually briefed on the project and reviewed all the material sent to participants. They also participated in an orientation session to help familiarise them with the nominal group process that was used during the meeting.

4. MEETING DAY FORMAT

Officials from the Departments of Home Affairs and Youth and Health as well as the Papua New Guinea Institute of Medical Research and UNICEF participated in the official opening and closing ceremonies. Dr. Naomi Martin, Chairperson for the Commission for Higher Education chaired the day. Ms. Margaret Nakikus opened the day by reviewing the process and summarising the key issues to be discussed. The majority of day was spent in small group discussions and group reports. Dr. Martin closed the day by summarising the reports of the groups and suggesting future directions.

STAGE 4: GROUP REPORTS AND RECOMMENDATIONS

The specific findings of the groups are listed in Appendix C. The list represents the key facilitating factors, barriers, strategies and projects identified in each topic area during the meeting. The list is comprehensive and includes recommendations for action at all levels. The time restrictions of the one day meeting did not allow for all groups to fully develop their project plans. In addition, some issues raised during the discussions did not lend themselves to the format as defined by the program. Therefore the discussions within some of the groups took a slightly different focus and this was reflected in their group report.

A review and summary of the individual group discussions has been done in an attempt to bring together the ideas of the participants and form a plan for future initiatives. In reviewing the reports from the groups, recurrent ideas have been identified and summarised here. While the individual group listings give ideas for specific actions, this summation gives an idea of the global directions that should be considered.

A. FACILITATING FACTORS

Group responses related to facilitating factors have been grouped into three categories. Though facilitating factors had originally been defined as current activities/resources, some groups defined them as any activity/resource that would be helpful in achieving the objective, even if they were not currently available.

1. EXISTING SUPPORT

It was generally agreed that there are currently in place numerous policies and programs as well as the infrastructure to assist in improving both the health status of women and the situation of women in general. This is especially true in the areas of education (formal and non-formal) and health services. In addition there exists the infrastructure to train people in these areas (e.g. teachers, health care workers).

The National Women's Policy, passed in early 1991, provides a basis and a mechanism for an increased emphasis on women, their value and their needs. The existence of the Women's Division(though there was strong support for an independent Ministry for Women's Affairs), provides an avenue for input to political decision making that can be used to improve the current situation. It was also felt that there exists a rising community awareness of the problems faced by women. The existing community structures also provide an avenue for improving the current situation.

2. EXISTING COMMUNICATIONS NETWORKS

These communication networks were discussed in broad terms. They included the expanding road and transportation systems in the country. They also included the increased availability of media resources such as television, radio and newspaper that enable rapid, country-wide communication. There are well-established formal and informal communication networks formed by community groups, women's groups, church groups, NGOs and existing government departments.

3. AVAILABILITY OF FINANCIAL RESOURCES

Though there have been budget cuts in all government departments over the past few years, it was felt that money is available to at least partially service the existing departments and projects.

There was also a general feeling that the amount of aid money may be decreasing somewhat and that the conditions for use of this money is becoming less flexible. It was the general consensus, however, that there is still aid money available to support innovative projects throughout the country.

B. BARRIERS

There were a number of barriers identified as major impediments to improving the current situation. These have been summarised into 5 categories.

1. ATTITUDES TO WOMEN AND THEIR ROLE

Attitudes to women and their role were discussed in four areas:

a. Government to Women

There exists in the country the policies and infrastructure to implement the changes necessary to improve the situation and the health status of women. There does not exist the political will to implement these policies and make equal participation by women a reality. This lack of political will is demonstrated in a number of ways. These include: the low priority given to projects designed for women; the lack of the evaluation of the impact of development projects on women; the lack of funds designated to women's projects; and the withdrawal of funding for many projects that benefit women. There is also a lack of specialised training for personnel responsible for implementation of the policies and programs that directly affect women. In addition there is a lack of involvement of women in policy and program decision making. A concern was also raised that active discrimination against women continues to be a real problem within the government sector.

It was mentioned that many of these problems have occurred as a result of decentralisation and that the decrease in funding to projects that benefit women has occurred within the provinces. This is especially true in the case of decreasing health services (especially MCH services) in many provinces.

b. Men to Women

There was a general feeling that the value of women and their input to the community and the country are underestimated by men in general. Women have therefore not been allowed to participate as equal partners within the family, the community or the country. Women are considered to be subordinate to men and this perception affects their access to basic needs such as food and shelter. In addition this attitude has limited their access to the benefits of development. This is specially true in relation to education and health services where the decisions as to who can access the services are for the most part made by men.

c. Women to Women

There is a general lack of support for women by other women. This is especially true as women begin to take on leadership roles. This area was not discussed in depth during this meeting.

d. Women to Themselves

The general low self-esteem of women in Papua New Guinea decreases their belief in their right to participate in decision making on personal, local and national levels. They are therefore reluctant to put their needs and opinions forward.

The reasons given for these attitudes were numerous, but were based in the traditional/cultural background of the people of Papua New Guinea, the lack of available information and the general lack of education, especially for women.

The result of these pervading attitudes is to dramatically decrease opportunities for women. This includes opportunities in the areas of education, employment, access to health and other services and in decision making at all levels.

2. LACK OF COORDINATION

It was felt that there was a lack of a mechanism for overseeing and coordinating projects that directly and indirectly affect women. This lack is reflected in a number of areas.

a. Planning

There does not appear to be an overall plan for improving the current situation. There is limited assessment of new projects with regards to their impact on women. There is often program duplication and some new projects actually hamper the effectiveness of existing projects, while existing projects hamper the effectiveness of new initiatives.

b. Implementation/Evaluation

There are numerous projects that have been recommended but have never been implemented. Similarly there are numerous projects that were started and did not receive adequate support to continue. In another context, there are projects that clearly are not effective, have not been evaluated and continue to receive support.

The result of this lack of coordination, planning and evaluation is seen in the duplication of projects, the implementation of projects that are actually detrimental to women and a lack of support for projects that could benefit women.

3. INADEQUATE TRAINING/LACK OF EXPERTISE IN PERSONNEL

This was discussed in the context of training of personnel not only in relation to the specific needs of women, but also in the areas of leadership and supervision. It included such things as the lack of training of health care workers to deal with women's health problems and the lack of appropriate training of teachers and literacy workers. Included also was the continued training of inappropriate personnel (e.g. male health workers) and a lack of leadership and supervisory training.

There is also a lack of leadership training for both men and women at the village level. Such training would give them the expertise to implement programs that will assist women.

On a more global basis it was felt that much of the problem arises from the lack of appropriate curriculum and education and training materials. Available materials do not adequately reflect the importance of women, their roles and their special needs, especially in the area of health. This lack of materials was noted at ALL educational levels and within both the formal and non-formal education networks.

4. COMMUNICATION BARRIERS

Language was identified as a major barrier in communication at all levels. It was pointed out that many women are unable to communicate in any of the three major languages and are therefore at a great disadvantage. Even if education programs reach their villages, often the educators are unable to communicate with these women.

Geographical barriers and limited access to many rural areas were seen as a major obstacles to communication as well as to the distribution of services and information.

5. LACK OF BASIC NEEDS

The fact that a majority of the people of the country do not have access to safe drinking water or have inadequate sanitation facilities means that most families lack basic needs and are living in unhealthy environments. Until this situation is improved, it was pointed out that dramatic improvements in the health status of all members of the society, not just women, will not occur.

C. GLOBAL STRATEGIES

Specific strategies were identified in each discussion topic area. A review of these can be summarised into 5 global strategies.

1. CHANGE IN ATTITUDE TO WOMEN

Strategies for changing the current attitudes toward women were discussed. Strategies for use at the government level included: a general effort to increase government support for the implementation of existing policies and projects that directly affect women; an increase in educational opportunities at the formal and non-formal level for women and girls; and an increased emphasis on the health needs of women within the National Department of Health and within the Provincial Divisions of Health. In the area of individual attitudes there were suggestions for: the integration of activities for women and men at the community level; support of existing and promotion of new women's networks; and an emphasis on the inclusion of women in the processes of decision making at all levels.

The incorporation of information on women's roles, issues and concerns within both formal and non-formal education materials was seen as fundamental to affecting a change in attitudes.

2. COORDINATION/INTEGRATION

There needs to be mechanism to coordinate/integrate existing activities as well as to assess their appropriateness and their impact on women in Papua New Guinea. This mechanism should also include the pro-active identification of new projects, as well as identification of sources of funding for such projects. In addition there needs to be assessment of other proposed projects to ensure their appropriateness and their impact on women.

There was discussion as to a number of ways this mechanism could be established. It could for instance take place within the current committees established as a part of the Women's Policy; as a part of the steering committee for the new Population Policy Unit; or through an independently established task force/advisory committee. There was consensus that this coordination/integration is absolutely essential if improvement is to be made in the current situation of women in general and women's health in particular in the country.

There was also consensus that this coordination must include ongoing supervision and evaluation of projects.

In addition it was strongly felt that the Women's Division be strengthened, in its current form or as a separate Ministry.

3. IMPROVED COMMUNICATION

This area includes such activities as the improvement of the transportation systems, increased availability ofinformation and the increased use of media to reach the rural populations of the country. Most recommendations centred on non-formal and formal education and education materials.

Included were recommendations to develop "Women's Information Centres". Such centres would utilise the services of the formal and non-formal education systems as well as the National Library Service. They would assist women to increase their knowledge and self-esteem and would also provide them with the information and support they need to deal with the current rapid social change occurring in the country.

There was a call for an updating of school curricula and education materials as well as making up-to-date materials available for use by the mass media. These materials should provide information on the value of women to the community and the country, the changing roles of women and the special health needs of women and girls.

The importance of making literacy and literacy training available to more women was emphasised. It was also suggested that the materials used in such programs contain up to date information on health and preventive health measures, with an emphasis on the special needs of women and girls.

4. TRAINING

Training programs in all areas need to be re-evaluated and if necessary updated to be certain that:

1. Curricula contain appropriate information on the importance and value of women to the country; the unique needs of women and girls; leadership training; and training in evaluation and supervision.

2. Appropriate workers are being trained. This included the training of more women in the health care field. There was also a call for the expansion of current training programs to include village level workers, especially in the areas of health care delivery and literacy training.

   In addition current personnel will also require upgrading of their knowledge related to women's health and the their health care needs, as well as strengthening of their leadership and supervisory skills.

5. IMPROVED WATER AND SANITATION FACILITIES

The supply of these basic facilities was seen as key to allowing women to improve their health and the health of their families. A recommendation was made for the creation of a rural/urban water body, with funds and capability, to oversee the supply of these services throughout the country.

CONCLUSION

All groups emphasised the need for local level involvement in the implementation of any of the strategies. Improvements must be seen as necessary at the local level and all permanent change must occur with the support of the community as a whole.

The discussions reinforced the key message underlying the working document, that the poor health status of women in Papua New Guinea is influenced by a number of factors, including the social, economic, political and legal status of women. This means that improving the health of women is not a health issue alone and must be addressed from the broadest perspective and include all aspects of life and development in the country.

Though two discussion groups specifically discussed access and appropriateness of health care, their recommendations coincided with those of the other groups with regards to: the need to change negative attitudes towards women; to better coordinate activities, to improve communication; to improve education materials to include more emphasis on the health needs of women and to adequately train appropriate staff to look after the health needs of women.

THE NEXT STEP

Participants in the meeting were asked to take the information from the meeting back to their respective departments/agencies and to consider this information in their future policy and program planning.

There was a commitment made at the meeting by the leaders in various government departments and non government agencies to follow through on the strategies/projects suggested at the meeting. There was also a commitment to continue the dialogue that was started at this meeting to encourage more inter-departmental/agency cooperation. In addition there was a call to formalise this process of cooperation.

The steering committee agreed to meet in the next month to discuss the best means to ensure follow-up on the discussions of the meeting. As of October 1991, this committee has drafted Terms of Reference for the inter-disciplinary task force/advisory committee that will be responsible for evaluating and initiating the strategies and projects identified at this meeting. They have approached funding agencies to support such a group and have begun contacting individuals/departments who, at the time of the meeting voiced their support for such action.

The real work of this project has not yet begun. The steering committee would however like to thank all those individuals, departments and agencies who have supported this project to date and encourage their continued support in the goal of improving the health of women in Papua New Guinea.

APPENDIX A

NATIONAL STRATEGY MEETING ON THE HEALTH OF WOMEN IN PAPUA NEW GUINEA

MEETING PARTICIPANTS

Dr.	Dennis	Ahlburg	University of Minnesota
Ms.	Louise	Aitse	Women's Division
Dr.	Isaac	Ake	Department of Health
Mr.	Clant	Alok	Department of Home Affairs and Youth
Ms.	Marilyn	Alok	Department of Education
Dr.	Michael	Alpers	PNG Institute of Medical Research
Ms.	Cecilia	Apini	CHW Training School
Miss	Helen	Ashwell	Salvation Army
Mr.	Peter	Baki	in-Service College
Mr.	Allan	Bass	Child Survival Project
Dr.	Elvira	Beracochea	UPNG - Community Medicine
Mr.	Martin	Bonai	Provincial Affairs Department
Br.	Mathew	Bouton	Church Medical Council
Dr.	Gilbert	Bukenya	UPNG Faculty of Medicine
Dr.	Jack	Caldwell	Health Transition Centre ANU
Mrs.	Pat	Caldwell	National Centre for Epidemiology- ANU
Mr.	Ron	Corden	National Waterboard
Mr.	Nick	DeGroot	The Melanesian Institute
Ms.	Pauline	Doonar	Department of Education
Dr.	Tim	Dyke	PNG Institute of Medical Research
Mrs.	Jane	Earland	Save the Children Fund
Dr.	Keith	Edwards	Child Survival Project
Mrs.	Alice	Erai	Melanesian Council of Churches
Ms.	Dorothy	Fernando	World Vision Australia
Mrs.	Barbara	Freeman	Islander Hotel
Ms.	Cherry	Galo	Solomon Islands Planned Parenthood
Ms.	Muwete	Gatsia	Project Concern
Mrs.	Josephine	Gena	Department of Home Affairs and Youth
Ms.	Susan	Haroe	PNG Nursing Association
Mrs.	Maria	Hayes	Women's Secretariat - Momase Region
Ms.	Hetra	Hekele	
Ms.	Vanessa	Howe	Save the Children Fund
Mr.	Davis	Iwuga	Milne Bay Division of Health
Mr.	Arietta	Kairey	Department of Home Affairs and Youth
Ms.	Marylene	Kajoi	Dept. of Home Affairs and Youth

Ms.	Leah	Kalamoroh	UPNG-Library and Information Studies
Mr.	Francis	Kambu	Oro Division of Health
Mr.	William	Kaptigau	Kimbe Hospital
Mrs.	Harumi	Karel	Project Concern
Dr.	Barry	Karlin	World Health Organization - PNG
Mr.	Kelly	Kewa	Western Highlands Division of Health
Mrs.	Rai	Kila	UPNG
Ms.	Delilah	Kila	Salvation Army Health Services
Mr.	Joseph	Klapat	Department of Home Affairs and Youth
Dr.	Cecil	Klufio	UPNG Faculty of Medicine
Mrs.	Maria	Kopkop	National Council of Women
Mr.	Gabriel	Kulwaun	Department of Manus
Mrs.	Macrine	Lavi	Catholic Family Life Office
Sr.	Cabrini	Lemeki	Milne Bay Church Health Secretary
Mrs	Jennifer	Litau	National Research Institute
Ms.	Susan	Maiasa	UPNG
Mrs.	Mioko	Manoa	Health Media Curriculum Unit
Mr.	Benedict	Mboya	UNICEF
Dr.	John	Mills	World Health Organization - PNG
Ms.	Florence	Mokolava	
Dr.	Glen	Mola	UPNG Faculty of Medicine
Mr.	James	Mulally	World Health Organization - PNG
Ms.	Margaret	Obi	UPNG - Library Sciences
Ms.	Matilda	Philemon	Division of Health - Milne Bay
Ms.	Andonia	Piau-Lynch	PTC
Ms.	Betty	Pilisa Lovai	UPNG-Anthropology/Sociology
Ms.	Balim	Pokpok	Department of Madang
Ms.	Hanna	Polume	Division of Health-Southern Highlands
Dr.	Timothy	Pyakalyia	Department of Health
Mr.	Renagi	Raga	Department of Home Affairs and Youth
Ms.	Glenda	Rattray	Salvation Army
Ms.	Mary	Rorcei	Health Training - Nursing Education
Dr.	Jerry	Russell	Child Survival Project
Dr.	John	Sairere	East Sepik Division of Health
Ms.	Elizabeth	Sakaiya	Alotau Provincial Hospital
Dr.	Frank	Schofield	University of Queensland
Dr.	Levi	Sialis	Department of Health
Ms.	Kathy	Simmons	United States Agency for Intertnational in Development
Dr.	Norma	Simpson	Goroka Teachers' College
Ms.	Ruta	Sinclair	UPNG - Anthropology/Sociology
Ms.	Mary	Soondrawu	East Sepik Women's Resource Centre
Ms.	Margaret	Street	Child Survival Project
Mrs.	Leontine	Tamate	UPNG - Faculty of Medicine
Ms.	Lois	Tanimia	SDA Church
Dr.	Reia	Taufa	NCD Division of Health

Mrs.	Carol	Taylor	Australian High Commission
Ms.	Kathy	Thomas	Australian High Commission
Dr.	Sue	Thornton	Menyamya Health Centre
Ms.	Yvonne	Underhill	UPNG - Geography Department
Mr.	Tavu	Vaira	Department of Central Province
Ms.	Sonia	Vano	UPNG
Ms.	Jossie	Villacorta	Department of Education
Ms.	Teresa	Waimani	Catholic Women
Mr.	Ricahard	Waive	Department of the Prime Minister
Sr.	Chanel	Williams	Hohola Youth Development Centre
Dr.	Marcus	Woibun	West Sepik Division of Health
Ms.	Brenda	Woods-Francis	Johns Hopkins University
Mr.	Micah	Yawing	Morobe Division of Health
Ms.	Ruby	Zarriga	Department of Finance and Planning

APPENDIX B

NATIONAL STRATEGY MEETING ON THE HEALTH OF WOMEN IN PAPUA NEW GUINEA

MEETING FACILITATORS

Dr.	Bill	Alto	University of Colorado
Ms.	Ulato	Avei	Prime Minister's Office
Mrs.	Gita	Badiyan	University of Papua New Guinea
Ms.	Veronica	Bagasell	Administrative College
Mr.	Edgar	Callanta	UNICEF
Ms.	Molly	Daure	Dept. of Youth and Home Affairs
Ms.	Regina	Kati	Department of Education-UNESCO
Ms.	Dora	Malum	Administrative College
Mrs.	Margaret	Misso	Department of Home Affairs and Youth
Ms.	Marie	Powell	UNICEF
Mrs.	Dorothy	Tekwie-Ortlauf	United Nations - UNDP

DISCUSSION GROUP REPORTS

TOPIC 1: EDUCATION

GROUP 1: INCREASED LITERACY RATES

FACILITATING FACTORS	BARRIERS	STRATEGIES	PROJECTS
1. Tok-ples and vernacular pre-skuls 2. Community awareness at all levels 3. Non-formal education	1. Attitudes: parents; cultural taboos; women's low self-esteem; men's attitude 2. Finance/resources - low government priority 3. Untrained/unskilled literacy personnel	1. Mass campaign to change attitude of community at large 2. Obtain total government support/ commitment to a broader spectrum of education — health education — training — tok ples preskul and adult women's programme. Extension programmes 3. Increase Accessibility: 1. Decreasing education costs 2. Having schools in more locations	1. Mass campaign to change attitude of community at large Components: Mass media — campaign to change attitude Production of awareness materials in 3 main languages Effective mobilisation of Women/ Community groups Establish national women's resource centres Sensitise men Theatre groups 2. Encourage Total Government Support/ Financial Commitment to a Broader Spectrum of Education — Tok Ples PS, Adult Women's Programme, Health Education and Training Components: Formation of a working group to prepare policy paper requesting government support for implementation of literacy programmes Form lobby groups to get government, politicians' and agencies' support Government to establish a body responsible for non- formal education. 3. Increase Accessibility: Free Schools Georaphically better placed schools that are available to both children and adults Components: Establish women's research centre in provinces Establishment of more central community schools Lobby government for free education up to grade 8 Train women to be women's literacy teachers Coordination of material production a village level Encourage village reading centres and libraries

GROUP 2. INCREASED HEALTH-RELATED KNOWLEDGE

<table>
<tr><th>FACILITATING FACTORS</th><th>BARRIERS</th><th>STRATEGIES</th><th>PROJECTS</th></tr>
<tr>
<td>1. Current education system both formal and non-formal
2. Church agency and N.G.O. project infrastructures
3. Media
4. Women in positions of power</td>
<td>1. Lack of access to information and education and lack of coordination and collaboration by all parties
2. Lack of prioritization for Funds/Resources
3. Traditional attitudes between men and women</td>
<td>1. Coordination of all information and activities by agencies and government departments
2. Identify lobbyists for Women's Health issues to secure funds and resources
3. Include men in women's activities</td>
<td>1. Annual Health Fair
Components:
Large scale fair might include booths on antenatal care, STD, malaria, family planning, sanitation, visual care, dental care, CDD, EPI. Also could be small scale village level fairs.
2. Educate the Community to Support Village Health Workers and to Take Responsibility for their own Health
Components:
Training of village health volunteers
Support services
3. Implement Women's Lobbyist at National and Provincial Levels
Components:
Establish job description
Select appropriate training
Identify appropriate persons
Seek clarified women's goals
Repr. National Women's Health Plan
Repr. Provincial Women's Health Issues.
3. Development of a directory of Health Activities
Aim:
Directory of Information/Health Education on programmes offered by all agencies and government bodies throughout PNG
Components:
Getting and collating information
Production of directory and updating system
Sources of funding to cover cost
Distribution
Promoting its existence</td>
</tr>
</table>

TOPIC 2. SOCIAL/CULTURAL:

GROUP 3. IMPROVED STATUS OF WOMEN

FACILITATING FACTORS	BARRIERS	STRATEGIES	PROJECTS
1. Equality and participation of women in decision-making at all levels 2. Policy directives, development priorities and legislative reforms 3. Existing programmes and projects	1. Cultural attitudes/behaviour 2. Lack of political will and commitment 3. Lack of continuity of services and support given and dependency on borrowed resources 4. Lack of access by women to information and resources	1. Relevant education Compulsory education on gender roles at all levels Education on appropriate skills for women in rural areas Compulsory education for children at community and high schools An increase in general awareness education on all matters including women's rights, health, literacy, business etc. 2. Equal responsibilities and opportunities for women Need to encourage and promote resources to ensure: A decrease in the workload for women at home Recognition of the value of women's work Equal emphasis on male and female children Equal pay for equal work for women and improvement in working conditions 3. Effective utilisation of local resources. The group felt that there should be greater emphasis: On use of existing resources and strengthening of ongoing projects and initiatives; On use of local financial and technical resources and less dependence on outside; On lobbying by women leaders and organisations for change 4. Education awareness While cultural and traditional practices and attitudes influence all aspects of development, the group felt that education plays a very important role. It emphasised that while legislative interventions are encouraged, major education awareness programmes are needed. This awareness should include women's roles and rights, health and family planning information, family life information, etc.	1. Development of Equal Responsibilities and Opportunities Components: Legislative reforms National women's policy 2. Effective Utilisation of Existing Resources Components: Strengthen existing women's development projects 3. Relevant Education Components: Community and high school expansion program Education awareness on women's role (Gender role)

GROUP 4. DECREASED WORKLOAD FOR WOMEN

FACILITATING FACTORS	BARRIERS	STRATEGIES	PROJECTS
1. Shared home and domestic responsibility 2. Improved public transport and water sanitation 3. Support for existing women's activities and groups	1. Lack of education 2. Lack of appropriate government system/s 3. Lack of proper communication and information services	1. Education of women and men on caring and sharing responsibilities 2. Support of women's groups and cooperatives 3. Improve water supply and transport and communications systems	1. Improved Water Supply and Sanitation. Components: Create a rational urban/rural water body with powers and funds, aimed at women's, youth's and children's welfare 2. Improve Communication System Components: Communication Policy — Road Network Improvement Radio Network Improvement Information services — for urban and rural areas aimed at youth, women and illiterates

TOPIC 3. HEALTH SERVICES

GROUP 5. IMPROVED ACCESS TO SERVICES

FACILITATING FACTORS	BARRIERS	STRATEGIES	PROJECTS
1. 3-Tier organisation. Aid-post — Health Centre — Hospital 2. Training of village aides is now being done 3. MCH (Ante-natal) services do exist	1. Geographic obstacles — distribution of facilities 2. General lack of knowledge and awareness 3. Lack of supervision and support	1. Better supervision/support of services 2. Availability of community based health workers 3. Health education of children and adults	1. Health Education Components: For children and adults All forms of media — Newspaper Video, TV, Radio Deal with various aspects of health - Hygiene, Family Planning Safe delivery - Antenatal care

FACTORS RELATED TO VILLAGE HEALTH AID PROJECT	BARRIERS RELATED TO VILLAGE HEALTH AID PROJECT	STRATEGIES FOR VILLAGE HEALTH AID PROJECT	PROJECTS FOR VHA
1. People want improved MCH services and easier access 2. Many educated women and men in community now 3. People are willing to volunteer for training 4. Some positive experiences already in PNG and neighbouring countries 5. This approach is consistent with Integral Human Development philosophy	1. Need to overcome compensation issue 2. Need to support, not compete with, existing 3-tiered system 3. Need to reverse thinking that Government give health services 4. Resources will be required for training, supplying and supportive supervision and simple management skills	1. Hold National Workshop with selected international guests on VHA, concepts and guidelines 2. Selected preliminary areas for its introduction 3. Develop suitable training system with materials 4. Plan evaluation component	1. Development of Management Skills Components: Train nurses, HEOs and Doctors in management skills at provincial and district levels 2. Training of Village or Community Health Aids Components: Utilise community voluntary helpers Train village birth attendants Need to include health education Need to provide a referral service

GROUP 6. IMPROVED APPROPRIATENESS OF SERVICES

FACILITATING FACTORS	BARRIERS	STRATEGIES	PROJECTS
1. Existing health infrastructure and labour wards in Health Centres 2. Availability of mobile health teams promoting MCH and FP services in HC 3. Availability of funds and technical assistance 4. Availability of trained health workers	1. Cultural factors 2. Shortage of female health workers in the rural areas 3. Health policy: Least regard for MCH 4. Inadequate delivery of health services and lack of appropriate health education	1. Use more trained community women to provide health services (community based) 2. Use more trained government health workers (women) 3. Improve training capability of front-line health workers on MCH 4. Use of incentives to upgrade/maintain rural health services	1. Appropriate Training in Maternal/Infant Health Components: To review current Health Workers' curriculum to ensure: Proper emphasis on maternal/infant health Community support/identifying needs Cultural aspects of women's health 2. Use of Trained Community Women to Improve Health Services Components: Study on use/training/remuneration of village women to provide basic health care Implementation of findings 3. Use of Incentives to Upgrade/Maintain Rural Health Components: Study of present conditions and incentives for rural health workers e.g. pay, promotion, training, support

TOPIC 4. GENERAL ISSUES

GROUP 7. IMPROVED COORDINATION/INTEGRATION OF ACTIVITIES

FACILITATING FACTORS	BARRIERS	STRATEGIES	PROJECTS
1. Existence of plans in each department 2. Coordination between departments 3. Health delivery system is in place	1. Lack of political will, commitment and priority 2. Physical and cultural barriers 3. Inadequate/lack of sensitivity to women's issues	1. Increase prominence and status of Division of Women's Affairs 2. Planned and active mass media and literacy awareness campaign 3. Strengthen Women's Advisory Committee 4. Research into cultural barriers 5. Ombudsman for women	1. Increased Prominence and Status Division of Women's Affairs Components: Submission to NEC to increase capacity by increasing staffing and funding in Women's Division at national and provincial levels. 2. Strengthen Women's Advisory Committees Components: Need to supply staff and support to the committee - needs an executive officer and assistant and support staff 3. Planned and Active Mass Media and Literacy Awareness Campaign Components: Staff training in media techniques Changes to the education curriculum Coordinated us of Mass media

GROUP 8. IMPROVED WOMEN'S MANAGEMENT OF SOCIAL CHANGE

FACILITATING FACTORS	BARRIERS	STRATEGIES	PROJECTS
1. Existing government policies/programs/projects (population, women's health, education, agriculture) 2. Existing network/structures (Government and NGOs) 3. Existing internal and external funding	1. Inadequate funding/essential services for all 2. Negative attitudes and low status of women 3. Lack of participation in planning management of projects/programmes related to women	1. Strengthen/encourage existing lobby groups to ensure government commitment on basic human rights 2. Commit participants to socially mobilise the community about issues of the seminar 3. Remove existing women's division from Dept. of Home Affairs and Youth and create Department of Women's Affairs	1. Creation of Department of Women's Affairs Components: Structural design of the department Policy design/implementation Monitoring all impacts Needs research 2. Central Women's Resource and Information Centre Components: National directory of groups Co-ordination of resources and services

Many of the discussion groups identified possible lead and support agencies for the strategies and projects. Some groups were even able to do more detailed planning related to timelines and budget needs. This information has not been included in this paper but is available on request.

FAMILY PLANNING, FAMILY HEALTH, HEALTH AND DEVELOPMENT

The papers in this section cover many aspects of the theme; the role of women and the family, family planning, sexually transmitted disease, antenatal care, smoking, drug abuse and suicide.

The role played by women in the rural development of Papua New Guinea is presented by **John Sairere** with a case in East Sepik, and by **Josephine Gena** who outlines the Women's Division of the Department of Home Affairs and Youth's plans, programmes and challenges in promoting women's issues in development programmes. **Maria Kopkop** discusses the National Council of Women's successes, and also the duplications, politiking and rivalries that hinder women's organisations in Papua New Guinea.

The rapid changes in the country have brought changing attitudes to the family, to marriage, and to the social structure of Papua New Guinea. The stresses invoked by such change are discussed by **Felix Johnson** with data on suicide and drug overdose, **Paul Freeman** on cigarette smoking, **Jenny Hughes** and **Timothy Dyke** on the incidence of sexually transmitted disease, and **Andonia Lynch** on the abuse of women within the family and in the workplace.

Family Planning utilization, distribution, and services are comprehensively covered. The National Department of Health's policies and plans for Family Planning are outlined by the Secretary for Health, **Dr Levi Sialis**. The Social Marketing of Contraceptives in Papua New Guinea is described by **Andy Piller. Cecil Klufio** discusses the risks to child bearing women who do not utilize family planning services. The Seminar was aptly reminded by **Graham Tucker** that Family Planning is for both sexes with his paper on vasectomy. International agencies' support for Family Planning in the region are outlined by **Joseph Sukwianomb.**

The problems facing the Maternal and Child Health Services in Papua New Guinea and the importance of prioritizing them and encouraging their utilization are described by **John Biddulph** and by **Cecil Klufio** and **Grace Kariwiga.** Programmes to promote safer child birth in the rural areas are discussed by **Margaret Street, Frank Schofield** and **William Alto. William Alto** also describes a rural scheme to monitor infant and child mortality. To highlight the importance of education in family health matters within Papua New Guinea **Norma Simpson** discusses a curriculum for teaching home economics teachers, and **Kerry Pataki** describes the teaching of demography to medical students within the context of maternal and child health.

A global view covering many of the issues in an international context is given by **John** and **Pat Caldwell** and the section is concluded by **Jennifer Litau** with a discussion of the Papua New Guinea Population Policy.

....

TUKUTAU TAUFA
Technical Editor
Chairman, 19th Waigani Seminar
Department of Community Medicine
University of Papua New Guinea

KEYNOTE SPEECH BY DR LEVI SIALIS

It is a great pleasure for me to be given this opportunity to give some opening remarks at this very important session of the 19th Waigani Seminar.

Family planning is not a new concept or practice in Papua New Guinea. Traditionally, children were planned for and valued for a wide variety of cultural, social and political reasons. In our traditional society, children grew up to provide support and care for aging parents and the extended family. Sons usually remained at home after marrying, while daughters moved away.

A common traditional motivation for having many children, especially boys, was to strengthen and continue the tribe. Often a man married simply to gain children. An increase in the numbers of a group meant prosperity, power and security against enemies. The individual prestige and power of a man was enhanced by having many children. Children validated adult status, and provided opportunities for exchange and transactions.

In most parts of Papua New Guinea, there was some control over the number and spacing of children. To a greater or lesser extent three direct methods have been used.

1. The institutionalized restriction of sexual intercourse,

2. The knowledge and use of techniques to avoid conception,

3. The practice of abortion and infanticide.

These cultural practices determined when children were born into a family, the spacing between children and the total number of children borne to a woman.

Overall, the postpartum sex taboo during a prolonged period of breastfeeding was probably the single most important factor which controlled family size and fertility.

Little is known of the use of traditional herbal contraceptives, as often it is a secret or taboo. Perhaps, this is one area where research efforts should be encouraged.

[1] Department of Health, Papua New Guinea

Changes in rural areas of Papua New Guinea during the past thirty to forty years have affected mortality and fertility. Death rates, especially infant mortality rates, have fallen and more children are surviving into adulthood. This is due to the increased availability of health services, including maternal and child health programmes, aidposts services, malaria control, and other related programmes. Improved social and environmental conditions have also contributed to this drop.

Traditional practices which control fertility are gradually breaking down. Beliefs which placed limits on sexual relations to protect breastfeeding or to avoid harmful effects to husbands are disappearing. Traditional periods of breastfeeding and sexual abstinence are shorter, which has resulted in more frequent pregnancies and larger family sizes. Traditional abortion and infanticide have been suppressed. Changes in living patterns now places husband and wife together, instead of apart as was the traditional practice. The main reason for continuing to have many children in our traditional society is to have some form of security and insurance. This is unlikely to change and will remain a strong motivation for many of our people.

Population growth is equated with political strength. In some areas, this is a major inhibiting influence on the implementation of family planning programmes. In some parts of our country, many people believe that there are large areas of land which could support a greater population then at present. Many areas, however, are unsuitable for agriculture. Already many of us are aware of certain areas of the country where there is a growing land shortage, leading to land disputes and other law and order problems.

It has been argued that people are needed to exploit the rich natural resources of the country. However, Papua New Guinea lacks skilled manpower and infrastructure. A sharp increase in the number of young people without a concurrent capacity to provide not only primary but higher education, and health services, will create more serious problems of unemployment, growing inequalities and law and order breakdown.

When it comes to family planning, there is often a conflict of interest between the husband and wife. Women often desire fewer children than men because of the additional work to feed and raise them. The problems of pregnancy and births, taboo and the possibility of pain or death for the woman herself. A great deal of fear and anxiety is often associated with childbirth among women. On the other hand in many traditional societies, the main purpose of marriage is to produce children. Women may desire family planning but their husbands may view it as a threat.

Children cost money to raise and educate. When people are aware of this economic factor it will influence their family size.

The recent endorsement of a National Population Policy by Cabinet highlights the commitment by the Government to the issues of population growth and high fertility in this country.

Modern family planning in Papua New Guinea is primarily concerned with the health and welfare of the family through the planning of pregnancies. This includes spacing child birth, regulating the size of family, helping sub-fertile couples to have children, and providing information and counselling to couples on matters related to parenthood.

Health facilities at hospitals, health centres and sub-centres, and some aidposts, urban clinics, private clinics and mobile clinics are participating as outlets for family planning services. Other services include the community based distribution programme of the privately run Family Planning Association of Papua New Guinea operating in Central, Morobe, and East Sepik, and private doctors and chemists.

The use of contraception may be looked upon as a licence for promiscuity or as a way of depriving the husband and family of offspring. The economy of Papua New Guinea cannot meet the needs and demands of our people. This is the major crisis facing Papua New Guinea today, and is caused by the uncontrolled population increase, particularly in the urban areas.

The population of Papua New Guinea is growing at well over 2.5 percent per year. The size of the population and the growth rate has created some development problems that have made it difficult for our country to achieve all our development goals. It is also causing major social problems.

The fertility rate is highest in the islands region of the country with an average of more than six births per women. It is lowest in the highlands with an average of just under five births per women.

Because of the rapid population growth, there is a high dependency ratio. That is, there are more people unable to look after themselves and who rely on others for support. For each dependent child, there is approximately one adult of working age. By the year 2000, there will be approximately two dependent children to one working age adult. In comparison for each dependent child, there are two or three working age adults, in industrialized countries.

The first family planning clinic was established in 1962 in Port Moresby as part of the maternal and child health services of the Department of Health, and issued oral contraceptives. The IUD was first used in 1965, and the Lippes Loop became freely available in 1967. During the early 1970s, the rate of annual new acceptors was small until an additional family planning programme was started in 1987 with the support of international agencies. The number of new acceptors of family planning reached 22,000 by 1980. However, with the decentralisation of the programme to the provinces, much of the impetus was lost and the number of new acceptors declined to about 15,000 in 1984. Since then, there has been a slow increase and by 1990 nearly 26,000 new acceptors of family planning have received services through the government and the churches health services.

Despite that slow increase in the new acceptors of family planning methods, the availability and use of family planning in Papua New Guinea remains limited, although there are increasing numbers of requests in urban areas, especially in Port Moresby where the economic necessity for family limitation is obvious.

There are many reasons for the limited use of family planning. Many village men are opposed to modern family planning. Many couples have little knowledge of the variety of methods available. Some women may experience unpleasant side effects and fear subsequent infertility. Others are shy to approach health workers for information. In many areas the use of contraception was traditionally associated with promiscuity, an attitude which is still common today. Finally, even though couples may wish to practise modern family planning, often contraceptives are difficult to obtain, especially in rural areas.

Modern family planning methods in order of their effectiveness are:-

Male sterilisation (vasectomy)	99%
Female sterilisation (Tubectomy)	99%
Depo Provera	99%
Lippes Loop (IUD)	92%
Oral contraceptives	95%
Minipill	90%
Condoms	85%
Natural methods	70%

The pill and depo provera are the Family Planning methods readily available. The IUD is not commonly used. The ovulation method continues to be the method of choice in many of the clinics operated by the Catholic Family Services. The use of female sterilisation is increasing slowly, whereas male sterilisation is not popular.

The Institutions that provide family planning services in Papua New Guinea are:-

Hospitals	100%
Urban Clinics	100%
Private Clinics/Chemists	100%
Health centres	90-94%
Health sub-centres	60%
Aidposts	23%

Due to high maternal morbidity and mortality, there is a need to encourage and promote family planning programmes in Papua New Guinea today. In fact, this is a major thrust of the 1991-95 National Health Plan, which aims to reduce the current maternal mortality rate from 7/1000 to 5/1000 by 1995.

A high maternal mortality rate makes it difficult for families to support their children, educate them, and grow enough food and earn money. Lack of family planning leads to frequent pregnancies, closely spaced childbirths, unhealthy children and a poor standard of living. This means that women are further burdened and are often too weak to have a healthy pregnancy.

There are many gaps in the actual delivery of family planning services in Papua New Guinea. Lack of community involvement in the provision of health services including family planning is one such gap. Most people believe that the government will provide these services and that they have limited responsibility. This is wrong thinking. The government needs communities to participate in various health services if they want to improve their standards of living.

The Department of Health has recognised these important issues and is now committed to addressing some of them. A number of important initiatives are being planned in close liasion and collaboration with provinces, the private sector, and communities, with technical and financial support from a number of international agencies to address some of these issues.

Special attention will be given to the following areas:-

1. Development of information, education and communication materials (IEC) for maternal care and family planning, to address the issue of lack of public awareness and poor knowledge about family planning methods and services;

2. Due to poor management of programmes, guidelines and information procedures will be developed;

3. Curriculum development and on-the-job training for family planning service providers to address the lack of knowledge and skills in the provision of quality family planning services; and

4. Social marketing of certain contraceptives through the private sector, and expansion of community-based distribution (CBD) programmes to address the issue of lack of private sector and community involvement and poor accessibility to family planning services.

Finally, ladies and gentlemen, I want to emphasise here that family planning is not the responsibility of the Government. It is everyone's business - political leaders, teachers, health workers and parents. If everyone takes part in family planning, then Papua New Guinea can achieve a population of about seven million commensurate with available agricultural land. But if the present growth rate continues to rise, Papua New Guinea will be well over this figure and will increase to 7.4 million by the year 2015.

Even if the Government starts a population programme immediately, and achieves an average of three children per woman by the year 2015, there will be about six million Papua New Guineans by 2015, with around 1.9 million living in urban areas, and approximately one quarter of these people being urban youths. This population growth will have considerable effects on the physical, mental and social well-being of our countrymen and women. If the growth continues in an uncontrolled manner, much of the new resources of the country will be spent just in trying to keep up present standards of living.

Major elements in the implementation of the population policy should be:-

1. Population growth should be slowed by reducing levels of fertility. Currently, the crude birth rate in Papua New Guinea is 35 percent per 1,000 and the government has established a target of reducing the crude birth rate to 30 percent per 1,000 by 1993. This would have significant impact on the rate of population growth. In order to achieve this, three approaches in particular should be utilized:-

   a) The length of a woman's fertility career should be shortened, and the total number of births per woman should be reduced through ensuring greater educational opportunities for women.

b) Contraceptive knowledge, attitude and practices should be improved at all levels. It has been clearly demonstrated that there is a direct relationship between information and contraceptive availability to women and reduced levels of fertility.

c) Motivation of men to take a leading role in properly planning their families.

2. Increased understanding of the implications of population dynamics for social and economic development should be promoted among decision-makers and opinion leaders at the national, provincial and local levels, and the people at large.

3. Government should promote and expand the primary health services, maternal and child health care, and the family health services, including efficient and accessible family planning services.

4. Information and education on the advantages of child spacing and on the means to achieve this should be widely disseminated.

5. Living conditions in the rural areas should be raised, and objective information provided on urban living conditions to prospective migrants, who may then pass this information on to the future generations.

FAMILY PLANNING AND FAMILY HEALTH

CECIL A. KLUFIO[1]

Family Planning improves the health and saves the lives of women and their children. This fact is well known and has been repeatedly stated by earlier speakers. But I have chosen to address it for the benefit of some of our non-medical audience, and because the statement bears re-emphasis. I propose to look at the causes of maternal death in this country and to show how family planning can prevent some of our maternal deaths. I will also touch of the influence of family planning on child mortality.

Dr Malcolm Potts, the immediate past President of Family Health International U.S.A, vividly described the global tragedy of maternal death and the world's nonchalant attitude to it as follows: "Every four hours, day in, day out, a jumbo jet crashes and all on board are killed. The 250 passengers are all women, most in the prime of life, some still in their teens. They all are either pregnant or recently delivered of a baby. Most of them have growing children at home, and families that depend on them. "(1). The vast majority of the half million maternal deaths which occur each year in the world happen in the developing world. The maternal death rate for Papua New Guinea is estimated at 7/1000, ranging from 2/1000 in the urban areas to 12/1000 in rural areas that have no access to health services. It has also been estimated that about 1000 maternal deaths occur in PNG each year (2,3,4,). Taking a cue from Potts, Mola likened the situation in PNG to an F28 full of women of reproductive age, crashing every month of the year and killing all on board (2).

It has been estimated that during her lifetime the average woman in Papua New Guinea has a 1 in 26 chance that pregnancy or childbirth will cause her death. By contrast, for the developed world, the lifetime maternal death risk is 1 in 1500 (4,5). The maternal mortality rate in the developed world is less than 1/10,000 livebirths compared with the 70/10,000 for Papua New Guinea.

Why is our maternal mortality rate so much higher than that of the developed world?

[1] Professor of Obstetrics and Gynaecology,
Medical Faculty, University of Papua New Guinea

The reasons may be summarized as follows:-

1. The general health of our women is poor. The main contributors are: malnutrition, malaria, hookworm infestation, and too many and too frequent pregnancies. Anaemia may be used as a rough measure of health. Defined as Hb level below 10g/dl we consistently find that about 40% of the women delivered at the Port Moresby General Hospital are anaemic at some time during their pregnancy; and that over 10% are below 8g/dl(7,8). The situation in some rural areas is worse.

2. The level of education and social status of our women are low. Education is more than a halfway house to health. The educated person is more likely to lead a healthy life-style and to make use of available health services. The higher the status of women, the more care society gives them. Longer schooling reduces the risk of pregnancy at very young ages.

3. Health services are inadequate and inaccessible in some areas.

4. Failure to make use of available MCH services. Low or non-education of women, and probably more important, of their husbands is a major factor in the utilisation of services.

5. Inadequate social services e.g. potable water, good housing etc.

6. Dangerous reproductive health behaviour. The reproductive characteristics of our women are hazardous.

   a) They start their families when they are too young ie. less than eighteen years. In some areas marriage is allowed at the commencement of menstruation.

   b) They have too many children ie. more than four.

   c) They have children too close together ie. at less than two year intervals.

   d) They continue to have children when they are too old to safely do so ie. after the age of thirty five. Apart from failure to make use of available services, reproductive behaviour is the only variable which lies within the power of the couple to control. Couples need to have access to family planning information, education, counselling and methods.

To see how family planning can reduce maternal deaths let us look at the immediate causes of maternal death in this country. These are in descending order of frequency:

i) puerperal sepsis (infection of the womb);

ii) post-partum haemorrhage (excessive bleeding after delivery);

iii) medical conditions such as pneumonia, malaria, anaemia;

iv) obstructed labour and ruptured uterus;

v) abortion.

All these conditions are more dangerous when malnutrition and anaemia are present. As we all know the beginning of a baby is the fertilized egg; and this egg is so small that it cannot be seen by the naked eye. Whatever the baby takes to grow from this invisible speck to the bouncing three kg baby at term, is supplied by the mother's body. Breast-feeding is as demanding. To supply the baby's needs without damaging her own health, the mother's diet must be adequate before and during the pregnancy and during lactation. We all know that the diet of many of our women is not adequate and is not balanced. They start pregnancy in deficit, and the situation worsens as pregnancy progresses. Frequent and repeated pregnancies make things far worse.

Postpartum haemorrhage (excessive bleeding after delivery)

The most common cause of this is failure of the uterus to contract and retract firmly after delivery ie. atony of the uterus. A second important cause is retained placenta (failure of the placenta to separate and be expelled). Whilst it is true that any woman may bleed excessively at delivery, for some categories of women the risk is particularly high. These risk categories include those who have already had four deliveries (grand multiparae), and those who have had postpartum haemorrhage or a retained placenta in a previous delivery. A retained placenta is more likely in a woman with many children. Family completion for these high risk groups can prevent these deaths.

Puerperal sepsis (childbirth womb infection)

The risk factors for this complication include: prolonged labour and retained placenta. Labour may be prolonged because the baby's head is too big for the maternal pelvis (CPO=cephalopelvic disproportion). CPD is likely in a girl who becomes pregnant before her pelvis is fully grown. Grand multiparity is a risk factor for retained placenta. Delaying first births and avoiding grand multiparity should reduce deaths due to puerperal sepsis.

Obstructed Labour and Ruptured uterus. This may occur when the baby is too big for the mother's pelvis, or when the baby is not coming head first (malpresentation). Malpresentation is more likely to occur in a grand multipara. Family completion to prevent grand multiparity should reduce these deaths.

Abortion. This is more likely to result in death when it is criminally induced. A woman whose pregnancy is unplanned and unwanted is the woman who is likely to turn to criminal abortion. The woman may be young and unmarried or a married woman who has more children than she can look after. In fact it can be any woman. In some countries criminal abortion is among the first three leading causes of maternal death. And in these countries, up to 50% of emergency gynaecological beds are occupied by women suffering from complications of abortion. Fortunately abortion is not yet a big problem in this country. But it must be noted that in 68% of the deaths from abortion reported in 1984-1986, the death certificate mentioned that the pregnancy had been interfered with. We can prevent these tragic deaths through family planning.

FAMILY PLANNING, CHILD HEALTH AND CHILD SURVIVAL

Birth-spacing:

That birth-spacing has a beneficial influence on child health has been known for a long time, and through the ages many societies have evolved obligatory customary behaviour patterns or taboos, which ensure long birth intervals, and thereby protect their children. Unfortunately, in many of these societies urbanization has eaten away at these traditional beliefs, and these beneficial taboos are dying out. Short birth intervals affect both the index child and the previous child.

It has been shown that throughout the developing world children are more likely to die if they were born less than two years after their mother's previous child was born, than if the birth interval was longer (9). In a survey of 6,000 women, the World Health Organization found that the infant death rate was 200/1000 livebirths if the birth interval was up to 1 year, 100 if it was 2-3 years, and 80/1000 livebirths if it was 3-4 years. It has been estimated that spacing births at least two years apart can contribute to a 10-20% reduction in infant and child mortality (10,11,12).

Many studies have established that low birth weight is associated with short birth intervals. The risks of both small-for-gestational age and preterm delivery are increased (12,13). The association of small for gestational age and short birth intervals still holds true when confounders, such as preterm deliveries, and patients whose last babies are not alive at the time of the birth of the index child, are excluded. A preliminary analysis of low birth weight, a study we are conducting at the Port

Moresby General Hospital, has shown this association.

Maternal Age

There is an association between maternal age and fetal and infant mortality. The relationship is roughly U-shaped. Death rates are highest when the mother is under 18 or over 35 years.

Parity (Birth Order)

Perinatal and infant deaths are high in first births, lowest in second births, and rise sharply after the fifth birth. We cannot prevent first births; we can make them safer by delaying them until after adolescence. And surely we can help women to avoid grand multiparity!

It must be noted that short birth interval, maternal age, and high parity, each independently increases the risk of perinatal, infant and child death. The effect is magnified when two or all three factors are combined.

Madam Chair, I have attempted to show that: the parents who understand the influence of birth interval, parity, and maternal age on the health of mother and child; the parents who are within reach of family planning services; the parents who make use of these services to avoid high risk pregnancies: these parents will have a family which is psychologically, emotionally and physically healthy, in short a happy family. The children are not likely to be born with low birth weight, or have poor nutrition, or suffer frequent infections, poor physical growth, low intelligence and poor academic performance. The mother is not likely to die in pregnancy or childbirth.

In conclusion, Madam Chairperson, I am convinced that if we do not make the best the enemy of the good, and if we are prepared to use the resources we have, within a short period of time we shall be able to provide family planning information, education, counselling, and methods to the majority of our people. I do not for example see why we cannot identify village female school teachers who are interested, and train them to dispense the progestogen-only pill (Microlut) and low dose combined oral contraceptives. They can easily be taught to use a risk check list to identify clients for whom these methods may not be suitable. They can be taught to take blood pressures. My point is that we do not need doctors or nurses to provide these services at the village level. If we were to wait for doctors and nurses to provide these services we would have to wait a very long time! Please let us not make the best the enemy of the good! Thank you.

REFERENCES

1. World Health Organization. Maternal Mortality: Helping women off the road to death. WHO Chronicle 1986; 40: 173

2. Mola G. Maternal death in Papua New Guinea, 1984-1986. PNG Med J 1989; 32: 27

3. Department of Health. Papua New Guinea National Health Plan 1991-1995. Department of Health 1991

4. Gillet JE. The Health of Women in Papua New Guinea. PNG Institute of Med Research Goroka, 1990 pp180

5. Mahler H. The safe motherhood initiative: a call to action. Lancet 1987; 1:668

6. Rinehart W, Kols A, Moore SH. Healthier Mothers and Children through Family Planning. Pop Reports, Ser J No. 27. Baltimore, John Hopkins Univ. Pop Information Program 1984; p40

7. Sill PR, hILL AVS, Igo JD. Multifactorial aetiology of anaemia of pregnancy in Port Moresby, Papua New Guinea. PNG Med J 1987; 30:193

8. Division of Obstetrics and Gynaecology, PMGH. Annual Reports. Port Moresby General Hospital.

9. Pebley AR, Millman S. Birthspacing and child survival. Intern Family Planning Perspectives 1986; 12:71

10. Hobcraft JN, McDonald JW, Rutstein SO. Demographic determinants of infant and childhood mortality: A comparative analysis. Pop Studies 1985; 39:363

11. Trussel J, Pebley AR. The potential impact of changes in fertility on infant, child, and maternal mortality. Studies in Family Planning 1984; 15:267

12. Fortney JA, Higgins JE. The effect of birth interval on perinatal survival and birthweight. Pub Health (London) 1984; 98:73

13. Lieberman E, Lang JM, Ryan KJ, Monson RR, Schoenbaum SC. The association of inter-pregnancy interval with small for dates gestional age births. Obstet. Gynaecol. 1989; 74:1

FIG 1. FACTORS WHICH CONTRIBUTE TO HIGH MMR IN PAPUA NEW GUINEA

1. GENERAL HEALTH OF OUR WOMEN IS POOR.
2. THE EDUCATION LEVEL AND SOCIAL STATUS OF OUR WOMEN ARE LOW.
3. HEALTH SERVICES ARE INADEQUATE OR INACCESSIBLE.
4. FAILURE TO MAKE USE OF HEALTH SERVICES.
5. SOCIAL SERVICES ARE INADEQUATE.
6. REPRODUCTIVE CHARACTERISTICS ARE HAZARDOUS.

FIG 2. DANGEROUS REPRODUCTIVE CHARACTERISTICS

1. PREGNANCY WHEN LESS THAN 18 YEARS OF AGE.
2. TOO MANY BIRTHS - MORE THAN 4
3. BIRTHS TOO CLOSE TOGETHER - BIRTH INTERVAL < 2 YRS
4. BIRTHS AFTER AGE 35 YEARS.

FIG 3. CAUSES OF 304 MATERNAL DEATHS REPORTED IN 1984-86 (2)

PUERPERAL SEPSIS	77 DEATHS
(CHILDBIRTH WOMB INFECTION)	
POSTPARTUM HAEMORRHAGE	66
(EXCESSIVE BLEEDING AFTER DELIVERY)	
MEDICAL CONDITIONS	60
(PNEUMONIA, TB, ANAEMIA, HEART DIS.ETC)	
OBSTRUCTED LABOUR AND RUPTURED UTERUS	21
ABORTION	20
OTHERS	51

FIG 4. COMMON CAUSES OF DEATH AND RISK FACTORS WHICH FP CAN PREVENT

1. EXCESSIVE BLEEDING AFTER DELIVERY (PPH).

   CAUSES i. ATONY OF UTERUS-POOR CONTRACTION/RETRACTION

   ii. RETAINED PLACENTA

   RISK FACTORS TOO MANY BIRTHS (> 4)

2. PUERPERAL SEPSIS.

   CAUSES i. PROLONGED LABOUR

   ii. RETAINED PLACENTA

   RISK FACTORS PREGNANCY < 18 = SMALL PELVIS = PROLONGED LABOUR

   TOO MANY BIRTHS = RETAINED PLACENTA

3. OBSTRUCTED LABOUR AND RUPTURED UTERUS.

   i. SMALL PELVIS

   ii. ABNORMAL PRESENTATION

   RISK FACTORS PREGNANCY < 18 YEARS = SMALL PELVIS

   TOO MANY BIRTHS = ABNORMAL PRESENTATION

4. ABORTION

   CAUSES CRIMINAL INTERFERENCE

   RISK FACTORS UNPLANNED PREGNANCY

   UNWANTED PREGNANCY

SOCIAL MARKETING OF CONTRACEPTIVES IN PAPUA NEW GUINEA

ANDREW PILLER[1]

During the course of this year's seminar, there has been frequent mention of the importance of family planning. An essential requirement for family planning programmes is to ensure that contraceptives are close at hand and accessible. Put simply, the easier it is for people to get contraceptives, the more likely they are to use them. One of the key strategies to making contraceptives more available is to create more than one source of supply so that people can get them easily.

Currently in Papua New Guinea, contraceptives are available only through a limited number of sources. These include health facilities, the Family Planning Association, urban based pharmacies and a few other urban outlets.

In an effort to increase the availability of contraceptives to the public, the National Department of Health requested assistance from SOMARC, a USAID (United States Agency for International Development) sponsored programmme. SOMARC (short for Social Marketing for Change) is managed by the private company, The Futures Group, which is working in thirty four countries developing the social marketing of contraceptives. SOMARC began preliminary work in Papua New Guinea in 1989 and the decision was made to introduce a pilot programme here, initially in four provinces along the highlands highway, Morobe, Eastern Highlands, Simbu and Western Highlands.

Social Marketing uses techniques developed by companies marketing a wide range of products. These techniques have their roots in sociology, anthropology and other social sciences. These methods have been refined so that they focus on the consumer. What information, ideas or products must programmes offer to satisfy consumers? Some people question the idea of treating public health programmes like toothpaste or soft drinks, but marketing principles are not product specific, they apply to any products.

[1] Service Expansion and Technical Support,
Department of Health, Papua New Guinea

Another question raised is why would someone pay money for something they can get for free? The answer has to do with costs, and not all costs are measured in Kina or Toea. True, one can go to a health centre in Papua New Guinea and get contraceptives for free. But you might have to wait for some time and there is a cost for time as well as the cost of transportation, and then they might not have any in stock. They may not be free either - some health facilities now charge for various services. Many people like convenience and are willing to pay for it. The purpose of social marketing of contraceptives is not to eliminate other sources of contraceptives, but to complement them, giving the public options so they can make their own decisions, and ultimately making it easier for people who want to plan their family to have access to family planning methods.

The method works. In many countries where social marketing programmes have been established, retail sales of contraceptives (condoms and pills) account for 50% or more of the total contraceptives (condoms and pills) distributed.

At this point, instead of talking generally, I'd like to present what has been happening here in Papua New Guinea over the last several months.

The specific objectives of the pilot project are as follows:

- To distribute and promote contraceptives in selected test market areas, in order to determine the feasibility and logistics required to expand the test market activity into a national social marketing intervention;

- To distribute and promote condoms in the selected test market areas to assist efforts in the prevention of the transmission of AIDS and other STDS; and

- To assist in increasing the awareness, knowledge and usage of these contraceptive products in the test market areas during the period of the pilot project.

To achieve these objectives, SOMARC has been involved in a variety of social marketing activities prior to actually introducing products. These activities include;

- A recently completed summary of previous research and distribution information concerning family planning throughout the country. While not comprehensive, there has been quite a bit of research and other information collected about family planning in Papua New Guinea.

- A baseline survey has recently been conducted. This is sometimes referred to as a Knowledge, Attitude and Practice (KAP) survey. This survey will give us general information about how much people know, what they believe and what they actually do about family planning. This is done before the marketing of contraceptives begins. In about two years the survey will be repeated. This will tell us roughly how much knowledge, attitudes and practices regarding family planning have changed since we began the project.

  SOMARC contracted with researchers from the Institute of Medical Research and the Medical College to conduct this research. The final report is being worked on now. UPNG medical students were hired and trained to conduct the survey.

- Along with the KAP survey SOMARC also conducted a series of discussion groups with single and married men and married women in Lae and Goroka. Known as 'focus' groups discussions, they provide descriptive information that we don't get from the quantitative KAP survey. Together these two types of research (plus the summary of previous research) provide us with a good foundation of information on which we will develop a marketing strategy to promote the use of condoms for both family planning and the prevention of AIDS and other STDs, and oral contraceptives.

HRD, a private marketing company, was contracted to conduct the focus group research. HRD has also conducted research to develop product names, packaging and instruction leaflets appropriate for PNG.

All this research has been compiled and is being used to develop a marketing plan which will lay out the strategies for sales, distribution, demand creation, usage information and project evaluation. Initially, the pills will be distributed in approximately seventy five specially selected trade stores and pharmacies whose staff will be provided with training in contraceptive technology. The product will be sold for K1.70. The condoms will be initially distributed in approximately two hundred retail outlets including pharmacies, trade stores, gas stations and bars, and will be sold for 75 toea for a box of three.

The income generated from the sale of the products (approximately 30% of what the consumer pays) will be deposited into a fund which will be reinvested in sustaining the marketing and promotional activities. In so doing, the project has a built in cost recovery mechanism which leads to autonomy and sustainability in the long run.

Both products will be promoted to encourage continuous and correct usage. This will include things like the use of Wokabout Marketing (a travelling theatre group), radio advertisements and dramas, posters, displays for use in stores and other advertising materials. The principal objective of the promotional campaign will be to establish a better understanding of the product and product usage amongst our primary target audience - young married couples.

The result of all these strategies is that in July we plan to launch the Protector Brand of condoms in the four pilot provinces. In October we plan to launch the low dose pill known as Microgynon 30.

Our target is to produce five thousand new acceptors in the four provinces over the next eighteen months. This will mean distributing approximately two hundred and ten thousand condoms and approximately forty thousand cycles of pills over that period. If we are successful, we would have assisted in increasing contraceptive prevalence in these provinces from 3% to 5%, an improvement of 40% in less than two years.

In addition to these activities, SOMARC has worked closely with the government to change policies that would encourage increased distribution of contraceptives. Last year, the oral contraceptive (the pill) was changed from a prescription to an over-the-counter drug. About the same time, the Department of Health regulation requiring a husband's signature for using contraceptives was dropped. More recently, the duty for importing condoms for private sector distribution was dropped from 7% to nil.

VASECTOMY AS A METHOD OF FAMILY PLANNING IN PAPUA NEW GUINEA

G. S. TUCKER[1]

INTRODUCTION

This paper is based on my experience as Medical Superintendent and Surgeon at the Balimo Health Centre working among the Gogodala people of the Western Province, since 1985.

The Balimo Health Centre seeks to provide primary and secondary health care for approximately 25,000 Gogodala tribal people living on the alluvial flood plains of the Aramia river some 40 kilometers north east of the Fly river. The region is well endowed with food, consisting of sago, fruit, fish and game, so nutrition is usually adequate.

The normal family size has tended to be in double figures in the past, because this appeared to be necessary to off-set the high infant mortality rate and the low life expectancy of adults.

When I started working at Balimo I was immediately impressed by the large number of young children around the place. A visit to the National Statistics Office in 1985 revealed that this area has an annual birth rate of 2.576%. Thus in the 5 year period 1985 - 1990 the population was expected to increase from new births by 3,143. Good health care has now significantly reduced infant mortality amongst the Gogodalas, and it became clear that such a high birth rate could not be sustained indefinitely before food shortages would become a problem. Unemployment is already a problem and is rapidly getting worse.

A family planning clinic had been available at Balimo Health Centre since 1967 but this appeared to be having little real effect on the population explosion. Oral contraceptives, Depo Provera and Intra Uterine

[1] Balimo Health Centre, Western Province
Papua New Guinea

contraceptive devices were readily available and in regular use but there were many failures as well as non-users. Coupled with that was the fact that a large family was still thought to be a desirable insurance policy for old age.

In 1985, when I commenced the vasectomy programme at Balimo, no one told me that the method might be unacceptable to the men, so I just went on in ignorance and did it. The theoretical objections to being permanently sterilised by an operation have never really surfaced to any extent, and as the message got passed by word of mouth from one satisfied customer to another, it appears that vasectomy has become a completely acceptable and even desirable method of family planning in this area.

In each case the procedure and it's sequellae are explained to the couple in their own language and a consent form is signed by the husband and wife.

METHOD

The operative procedure itself is simple and safe and can easily be taught to doctors and HEO's. It is done painlessly under local anaesthetic and requires only a minimum of instruments. It takes about 10 minutes. A short description and video are available for anyone wanting technical details.

POST OPERATION

The only significant complication we have encountered is a scrotal haematoma. This can be a frightening problem but has been almost completely avoided by a twelve hour period of compulsory bed rest after the operation. The patient is sent home the following day and can return to work immediately.

We do not routinely give antibiotics or analgesics. The skin sutures are removed on the seventh day and the patient is normally not seen again after this.

The only absolute proof of sterility is a negative sperm count six weeks after the vasectomy, but we do not routinely do this because of the logistic difficulties involved. Instead we advise the couple to continue normal sexual relations using alternative contraception. After six weeks or eighteen ejaculations the seminal fluid will be free of spermatazoa, and we are confident that no pregnancies will occur.

DISCUSSION

We have now carried out over two hundred vasectomy procedures since April 1985. Many men are now requesting the operation. In other cases the initiative comes from the nursing staff of the obstetric ward. We suggest, and in some cases strongly advise, the operation where there are four children. We find that it is usually easier to sell the idea to a post partum wife who then talks her husband into it. This obviously works best when there is a strong matriarchal dominance in the society.

The scheme has not been entirely without opponents. Some of the older men, especially those with two or more wives, are naturally highly resistant. A few of the local pastors have also spoken against it and quoted bible verses such as Genesis 9:1, where after the flood, God blessed Noah and his sons and commanded them to be fruitful and fill the earth.

We replied to that by explaining that the command has now been abundantly fulfilled by their fathers, and does not need to be pursued so vigorously. Perhaps of even more importance is the statement in Paul's letter to the Ephesian church, where husbands are commanded to love their wives just as they love their own bodies.

We make a policy of not sterilising single men inspite of receiving some requests. Otherwise our selection criteria are quite loose. Couples with two or more children are eligible, but even couples with less than two children are still eligible when there are medical or other indications.

I cannot provide hard statistical data that the programme is reducing the birth rate at Balimo. The recent census figures will need to be analysed when they are published. We have however seen a levelling off in the number of births at the health centre over the last two years which is a promising sign.

CONCLUSION

In conclusion I present to you the concept of vasectomy as a viable alternative to other methods of fertility control at present in common usage in Papua New Guinea. Because vasectomy is an invasive and slightly more aggressive approach, it is likely to be resisted more by staff than by patients. It needs to be sold to both, and with promotion and commitment, I believe it could become an important part of population control programmes in Papua New Guinea, as it is elsewhere in the world.

STRENGTHENING FAMILY PLANNING PROGRAMMES IN THE SOUTH PACIFIC

JOSEPH SUKWIANOMB[1]

There are many factors that affect the strength of a family planning programme. In this paper I will only highlight a few that we are focusing on at SPAFH. SPAFH is a regional, nongovernmental, nonprofit organisation, that seeks to support the development of quality family health programmes compatible with the culture and customs of the people of the South Pacific. We do not provide health or family planning clinical services, but work to strengthen the provision of these services in the region. We do this by:

* offering technical and financial assistance to member country organisations;
* assisting in raising awareness of population and family planning issues;
* assisting in identifying and developing innovative family health programmes; and
* serving as a resource centre on family health issues for the South Pacific.

SPAFH is staffed by citizens of the South Pacific member nations, which helps SPAFH to effectively identify needs and develop appropriate programmes for the region. The ten current member countries of SPAFH are the Cook Islands, Fiji, Kiribati, Niue, Papua New Guinea, the Solomon Islands, Tonga, Tuvalu, Vanuatu, and Western Samoa. SPAFH hopes to serve additional member countries as funding allows. SPAFH currently receives core support from the United States Agency for International Development, but also receives support from other bilateral donor agencies and private foundations.

SPAFH has identified a few strategies for strenthening family planning programmes in our region, which I will briefly discuss today. These include:

* public education and outreach
* ensuring high quality services
* better programme management
* more grass roots level programming
* increased private sector involvement
* increased male motivation
* governmental support for family planning

[1] Secretary General, The Regional Secretariat of the South Pacific Alliance for Family Health (SPAFH), Tonga

Public Education and Outreach is especially important because many studies as well as our experience show that awareness of the benefits of family planning is very low in our member countries, especially in more rural areas. There is a scarcity of information, education and communications materials, such as family planning brochures, posters, or videos, in the region. The materials that are available are not always culturally appropriate. They may not reflect the methods available in our clinics or they may not be written in our native languages, or the pictures and language used may not be clear and easily understood by our people. This means they are less effective.

Another area that we need to focus on in this region is ensuring that the **services offered are of high quality.** If a potential family planning user receives poor quality care, he or she will not only discontinue using family planning but will probably discourage many others from using family planning. It has been shown by many studies that important service features include:

* low cost
* convenient location
* convenient hours of operation
* short waiting period
* courteous service
* high quality counselling
* confidentiality
* good follow up programme

High quality services will not only attract more new users of family planning, but will help us to keep existing users. Discontinuation rates appear high in this region, and attention to the quality of the services we offer should help in this area.

Better family planning programme management is needed to ensure that quality standards are met, and for other reasons as well. One key need is for programme managers to ensure that accurate family planning clinic records are kept. It is through these records that we can learn which efforts are successful and which are not. Accurate clinic records are also needed for good patient follow up, selecting areas to target for future programming, and evaluating the success of a programme. Family planning data in this region is scarce and good basic record keeping in clinics is essential to improve it. At the national level, good management would include a clear division of labour. Ministries of Health should attempt to clearly define the roles of their family planning personnel to avoid inefficiency.

We also feel that **grass roots or community level programming** can improve family planning use in the South Pacific. Such programmes are usually more sensitive to the actual needs of people. Small grants programmes are often more successful than larger programmes because they fund projects that are designed by the community members themselves in response to their most basic problems. Involving members of the target community in planning and implementing a project almost always improves the effectiveness of the project.

Involving the private sector is another strategy that would help to increase family planning use and effectiveness. There is a definite role for IPPF affiliates, other private clinics, pharmacies, and even businesses to play. Most of the burden of providing family planning services now rests on the public sector. But these days there are more and more demands being placed on public sector resources and the two sectors will need to work together toward the goal of improved health and well being for our people. For example, pharmacies could more actively promote family planning and relieve the public sector of some pressure. Businesses could offer family planning services to their employees along with other basic health care, which would not only result in benefits for the employees but also for the employer. Providing family planning services can help decrease employee turnover and the number of sick days and leave days taken by employees, and it can improve employee productivity, job satisfaction, and community relations.

Male motivation is also needed to strengthen family planning in our area. Males need to be educated about the many benefits of family planning. Their support for family planning is vital. It needs to be made clear that family planning does not go against the traditional role of men, in fact being responsible and caring for the family is a traditional male role. The condom and vasectomy are two excellent family planning methods, and males should be encouraged to <u>use</u> family planning more frequently, in addition to supporting women's use of family planning. We are lucky to have a good model programme to refer to in Kiribati. The Ministry of Health in Kiribati has been quite successful with a national vasectomy programme.

Finally, **government support** is crucial to the success of any national family planning programme. Without governmental commitment, services will be underfunded and unsuccessful. A national population policy and family planning strategy are two important components of this support. We are pleased to note that in recent years two South Pacific countries have been leaders in this area. Both the Solomon Islands and Papua New Guinea have adopted official population policies and are implementing strategies to meet set family planning goals.

To conclude, I would like to mention that we at SPAFH are currently working in many of these areas as a part of our attempt to help strengthen family planning programmes.

*We have supported both the Solomon Islands and Papua New Guinea in their efforts to develop population policies, through financial support to governmental seminars.

*We have recently received funding from AIDAB for a private sector programme, to encourage pharmacies in Fiji to more actively promote family planning. This programme should begin within a few months.

*Over the past few years we have funded over twenty small grass roots family planning projects.

*Several of these projects have supported public education campaigns and the development of IEC materials. We are also currently conducting a programme to collect IEC materials and distribute them to family planning groups so that they can use them as models for developing their own appropriate materials.

*Finally, we are working with clinic managers on such issues as supply management and record keeping through technical assistance visits and training workshops.

I have mentioned just a few ideas on how to improve family planning programmes. Other groups are making great contributions in these and other areas. It is our hope at SPAFH that we can be a part of this important work. If all of the concerned groups work together, I am sure that we can see a great increase in the use of family planning in this region and a corresponding increase in the health and well-being of the people of the South Pacific.

PRIORITIES FOR EMERGING PROBLEMS IN MATERNAL CHILD HEALTH IN PAPUA NEW GUINEA

JOHN BIDDULPH[1]

MATERNAL MORTALITY

The infant mortality rate (deaths in children under 12 months of age per 1000 live births) in Papua New Guinea (PNG) has fallen from approximately 140 in 1970 to about 60 in 1990. No such dramatic fall has occurred in maternal mortality. The maternal mortality ratio (deaths of women from pregnancy related causes per 1000 live births) remains among the highest in the world (1).

Statistics from the UNICEF 1990 Report (2) are shown in Table 1. PNG has a GNP/capita at least double and an infant mortality rate approximately half that of many African countries. Yet PNG's maternal mortality ratio is higher than many of these countries. PNG ranks 70th highest out of 131 countries for infant mortality, 60th highest out of 121 countries for GNP/capita, but 5th highest out of 101 countries for maternal mortality (30 countries did not have a figure given for maternal mortality). Compared to developed countries, PNG has an infant mortality rate less than ten times greater but a maternal mortality ratio at least 100 times greater.

The situation is, in fact, even worse because the maternal mortality ratio only relates to one pregnancy. While a woman in a developed country has a total fertility rate (average number of expected live births per woman) of less than 2, the total fertility rate in PNG is 5.7 (2) which is at least 3 times higher. The risk of maternal death during a woman's lifetime is estimated by multiplying the maternal mortality ratio by the total fertility rate. Table 2, using data from the UNICEF 1990 Report (2), shows that the life time risk of maternal death to a PNG woman is 1 in 20, compared to 1 in 7,000 for an Australian or USA woman. Thus a PNG woman has a 350 times higher risk of maternal death compared to an Australian or USA woman.

[1] Emeritus Professor of Child Health, University of Papua New Guinea. SSMO Child Health, Department of Health, PNG up to 1990. Now retired and lives in Brisbane, Australia

While PNG's infant mortality rate of 57/1000 approximates that of the UK for 1940 (50 years ago), the maternal mortality ratio of 900/100,000 is higher than the UK figure for one hundred years ago - 549/100,000 for 1891-95 (3).

Estimates of maternal mortality ratio in PNG since 1970 have shown little improvement. Table 3 shows the various estimates made (4-8). An estimate of 9/1000 was made by Bell in the early 1970s (9) and also by the UNICEF 1990 report (2) for the period 1980-7. Everett (10) estimated that nearly 90% of babies born in 1985 in Central Province and National Capital District were delivered in Port Moresby General Hospital. Only 6.6% of the nearly 8000 births were unbooked (i.e. had not received any antenatal care). The maternal and perinatal rates were 0.9 and 29 per thousand respectively. She estimated the maternal mortality rate to be about 10 and the perinatal mortality rate to be about 60 per thousand respectively in the rest of Papua New Guinea.

A critical factor affecting maternal mortality is the availability and acceptance of antenatal care. At present only 68% of women who deliver in PNG have received any antenatal care (1). The three essential components of good antenatal care are listed by Everett (10) as follows:

"1. The selection of high-risk women for institutional delivery

2. Prophylaxis for anaemia, malaria and tetanus.

3. The early recognition and correct management of maternal disease and obstetric abnormality".

Everett found that good antenatal care was relatively neglected by maternal child health clinics. Gillett (1) comments "Often antenatal care is superficial and little effort is made to identify high-risk pregnancy women or to persuade them to deliver at hospital or health centre". Yet Lennox (11) found that about 90% of high-risk women can be detected by history alone at one antenatal visit. Clearly the coverage and quality of antenatal care need to be improved if maternal mortality is to be reduced. Studies from all continents have shown that 80% of maternal deaths occur in women who have never received any antenatal care (12).

The risk approach, however, will only succeed if there is an efficient referral system. Credibility in primary health care will be lost if it is not backed up by an efficient referral system. The reduction of maternal mortality requires good antenatal care linked in with a first referral level which can provide the essentials for obstetric emergencies. Life saving obstetric facilities are required as close to people's homes as possible and at the most peripheral level at which they can be undertaken safely and effectively (12).

The essential obstetric functions at the first referral level which are indispensable for the reduction of maternal mortality and morbidity have been detailed by WHO as follows (13):

1. Surgical: caesarean section.

2. Anaesthetic

3. Blood transfusion

4. Medical treatment: for shock, sepsis

5. Manual and assessment functions: manual removal of placenta, vacuum extraction, use of cervicograph.

6. Family Planning: surgical methods

7. Maternity waiting houses.

These essential functions at first referral level require specific skills of health staff, physical facilities, special equipment, essential drugs and supplies. They form a link between good antenatal care delivered by primary health care in the community and the tertiary level of care provided by provincial hospitals with their specialist staff. The first referral level must be adequately supported and supervised by the provincial hospital and its staff. In PNG the first referral level is the health centre. These require urgent upgrading if maternal mortality is to be reduced. Staff at health centres, such as HEOs and midwives, need to be trained to provide competently and safely the necessary obstetric skills. This will need changes in curricula as well as inservice training, changes in regulations, political will and policy commitment. At present health centres are, in almost all cases, totally unable to provide the services required of a first referral centre in terms of maternal survival - caesarean section, safe anaesthesia, cross matching of blood, manual removal of placenta, tubal ligation and a maternity waiting house.

Only 43% of deliveries in PNG receive any medical or nursing supervision (1). Yet the number of women seeking supervised institutional deliveries has risen dramatically over the past thirty years and is the fastest growing area of demand for health services. Admissions to health institutions for obstetric conditions has risen from 6% of total admissions in 1960 to 20% in 1988 (1). Urban and periurban women are flocking to hospitals for delivery. But health centres and subcentres are considerably underutilised. A sample survey of rural health facilities in 1988 found the health centres had only an average of 1.1 deliveries per week, and subcentres only an average of 0.6 deliveries per week (14). Clearly, rural women are not impressed by the obstetric services offered by the health centres. This is not surprising. A quality assessment of health centres and subcentres in 1988 found that almost half of the 71 centres sampled were deficient in basic delivery facilities (no oxytocic drugs readily available or no suction ready or no delivery ward) (15). This study also found that nearly one-third of the centres had not received any clinical supervision in the preceding twelve months, and 20% of centres did not have any chloramphenicol or quinine.

There are isolated instances in PNG where rural health staff have tried to provide some of the essential obstetric functions at a first referral level. An Aidpost Orderly at Kainantu was very skilled at tubal ligations (personal communication, Dr Paul Crouch), some HEOs and nurses have learnt surgical and anaesthetic skills. A maternity waiting house adjacent to Alotau Hospital has even been used successfully for grand multiparous women in Milne Bay (16). The importance of this strategy for reducing maternal mortality is highlighted by Mola and Aitkin's finding that grandmultiparas (para 5 or more) accounted for one-third of maternal deaths (7).

Maternal mortality is exacerbated by low contraceptive use. PNG has poor access to and use of family planning. In 1987 less then 3% of women of childbearing age (15-44 years) were new acceptors of family planning (1). Effective and accessible family planning services are vital to reducing maternal mortality.

In summary, a reduction of the maternal mortality ratio in PNG to a more acceptable level below 5/1000 will require the following:-

1. **Primary health care level:** Increase coverage and quality of antenatal care.

2. **First referral level:** Upgrade facilities and improve quality of care at health centres so that they can provide the essential obstetric functions of a first referral centre.

3. **Provincial hospital level:** Improve support and supervision given to health centres.

4. **Family Planning:** Increase utilisation by making the services more accessible and acceptable to the community.

5. **Community education:** Information and education on all the above.

Fundamental to all the above is political will and policy commitment. Improving the social and economic status of women and increasing the awareness of women's health issues at national, provincial and local levels is also required.

DISABLED CHILDREN

As the infant mortality rate falls to 50/1000 or less there will be increasing community concern for the quality of the survivors and less focus on quantity. The prevalence of major disabilities in PNG has been roughly estimated as 25/1000. The most common disabilities reported in the few surveys done were deafness, blindness and lameness, each at 4/1000 (17).

Deafness is common among children in PNG. One survey found 6% of students in 4 Eastern Highlands high schools had significant hearing loss. A national epidemiological survey indicated that 26/1000 children aged 5-14 years had mild deafness (20-25 decibels hearing loss) and a further 4/1000 had severe deafness (40-50 decibels hearing loss) requiring a hearing aid (18).

Eye problems in PNG affect adults more than children. Only 1.4% of Madang school children had a significant refractive error requiring spectacles (17).

The main causes of lameness in school children are polio, talipes (club foot), trauma and arthritis (17). This disability has decreased in recent years due to polio immunisation.

Mental retardation has only been reported at a rate of 1/1000 in limited surveys done in PNG. From clinical observations as well as world-wide experience that at least 0.1% of the population are severely retarded and a further 0.4% are moderately-mildly retarded, this is a gross underestimate.

It is increasingly accepted that the disabled have the same rights as the rest of the community, but in addition have special requirements. As budget constraints limit the ability of the government to meet these special needs, close co-operation with non-government organisations is essential if these requirements are to be met.

Programmes for the disabled need to be community-based and not institutionalised.

SOCIAL PAEDIATRICS

Certain groups of disadvantaged children will become more evident and require imaginative, low-cost, community-based interventions. These groups will include:

1. **Motherless children.** The rising tide of human immunodeficiency virus (HIV) infection will take its toll of mothers, leaving behind an increasing number of motherless children. Only 30-40% of HIV-infected mothers transmit the infection to their babies either intrauterine or perinatally. Social attitudes to HIV infection may make it difficult to obtain adequate substitute care for these children.

2. **Children whose mothers are in paid employment.** Creches and child minding facilities will be increasingly in demand and will require adequate control.

3. **Children not in school.** The worsening economy in the short term will not improve this situation despite the Government's goal of universal primary education.

4. **Unemployed youth.** Each year a fresh cohort of pushouts from the education system adds to the already swollen ranks of the unemployed youth. This is a socio-political time bomb.

5. **Child victims of accidents,** especially from motor vehicle accidents and industrial pollution.

6. **Victims of child abuse and child sex abuse.** This problem, particularly child sex abuse, is being increasingly recognised in PNG (19).

7. **Teenage prostitution and sexually transmitted diseases including HIV infection.** Increased numbers of unemployed urban youth will inevitably lead to an in crease of this problem.

8. **Drug abuse problems.** The main drugs are tobacco, alcohol and marijuana. Tobacco and alcohol are more deadly but are legal drugs. Marijuana, although less dangerous than either tobacco or alcohol, is an illegal drug. It therefore brings its users into potential contact with criminal elements and into conflict with the law.

In the next few years doctors and other health workers will need to become more vocal advocates for these disadvantaged groups of children.

REFERENCES

1. Gillett J E. The Health of Women in Papua New Guinea, Kristen Press, Madang, 1990

2. UNICEF. The state of the World's Children 1990. UNICEF, New York, 1990.

3. Campbell J M. Maternal Mortality. Reports on Public Health and Medical Subjects No. 25. HM Stationery Office, London, 1924.

4. Johson D G. Maternal mortality in Papua New Guinea. Papua New Guinea Med J 1971; 14: 133-5

5. Babona G, Bird G C, Johnson D G. Maternal mortality in Papua New Guinea 1971-72. Papua New Guinea Med J 1974; 17:331-4.

6. Vacca A, Bird G C. Maternal mortality in Papua New Guinea 1973-75. Papua New Guinea Med J 1977; 20:180-6.

7. Mola G, Aitken I. Maternal mortality in Papua New Guinea 1976-83. Papua New Guinea Med J 1984; 27: 65-71.

8. Mola G. Maternal death in Papua New Guinea 1984-6. Papua New Guinea Med J 1989; 32:27-31.

9. Bell Co. The diseases and health services of Papua New Guinea. Department of Health, Port Moresby, 1973.

10. Everett V J. The M of MCH. Papua New Guinea Med J 1987; 30:121-5.

11. Lennox C E. An action-orientated antenatal card for Papua New Guinea. Papua New Guinea Medical Journal 1981; 24:280-5.

12. Kwast B E. Maternal mortality: levels, causes and promising interventions. J Biosoc Sci., Suppl. 1989; 10:51-67.

13. WHO. Essential obstetric functions at first referral level. Document FHE/86.4. WHO, Geneva, 1986.

14. Mitchell M, Donaldson D, Thomason J. Papua New Guinea rural health services cost study. Boston, Management Sciences for Health, 1988.

15. Garner P, Thomason J, Donaldson D. Quality assessment of health facilities in rural Papua New Guinea. Health Policy and Planning 1990; 5:49-59.

16. Barss P, Blackford C. Grand multiparity. Benefits of a referral program for hospital delivery and postpartum tubal ligation. Papua New Guinea Med J 1985; 28:35-9.

17. Government of Papua New Guinea and UNICEF. An analysis of the situation of children and women in Papua New Guinea. Port Moresby 1987.

18. Vines A P. An epidemiological sample survey of the highlands, mainland and islands regions of the Territory of Papua New Guinea. Department of Public Health, Port Moresby, 1970.

19. Vince J. Child abuse. Papua New Guinea Med J 1990; 33:1-4.

TABLE 1. BASIC DEMOGRAPHIC DATA

COUNTRY	POPULATION (MILLIONS, 1988)	GNP/CAPITA (USA$ 1987)	INFANT MORTALITY RATE (PER 1000, 1985)	MATERNAL MORTALITY RATIO(PER 100,000 1980-7
Sierra Leone	3.9	300	153	450
Burkina Faso	8.5	190	137	810
Niger	6.7	260	134	420
Central African Rep	2.8	370	131	600
Somalia	7.1	290	131	1100
Zambia	7.9	250	79	150
Botswana	1.2	1050	66	250
Papua New Guinea	3.8	700	57	900
USA	245	18500	10	8
UK	57	10400	9	9
Australia	16.5	11000	9	8
Singapore	2.6	8000	9	5
Sweden	8.3	15500	6	5

Source: UNICEF, The State of the World's Children 1990

TABLE 2. LIFETIME RISKS OF MATERNAL DEATH

COUNTRY	MATERNAL MORTALITY RATIO (100,000, 1980-7	TOTAL FERTILITY RATE (1988)	LIFETIME RISK OF MATERNAL DEATH
Sierra Leone	450	6.5	0.029 = 1 in 35
Burkina Faso	810	6.5	0.053 = 1 in 19
Niger	420	7.1	0.030 = 1 in 33
Central African Rep	600	5.9	0.035 = 1 in 29
Somalia	1100	6.6	0.073 = 1 in 14
Zambia	150	7.2	0.011 = 1 in 91
Botswana	250	6.2	0.015 = 1 in 64
Papua New Guinea	900	5.7	0.051 = 1 in 20
USA	8	1.8	0.00014=1 in 7000
UK	9	1.8	0.00016=1 in 6000
Australia	8	1.8	0.00014=1 in 700
Singapore	5	1.6	0.00008=1 in 1200
Sweden	5	1.6	0.00008=1 in 120

Source: UNICEF, The State of the World's Children 1990.

ABLE 3. ESTIMATES OF MATERNAL MORTALITY RATIOS MMR IN PNG SINCE 1970

EAR	AUTHOR	REF	ESTIMATED MMR/1000 BIRTHS			
			URBAN	RURAL	TOTAL	FRACTION REPORTED
70	Johnson	4	2	20	10	1/6
71-2	Babona, Bird Johnson	5	2	7	6	1/4
73-5	Vacca, Bird	6	2	8	7	1/5
76-83	Mola, Aitkin	7	2	20	8	1/10
84-6	Mola	8	2	12	7	1/10

AN ALTERNATIVE TO UNATTENDED DELIVERY - A TRAINING PROGRAMME FOR VILLAGE MIDWIVES IN PAPUA NEW GUINEA

WILLIAM A ALTO[1], RUTH E ALBU[2], GARABINU IRABO[2]

INTRODUCTION

Childbirth is a life crisis that is rarely approached alone. Most societies have included the role of a traditional birth attendant as an assistant to support and care for the labouring mother and newborn infant. However, several language groups in Papua New Guinea are without indigenous birth attendants. The Angal Heneng are one of these groups who still maintain the custom of unattended delivery. Local Angal Heneng women have recently been trained as village midwives and their role has been integrated into their culture, contributing to an improved maternal and perinatal survival.

The Southern Highlands Province is located in the centre of the island of New Guinea. Within the Nipa District of Southern Highlands reside the 30,000 people of the Angal Hengeng language group. They live in scattered hamlets in the intermountain valleys of 1500-1800m elevation. Their houses are constructed of local wood, bark and grasses with an earthen floor and a central firepit. The staple diet consists of sweet potato and greens with occasional pig meat and, for those with a cash income, tinned fish or meat and rice. First contact with Westerners was in 1935, although modern health services did not become available in Nipa until the 1960s.

LOCAL CUSTOMS

Due to cultural prohibitions the Angal Heneng-speaking woman is expected to deliver alone [1]. Woman's blood is considered dangerous and contact with blood is believed to result in illness or death. Other village women are not willing to assist one another in labour or delivery for

1 Saint Mary's Family Practice Residence Program, 233 North Sixth St, Grand Junction, Co. 81501, USA

2 Nipa Health Centre, Nipa, Southern Highlands Province, Papua New Guinea

fear of becoming contaminated. Conception and pregnancy are forbidden topics of discussion between men and women and a source of embarrassment even between women themselves. Congenital defects are believed due to a cultural infraction by the mother, and twins are often attributed to maternal adultery. Infanticide has been practiced rather than returning in shame to the village with such infants.

When confinement draws near, the husband builds a small delivery hut in a nearby garden. As labour commences, the parturient retires alone to this hut to await delivery. Custom allows another woman to call out to her but not to actually enter the delivery hut. Only after one or two days of unsuccessful labour might a decision be reached by the village women to seek assistance at a health centre. The husband may assist in arranging transportation but rarely accompanies his wife to the health facility.

MATERNAL HEALTH SERVICES

Through the efforts of the local churches and the Division of Health, the percentage of Angal Heneng women who attended antenatal clinic at least once during their pregnancy has increased from 73% in 1979 [2] to 98% [3], although many women visit only a single time in the second trimester to have the pregnancy medically confirmed. The percentage of deliveries that are supervised in the health centre has increased from 35 to 45% over this same time period [2, 3]. A number of measures have been instituted to increase the rate of supervised deliveries. A traditional bush material house and garden have been provided at Nipa Health Centre for high risk women to live in while they await delivery. Around-the-clock transport to the health centre is offered to any woman in labour. Women who deliver their infants at the health centre or who are supervised by a village midwife receive a free 'road to health' book and birth certificate. Those who deliver their infants in the village in the traditional manner are required to purchase the book and certificate.

This improvement in antenatal coverage has approached the maximum contact the health service can establish with the pregnant population because of the remoteness of the region and the scarcity of roads. Prior to 1985, 25% of all Angal Heneng women lived within a one hour walk from the health centre [3] at Nipa; this figure improved to 31% in that year with the opening of a new health facility at Karinja. A one hour walk is believed the longest a labouring woman might undertake, although it is unlikely that even this distance would be attempted after dark. Expectant women are reluctant to be admitted to the health centre prior to the onset of labour because of their responsibilities at their homes and gardens. The 17 aidposts in the area serve out-patients exclusively and are staffed by male orderlies which renders them culturally inaccessible for obstetrical care even in an emergency. Thus for many, culture and distance combine to limit access to a supervised delivery. It is because of these constraints to supervised delivery and the subsequently high maternal and perinatal morbidity and mortality that a village midwife programme was started in 1981 at Nipa Health Centre.

The maternal mortality rate for the Angal Heneng is unknown, but the Huli language group with whom they share a common border had a maternal mortality of 4.6/1000 during the period from 1977 to 1983 [4]. The Huli culture encourages delivery in a health facility and a majority of their births are supervised so that it is unlikely that the maternal mortality of the Angal Heneng is considerably lower. There were no Huli village midwives in the study area over this time period. In the Southern Highlands Province, maternal mortality was reported as 9.0/1000 in 1984 [5] and 15.6/1000 in 1986 [6]. However, communication of maternal deaths to health officials is sporadic and incomplete, and the actual figures are probably much higher. About 50% of all maternal deaths in Papua New Guinea have been reported to be due to haemorrhage or sepsis [7].

Infant mortality was reported as 116/1000 in the Southern Highlands Province in 1980 [8] which was the highest in all of Papua New Guinea, and it was estimated to be 68/1000 in 1986 [9]. The infant mortality rate among the Angal Heneng language group's area is unavailable for 1980 and was estimated as 62.3/1000 in 1986 [9] using the method of determining the survival of previous infant at the time of birth registration and life tables [10]. No accurate data are available concerning perinatal or maternal morbidity of the Angal Heneng.

Because of the inability of the government and church health services to further extend maternal child health services to this remote population, a village midwife training programme was restarted in 1986 after a lapse of 5 years. The programme was based on a pilot project conducted in 1981 that trained the initial four Angal Heneng village midwives. Funding was provided in part by the Asian Development Bank Rural Health Improvement Loan II which purchased a vehicle and paid the salaries of its driver and a village midwife tutor. The total grant for the 5 year programme was 70,000 U.S. dollars.

METHODS

Beginning in 1981 and continuing through 1989, 32 Angal Heneng women have received instruction as village midwives (VMW) at Nipa Health Centre (Table 1). The 1981 class were midwives number 1-4 while the others were trained during the years 1986-1989. As is the traditional custom, they were chosen as VMW candidates by the men of their community after discussion with the midwife trainer. The would-be students were enrolled into the course only after the local men had built a delivery house with a pit latrine and rubbish hole. None of the women had more than a grade 6 education and most were illiterate. Only older women with several children were accepted for training. For the most part, the VMWs were the wives of indigenous pastors, headmen or health workers. They undertook their studies and conducted their work as a Christian duty to serve the women of their village and relied on their faith to overcome the traditional taboo against becoming soiled by women's blood. All of the VMWs were unpaid by the Health Department.

The curriculum of the course has been described previously [11] and is briefly presented here. During a 4-week course, VMW students were instructed in basic anatomy, the normal progression of pregnancy and how to determine foetal lie. Each student conducted five normal deliveries and had the opportunity to observe several complicated deliveries. They were taught what is an appropriate obstetrical referral. All women that are nulliparous, grand multiparous, non-cephalic lies, in premature labour, have multiple pregnancies and those with previous obstetrical complications were to be sent to the health centre for delivery. Umbilical cord care and general hygiene and sanitation were also included in the course syllabus. The teaching was non-formal in style and much of the curriculum was taught through plays and skits rather than classroom lectures. The utilization of these teaching techniques avoided the student embarrassment that would have resulted from a more direct discussion of reproductive function. The students lived in a traditional house on the health centre grounds and were on call and available for all deliveries.

A delivery kit consisting of a sharp knife, cotton cord ties, gentian violet for umbilical cord care and ergometrine tablets were supplied. New banana leaves provided a clean delivery area and moss was used as surgical sponges. A fire or a kerosene lamp furnished light.

Supervision of the VMWs is carried out at monthly MCH clinic sites by the neighbouring health centre clinic sisters. They reviewed the past obstetrical history of potential VMW clients and together they examine the antenatal women. The nurses also conduct a verbal history of the VMW's recent deliveries and record them in a permanent record book that is kept by the VMW as well as on the routine Department of Health reporting forms. The VMW tutor visits the VMW at her delivery house at 1,2,6 and 12 months after completion of the training course and then again at 6-12 month intervals thereafter or whenever the need arises. In addition a yearly one week inservice training course is held for all the VMWs. The tutor also maintains contact with the male leaders of the village, encourages their continued support and intervenes on behalf of the VMW if necessary.

Remuneration to the VMW is primarily through an increase in status within the community, although food or firewood are often offered by the patient. The VMWs also receive a tin of fish and a bar of soap, or similar pay, for their assistance at the MCH clinics.

RESULTS

Deliveries and referrals

During the period 1981 through 1987 there were 254 deliveries supervised by 3 VMWs with no maternal deaths (Table 1). At least 10 of these deliveries were of primigravida, and an unknown number were grand multiparous women who went to the village midwife rather than risk a long walk to a health centre and a possible delivery enroute. Thus, although an effort was made by the MCH-VMW team to deliver all 'high risk' parturients at the health centre, this proved impossible due to distance and the woman's preference.

In 1987, the first year complete data was collected, 23 VMWs supervised the deliveries of 121 infants. Eighteen antenatal referrals (12.9%) of high risk women were sent to the health centre from a total of 139 VMW clients. Details of the reasons for referral are shown in Table 2. There were no deaths among these antenatal women or of an additional 4 postpartum women who were also referred. VMWs attended 121/429 (28%) of all supervised deliveries in 1987, or 121/838 (14%) of all deliveries.

Table 1. Deliveries supervised by Angal Heneng village midwives

Midwife number	Village	Date trained	Deliveries through 1986	1987	1988	1989	Total	Still Births
1	Songura	1981	112	14	15	6 "	147	0
2	Kanj	1981	91+	3	3	0 "	97	2
3	Obal	1981	49	3	4	4 "	60	0
4	Hebinja	1981	0#	0	0	0	0	0
5	Semin	1986	0	5	3	6	14	0
6	Semin	1986	0	11	15	6	32	0
7	Semin	1986	0	11	4	6	21	1
8	Tegipo	1986	0	8	1	0*	9	0
9	Montanda	1987	-	2	4	0*	6	1
10	Ungubi	1986	0	5	5	4	14	0
11	Ungubi	1986	0	6	9	4	19	1
12	Ungubi	1986	0	6	5	3	14	0
13	Haralenja	1987	-	2	6	4	12	0
14	Haralenja	1987	-	2	4	4	10	0
15	Ingin	1986	0	3	4	2	9	0
16	Ingin	1986	0	1	5	2	8	0
17	Suma	1987	-	0	11	3	14	0
18	Sekib Te	1987	-	14	13	5	32	1
19	uma	1987	-	0	6	2	8	0
20	Lloab	1986	0	2	1	4	7	0
21	Solbaem	1986	2	6	8	1	17	0
22	Kabendaka	1986	0	9	6	4	19	0
23	Imilhoma	1987	-	3	6	9	18	0
24	Tiwao	1987	-	3	10	5	18	0
25	Sumbi	1987	-	1&	2&	0&	3	0
26	Sumbi	1987	-	1&	1&	0&	2	0
27	Salenda	1987	-	0	2	1	3	0
28	Salenda	1987	-	0	1	2	3	1
29	Songura	1989	-	-	-	3	3	0
30	Obal	1989	-	-	-	3	3	0
31	Wara Wagi	1989	-	-	-	1	1	0
32	Wara Wagi	1989	-	-	-	0	0	0
Total VMW-supervised deliveries			254	121	154	94	623	7
Estimated Angal Heneng births				838	856	875		
Percentage of births supervised by VMWs				14%	18%	11%		

*Resigned, no village support, still evaluating and referring women.
+Employed at Karinja Health Subcentre
#Resigned, no support by husband.
&Tribal warfare in area.
"Retired and replaced by younger VMW.

Table 2. Reasons for referral by all Angal Heneng village midwives in 1987 and 1989 and by village midwives from the Nipa Health Centre Area in 1988

	1987	1988	1989
Antenatals:			
Nulliparity	4	7	13
Grand multiparity	11	9	17
Medical illness with pregnancy:			
Anaemia	1	1	1
Malaria	0	1	0
Pneumonia	1	1	0
Complications of pregnancy:			
Twins	0	1	0
Oedema	1	1	0
Previous delivery with retained placenta	0	1	0
Complications of labour and delivery:			
Retained placenta	1	1	0
Premature labour	0	1	0
Postpartum haemorrhage	0	2	0
Perineal tears	0	2	0
Prolonged labour	1	1	1
Postpartum fever	4	0	0
Other	0	0	2
Gynaecological:			
Threatened abortion	0	2	2
Incomplete abortion	0	0	1
Total:	24	41	37

Table 3. Mortality rates of the Huli People (Tari) compared with the Angal Heneng village midwife-supervised deliveries.

	Tari 1984*	Angal Heneng-VMW 1981-1989
Stillbirth rate	16.3/1000	11.2/1000
Neonatal mortality	19.4/1000	4.8/1000
Perinatal mortality	31.0/1000	12.8/1000
Maternal mortality	4.6/1000	1.6/1000

*59.5% of all deliveries attended by a health worker.

In 1988 there were 27 VMWs in independent practice, another was employed at Karinja health subcentre, and one was inactive. Detail of the numbers of supervised deliveries in that year are presented in Table 1. Midwife number 4 never practiced in her village. She had been chosen by her village headmen while her husband was away and when he later returned he forbid her working. Midwives 25 and 26 lived in an area that was engulfed by tribal fighting late in 1987, and their houses and gardens were destroyed as was the local school and health aidpost. The people affected moved off to the bush, and all government services have ceased since then. In 1988 the reporting of referrals and delivery complications was available only for the Nipa Health Centre administered VMWs (numbers 5-19). These 16 VMWs referred 41 antenatal or postpartum women. Thirty-two of these were antenatal complications or high risk patients; 7 were complications of labour or delivery; and 2 were threatened abortions. The reasons for referral to the health centre are listed in Table 2. There was one maternal death of a woman from the Nipa area as a result of a postpartum haemorrhage. The VMW who was helping the haemorrhaging woman was unable to find transport to carry her to the health centre. This was the only maternal death of a VMW-supervised delivery since the programme's inception. Seven other women, out of a total of 155 (4.5%) women in labour, required referral to a health centre for peripartum complications. Village midwives attended 26% of all supervised deliveries and 18% of an estimated 856 total deliveries in 1988.

In 1989 the number of supervised deliveries declined to 94 or an estimated 10.7% of all Angal Heneng deliveries. There were 37 maternal referrals and no maternal deaths. Twenty-five VMWs were supervising village deliveries, 2 VMWs were only evaluating and referring pregnant women, and the 3 older VMWs trained in 1981 retired after 10 years of service. Two of the three retirees were replaced by recently-trained VMWs from the same area.

The maternal mortality of the first 623 VMW-supervised deliveries over the period 1981-1989 was 1.6/1000 compared to 4.6/1000 in Tari in 1984 (4). Each midwife who ever practiced has averaged 5.7 deliveries per year of service.

Perinatal complications

Two stillbirths and no neonatal deaths of VMW-supervised deliveries were recorded prior to 1987. In that year there were 1 macerated stillbirth and 2 obstructed breech presentations that sought assistance too late with dead foetuses.

Neonatal complications occurred in 5 of 166 (3.0%) VMW-supervised deliveries from the Nipa Health Centre area in 1988 (midwives 5-19, Table 1). There was 1 premature infant that died shortly after birth and 1 stillbirth. A second premature infant died at 2 weeks of age of an unkwown cause. Two neonates received respiratory resuscitation by a VMW and survived. Karinja Health Subcentre and the other VMWs reported perinatal and neonatal mortalities of zero in 1988.

In 1989 there were 1 neonatal death of a premature infant and 1 stillbirth of all VMW-supervised deliveries. Table 3 presents the comparison between the mortality rates from the 1981-1989 VMW-supervised deliveries with that reported in 1984 for all health centre and unsupervised village deliveries occurring in the neighbouring Tari Basin (4). The two groups are not identical, as the majority of the VMW-supervised deliveries were from a low risk maternal group. Therefore the results cannot be compared statistically. The difference between the neonatal mortality rate in the Tari Basin and the lower rate of the VMW infants is considerable. The perinatal mortality rate is also lower for the VMW-supervised deliveries in comparison with the Huli. Table 4 shows the comparison between infant mortality rates between the Tari Valley (Huli language) with that of the Angal Heneng group. The Angal Heneng have a lower infant mortality rate.

Table 4. Estimated infant mortality in the Tari District and in the Angal Heneng Linguistic group in 1986*

Tari	Angal Heneng
83.7/1000 n = 942	62.3/1000+ n = 757

*Using method of Hill and Macrae (10) and Coale and Demeny life tables of the West model.

+Chi squares = 5.99; P = 0.01437.

DISCUSSION

Despite customary prohibitions, it has been possible to train village midwives to provide obstetrical services in a remote part of Papua New Guinea where there was previously no cultural role of traditional birth attendant. Extensive preliminary health education of village headmen and careful selection of VMW trainees has allowed the development of an accepted and accessible maternity service to women who would otherwise have delivered their infants unattended. Of greater significance has been the relative safety of VMW-supervised deliveries both to the mother and her newborn. The single maternal death that occurred in 1988 might have been prevented had the delivery occurred at a health centre that had transport available. Nipa Health Centre is one and one-half hours by road from the Provincial Hospital at Mendi where transfusion services are regularly available. However, as the woman who died was at low risk for perinatal complications and she lived a considerable distance from a health centre, it is likely that she would have delivered in the traditional manner and died alone.

The neonatal mortality rate of infants delivered of mothers under the care of VMWs is less than that in Tari, a well studied and adjacent area; and there was a lower perinatal mortality rate among the infants of VMW-supervised deliveries. Although the VMWs cannot be solely credited with the lower infant mortality rate among the Angal Heneng people compared with that of their neighbours, these better MCH health indicators are of considerable interest. Perhaps the community support of the VMWs is a reflection of greater health consciousness of the Angal Heneng as compared to the Huli. In other health and social-economic indicators the two groups are similar.

Access to health services is better among the Huli than in the Nipa area. Nutritional status of Huli children is superior to those in the Nipa District (3), which has one of the most serious malnutrition problems in the nation. Maternal education levels, birth spacing and per capita income are approximately equal in both areas where subsistence agriculture is universal and small coffee gardens provide a small cash income. A majority (86.7% in 1987) of Huli women deliver in a health centre or hospital compared with the Angal Heneng (64.0% in 1987). The percentage of women of childbearing age that use artificial methods of contraception is similar in each area and less than 7% (3). Antenatal clinic registration is nearly 100% in both groups but attendance after the first visit is equally poor averaging 2.3 additional attendances per woman in Tari and 1.2 in the Nipa area in 1987 (3).

The maternal and infant health of the Angal Heneng appears to be superior to that of its neighbours, the Huli, although there are differences between the two populations studied. The reasons for this difference are uncertain, but the village midwives have probably contributed to the reduced mortality by encouraging antenatal care, referring high risk pregnancies to deliver in health facilities, and providing delivery services for women who are too distant from health centres. The VMWs are believed to have contributed to the improved neonatal survival and have enhanced attendance of infants and children at MCH clinics.

Although the number of VMW-attended deliveries is small and the women they serve are in a relatively low risk group, there would have been at least 2 maternal and 19 neonatal deaths expected (using Tari Research Unit's maternal and neonatal mortality rates) rather than the 1 or 3 observed. Frequent supervisory visits and inservice training along with VMW-MCH clinic staff cooperation have allowed identification of women with potentially high risk deliveries and facilitated timely referral to a health centre. This teamwork has contributed to the relative safety of a VMW-supervised birth.

The programme has been enthusiastically supported by most of the communities and a waiting list of villages and their trainees has developed. Only two women have stopped providing midwifery services because of the loss of village support although this continues to be a hindrance to another VMW (No. 15). Two other VMWs have curtailed their services because of a prolonged tribal war in their area. The Kanj VMW (No. 2) was offered employment at Karinja Health Subcentre after it opened near her village in 1985. The deliveries she conducted at the health centre were not counted as VMW-supervised although she also continued to attend a few deliveries outside the health centre. Three VMWs have retired after 9 years of service having supervisied 304 deliveries in all.

Four community councils have offered cash financial support to their midwives. Other VMWs are rewarded directly by their clients. It is surprising that the VMWs who have been paid have supervised 4.7 deliveries per year as compared with the 7.3 deliveries per year conducted by the midwives who did not receive any form of payment. The increase in social status and doing one's Christian duty appear to be the motivating force behind these women. No midwife has been approached to pay compensation for a delivery-related complication. The attrition rate of the VMWs for all causes has been 8 of 32 (25%).

Over 80 VMWs are now working among 8 different language groups in the Southern Highlands (11). They have been trained in Nipa and Tari by two VMW tutors and two assistants and at a third ad hoc programme in the Koroba District. Several other VMW training courses are currently in operation in Papua New Guinea including one in Morobe Province (12) while other programmes are in the planning stages.

CONCLUSION

In rural areas of the less developed countries of the world, health services are often inadequate because of financial constraints and inaccessibility of the people to health facilities. In many societies, the traditional birth attendant fills this gap in the provision of maternal-child health care. There was no cultural role for the TBA in the Angal Heneng community, and the village midwife has now filled this void. The VMW's geographic accessibility in the village and their sharing of the same cultural orientation as their clients have permitted their easy integration into the birth practices of the women. Their presence has contributed to the increased number of supervised births and is believed to have contributed to the decreased neonatal and infant mortality of the Angal Heneng.

Acknowledgement

We wish to thank Sr Elsie Schlatter at Karinja Health Subcentre for her assistance in providing follow-up information on the village midwives.

REFERENCES

1. Townsend P K. Traditional birth attendants in Papua New Guinea. IASER Discussion Paper No. 52, p. 21. Papua New Guinea Institute of Applied Social and Economic Research, Boroko, Papua New Guinea, 1985.

2. Clark L. Extracts from the Southern Highlands Province official briefing paper 1979. For the SHP Rural Development Project. Mimeograph, Division of Health, Mendi, Southern Highlands, Papua New Guinea.

3. Division of Health Annual Report 1987. Provincial Printer, Mendi, Southern Highlands, Papua New Guinea.

4. Lehman D. Summary of Financial Report, Tari Research Unit. Provincial Printer, Mendi, Southern Highlands, Papua New Guinea, Nov. 1984.

5. Division of Health Annual Report 1984. Provincial Printer, Mendi, Southern Highlands, Papua New Guinea.

6. Division of Health Annual Report 1986. Provincial Printer, Mendi, Southern Highlands, Papua New Guinea.

7. Mola G and Aitken I. Maternal morbidity in Papua New Guinea. Papua New Guinea med J. 1984 27, 65.

8. National Statistical Office. 1980 Census, Government Printing Office, Port Moresby, Papua New Guinea.

9. Prybylski D. Division of Health, Mendi, SHP. Personal communication.

10. Hill A G and Macraè S. Measuring childhood mortality levels: a new approach. UNICEF Soc. Statist. Bull. 1985 8, 1.

11. Albu R and Alto W. Training of village midwives in the Southern Highlands Province. Papua New Guinea med. J. 1989 32, 89-95.

12. Schumacher E. Village midwife training on the Huon Peninsula. Papua New Guinea med. J. 1987 30, 213.

BOOKED AND UNBOOKED MOTHERS DELIVERED AT PORT MORESBY GENERAL HOSPITAL: A RANDOMISED CASE CONTROL STUDY OF THEIR SOCIODEMOGRAPHIC AND REPRODUCTIVE CHARACTERISTICS

CECIL A. KLUFIO[1]
GRACE KARIWIGA[2]

It is well known that antenatal care is good for the mother and for her baby. A woman who does not attend for antenatal care in her pregnancy is more likely to suffer serious complications during her pregnancy and delivery than a woman who attends (1,2,3). Some of these complications may kill the baby or the mother. It is also known that when we look at women with the same number of deliveries, the more antenatal visits a woman makes, the higher the chances of survival for her baby (1,4). These observations are especially true for deprived communities and for the developing world where pregnant women suffer from conditions or circumstances which increase their chances of complications. Antenatal visits also give us the opportunity to teach women about family health.

The Port Moresby General Hospital (PMGH) delivers around 8,000 women a year. About 500 (6%) of these are women who never attended for antenatal care in the index pregnancy. These unbooked mothers have a perinatal death rate (stillbirths & 1st week deaths) per 1000 total deliveries (ie. livebirths and stillbirths) which is four times higher than that of mothers who attended antenatal clinics. For example, for the year 1989, the perinatal death rate (PNDR) was 20/1000 deliveries for the booked as against 82/1000 for the unbooked.

The aim of the study was to find out if women who do not attend are different from the attendants in some selected characteristics. For the purpose of this study we defined an "unbooked" patient as one who never attended for antenatal care in the index pregnancy; and a "booked" patient as one who attended at least three times, the first attendance being at less than thirty weeks pregnant.

The labour ward nursing staff record the particulars of all patients in the labour ward register in the chronological order in which the patients were delivered. Each morning during the period of the study, the researchers consulted the labour ward register and noted the names and parities of the cases. For each case, the control was the first booked patient of the same parity as the case, to deliver after the

[1] Professor of Obstetrics and Gynaecology, Medical Faculty, University of Papua New Guinea.

[2] Registrar, Obstetrics and Gynaecology, Port Moresby General Hospital

case. To assess the influence of parity, the cases were compared with all patients delivered in 1989. This was a case-control survey of 136 unbooked mothers (cases) and 136 parity-matched controls, delivered at the PMGH between December 1989 and April 1990. A pretested questionnaire was administered to each subject after her delivery and before her discharge from the hospital. The chi square test was used to determine the significance of differences between the groups.

The results are summarized in Tables 1-4:

AGE: (Table 1). There was a significant difference between the cases and controls when age groups were compared. The unbooked were more likely to be under 20 years i.e. adolescents.

EDUCATION (Table 1). This was measured as the total number of education years completed.

PATIENTS' EDUCATION: The mean was 5.8 years (st dev 3.6) for the booked as against 4.6 (st dev. 3.4) for the unbooked. The difference between the means (1.2 years) was three times the standard error and therefore significant. When categorized as shown in the table the difference was just significant (p=0.0491).

HUSBANDS' EDUCATION: On the other hand, for the husbands, the differences between the means (8.3 vs 6.6) and the categories were both highly significant.

SOCIAL CLASS (Table 1). This was scored as a composite variable using the following: area of residence, type of house, ownership of house, occupation of husband, whether the husband was employed, and sum of education years of the patient and her husband. As the table shows the unbooked were more likely to belong to a lower social class.

CLINIC ATTENDANCE IN PENULTIMATE PREGNANCY (Table 1). The difference between the two groups was significant.

The following variables which had been found to be of significance in other studies, or which we thought should make a difference, were not found to be so in this study (Tables 1-4): previous perinatal death; distance between present residence and nearest clinic; patients' impression of clinic attended in penultimate pregnancy; and women's appreciation of the benefits of antenatal care (5,6, 7, 8). There was no significant difference in marital status between the groups. The numbers of "not currently married" in the booked and unbooked were 5 and 7 respectively.

PARITY (Table 4). When the cases were compared with the 1989 deliveries, significantly more of the unbooked were found to be para 5 or higher (18.4% vs 7.9%; p<.005).

COMMENTS

The results of this study identify the following important factors: maternal age under 20 years, social class, attendance in previous pregnancy, husband's education, and high parity. Patient's education deserves comment. The difference between the means was significant at the 95% confidence level whereas when categories were compared, it was just significant. We considered the categories more useful than the means as a few women with university education in one group could unduly influence the mean. The high significance of the husband's education is important. It is not surprising in a male-dominated society such as ours. Although we tested formal education, we think that it is the husband's appreciation of the importance of antenatal care which is the determinant. Educating husbands, whether they are literate or not, on the benefits of antenatal care should achieve the same result. The implication is clear. As in the case of family planning, to promote antenatal care we must educate our men about its importance.

It is an objective of the 1991-1995 National Health Plan to increase the number of pregnant women attending antenatal clinics three or more times as a proportion of all pregnant women to 60% by 1995 (9). We may need to take the findings of this study into consideration in our strategies.

REFERENCES

1. Janowitz B, Lewis JA, Burton N, Lamptey P. Reproductive Health in Africa: Issues and Options. Family Health International NC U.S.A. 1984:64

2. Gortmaker S L. The effects of prenatal care upon the health of the newborn. Am J Public Health 1979; 69: 653.

3. Greenberg R S. The impact of prenatal care in different social groups. Am J Obstet Gynecol 1983; 145: 797.

4. Caldwell P, Caldwell J C. "The function of Child-spacing in Traditional Societies and the Direction of Change." In: Page and Lesthaeghe (eds), Child-spacing in Tropical Africa: Traditions and Change. London: Academic Press, 1981.

5. Ray S K, Mukhopadhyay B B, Das R, Ganguly M M, Mandal A, Roy S C. Extent of utilization of maternity care services of PHC by the families of a rural area. Indian J Public Health, 1984; 3: 122.

6. Abbas A A, Walker G J A. Determinants of the utilization of maternal and child health services in Jordan. Int J Epidem. 1986; 15:404.

7. Wong EI, Popkin B M, Guilkey D K, Akin J S. Accessibility, quality of care and prenatal care use in the Philippines. Social Science and Medicine 1987; 24: 927.

8. Williams C D, Baumslag N, Jelliffe D B. Mother and Child Health: delivering the services. 2nd ed. London, Oxford University Press, 1985: 316.

9. Department of Health. Papua New Guinea National Health Plan 1991-1995. Department of Health 1991.

Table 1. Selected Characteristics of Mothers.

Characteristic	Booked	Unbooked	Chi sq	p value
Age Group:				
< 20	8	23		
20-24	54	49		
25-29	38	27		
30-34	25	23		
35+	11	14		
Total	136	136	9.806	<.05
Age Group:				
< 20	8	23		
> 20	128	113		
Total	136	136	8.192	<.005
Education of patient in school years completed:				
0	25	37		
1-3	11	16		
4-6	51	53		
7+	49	30		
Total	136	136	7.857	=.0491
Education of husbands in school years completed:				
0	11	31		
1-3	4	10		
4-6	30	37		
7-10	68	42		
11+	17	12		
Total	130*	132**	19.820	<.005
*Dont know=6	**Dont know=4			
Social Class:				
High	11	13		
Middle	63	34		
Low	62	89		
Total	136	136	13.665	<.005
Antenatal clinic attendance in last pregnancy:				
Attended	86	69		
Did not attend	11	28		
Total	97*	97*	9.275	<.005
*Number of para 0 in each group=39				
Previous Perinatal Death (PND):				
Previous PND*	9	7		
No previous PND	88	90		
Total	97	97	.272	Not significant
*PND = stillbirth or first week neonatal death.				

Table 2. Distance between present Residence and nearest Clinic.

Distance	30min walk	15min PMV**	16-60min PMV	60min+ PMV
Booked	50	35	30	21
Unbooked	43	40	22	31

* Distance measured in travelling time between clinic and residence.

**Privately owned motor vehicle for mass transit.

CHI-SQ. = 0.14 DF = 3   Not significant.

Table 3. Patient's impression of clinic attended in penultimate pregnancy.

Characteristic	Booked	Unbooked	Chi sq	p value
Assessment of waiting time at clinic before being attended to:				
Short	9	7		
Reasonable	42	39		
Too long	31	23		
Total	82*	69	.45	Not Significant.
*Dont know=4				
Was clinic of benefit?				
Useful	71	56		
Not useful	10	7		
Total	81*	63**	.052	Not significant.
*Dont know=5	**Dont know=6			
Did patient like clinic?				
Yes	73	58		
No	11	9		
Total	84*	67*	.004	Not significant.
*Dont know=2.				

Table 4 Parity of Cases compared with 1989 Deliveries

Parity	1989 deliveries	Unbooked
0	2265	39
1-4	4923	72
5 & higher	613	25

Chi square = 20.620 df=2 p<.005. Significant.

THE NEED FOR VILLAGE MIDWIVES

A POLICY FOR RURAL SOCIAL DEVELOPMENT

FRANK SCHOFIELD[1]

Recent documents and publications, and Jane Thomason's careful analysis yesterday and John Biddulph's today show that the indicators for maternal care and protection of the newborn in rural Papua New Guinea are all static or in some respects are worsening. These include:-

- Social indicators, the utilization rates of pre- and postnatal delivery and family planning services.
- Service indicators, such as geographical coverage at a defined standard.
- Economic indicators, such as the ratio of unit output work to resource input costs; and
- Epidemiological indicators, such as estimates of rural maternal death rates. (The much more sensitive perinatal and neonatal death rates are not yet being measured, which in itself indicates a big gap between the basic MCH services and rural mothers.)

These inevitable problems of basic health services have caused many other countries to adopt the Primary Health Care (PHC) strategy. But in spite of such manifest problems there appear nevertheless in PNG to be donor-driven MCH Projects which hope over the next five years greatly to improve provincial rural basic MCH services cost effectiveness, and simultaneously to recruit enough rural couples into the National Family Planning Programme to begin to have a significant effect.

Before they can accept these hopes as feasible of achievement, realistic health planners and policy-makers in duty bound must ask "where is there any other country in the world which lacked rural primary health care, as rural PNG still does, and yet was able to achieve these rural goals?"

The answer is certain: there are none.

1 Visiting Professor of Community Medicine, Medical Faculty, University of Papua New Guinea

Policy in PNG seems confused on this most important issue, as shown by the nomenclature now in use. Entirely "top-down" basic health services are being labelled as "Primary Health Care"; and a cadre of government-paid health workers are, very misleadingly, being called "Community Health Workers" although they are not controlled or supported by Communities.

Let us look again at the unequivocal definitions of PHC laid down at Alma Ata in 1978 by the governments of PNG and 133 other countries, plus UNICEF and WHO: Extracts are quoted:

> "The people have the right and duty to participate individually and collectively in the planning and implementation of their health care"
>
> "PHC is essential health care based on socially acceptable methods made universally accessible to individuals and families in the community through their full participation and at a cost the community can afford"..."It brings health care as close as possible to where people live"...."It includes maternal and child health care and family planning".
>
> "PHC evolves from the economic, socio-cultural and political characteristics of the country and of its communities,"..."It requires and promotes maximum community and individual self-reliance and participation in the planning, organization, operation and control of PHC, making fullest use of local and other available resources".

SOME COUNTRIES' EXPERIENCES OF TRAINING TRADITIONAL BIRTH ATTENDANTS (TBAS) AND/OR <u>COMMUNITY MIDWIVES</u> DE NOVO

SUDAN	FIRST: IN 1920S. Very successful socially; on MM & IM. independent of Government except for training, "Refresher" & Certification.
PAKISTAN	Midwives gone "Private", with "Dais", now serve 83% of all pregnancies.
PHILIPPINES	"Barangay" midwives & trained "Hilot". Variable success: M.M. 1-4 per 1,000 LBs F.P. variable.
VIETNAM	"Sage Femme". No training for the last 15-20 years.
CAMBODIA	Ignored by Governments. Do 85% of rural prenatal care and deliveries, all alone.
THAILAND	"Mohtamyae" trained. Very successful on MM; TM; IM and with Family Planning; helped by the "Village Health Communicator".
MALAYSIA (Peninsula)	"Bidan Kampong" trained. Did 95% of prenatal care, 57% of deliveries in 1970's.

BANGLADESH 1979-82

"Almost all the births in rural Bangladesh are attended by untrained Birth Attendants - neighbours or mothers-in-law".

Exp:Gp. "Train Villagers as TBAs"		Control Gp "No Villagers Trained"
No of deliveries	713	998
Median age	25.9yrs	25.5yrs
Median no. children living	1.69	1.86
Previous pregnancies/ mother	3.35	3.72
"Pregnancy wastage"	1.66	1.86
Median age last child	1.38	1.92
Deaths B.I.) Neonatal + R.D.S)	7.02*	25.05/1,000 live birth
N.Tetanus - "	5.61*	24.24 " "
Resp: Infection - "	5.61*	17.03 " "
All Causes - "	23.84*	85.17 " "

*All statistics significant at 5% level

THREE ESSENTIAL SOCIAL CONDITIONS FOR EFFECTIVE RURAL COMMUNITY MIDWIFERY

1. She must be married, living in the Community and preferably has children of her own.

2. She is chosen for training by her future clients, the mothers in her community.

3. She is economically supported by her clients' families and by her community.

TWO MODERN ADMINISTRATIVE CONDITIONS

4. Her essential supplies must reach her community independently of the Basic Health Services' supply system.

5. Her community must agree to pay the transport costs of any patient she refers to her nearest competent obstetric service.

TWO MODERN PROFESSIONAL CONDITIONS

6. She must be trained well enough to recognize high risk pregnancies in good time, and should receive official certification.

7. She should be given professional advice and encouragement at least once a year by a senior professional visitor from the nearest competent obstetric service who has also obtained "feedback" from the community on her performance and on its unmet perceived needs in MCH.

How is a successful community midwife professional initiated by rural populations? The process consists of three continuous stages: Community diagnosis, community participation and organization, and community and local health planning, as outlined below:

1. **COMMUNITY DIAGNOSIS** (S. Kark) is a bottom-upwards, community self-help process of identifying each community's:-

   - Relevant societal needs.
   - Relevant social organizations and structures
   - Relevant other resources potentially adaptable to meet those needs

2. **THE PROCESS OF COMMUNITY PARTICIPATION:**

   - Setting-up the clients' own organization
   - Selection by it of one or more candidate community midwives (CM)
   - Definition of its own and the CM's responsibilities her fees, necessary transport arrangements etc.

   (Note: The above social processes all need to be facilitated by socially appropriate behavioural scientists (not official) who are female.)

3. **THE JOINT COMMUNITY & HEALTH PLANNERS** decide together:

   The CMs Training; her Professional Monitoring & Supply Arrangements; "Feedback" to and by the Community (Independant of the Local Health Services.)

PNG does not need to "reinvent the wheel", nor need we rediscover the well described methodological pitfalls, constraints and successful approaches already discovered in other countries. But PNG does need a clearly stated policy and the political will to implement the well tried practical programme steps to achieve safe maternal and neonatal care, and healthy planning by families through the PHC social approach. That means a participatory "bottom-up" strategy of mother's self-help will need to be facilitated by this programme village by village in every rural population in need of it.

BARRIERS AND BRIDGES TO THE SPREAD OF SEXUALLY TRANSMITTED DISEASES AMONG THE HULI OF SOUTHERN HIGHLANDS PROVINCE, PAPUA NEW GUINEA

JENNY HUGHES AND TIMOTHY DYKE[1]

INTRODUCTION

There were nearly 1400 reported cases of sexually transmitted disease in Southern Highlands Province in 1987. In the same year there were 428 attendances at the Sexually Transmitted Diseases or STD clinic in Tari Hospital. By 1988, however, attendances had increased to 620 and over 900 in 1989. That the numbers had doubled in two years cannot be taken lightly.

The reason that the graph did not continue climbing was that the clinic had to be closed because it ran out of drugs.

The social and economic environment of Tari is changing rapidly. The next few years will see an increasing number of mineral development projects in the surrounding district. The jobs created are likely to put more cash into the area than there are currently consumer goods to be bought. Money as compensation for land used for the siting of electricity pylons as part of the Hides Power generation project has recently been paid. These payments are seldom distributed in a way which encourages long term investment but is more than sufficient for large parties. Alcohol, in which traditional taboos and restraints are easily soluble is freely available, and sexual services are increasingly on offer.

A forty five year old male attender at the Tari STD clinic said that he had caught gonorrhoea from a paid participant at such a party. On an earlier visit to Moresby, he had been with prostitutes and had suffered the same symptoms but was surprised to have contracted gonorrhoea from a Huli woman. There is every reason to think that there is now a well established pool of infection within Tari district.

The question we ask in this paper is whether traditional methods of maintaining good spiritual health in the highlands may be re-inforced with contemporary health promotion to provide barriers to the spread of STDs amongst highlands communities.

[1] Tari Research Unit, Papua New Guinea Institute of Medical Research

So what sort of a problem are STDs in the Tari area?

STD clinic figures since 1983 indicate that over 80% of all patients are married adults between the ages of 25 and 40. This suggests that pre-marital promiscuity is less significant than extra-marital liasons.

90% of male attenders give their contacts as other than their spouses. The figure amongst female attenders is a little over 50%. These proportions have been consistent for the past seven years.

There is a strongly held belief among the Huli that STDs are spread from men's illicit contact with a small infected group of prostitutes or pasendia meri. Both men and women find this group a convenient scapegoat on which to lay responsibility. This has resulted in a casual attitude to preventative measures and the view expressed by men is that their contacts do not fall into this category so they are not at risk. This myth hides the reality that some women, for a multitude of reasons, will make their services available in certain circumstances.

Sexually transmitted diseases do not conflict with the traditional health beliefs of the Huli as they are seen as new diseases for which no traditional treatment exists. But they have a well-defined sense of what is correct behaviour between the sexes. Older men are troubled by the new relaxation of relations with women and view STDs as a new and virulent form of an old spiritual enemy which they traditionally guarded against.

The traditional health beliefs of Hulis are based on the concept that women are dangerous to males. Whilst fulfilling their functions within the society they are best avoided by men, especially during menstruation. This concept was taught to both males and females from an early age and was supported by elaborate rituals and spells. Traditional beliefs concerning intercourse at this time are still very strong among Huli men and women of all ages. All the restrictions mentioned above place responsibility on women, which may be seen as risk - taking behaviour on the part of men!

Extra-marital and pre-marital liaisons undoubtedly occurred in pre-contact times but the concept of a woman selling her sexual services was unknown. To the observer in the early contact period women's lives appeared to be heavily circumscribed by restrictions. Today there are opportunities for education, work and travel albeit for only a limited number of women. Adult female literacy is still unusual, and despite the efforts of the missions, polygyny is still not uncommon.

METHOD

To investigate the circumstances of STD transmission in the Tari district part of the research for this study was by way of semi-structured interviews amongst attenders of the STD clinic at Tari Hospital. This was supported with focus group interviews with different sectors of the Huli Community. The interviews with clinic attenders were held in a separate room to the clinic.

A specially tutored female research assistant who was a registered nurse acted as translator into tok ples. 25 men and 35 women were interviewed; 80% of whom were attending for follow-up having had a definite diagnosis of an STD made at a previous visit. 50% of attenders had one or more marriage partners either at the time of interview or in the past. Only one man was living with more than one wife, although seven women attending alone had one or more co-wives.

RESULTS

Over 80% of male attenders interviewed had at one time travelled beyond Southern Highlands and had seen "life" as it may be experienced in Mount Hagen, OK Tedi and in Port Moresby, compared to only 5% of the women.

Male clinic attenders were found to have much clearer ideas of STD transmission than women, but self-delusion was common among both men and women. 70% of the male clients interviewed were aware of the method of transmission of STD although the actual source of the disease was not always known. Most men had attended local courting parties, known locally as dawanda, but were reluctant to connect their infection with intercourse with women whom they met there. Their preferred belief was that the disease was contracted whilst staying outside of Tari; reinforcing the myth that STD is still an imported product.

Female attenders were found to be much less prepared to discuss their knowledge of STD transmission. Only 55% appeared to have had full knowledge of the means of transmission. As it is a popular belief that women, other than pasenda meris, do not contract these diseases and therefore would not know anything about them; there might have been an effect which inhibited women from talking about it.

Knowledge of transmission cannot be assumed to be the same as knowledge of prevention. Half of the female clients identified dawanda attendance as a factor and spoke of their opposition to their husband's attendance, but condoms were mentioned by only four of the twenty five male patients as a means of preventing transmission. No one had the opportunity to use them because of their unavailability.

It was evident from the focus group interviews that members of the larger Huli community are less well informed than clinic attenders, although it was evident that STDs were a frequent topic of conversation. The issue of condom availability and use was raised with community groups of both men and women in single sex groups and met with diametrically opposed attitudes. Women were opposed as they said that without the fear of contracting STD, men would "go wild"; men thought it would be the other way around! Concern was expressed that condoms or gumis in pidgin would become lost inside women and babies would be born intertwined in them. When canvassing opinion among women who did not oppose in principle the distribution of condoms; STD and Family Planning Clinics were the only outlets deemed acceptable by even the most liberal minded, and the suggestion that trade stores could sell condoms was greeted with universal disgust. As a result of this the opinions of trade store owners themselves were sought. Visits were made to seventeen trade stores around Tari district and the views of the owners surveyed. Eleven owners said that they would be prepared to sell them if a wholesale supply could be arranged, four would not, and two were undecided.

Men were not altogether in favour of ready availability of condoms but almost all knew of their existence and purpose. Fears concerning the probable "wild" sexual behaviour on the part of some younger males were expressed by older men which reflected women's anxieties. It is striking that men's traditional anxieties about sexual contact with women and the contraction of STDs have not converged into an association that condoms might protect against the polluting consequences of intercourse.

DISCUSSIONS

What are the longer term implications of STDs?

Apart from the obvious reduced quality of life which a person suffers from an untreated STD, there will be two major concerns for the Huli community if STD continues to spread widely through the population. The first is the problem of infertility which seems to be recognised by those attenders of the clinic. The second is, of course, the role STDs play in the transmission of HIV.

Gonorrhoea is a major cause of infertility among women in developing countries. The symptoms of gonorrhoea are frequently mild and detection is often delayed. This can result in damage to the fallopian tubes and subsequent pelvic inflammatory disease which is associated with ectopic pregnancies and infertility. Evidence from Africa suggests strongly that men also may become sterile through delayed or inadequate treatment.

60% of those interviewed said that they were very concerned that they were apparently unable to have children and associated this with STD. Twenty respondents had no child from their current marriage and a further nine, who still desired more children, had not had a child for at least five years. Perceived infertility seemed to be as much of a concern as the presenting symptoms. The tragedy for these patients is that they have discovered the cause long after any hope of preventing the effect. When considering the emphasis that might be placed in health education, it is likely that the possible consequences in terms of infertility as a result of STD infection may prove a powerful carrier for promoting healthier behaviour.

CONCLUSION

In conclusion, in pre-contact Huli society sexual contact was kept to a minimum and all activities involving both sexes were hedged with restrictions and ritual. The absence of sexually transmitted diseases in those times meant that ritual was adequate to restore balance and alleviate the illnesses which were believed to be caused by improper sexual conduct. Traditional barriers served the Huli well, at least in their psychological well-being. Today, however, the barriers have proved to be more permeable than in the past so that new barriers to the diffusion of sexually transmitted diseases must be constructed.

PROMOTING INFLUENCES TO THE SPREAD OF SEXUALLY TRANSMITTED DISEASE

- DIMINISHING INFLUENCE OF TRADITIONAL TABOOS
- INCREASING AFFLUENCE
- INCREASING ALCOHOL CONSUMPTION
- DAWANDA ATTENDANCE
- POLYGAMY

POSSIBLE PATHS FOR HEALTH EDUCATION MESSAGES

- CONDOMS AS A MEANS OF PREVENTING "POLLUTION"
- EMPHASISING INFERTILITY AMONGST THE CONSEQUENCES OF STDS

"REASONABLE KNOWLEDGE" OF THE CAUSES OF STD

	Men	Women	
Yes	18	19	37
No	7	16	23
	25	35	60

PROMOTING SAFE CHILDBIRTH

MARGARET R STREET[1]

The health of the rural family in Papua New Guinea is closely related to the quality of family life style, customs and values, the health and education of both parents and more especially that of the mother. The birth of a new member of the family should be a happy, normal, family centred event and an occasion for celebration.

I have lived and worked in Papua New Guinea since 1963 and until 1976 was involved in promoting safe childbirth at community, provincial and national levels. At present I am working with the National Department of Health (NDOH) in the Child Survival Support Project (CSSP). In this capacity there has been opportunity to assess the present situation in relation to safe childbirth for rural women. In many provinces there is a lot of activity to promote safe childbirth and this is encouraging. There are new innovative initiatives taking root from pilot studies in the last few years and this is exciting. But there are four facts that are disturbing.

1. Four Disturbing Facts

1.1 Everyday in 1991 in PNG, three women die because they are pregnant. This means everyday three families lose their mother. For them the birth of a new member of the family is a sad event that tears apart the very fabric of family life and puts the lives of young children in great danger. They are deprived of the one person responsible for their health and well being. this first fact is taken from National Health Statistics. WHO indicators estimate that only 10% of maternal deaths are reported.

1.2 The second disturbing fact is also taken from NationalHealth Statistics and relates to the percentage of births that are supervised by health workers or trained village birth attendants. The fact is that only 57% of all births in 1989 were supervised. 43% were not supervised. These village births may be attended by female family members who support the labouring woman and stay with her during her time of pain, fear and dread of the eventual outcome. In recent months my interactions with these family birth supporters have been most revealing. They have shared their experiences of prolonged labour, abnormal presentations, women dying of haemorrhage, of difficulties in finding affordable transport and the inadequacies of male health workers to save the life of the mother.

[1] Community Health Nursing Adviser, Child Survival Support Project, National Department of Health

MATERNAL HEALTH COVERAGE 1989

RECE. PROVINCE COVERAGE	ANC % COVERAGE	SUP. DEL. % COVERAGE	NEW FP %
Western	65	28.6	5
Gulf	67	79	2.4
Central	48	51.5	3.8
N C D	153	109	6.8
Milne Bay	59	44.2	2.6
Northern	57	78.5	2.8
Southern H	61	33	1.9
Enga	58	33	1.8
Western H	63	42	1.6
Simbu	80	51	1.9
Eastern H	67	42	4.3
Morobe	56	46	3.5
Madang	49	36	1.8
East Sepik	61	35	1.2
West Sepik	52	26	1.8
Manus	101	75.2	3.7
New Ireland	58	88.6	0.6
East New B	102	85	6.0
West New B	73	50.9	3.0
N Solomon	74	19.4	1.4
TOTAL	67	57.8	2.8

Source: National Health Statistics 1989.

1.3 The third fact I discovered at a recent National Workshop for Village Birth Attendants (VBA) conducted by NDOH with funding and support from CSSP. Forty three percent of rural women who deliver in the village without trained supervision do so alone. They endure a private hell, alone in the bush, the garden or a special temporary shelter. There are no female family supports. A neighbour may drop by, after 24 hours or so to check if the woman is still alive. Twenty percent of the children born in this country in 1991 are born in these circumstances. Table I gives the details of this for 1989.

1.4 The fourth fact I observed when visiting Provincial and NCD obstetric units. A village woman may decide to go to the obstetric unit for her delivery. She hopes this will be a safe place, but it may be a nightmare experience. She, and she alone, is often separated from her relatives and taken to a large, impersonal, sterile, strange, busy, bossy place filled with machines. There she is treated as an impersonal machine. The operators of these highly productive units are knowledgeable, skilled, efficient and poor communicators. They expect the passive, inert patient to accept and cooperate with all their expert decisions without question. There are usually no family supports, no respect for local language, customs and values and the woman is so intimidated she suffers, for the most part, in silence. In the past I have helped to train many midwives in this country. Today, I find this fact very sad.

2. The Choices for the Pregnant Woman

2.1 The choices for the pregnant woman are difficult. Her personal decision making about where to go to have this next child are crucial to her future life, health and well being.

She will assess her options, depending on where she lives and her life circumstances, knowledge and education. Then she will plan what she thinks is the best alternative from her understanding of her situation. Later she will try to take action to make her plan work. The support of her husband and family to take wise actions will be very important. Later, hopefully, if she is still alive, she will think about what happened and what she would like to happen next time. (see Diagram I)

The mother's decision making will be influenced by many factors.

2.2 Basic Education and Literacy

The links between the level of literacy and decision making related to health have been the subject of significant overseas study in recent years.

Literacy in Papua New Guinea is estimated to be 33%. Primary education provided in community schools is not universal and 28% of children never enter school. Of the age group 7-12 years, 64% were enrolled in school in 1983. Of this only 46 completed community school and 16% go on to high school.

There is considerable provincial variation in the proportion of girls in school. For example in 1988 54% of school age girls enrolled in school in West Sepik while 86% enrolled in Manus. Overall between 1971 and 1988 the % of females at school entry increased from 37% to 44%. There continues to be a gap between grade 6 and high school; overall 31% of the available girls were selected for grade 7 compared with 40% of the boys. That is a 22% advantage to the male sex. At present 80% of the women in PNG are illiterate.

The constraints for females in pursuing an education include:

* The labour of daughters to care for younger siblings.
* Early marriage customs.
* Fear of sexual harassment.
* Women's role is seen in subsistence agriculture and child bearing.
* Low self-esteem and aspirations of girls.
* Parental control of teenage daughters in relation to brideprice and marriage relationships.

These same constraints influence her decisions about health issues including safe childbirth.

With the slowly changing attitude towards female schooling has come the desire by unschooled women to be able to read and write. This is often expressed as a key to being able to take more control of their own lives and increase their status in their own society. Women who read and have some education are in a better position to make a wise decision about safe childbirth. Of course they will be helped by written materials about the reproductive process and family planning.

Table 2 Enrolment rates, grades 1 to 6 by province and sex, 1982-1988.

Province	1982		1985		1988	
	M	F	M	F	M	F
Western	74	62				
South Fly			83	78	88	81
North Fly			92	64	96	79
Gulf	75	39	79	59	81	61
Central	75	64	86	77	92	81
NCD	80	77	77	76	83	81
Milne Bay	71	55	74	72	75	74
Oro	68	57	75	64	76	68
S. Highlands	65	39	64	45	69	47
W. Highlands	51	42	56	48	68	58
Simbu	60	43	69	54	102	80
E. Highlands	58	47	70	60	82	68
Morobe	67	52	70	54	73	58
Madang	64	45	69	52	71	56
East Sepik	71	53	82	67	75	69
West Sepik	71	45	73	40	77	54
Manus	90	83	94	83	93	86
New Ireland	80	73	89	89	88	85
East New Britain	82	81	82	79	84	82
West New Britain	80	72	82	74	80	70
North Solomons	72	67	74	74	74	74
Papua New Guinea	67	51	72	61	77	65

Sources: Webster 1989: Table 7
Asia and Pacific Program of Educational Innovation for Development (APEID) 1989: Table 2.1

Recently, I did some pretesting of forty drawings and diagrams for booklets for new adult readers on pregnancy, delivery and family planning. The results were very interesting and revealed a lot about what rural women in PNG see in pictures. Simple clear illustrations with words that reinforce the main message were well understood. A series of drawings that illustrate a process or an abstract concept were not understood. Three drawings of the stages of pregnancy were rightly seen as three young women who were pregnant! Of course these drawings are useful in a flip chart with an explanation of points to discuss. I concluded that the readability of pictures is tricky and pretesting is never a waste of time and effort.

2.3 Family Status, Responsibilities, Obligations and Supports

These are significant factors in a woman's decisions in relation to a safe childbirth. The wife of the village magistrate is in a stronger position than most to have cheaper access to village transport both to attend antenatal care and to organize a supervised delivery if that is her choice. The extended family obligations to provide money for male oriented projects or schooling or trips to the urban centre will influence the money available to the woman for transport or to recompense a village birth attendant. Again the rural mother is responsible to produce, harvest, prepare and cook the food the family eat. Where there is no help from the husband or other extended family with these responsibilities the mother may be very reluctant to leave the village to provide herself with a safer place for childbirth.

2.4 Support from Primary Industry

This will influence the economic factors within the family situation, and the mother's involvement in the daily grind of subsistence agriculture. Agricultural development projects aimed at helping the women, who do 80% of the work in such projects, need to be increased. This in turn would give women more time, energy and resources to control their own lives.

2.5 Support from Women's Organizations

Either a church womens group or a Council of women group can have a significant influence on a woman's decision about safe childbirth. As she interacts with others and becomes aware of her own self worth and the opportunities for help that are available to her, so the options she uses to make her decisions are increased.

2.6 **Information, Awareness and Communication Networks**

These too may come through affiliation with a womens group or via the radio, doctor or other health programmes. The National Womens Training Project is active in this area and such initiatives need to be strengthened with grassroots programmes that are positive, practical and enable rural women to become equal partners in development and in family decision making.

2.7 **Customs, Practices and Values of her Ethnic Group and that of her in-laws**

This includes the family birth supporters and the ethnic customs and practices that will influence the rural woman's perceptions of the way childbirth should happen and the reasons why she may encounter difficulties. This aspect of child birth needs to be explored and discussed with rural women to gain an insight into practices that are beneficial and should be promoted at the health centre as well as those that are harmful and should be changed.

2.8 **Health Facilities Available**

The availability of affordable transport will be a major factor in her decision making. Of course it depends on how far she lives from the health centre, rural hospital or provincial obstetric unit and on the availability of a maternity waiting house, or affordable accommodation close to the birthing centre, if she makes the journey before labour begins. Maternity waiting houses are urgently needed in most districts and should be a subject on the agenda of Community District Councils.

3. **There are four ways that Safe Childbirth can be Promoted**

3.1 **No pregnant woman in PNG should deliver her baby alone**

Female family support should be available to all, during pregnancy, labour, after the birth and in the care of the newborn. This includes in obstetric units as well as for that 20% of women who currently deliver alone in the village.

3.2 **Every pregnant woman should be examined by a skilled female health worker at an antenatal clinic at least three times during her pregnancy**

I am aware that antenatal clinic attendance is difficult for many rural women. Distance, time, transport and other pressing family priorities come in the way. Mobile antenatal clinics seem to have faded away, or never really taken root in many Districts. Antenatal fixed clinics are most often held at a time and place to suit the health workers. As well as the time and place, the quality of the assessment depends on the knowledge, skills and attitudes of the staff, their ability to communicate across the language barrier and the equipment/supplies available to them.

3.3 **Every "at risk" pregnant woman should be attended in childbirth by a trained health worker.**

This objective is also difficult to achieve. Recently I checked the Antenatal Records of a Health Subcentre. At risk factors were documented for twenty women seen at the AN clinic in the past year but only three out of the twenty delivered at the HSC. There was no record of where the other seventeen delivered.

3.4 **Every woman of child bearing age should have access to information, interventions and health services that enable her to be in control of her own fertility**

Where children are born too close together their chance of a healthy childhood is reduced. The health of the mother is also more likely to be poor, particularly because of poor nutrition and chronic anaemia. Her chances of a safe childbirth next time are considerably reduced.

4. **Current Health Department Projects**

The NDOH and some provinces are currently involved in several projects and activities that address these four issues:

4.1 **VBA Programmes**

A large part of the work of trained Village Birth Attendants is to encourage and promote attendance at antenatal clinics where high risk factors that endanger the life of the mother can be attended to. As well as this VBA's have their own short list of "at risk" women they will not deliver. These include: first baby, after fourth baby, an abnormal lie and a woman who has had a previous problem in labour. The recent National VBA Workshop reviewed all the currently active VBA projects in PNG. The aim was to interact with current practising trained village birth attendants and the provincial health workers who are active in their supervision and training. As a result of this workshop the NDOH is writing guidelines to assist Provincial Health Divisions who want to put time, energy and expertise into community based village birth attendants programmes.

One of the key strategies to successful VBA programmes in PNG is the constant, ongoing, fulltime, monitoring, supervision support and encouragement needed from national midwives employed by the Provincial Division of Health, and VBA's who are linked to a skilled committed health team. Health workers need to be able to assess and deal with "at risk" pregnant women and provide a safe happy childbirth experience in a well equipped health centre with transport and radio links to the Provincial Obstetric Unit.

4.2 Rapid Evaluation Method of MCH Services

The NDOH is currently working with WHO and CSSP in assisting ten provinces to undertake a rapid evaluation of the quality of their maternal health and family planning services.

This will involve district health managers in working with a trained team to evaluate the quality of their services in terms of the outcomes. The methodology involved includes gathering information from village focus groups. This will form the basis for strategies to improve the services.

4.3 Home Based Mothers Health Record Book

The NDOH is also involved with CSSP in a pilot study to introduce a national home based mother's health record book. This provides the mother with her own record of her health history over a period of five pregnancies and includes sections on family spacing and health topics discussed with the mother. Two provinces have variations on this kind of health record. The aim of this project is to make it nation wide.

4.4 Information, Education and Communication Activities

The Family Health Division of NDOH is currently preparing a series of booklets for new adult readers, information for pregnant women and a flip chart on safe childbirth and family spacing.

4.5 Provincial DOH Planning Workshops

The NDOH is currently involved with eight Provincial Departments of Health who have been looking critically at their performance in 1990 and are now planning for the next five years. Antenatal attendance, supervised deliveries, and new family planning acceptors have been three areas where facilitating factors, barriers to achievement and innovative strategies have been under discussion. Hopefully improvements will occur in the life of the current Five Year Health Plan.

5. **Conclusion**

The key to promoting safe childbirth for rural women is to strengthen the decision making ability of the pregnant woman. She, and often she alone, makes the decision about where her baby will be born.

Of course it depends on her knowledge of her own health history, of the "at risk" factors that could cause her death, where she lives, her access to affordable transport, and relatives to provide housing near the birth centre.

Everyone in this room has the opportunity to influence her decisions and help her to achieve a safe birth in a happy family centred environment.

May I close with a Poem about a young pregnant woman from Manduwasa Village in Western Highlands Province.

FEARS OF A YOUNG PREGNANT WOMAN FROM MANDUWASA

How safe am I now I am pregnant?
How dangerous is it to have this baby?
Will I be safe? Will the baby?

How competent are the health workers to check my pregnancy?
Can they diagnose any problems?
Can they treat any problems they think they find?

How competent are the health workers to deliver my baby?
Will I be safe in their care? Private?
Get a hospital infection?
Will the baby be safe?

How far do I have to travel to a safe place?
For antenatal care? For child birth?
Is there accommodation for a wantok - for me to stay before the birth?

How likely is the baby to die in the first few weeks of life?
What should I do to keep my baby safe?
What should I do if my baby is born premature in the village?

Who cares if I die?
Blood pollution is much more a problem - men are more worried about blood taboo.
They do not really care about me.
They will not help me if I'm in trouble at the time of the birth.

Three women died today, they died because they were pregnant.
Three women died yesterday, and on Thursday, and on Wednesday.
Three women die in childbirth everyday of every week of every year.

I am just part of the throw away property.
If I die the man will just buy another wife.

Who oh who is strong enough to help me?
Is there any one out there who cares?

REFERENCES

Gillett, Joy E. The Health of Women in PNG, PNG IMR Monograph No. 9, 1990.

Jogo, Somere. Effects of Mining Development, A Women's Concern: The Ok Tedi Story, Pacific Workshop, 1989.

Royston E and Armstrong S. Preventing Maternal Deaths, World Health Organization, Geneva, 1989.

Street, Margaret R. Active Birth Attendant Projects in PNG in 1991, Paper presented at National VBA Workshop, April 1991.

Street, Margaret R. Pretesting of Pictures, Paper prepared for Child Survival Support Project, May 1991.

Tekwie - Ortlauf D. Gender Sensitivity in Development, Planning, Implementation and Evaluation Pacific Workshop, 1989.

Tekwie - Ortlauf D. Women and Literacy in PNG, Paper presented at Women and Literacy Seminar, 1990.

Literature for PNG Literacy Programmes, Literacy and Awareness Secretariat, N. Dep of Ed.

Handbook Health Statistics PNG 1989, N. Dep of Ed.

PNG Health Plan 1991-1995, N. Dep of Health.

PNG Integrated National Population Policy for Progress and Development, Dept of Finance and Planning, 1991

Provincial Health Department Guidelines for VBA Programmes, Nat. Dep. of Health

Health Implications of Sex Discrimination in Childhood, World Health Organization, Geneva, 1986.

Decision Making Related to Childbirth - Diagram I

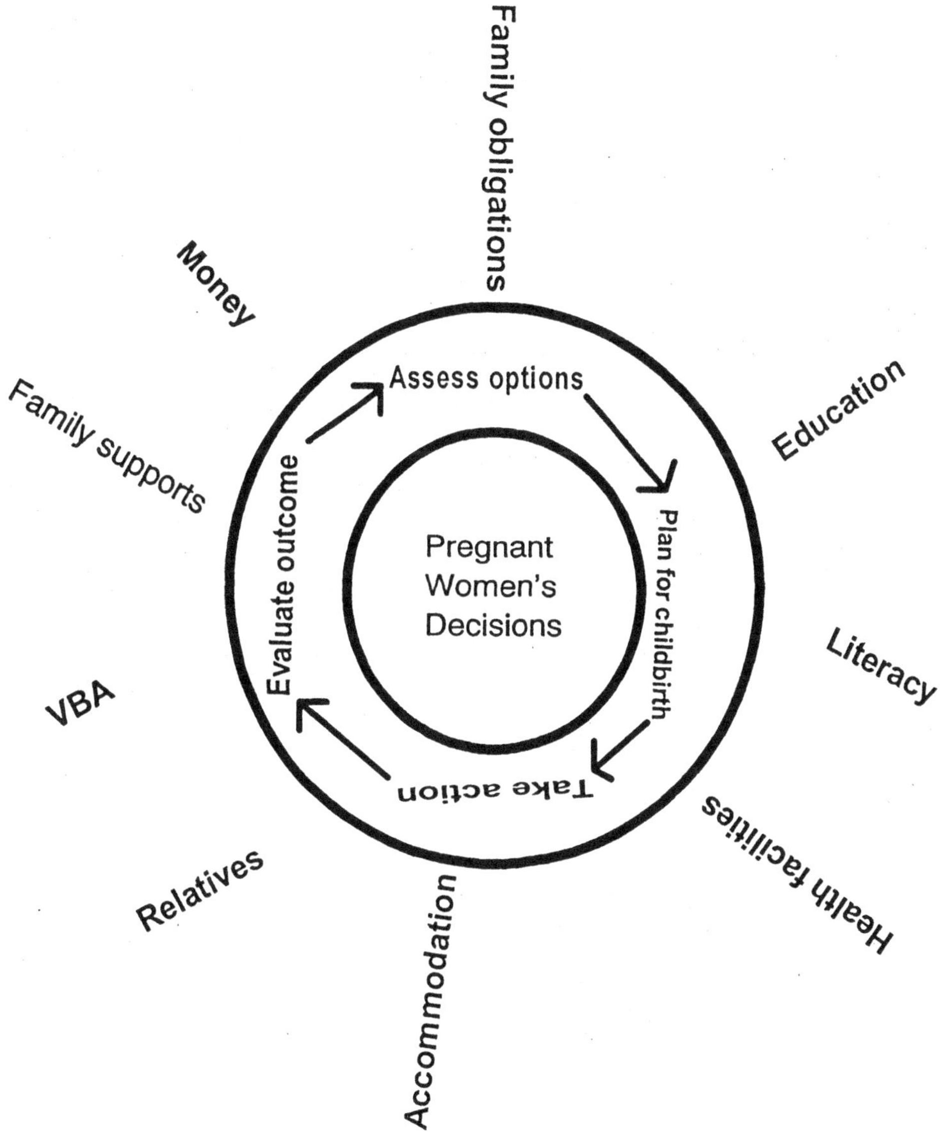

MEASUREMENT OF CHILD MORTALITY IN ASSOCIATION WITH A MULTIPURPOSE BIRTH CERTIFICATE PROGRAMME IN THE SOUTHERN HIGHLANDS PROVINCE OF PAPUA NEW GUINEA

DIMITRI PRYBYLSKI[1], WILLIAM A. ALTO[2], STEPHEN ROGERS[3], AND HELEN PICKERING[3]

INTRODUCTION

The registration of births and deaths in the less developed countries of the world is often of poor quality or non-existent. This deficiency of accurate information hinders health planners in decision making as to the best way to allocate scarce resources. It also limits their ability to evaluate interventions designed to improve infant and child mortality. A recently described method for monitoring childhood mortality levels (1) has been incorporated into a multipurpose birth registration scheme in the Southern Highlands of Papua New Guinea (PNG). Here we present the experience of the first year of data collection and the practical problems in the application of the programme along with some of the useful information already collected.

STUDY POPULATION

The Southern Highlands Province (SHP) had the highest infant mortality (116/1000) and 1-4 years of age (child) mortality (75/1000) rates in all of Papua New Guinea according to the 1980 national census (2). Two years before this period, in 1978, just 21 percent of all deliveries in the SHP were supervised at a health facility; 60 percent of children under 5 years of age were enrolled at a maternal-child health (MCH) clinic with only one-half of those registered attending on a regular basis (3).

1 Primary Health Care Assistant, Division of Health, Mendi, Southern Highlands Province, Papua New Guinea

2 Saint Mary's Family Practice Residency Program, 233 North Sixth St., Grand Junction, Co. 81501, USA

3 Papua New Guinea Institute of Medical Research, PO Box 35, Tari, Southern Highlands Province, Papua New Guinea

Over the next eight years the health services were expanded and a variety of new programmes introduced to improve child survival. The number of health facilities were increased by 21 percent; supervised deliveries doubled to 42 percent, MCH clinic registration approached 100 percent in most areas with the average under-5 year old child attending clinic 7.9 times in 1987 (4). Measles (5) and pig bel (enteritis necrotitans (6) vaccines, oral rehydration solution (7), a village midwifery training school (8), a malaria control spray programme, and rural health patrols (9) were all introduced into the province after 1980.

The Tari Research Unit (TRU), a section of the Papua New Guinea Institute of Medical Research, has since 1980 monitored the demographic characteristics of 30,000 people of the Huli language group who reside in the Tari Basin of the SHP (10). Natality and mortality information is collected on a monthly basis from this population and validated by periodic census (11). Analysis of health indicators derived from data collected by the TRU has allowed the Health Division to monitor the effect of health interventions on this select group of the Huli people and to direct resources to those identified as the most in need. But this monitored population includes less than 10 percent of the people living within the Southern Highlands and information from one language group is not necessarily transferable to the other seventeen distinct language and cultural groups living within the province.

In order to monitor the changes in early childhood mortality and to identify the cumulative effects of a new child survival project on these health indicators, plus identify the areas in greatest need for additional intervention, a new computerized health information system was established in 1988. Its introduction was supported by the success of a pilot study conducted at the TRU in 1986 that demonstrated the ability of a simple method to estimate childhood mortality from reports given by mothers near the time of a recent maternity (12). The method is known as the preceding birth technique (1,13,14).

A new birth certificate/registration form was designed to collect the childhood mortality data. Included in the same birth certificate were additional questions designed to monitor the number of supervised deliveries and to determine the mean birth interval. It was envisioned that the birth certificates would be attractive to mothers and, therefore, would promote supervised deliveries and encourage clinic attendance and immunization.

The project was funded in part by UNICEF as a means to monitor a Community Based Child Survival and Development Programme.

MATERIALS AND METHODS

Late in 1987 and through the first quarter of 1988, a new birth registration form was introduced to all of the forty three MCH nursing teams that delivered antenatal, postpartum, and well-child care at clinic sites throughout the province.

Each MCH team was visited by two volunteer medical students and a staff physician as part of a routine monthly or bimonthly supervisory visit. An in-service training session about the new birth certificate and registration was presented. It consisted of a short lecture and a series of scenarios with the MCH nurses questioning the mother (played by the medical student) about the circumstances of her recent delivery. Questions to be answered by the mother included: "Was the delivery supervised at a health facility, attended by a village midwife, or delivered unsupervised at home? What is the current status of the last live-born child prior to this current birth? Is this child now alive or dead, or was there no last live born child (if this was the mother's first live birth)?" The actual or estimated date of birth of the child born previous to this recent birth was also recorded and validated from the older child's clinic records when necessary. Other routine information collected included the mother's name, the child's name, this newborn's date of birth and place of birth, and the mother's home village at the time of birth.

Each registration form had a unique number and a self-carbonizing copy that was sent to the Provincial Health Office. The original copy was offered to the mother. She received it for free if she had a supervised delivery either in a health facility or by a village midwife, but was required to pay a small fee for it if she had delivered unsupervised in the village. The certificate was designed so as to appear official-looking and attractive to the mother. It was signed by the health worker who collected the information to facilitate follow-up.

All supervised births were recorded before discharge from the health facility or at the time of the infant's first visit to a well-child clinic. Clinics are held in a routine fashion on a 1-3 month basis.

The initial issuance of birth certificates began several days before the 1st of January 1988. The last of the MCH teams completed their training and began to issue certificates in April. Only those birth certificates completed between 1 January 1988 and 31 December 1988 on children less than 16 months of age at the time of birth registration are included in this study in order to minimize omissions due to poor recall by the mother of her previous birth (15). Incomplete or incorrectly completed forms were returned to the health worker who had filled in the original record for correction from MCH cards held at the health centre or by reinterviewing the mother at the next clinic. Refresher courses to review the proper method of completion of the form were conducted as needed.

The preceding birth technique was used to estimate the 0-2 year mortality risk [q(2) in lifetable notation]. It involves counting the number of mothers whose previous live birth had died by the time of the present delivery and calculating the ratio of that number to the number of mothers having had a previous live birth.

0-2 mortality/1000 = number dead/(number alive + number dead) where 'number dead' is the number of mothers whose previous live birth is now dead and 'number alive' is the number of mothers whose last live birth was still alive at the time of registration.

The retrospective mortality rate refers to a period approximately two-thirds of the mean birth interval prior to the date that the birth registration data was collected. For example, the 1988 data that are presented here provided the estimate of q(2) for 1986.

Information extracted from the completed and returned birth registration forms was entered onto a microcomputer. The estimated number of births in the province, used to calculate the coverage with the birth certificates, was based on the 1980 national census with an annual population growth rate of 1.8 percent. However, in the TRU surveillance area, mortality rates were based on their census data.

Infant mortality rates were estimated by abstracting expected values for q(1) from the observed q(2) values using Coale-Demeny model West standard life tables.

RESULTS

REGISTRATION

In 1988, 8,201 completed and correct birth registration certificates were collected within the Southern Highlands Province that met the study criteria. Seventy-seven percent of the estimated 10,611 total births in the province were registered; 99 percent of those infants registered had been delivered within the province and 51 percent of all birth registries were males. The age distribution of infants at the time of their registration is presented in table 1. 98 percent of registrations were in the first month of life. Enrolment of infants under 1 year of age at the MCH clinics varied from 46 percent to 156 percent, median 85.5 percent, for the 14 health districts. No instance of multiple registration of a single infant was detected.

MORTALITY RATES

For the Southern Highlands as a whole, 6,510 (79 percent) mothers reported having had a previous birth at the time of a current maternity in 1988. Of these 6,510 children, 592 were dead at the time of registration. This corresponds to a 0-2 year mortality rate of 91 per 1000 (1000 q(2) = 91) and refers to the year 1986. Using standard life tables, this value is equivalent to an infant mortality rate of 77/1000.

In the entire province, the estimate of q(2) for the previous child if the current infant was delivered by a health worker was 103/1000 (300/2905) while it was 81/1000 (293/3607) if the current child had been an unsupervised delivery.

Approximately 1,000 birth certificates must be registered in order to obtain reasonably stable estimates of q(2) (1), so only the larger districts in the SHP could be considered to have accurate annual mortality rates calculated from the data collected in 1988 (Table 2).

Comparisons between the TRU community surveillance survey data and that from the birth registration programme are shown in Table 3. In the entire Tari Basin, which includes the TRU surveillance area plus one other health centre (943 registries), and in the TRU area alone, where 745 birth registrations were collected, we found that the 0-2 mortality estimates calculated for 1986 were in close agreement with the rate generated from demography data of the Tari Research Unit.

BIRTH INTERVALS

Child spacing (mean live birth interval) information is available from age estimates of the previous last live-born child at the time of a current maternity. This calculation is based only on cases where there is a surviving previous birth because the estimated age is more likely to be accurate than if the previous birth is now dead.

The mean live birth interval for the entire SHP is estimated to be 40.8 months (SD 7.5 months) and 39.3 months (SD 4.6 months) for Tari District (excluding a health centre outside the TRU surveillance area). This mean birth interval derived from the certificates is similar to that found by the TRU in their surveillance area over the years 1984-1988 (37.0 months, SD 9.6 MONTHS) (16).

SUPERVISED DELIVERIES AND CLINIC ATTENDANCE

The percentage of health centre deliveries can be calculated from the registry; and the birth certificate derived provincial rate (48 percent) is similar to the standard MCH monthly health centre report calculations (45 percent). Health workers encourage nulliparous women to deliver their infants under medical supervision at a health centre, and 62 percent of the first time mothers followed this recommendation as calculated from the registry data.

Analysis is not yet available to compare MCH clinic attendance and the rate of supervised delivery between the pre-birth certificate (1987) and post-birth certificate periods (1989).

DISCUSSION

REGISTRATION

In general, the introduction of the birth registration programme was highly successful; however, in their enthusiasm to distribute the birth certificates, some of the MCH clinic staff gave them to children over the age of one year and some infants and children were registered prior to the official start of the collection period on 1 January. These certificates were entered into the registry and were included in our analysis as only seventeen records were involved. In the first year of the programme it would be expected that a number of older infants would be initially registered as there was a backlog of 0-1 year olds awaiting the new certificates. This would have increased the number of certificates issued in comparison to subsequent years. This did not appear to be a problem in our experience as 98 percent of all registrations occurred within the first month after birth (Table 1). It seems that the high rate of clinic enrolment (median 86 percent, range 46 percent-156 percent) in the province accounts for this finding. Mothers living in remote regions outside of a health centre clinic catchment area could not register their infants but infants who had access to MCH clinics were registered soon after birth. Furthermore, late registration was balanced somewhat by the delayed introduction of the programme to certain MCH teams who did not begin to issue certificates until April, or in the case of quarterly clinics, not until June or July. One small health centre did not issue birth certificates in 1988. The delayed introduction allowed a number of infants in these areas to achieve their first birthday prior to their next clinic visit, and they thus became ineligible to be registered. This delay helps account for the fact that only 77 percent of all infants were registered in the province where virtually every child is enrolled in a MCH clinic by the age of 1 year.

A number of mothers crossed district boundaries to attend a clinic that was closer or more convenient to their homes and this, along with in and out migration, variability of population growth, and under-enumeration at the 1980 census, explains why some clinic registrations exceeded 100 percent.

Some children who were village-born and died before their first clinic visit were also not registered and the mother's past maternity history was never recorded.

The neonatal mortality rate of the province is not known but it is probably similar to or less than the 19.4/1000 reported from TRU observations in 1983 (11). As nearly one-half of all registries occurred at the time of birth and most registries were recorded within one month of birth, the problem of not interviewing mothers whose infant had experienced a neonatal death was not as important as if registration had occurred later. Mothers who had delivered a stillborn infant would not register that birth and the status of their past child would not have been recorded. The stillbirth rate in the TRU area was 12.7/1000 in 1984-1986 (12). Having a stillbirth during the present pregnancy may be associated with a higher-than-average mortality of a previous birth. If this is true, it would lead to an underestimation of the mortality rates derived from the registry, as mothers are only questioned if they have had a live birth.

No certificates were known to have been lost since each had a consecutive number and each number group was distributed to a specific MCH team. An attempt was made to identify any missing numbers at the time of data entry. Certificates that were voided because of errors made at the time of completion were returned.

MORTALITY RATES

The birth registration programme provides reliable information on vital health indicators such as childhood mortality risks (q(2)). The estimated 0-2 year mortality figures in the Tari area (16) are in close agreement with those collected from the population under surveillance by the reporters of the Tari Research Unit. Estimates of q(2) from the other districts in the province cannot be validated as was done in Tari, but they should provide a reasonable estimate for planning purposes and, as several years of data are accumulated, these figures can be utilized in the evaluation of trends.

There was a very good agreement between our estimate of q(2) and those reported by Pickering et al. (12) who used the same preceding birth technique. Their study was limited to comparing the survival of the previous birth of only those mothers who had an attended delivery at a health centre or hospital (1000q(2) = 100.4) with those of the TRU surveillance population (1000q(2) = 113.2). These mortality figures are for 1984-86 as the health facility information was collected in 1986. The authors attributed the differences in 0-2 year mortality between the health centre and the TRU population surveillance area to selection bias and hypothesized that the lower mortality rates of the former existed because the mothers who gave birth in health centres or hospitals were better educated, younger, or lived closer to a health facility. They recognized that the opposite might be true on a province-wide basis; mothers who had their previous child die would be more likely to deliver the next child under medical supervision.

We found support for the latter hypothesis on a province-wide basis; mothers who delivered their current child at a health centre had a higher level of mortality for the previous child than those who had delivered their recent child without supervision. Another possible explanation for this finding is that more accurate maternal histories are likely to be recorded in obstetrics units than in MCH field clinics and hence, previous birth deaths are less likely to be missed.

However, in the TRU surveillance area, we found the opposite hypothesis to be true, with the probability of dying by age 2 of 1000q(2) = 93.2 and 1000q(2) = 188.7 for the two groups respectively. The results within the TRU surveillance area are based on 745 registries with 557 previous births of which only 53/557 (9.5 percent) occurred without medical supervision. Only ten of the next younger siblings of these 53 had died and this apparent difference between the Tari and the provincial mortality rates may be due to the small sample size and should therefore be interpreted with caution.

The surveys recorded a dissimilar number of multiparous births, 787/950 (82.8 percent) for the 1986 study and 557/745 (74.7 percent) for our 1988 study, but 55 records were incomplete in the Pickering study and were not included in their analysis. In addition, the increase in the proportion of supervised deliveries from 87% in 1986, at the time of the Pickering study, to 92% in 1988 may have included a disproportionate number of primiparous women.

In our study, only 745 registrations from within the TRU survey area were available for analysis, with 557 previous births, less than the 1000 registrations believed necessary to derive a reasonable estimate of q(2). Even when all the health facilities in the Tari District are included for analysis (942 registrations, from Table 2) the registry-derived mortality estimates are not significantly different.

The mortality rates derived from the registry should be considered as minimum estimates for a number of reasons. Some remote, sparsely populated regions of the province still have no access to health care and the estimate of q(2) in these areas are undoubtedly much higher. In addition, reports on the survival of the preceding infant are not recorded when the current delivery is a stillbirth. These women often have higher perinatal mortality risks. Moreover, it is probable that a certain proportion of neonatal deaths were reported as stillbirths in order to avoid the social stigma attached to the mother whose liveborn infant has died. Mortality is especially high during the neonatal period and hence q(2) would be underestimated. Finally, a maternal-infant death, while rare, is not an unusual complication and would result in under-reporting but this may not change q(2).

CHILD SPACING

The provincial mean live birth interval of 40.8 (SD +/- 7.5) months reported here is higher than that of many developing countries. It is also higher than most previous reports of birth intervals in the Highlands of PNG that ranged between 29.2 and 42.3 months (17). However, our reported birth interval is probably over-estimated because it is based only on cases where there was a surviving previous birth. It is well known that the birth interval is significantly shorter after the early death of a young child (15). Another reason why the birth interval reported here should be considered a maximum estimate is due to the delayed registration of some of the children. This effect is minimized by the fact that 98 percent of the births were registered within the first month after birth.

We measured the live birth interval because stillbirths are rarely medically attended or recorded in the SHP and are frequently forgotten. Highlands custom proscribes sexual intercourse with a lactating female and weaning does not usually occur until the child is two or three years of age. It is probably this social taboo and the high male absentee rate, rather than family planning acceptance (less than 7 percent) (4) that results in the long interval between births. A second cultural factor that might account for the long mean birth interval is that mothers may be reluctant to mention a previous birth who has died and instead give information concerning their last born living child. We attempted to avoid the bias by specifically requesting information concerning the last live-born child, even if this child may have already died. Many of the MCH clinic nurses are familiar with all of the children of a mother and would be aware of a death of a previous child and detect this error at the time of registration. But we were unable to estimate how many previous births reported were of an earlier child than the last child, a factor that would have distorted our mean birth interval figure upward. The mean birth interval derived from the registry was greater than the TRU census data probably because of this selective factor and perhaps because the Huli women who were surveyed were reluctant to mention the death of a child that had died prior to its first birthday when, according to Huli custom, it would have been named. The data collected by the recorders of the TRU is based on frequent household surveys and would be less likely to be biased by this recall error. Despite the extremely long registry-derived mean birth interval reported here, the preceding birth technique can still be utilized to estimate q(2) accurately (15).

A potential bias introduced into our estimation of mortality rates is that while the preceding birth technique is designed for the collection of information during a current maternity, some mothers were interviewed after this time. The effect of this is that their previous births were exposed to too long a risk of dying period. Nevertheless, this bias should be insignificant as 98 percent of births were registered within a month of delivery and additional months of exposure do not affect early-age mortality patterns greatly since all the preceding births have been exposed to the high mortality risks of the earliest part of life (15).

SUPERVISED DELIVERIES AND CLINIC ATTENDANCE

The registration programme slightly overestimated the percentage of health centre deliveries (48 percent) compared with the standard MCH reporting system (45 percent). This is probably because the registry was not operational for the entire twelve months of 1988 in all the districts of the province. Data collection first began in districts that had a higher rate of supervised deliveries (Mendi 161 percent, and Tari 82 percent) and started later in outlying districts with lower rates of health centre deliveries such as Kopiago (45 percent) and Pimaga (52 percent). These errors should not be present in the second year of the registry when both data collecting systems are in operation for a complete 12 months.

Only 40 percent of Huli women in the TRU surveillance area delivered their infants under medical supervision in 1984 (11). This had increased to 87 percent by 1986 (18). Yet there are no apparent change in infant mortality, 1000q(1) = 92.6 (12) and 1000q(1)=93.2 (16).

Supervised deliveries are specifically enumerated by the new system of birth registration. Mothers are encouraged to use and support the village midwives as birth certificates are provided free with any delivery attended by a health worker. Mothers who do not deliver under medical supervision are required to purchase their infant's birth certificate if they wish to receive it. This "fine" of the purchase price may be paid in the form of garden produce or a small amount of money, always less than one dollar. The proceeds collected are either given to a village midwife who is assisting at the MCH clinic or used to support a suplemental nutrition programme for health centre patients. If the mother is unable or refuses to purchase the certificate the back (carbon copy) information sheet is still forwarded to the Health Division for data entry and the front sheet held at the health centre in case she has a change of mind. Fines have proven successful in the modeling of maternal behaviour; the penalty of a 25 cent fine for a child's non-attendance at a monthly well child clinic led to a 46 percent increase in visits at one health centre (19).

It is impossible at this time to evaluate and quantify the effectiveness of the birth certificates as a motivational reward. Numerous health staff have reported that the certificates are highly valued by mothers and that this has encouraged them to deliver their infants at a health centre. More than this anecdotal evaluation should be possible by the analysis of future data.

OTHER USES

The registry has provided a confirmation of age for the 77 percent of infants that registered in 1988. Such age confirmation is required for school entry and public service employment. Prior to this registration scheme Southern Highlands infants rarely had their births registered because of the cost and the difficulty of completing the central registry application forms by a largely illiterate population. Village registries of births and deaths ceased to be kept in the province after the colonial period ended in 1975. This birth registry programme provides important information for the infant in later life. It has also been used by certain language groups, such as the Huli, as a permanent reminder for the celebration of the first birthday, a day when the infant is seen to be past the constant risk of death associated with early infancy and is officially welcomed into the family by finally being given a name. Names that are bestowed after registration can be easily added to the registry.

The birth certificate programme serves as a linkage to an Immunization Certificate Programme which, in cooperation with the Division of Education, requires children to receive a completed series of vaccinations in order to obtain an immunization certificate needed for admission to primary school. The birth certificate number provides a unique identification to an infant that can be updated on the computer registry when immunization is completed.

A master list of all registered children and those who are completely immunized will be offered to education authorities at each school prior to school registration day. This will provide planning information on school enrolment for local officials and allow the Education Division to identify incompletely immunized children and require their attendance at make-up clinics held at school during and after registration day. This part of the programme will not be tested until the first cohort reaches seven years of age in 1995.

CONCLUSIONS

The birth registration programmed has been easily introduced into the province and has been utilized to provide key health indicators for health planning and in the monitoring and evaluation of new interventions designed to promote child survival. The design is simple, requires minimal time to complete, and estimates of q(2) are easily and immediately accessible to any health worker with a hand-held calculator. Mothers are anxious to have a birth certificate and preliminary reports indicate that interest in antenatal and immunization clinics has increased. There was a close correlation between the information collected in this study and other independent and verifiable sources in the Southern Highlands.

This simple method should be transferable to any area where MCH clinic attendance or the percentage of supervised deliveries is high, thus insuring an adequate sample of the parturients. In districts where the population is small and annual mortality rates cannot be accurately determined, this method will still be valuable in estimating trends in mortality. In addition, several years of data may be combined to obtain a larger sample and an estimate of the 0-2 year mortality rate. Preliminary work is now under way to expand the programme to selected provinces in Papua New Guinea. This is of particular importance since the 1990 PNG National Census did not provide estimates of early childhood mortality.

ACKNOWLEDGEMENTS

We wish to thank Dr Sitaleki Finau for his invaluable assistance with statistical analysis, Dr Jan Pryor for computer analysis, Mr Stuart Harris for providing the Tari Research Unit mortality figures, and Cindy Parker, Dr Sarah Snell, Dr Eric Meyer, and Mr Allen Ziff who assisted with the training of the MCH teams. Ms Blonde Pope was responsible for computer data entry and for updating and checking records. Her skill and dedication are appreciated.

REFERENCES

1. Hill A. G. & Macrae S. (1985) Measuring childhood mortality levels: a new approach. UNICEF Social Statistics Bulletin Nairobi 1985; 8:1

2. Papua New Guinea Census. National Census Office, Port Moresby, Government Printer. 1980

3. Clark L. Brief for the Southern Highlands Rural Development Project. Division of Health, 1979; Mendi, Southern Highlands Province, Papua New Guinea. Mimeo, 1979.

4. Annual Report Division of Health, Mendi, Southern Highlands Province, Papua New Guinea, Provincial Printer. 1987.

5. Alto, W.A & Cutts D. Measles immunization and its effectiveness in the Southern Highlands. Papua New Guinea Med J 1989 32:45-49.

6. Davis M. V., Barker M. J., Griffiths C. J., et al. Active immunization decreases the incidence of necrotizing enteritis in Papua New Guinea. Department of Health; Madang. 1984

7. Frankel S. J. & Lehman D. Oral Rehydration Therapy: Combining anthropological and epidemiological approaches in the evaluation of a Papua New Guinea Programme. J Trop Med Hyg 1984 87: 132-42.

8. Albu R. & Alto W.A. Training of village midwives in the Southern Highlands Province. Papua New Guinea Med J 1989 32:89-95.

9. Buchanan A. & Maclauren G. Doctors health centre visits in the Southern Highlands Province. Papua New Guinea Med J 1987; 30:45-48

10. Tarr P. I. The Tari Research Unit morbidity surveillance system. Southern Highlands Rural Development Project; Mendi, Southern Highlands Province, Papua New Guinea. Mimeo. 1979.

11. Lehmann D. Summary of the final report of the Tari Research Unit for the Southern Highlands Rural Development Project. Provincial Printer. 1984.

12. Pickering H., David P H & Hill A.G. Continuous monitoring of child mortality from clinic records. J Tropical Med Hygiene 1989; 92:71-74.

13. Brass W & Macrae S. Childhood estimated from reports on previous births given by mothers at the time of a maternity. I. Preceding birth technique. Asian and Pacific Census Forum 1984; 11 (2):5-8.

14. Brass W & Macrae S. Childhood mortality estimated from reports on previous births given by mothers at the time of a maternity. 11. adapted multipling factor technique. Asian Pacific Census Forum 1985; 11:5-9.

15. Hill A.G & Aguirre A. Childhood mortality estimates using the preceding birth technique: some applications and extensions. Population Studies 1990; 44:317-340.

16. Harris S. Personal communication. Tari Research Unit, Tari, Southern Highlands Province, Papua New Guinea. 1989

17. Collins, A. Age determination in epidemiological studies in the Highlands of Papua New Guinea. Papua New Guinea Institute of Medical Research; Goroka. 1984

18. Annual Report Division of Health, Mendi, Southern Highlands Province, Provincial Printer. 1986

19. Nipa Health Centre Reports, as presented in Division of Health reports of 2 years, Mendi, Southern Highlands Province, Papua New Guinea. 1984-86.

TABLE 1. Age of Infants when Registered in Birth Certificate Registry, 1988 Data.

Age (months)	Frequency	Percentage	Cumulative Percentage
<1	8068	98.4	98.4
<6	61	.7	99.1
<12	55	.7	99.8
<16	7	.2	100.0
TOTAL	8201	100.0	100.0

TABLE 2. Indirect Mortality Estimates per 1000 live births from Birth Certificate Registry, 1988 Data.

DISTRICT	No.	A	D	N	0-2 MORTALITY	0-1 MORTALITY	MBI	HCD %
Tari	942	646	76	220	105.3	87.9	39.6	90
Koroba	813	590	73	150	110.1	91.7	40.8	51
Komo	218	164	23	31	123.0	101.7	42.0	59
Mendi	1364	940	97	327	93.6	78.9	40.8	64
Poroma	978	756	71	151	85.9	72.8	42.0	35
Munihu	330	223	32	75	125.5	103.6	42.0	51
Erave	149	98	9	42	84.1	71.4	38.4	63
Pimaga	95	63	7	25	100.0	83.8	38.4	34
Pangia	485	356	20	109	53.2	47.2	40.8	22
Nipa	589	452	27	110	56.4	49.7	43.2	49
Kagua	841	618	56	167	83.1	70.6	39.6	13
Ialibu	737	555	37	145	62.5	54.5	42.0	28
Kopiago	98	68	10	20	128.2	105.7	43.2	28
Margarima	562	390	54	118	121.6	100.6	42.0	57
SHP	**8201**	**5919**	**592**	**1690**	**90.9**	**76.8**	**40.8**	**48**

No. = Number of completed birth certificates

A = Number of mothers whose previous live-birth was "alive" at time of registration

D = Number of mothers whose previous live-birth was "dead" at time of registration

N = Number of mothers who did not have a previous live-birth at time of registration

MBI = Mean live birth interval (in months)

HCD% = Percentage of deliveries supervised by a health worker

TABLE 3. Child (0-2 year) Mortality per 1000 Live Births in Tari Research Unit Surveillance Area in 1986.

	Tari Research Unit Surveillance Data (July 1985-June 1986)	Birth Registration Programme Data (Referenced for 1986)
0-2 Year Mortality	112.0	102.3
Number of Children in Sample	857	557*
Percent Registered	100	86.9

* Mothers registered = 745, status of previous birth: alive = 500, dead = 57, no previous birth = 188.

Comparison between 0-2 year mortality: no significant difference, p = 0.567 (Chi squared test).

FAMILY AND MENTAL HEALTH: TRADITIONAL VERSUS MODERN CONCEPTS OF A FAMILY

ANDONIA PIAU-LYNCH

INTRODUCTION

It has been said that the only thing that we can count on in life, besides death and taxes - with the exception of the latter in Vanuatu - is change. For better or for worse, nothing ever stands still, and in today's world we are presented with more changes than ever before. We change everything rapidly, and, nearly everything around us changes <u>us</u> rapidly: where we live and work, our friends, our political affiliations, and even our spouses. It is unfortunate that, although some of these factors do change frequently, others, such as our attitudes to specific things, are so ingrained that it takes generations to change.

What I hope to cover in this paper is to support this idea about change and the fact that we cannot be expected to remain in a constant state. Being alive means we are in a constant state of change. The purpose of this paper is to highlight this statement, but in the process, to emphasise some of the stresses that we face in this world of ours where expectations are ever changing.

The ideas and cases that form the basis of my paper are those that I have come across and dealt with over the past twelve years as a psychologist, and, more recently, as a pseudo-welfare officer, social worker, and legal officer, during the past three and a half years in a statutory organization in Port Moresby. I will be referring specifically to a population who are educated, employed, and thus, wage earners in an urban situation. Although I may talk about the idea of a transitional period between traditional and modern changes in the concept of what constitutes a family and the problems that families are faced with in Papua New Guinea, I believe that those of you from other countries will find similarities in what we are experiencing.

Everyone of us has at one time or another talked about, or heard others speak of, the necessity of maintaining the family unit, whether it be at the village or at the urban level. We are constantly reminded that the family unit is the most important unit in our lives, that it is the future of our country and that we must ensure its well-being and continuity. But we do not often stop to think about what exactly this means. The mere fact that we are constantly reminded of it suggests that the family unit as it was some twenty or thirty years ago is indeed breaking down and that we must do something about it. But what?

Are we speaking about the breakdown of the family because of the incompatibility of the couples? Are we speaking about the breakdown of the family because of the non-recognition of the unit as a traditional or even a legal unit? Are we talking about the family breakdown as a result of the stresses which become part of us as a consequence of the modernization which is faced by the couples? Or are we just mouthing off something that is too basic and too near to us, so that we do not want to delve into it too deeply for fear that it might reveal our own problems? I am not here to ask these questions of each one of you directly, but I believe they are thoughts that we should entertain whilst we speak about the issue of health and, in this case, mental health and the family.

DEFINITION OF HEALTH

The World Health Organization defines health as a **"state of complete physical, mental, and social well-being"** and the absence of diseases, thus enabling the person to be able to live fully. Behaviours that are thus attributed to the mental well-being of a person can be described as those behaviours that the individual engages in which are culturally acceptable, as opposed to mental illness which occurs when an individual is unable to conform to or engage in those behaviours which are culturally acceptable.

The Pacific nations have in the past six decades faced changes that were, and probably are today, mind-boggling not only to our grandparents and our parents, but to us also. We have been introduced to technologies that surpass even the most imaginitive of minds. We have been introduced to ideas and concepts that would have cast doubts on our sanity had we not been "discovered" and "civilized" as part of another sovereign nation. Our "discovery" and "civilization" has meant that we are faced with additional stresses that we do not appear to be coping with too well: we as individuals, as parents, as couples, as workers and non-working individuals on the streets, and as men and women, are putting to the test the maxim of "the survival of the fittest". The mere fact that we are talking about it shows quite clearly that we today are facing so much pressure for change or to change that I am quite surprised that I can even talk about mental well-being or mental illnesses at all!

FACTORS AFFECTING THE MENTAL WELL-BEING OF FAMILIES

There are so many factors that affect the well-being of a person in today's circumstances that it would be impossible to cover them all. Some of these factors have been enumerated over and over again; for example, the pressure of land and its subsequent consequences like tribal fights, and the stresses and trauma that follow; the traumas of deaths due to alcohol-related accidents; the effects of a cash crop economy on the welfare of the family; the effects of education, and lack of education, and its effects on employment, unemployment, criminal activities, and so on.

There are, however, some factors which I believe are so central to the well-being of all our people that their mere existence is a hindrance to achieving that state of being healthy either physically, mentally or spiritually. What will be discussed below will be related to a small segment of our population, and as I have already mentioned above, to those who are employed, wage-earning and who live in an urban environment.

1. DIFFERENCES BETWEEN TRADITIONAL AND MODERN CONCEPTS OF A FAMILY

1.1 Marriages and De facto Relationships

There are two issues in our lives, that are so closely interwoven that we often neglect and fail to distinguish between them, and I speak about the institutions of customary and statutory marriages on one hand, and the de facto "marriages" on the other, and their associated effects. It appears to me that because we are in a transitory period of our development, what we consider to be traditional or custom, and what we consider modern are not mutually exclusive and, indeed, the attitudes accompanying such concepts are invariably confused.

In Papua New Guinea the law recognizes two types of marriages: traditional (including church marriages) and statutory marriages. What constitutes a traditional marriage is as diverse as our cultural and linguistic diversity but it had one thing in common: it was recognized as a marriage when gifts were exchanged between the bride's and the bridegroom's clans not only before the parties were tied to each other, but also after they tied the knots, so to speak, and when children appeared on the scene. In other words it was a contract. In statutory marriages, vows are made to "have and to hold until death do us part"; although vows were made before celebrants or a Registrar General or the kiap, exchanges were and still are a part of the ceremony that is supposed to link the parties for eternity. Again, it was a contract. Whereas the former did not have a piece of paper to tell the world that the parties were married, the latter did. Whether or not these two forms of marriages and their respective traditions actually maintain the family as a unit is I believe, becoming questionable.

In the last fifteen to twenty years, another type of 'marriage' has become quite popular and, indeed, is becoming socially acceptable in Papua New Guinea. I am referring to the de facto marriages, which are entered into because of circumstances, and not necessarily because the woman and the man want to be liberated and independent and 'free living'. What often necesssitates these de facto relationships is that a child happens to be begotten. In very few cases do couples live within these de facto marriages because they want to live this way, thus enabling each party the opportunity to leave when the going gets tough. However, in my experience over the past couple of years, a de facto relationship is basically a relationship of convenience, with the same meaning and flavour of the traditional "marriages of convenience" or "shotgun marriages". However, it is not a 'marriage' when problems arise as will be discussed below.

1.2 The Concept of "Bride Price"

Today, indeed, in the past decade or so, bride price has become an excuse to accumulate wealth. It has been commercialized, and girls and women are now a commodity to the extent that they might as well be included in the calculation of the CPI along with betel nut! In the past, it most certainly had some significance, in terms of establishing alliances between groups, strengthening alliances already in existence, and keeping that solidarity intact. As one author has put it, "the practice of presenting bride-wealth or bride price is believed to give the husband or husband's clan [the] rights over the woman's reproductive capacity and labour. This includes the right to physically punish [her] by beating her (according to customary law)....Traditionally, the payment of bride-wealth validates and cements the marriage relationship, symbolically binding together two clans"(1).

Today, however, I find it very difficult to see the significance it plays except as a means of accumulating quick riches. As far as I am concerned, it conveys very little of the traditional meaning of such a relationship and I believe that it is, and has been, abused to the benefit of the brides' relatives. It is a major stumbling block to enhancing and fulfilling marital obligations of couples both in the urban and rural setting. **I believe that the idea of paying brideprice should be totally discarded**.

The exchanges of goods and bridewealth in the forms of traditional items is still in existence in parts of the country. However, with the modernization of PNG and the modern items that now are becoming part of traditional exchanges, it places a heavy burden on the young couple, particularly the males, to meet the high demand of 'brideprice'. Prices of goods in the urban setting are now exorbitant. Added to these are pigs, chicken, cows, beer and the inevitable cash, even to the tune of K10,000 or more. Is a down payment on a woman a guarantee of a happy marriage? Surely not if the woman feels that she is being sold to the highest bidder!

1.3 De facto Marriages

I have mentioned previously that we are presently seeing more and more relationships which take on the guise of marriages but which in fact are not marriages either customarily or legally. These "marriages" resemble customary or legal marriages until the couple strike a problem, then everyone, including those who accepted the couple's living arrangements earlier, start questioning, abusing and accusing one or the other or both parties of infringing 'customs'! Many couples do live a happy 'married' life, but those who do not are faced with such debilitating consequences that you start to question who is 'marrying' whom! Some of the stresses that these couples face can be gauged by looking at Table 2, but not necessarily as couples but as individuals.

The use of traditional or customary reasons to justify and explain behaviour in a modern situation (for example, being "married" and having a de facto partner) is a point of contention experienced by many men and women today. It appears acceptable to the man if he wants to marry another woman, but when it comes to the woman wanting to leave her 'de facto' and "marry" another man, then all hell breaks loose. The justification that in his tradition or custom it is permissible to be married to two women is an abuse of custom which justifies an illegal and non-customary behaviour. For men to use the traditional behaviour and reasoning to hide behind a modern diversion is enough to make a woman want to go and get another man!

2. THE ROLE OF THE WORKING WOMAN

The role of a woman in today's world is as demanding as it was in the past. And in the urban, wage-earning sector, more so, especially if the woman is also a mother and a full-time worker. The work demands placed on her time are huge: she gets up in the morning, gets the kids ready, prepares breakfast for the kids and the husband, takes the kids to school, goes to work, goes to the market or does her shopping during lunchtime, picks the kids up, gets home to prepare the kids' bath and cooks, washes the dishes and she is now in a state of near collapse. If she is lucky she will get about five hours of sleep.

Many of these women also contend with a drunken husband who, after a night out with the boys, returns home, demands that the food be brought out immediately, and if by any chance it is cold, beware! Having filled his stomach with more solid substances, he then demands that the wife fulfils her womanly role and sleeps with him. If she does not because she is tired, or it is the wrong time of the month or whatever, then a little beating here and there might teach her that she must obey her man! But beware also if <u>he</u> is unable to get it up because then it will be her fault, never his! Again, if she is unfortunate enough to receive these assaults, she often receives extra punishment such as having to take time off work and in many cases termination of her employment.

There will be some amongst us who are unfortunate enough to have experienced these aggressive behaviours, of being assaulted, of being accused of adultery, of not being proper mothers and not good enough to be your husbands' wives! What is often accepted but not questioned is why it should continue. Why should women, and the men who are also sufferers of assaults, continue to take these batterings?

The Law Reform Commission must be commended and congratulated for its initiatives in passing legislation that aims to assist women, and men, who have suffered assault, as well as trying to place some semblance of responsibility on those who err. Although we are a long way from it becoming common knowledge and acceptance that assaults in the home and outside are criminal behaviour, at least it is a beginning.

We often understand the plight of, but find difficulty in assisting, those who do suffer from assaults in the home; for example, working men and women who have to take time off because they cannot physically come to work, or because they are hospitalized, or because the signs of assault are so obvious and are an impediment to their personal image and work, that they are better off at home.

There is a tendency in all sectors of our community to consider domestic problems as just domestic problems. The bosses either forget or ignore the fact that a happy man or women at home is <u>also</u> a happy employee. Often the sick leaves that are available are used up and employees are forced to take leave without pay. A more sympathetic approach in trying to understand the causes of such leave would, in my opinion, assist the sufferer to cope with one less stress: the possibility of termination because of too much sick leave or leave without pay.

It has been my experience that most assaults are received by women as a result of a domestic problem. In instances such as this, they are the ones who have to suffer the extra consequences of taking sick leave, not because they are physically sick, but because their illnesses and disabilities are the result of an attack by their partner. They are the ones to whom the employer gives extra punishment because they take time out. They are the ones who have to face the possibility of termination. But does anyone question the role of the assaulter in this case, and see if anything as drastic is happening to them? In my experience, in very few cases does this happen. This could be an avenue to look at in trying to decrease the added punishment and sufferings of the assaultee. We talk of equal opportunity. Is there anything equal about this situation?

3. **ABUSE OF ALCOHOL**

Many of us have had first hand experience of, or else have got to know through the experiences of others, the effects that alcohol can have on our lives. What is lacking at present is that we tend to ignore the small problems, such as late lunches. We tend to ignore assaults caused by drunken husbands; we tend to laugh when someone runs into the lights at Boroko at one in the morning. These are signs of a problem that we should take seriously.

At present we do not, and we let the problem accelerate. Some twenty years ago, there were recommendations that breathalysers be used to detect drunk drivers[(2)]. Ten years later, there was again a call for their introduction[(3)]. In 1991 calls to introduce breathalysers were made at the Lae Conference on Drug Related Crimes in PNG organized by the Foundation for Law Order & Justice in May[(4)] and also at the Forum in Port Moresby on Drug Education in PNG which was staged in June by the National Health Education Advisory Committee. One of the objectives of the PNG National Health Plan 1991-1995 is that "By 1995, the police should use breathalysers on drunk drivers"[(5)].

One of the papers which was given at the Lae Conference by the Department of Transport presented some sobering figures on trends of alcohol-related accidents. Out of 491 cases of casualties as a result of alcohol-related accidents in 1989, 49% (n=233) of people were seriously injured and 7% (n=61) of these were fatal. These casualties were a result of a total of 695 alcohol-related accidents. Twenty percent of these occured on Fridays whilst 13% occured on Saturdays. From Sunday to Wednesday the accidents varied from 5% to 13% [(6)].

Even more sobering are the results of the Alcohol Survey done in Port Moresby between 21 August and 23 September 1990 which aimed at finding the proportion of drivers who were drunk and driving, through the use of breathalysers, in a bid to provide evidence that legislation be amended to include a specific blood alcohol limit. (Most other countries have a legal limit of between 50 and 80 milligrams of alcohol per 100 milliliters of blood). Comparisons with two other test sites where similar surveys were done over the same period of time found that, of the 901 drivers tested in Port Moresby, 23% registered more than 80mg%, while 1.5% of drivers in the UK and 4% of drivers in Adelaide registered readings of over 80mg%. Readings made on Thursdays to Saturdays suggested that these days presented with more drivers recording over 80mg% than other days. The following table is the analysis from this study.

TABLE 1

Blood Alcohol Content Readings of Drivers in Port Moresby on Specific Days from 21 August-23 September 1990

	Number of Drivers				
BAC (mg%)	**Thursdays**	**Fridays**	**Saturdays**	**Sunday**	**Total**
0 - 5	99	158	167	136	560
10 - 40	12	23	25	7	67
45 - 80	16	25	22	2	65
85 - 115	13	19	18	4	54
120 - 150	10	19	15	2	46
155 - 180	7	16	15	2	40
185 - 215	8	14	8	1	31
>215	9	15	11	3	38
TOTAL	174	289	281	157	901
>80mg%	27.01%	28.71%	23.84%	7.64%	21.64%

Adapted from Department of Transport, 1991, Alcohol Suspected Accidents in Papua New Guinea, p. 6.

Excluding Sundays, 26.48% percent of drivers on the road from Thursdays to Saturdays are driving with a BAC level of over 80mg%! As the Department of Transport state, "...a good number of people were driving after drinking alcohol showing the general attitude of unconcern towards drinking and driving in PNG. Further, for every nine (9) drivers during the survey, 2 drivers were over the 80mg% and out of these 7.2% consumed excessive amounts over 190%mg..."(6).

It may be that there is a general lack of concern about drunk drivers, but when an accident happens to you or to the one you love, that lack of concern turns into bitterness, grief, blame and all the other negative thoughts and behaviours that occur at times like this. Alcohol as a substance is not in itself a cause of stress; often it is used to reduce stress, to make people feel comfortable, to make them feel superior or big (Karlin, 1991). However, the use of this substance excessively has caused many problems in the family as well as in the workplace, and it also has a ripple effect: assaults, road accidents, accidents at work and the like. As no indication is made in the Health Plan 1991-1995 (PNG, 1991, p. 198) of establishing a legal limit of blood alcohol content (BAC), except that breathalysers should be used to estimate blood alcohol levels of the drivers involved in crashes, I would suggest -

i) that breathalysers be introduced immediately, and

ii) that the legal BAC limit be .05mg%.

4. **LACK OF BASIC ESSENTIALS**

Increasingly, a source of stress is our inability to provide what are considered to be basic human rights: food, water and shelter. The lack of accommodation, for example, is an acute factor often causing families to split up and thereby breaking a unit that is considered to be important. If the family unit is important enough to be concerned about, then an attempt at assisting its continuation and well-being by provision of housing is imperative.

Below is a table showing some of the behaviours and associated symptoms that have been exhibited by clients that I have worked with. Many of the stresses indentified are presented by both men and women; some of the behaviours are exhibited by only one sex. Although it is not complete, it is an indication that, when we look at how our changing society is affecting us as a family unit, it is indeed all-encompassing and does not discriminate between the sexes.

TABLE 2

Some Symptoms and Accompanying Behaviours as a Result of Stress Within the Family

Symptoms & Behaviours	Experienced by Males	Females
Abortion*		x
Absenteeism	x	x
Accidents at workplace	x	x
Adultery	x	x
Aggression	x	
Alcohol abuse	x	x
Assault		
Bodily damage such as bruises		x
Bodily damage including broken arms, legs, ribs, hips		x
Bodily damage including biting		x
Bodily damages from dangerous weapons	x	x
Rape		x
Bride price (payment & non-payment of)	x	x
Death of family and friends	x	x
Financial difficulties	x	x
Loneliness	x	x
Sickness	x	x
Social isolation	x	x
Depression	x	x
Despair	x	x
Drug addiction	x	
Extra-marital affairs:		
Co-habitation with de factos	x	x
Financial needs &/or mismanagment	x	x
Gambling (cards)		x
(horses)	x	x
Habitual or Fortnightly Drunkeness including Thursdays-, Friday- and Monday-itis	x	
Incest	x	

* Indicates cognitive restructuring therapy to the effect that the pregnancy was completed.

Some Symptoms and Accompanying Behaviours as a Result of Stress within the Family (cont.)

Symptoms & Behaviours	Experienced by Males	Experienced by Females
Legal complications:		
Adoption	x	x
Custody	x	x
Divorce	x	x
Maintenance		x
Property distribution	x	x
Separation	x	x
Loss of friends and separation from families	x	x
Murder		x
Non-acceptance of being a step-parent	x	x
Non-acceptance of contraceptives	x	
Non-availability of basic human needs e.g., Food, shelter & water	x	x
Parent/child conflicts	x	x
Personality disturbance	x	x
Prostitution		x
Psychological disabilities		
clinical depression	x	x
suicide thoughts	x	x
anxiety reactions	x	x
jealousy	x	x
deteriorating health	x	x
lack of concentration	x	x
lack of sleep	x	x
poor eating habits	x	x
more susceptability to illnesses	x	x
sexual coldness	x	
poor working habits	x	x
guilt	x	x
Resignation/Retrenchment	x	x
Sexual harrassment		x
Sexual non-gratification	x	x
Sexual transmitted diseases	x	x
Single parenting		x
Termination of employment	x	x
Theft/Stealing	x	
Unequal employment opportunities	x	x
Unwed parenthood		x
Work or career disappointment/failure	x	x

5. EFFECTS OF NON-AVAILABILITY OF PROFESSIONAL COUNSELLING AND WELFARE SERVICES

There are only limited professional services available today to assist people with these kinds of problems. From my working experience, it is difficult to refer people to bodies that can assist people with problems. The Health Department has 32 psychiatric nurses throughout the country; in 1982, the Psychological Services Division of the Public Services Department was thought to be a non-essential service and was therefore disbanded; the Welfare Office is understaffed; the Mental Health Division of the Health Department is also understaffed, etc. etc.

In very few places is there a welfare and counselling service. To some this seems a luxury; however, in my opinion, as I have mentioned above, there is no better working man or woman than the one who thinks that he/she is being cared for.

If we are to seriously consider the mental well-being of our staff in a working environment, then we must take care of what is often described as the human resources. Without them, we won't have a department, or an organization, or a company.

Until and unless we recognize these symptoms for what they are, it would be very difficult and, indeed, hypocritical, to pontificate on the invaluableness of the family unit. We must accept that we are living in a climate of change, whether it be to the Ozone level, the Bougainville crisis or the family unit. When we start to accept that we cannot go back to what it was like when our grandparents were alive, and indeed to accept that we must change, then perhaps we may effect some change that will lessen the negative and often drastic effects that so-called progress and development has on the health of our people.

I believe that we can effect changes but, alas, I fear that those who are above us are either too selfish, or else are blatantly refusing to acknowledge, that we must change our approach with the changing of the tides. It is therefore up to us who are in this field to push these thoughts forward to a state of acceptability and accountability. If we, who are here to discuss the health of our people, just talk about it, then I fear that we too will have failed them.

CONCLUSION

There is not much that I would like to recapitulate on and emphasise except the following:

1. The environment in which we live today is filled with many stressful and traumatic elements that cause disharmony within and outside ourselves.

2. Much of the stress that we face today is a result of being and becoming modern.

3. The concepts or attitudes that we hold close to our hearts about being truly Papua New Guinean are dated.

4. The use of custom to justify modern behaviour is unacceptable, and specifically:

   4.1 The concept of brideprice should be done away with (I cannot accept any in between compromise, such as there being a limit to how much a woman should cost);

   4.2 In an urban setting, if custom is to be used, it should not be mixed with modern decorations;

   4.3 If we speak of being equal partners, and if the practice of bride price is continued, then there should be reciprocity in that there should be bride-groom prices as well.

5. Many of us talk about education for women on the basic human rights such as the decision to create or not to create life; we forget to educate the men that they too must respect these rights.

6. Many of us talk about education on the importance of contraceptives; but we forget that education is not only for women, but also for men; therefore we must educate, or in many cases, question why men do not want women to use contraceptives.

7. Many of us face stresses related to one of the basics of human existence: shelter. There should be more shelter provided at lower cost. The current high price of accommodation in Papua New Guinea is only making the rich get richer and the poor poorer.

8. The use of alcohol and its abuse is a cause of stress that many of us face; if we are to think about the health of this nation, then we should do something about it. In this paper, I have spoken about two issues that should be looked at immediately:

   8.1 The immediate introduction of breathalysers; and

   8.2 The introduction of a BAC level of .05mg%.

9. Equal opportunity in the workplace is questionable for both males and females; in today's world it appears to be not what you know, but who you know.

10. There are definitely insufficient resources to assist those with problems, such as counsellors in the social work, psychiatric, and marital fields.

REFERENCES

Gillett, J. 1990. The Health of Women in Papua New Guinea (PNGIMR Monograph No. 9). Madang: Kristen Press.

Royal Commission of Inquiry. Papua New Guinea, 1971.

Marshall, M., Piau-Lynch, A., & Sumanop, F.H. (1981). Conclusion and Policy Implications. In M. Marshall (Ed.) Through a Glass Darkly: Beer and Modernization in Papua New Guinea (Monograph No. 18, pp. 451-461). IASER: Port Moresby.

Karlin, B. Summary Points Re: Drug Education in PNG. Paper presented at the Conference on Drug Related Crimes in Papua New Guinea, Lae, 13-17 May 1991, and the Forum on Drug Education in Papua New Guinea, Port Moresby, 13-14 June, 1991.

Papua New Guinea National Health Plan 1991-1995. (1991). Port Moresby: Government Printer.

Department of Transport. Alcohol Suspected Road Accidents in Papua New Guinea. Paper presented at the conference on Drug Related Crimes in Papua New Guinea, 13-17 May 1991, Lae.

A STUDY OF COMPLETED SUICIDE IN THE NATIONAL CAPITAL DISTRICT AND CENTRAL PROVINCE OF PAPUA NEW GUINEA

FELIX Y. ATTAH JOHNSON[1]

INTRODUCTION

The Dictionary of Medical Ethics (1) defines suicide succintly as "an act of deliberate self-destruction". Camus (2) expressed the view that "there is only one philosophical problem and that is suicide". Suicide appears to be ubiquitous and as old as man. Duncan et al (I) commented that "The civil law has followed the ecclesiastical law, that against suicide being abolished first in France in 1790. It has been abolished, state by state, across the USA although several southern states still retain it. The Act against suicide in England was repealed in 1961, but it is still an offence to aid or abet suicide and survivors of pacts may be prosecuted. Nowhere has the existence of abolition of the law been shown to affect suicide rates though attempted suicide is another matter." In the independent state of Papua New Guinea the law against suicide is still on the statutes (3). It is important to understand the differences between people who commit suicide (completed suicide) and patients who survive after taking an overdose of drugs or harming themselves (deliberate self-harm). This difference is important for assessing patients properly and also for the purpose of research. According to Gelder et al. (4): "In general, compared with people who harm themselves and survive, those who commit suicide are more often male, and are suffering from a psychiatric disorder. They plan their suicide acts carefully, take precautions against discovery, and use dangerous methods. By contrast, among those who harm themselves and survive, a large proportion carry out their acts impulsively in a way that invites discovery and is unlikely to be dangerous. The two groups are not distinctly separate; they overlap in important ways."

1 Associate Professor of Psychiatry, Department of Clinical Sciences, Faculty of Medicine, University of Papua New Guinea

The purpose of the present paper is to report a study of completed suicide cases in the National Capital District (NCD) and the adjacent Central Province (CP) of Papua New Guinea. There have been a few studies of suicide in Papua New Guinea reported in the literature (5,6,7,8,9,10). In their paper Parker and Burton-Bradley (5) commented that "forty-one indigenous deaths attributed to suicide were officially reported during the five-year period from January 1961 to December 1965. We infer that, given the nature and terrain of the country with its difficulties of transport and communication, this figure is an underestimate. The true picture is unknown". Over the same period Parker and Burton-Bradley (5) reported eleven European deaths in Papua New Guinea attributed to suicide and "only one mixed race person killed himself". Burton-Bradley (11) wrote the following comment on indigenous methods of suicide: "From the reported incidence of indigenous suicide .... hanging is the most popular method favoured equally by men and women. From a total of forty-one suicides, thirteen males and fourteen females hanged themselves, three males shot themselves and one male and seven females ate derris root and three males used other methods." Derris root contains a strong toxin which is usually used to stun fish during fishing. The chewing of derris root was described as predominantly a female method of suicide in some provinces of Papua New Guinea. Stanhope (7) was very critical of the paper by Parker and Burton-Bradley, especially their statement that suicide is "not common" and the supporting evidence that "During the five-year period from January 1961 to December 1965, there were 41 deaths from suicide among indigenous people, representing a rate of 0.7 per 100,000". He reported that the New Guinea Mortality Survey for 1966 had shown five suicides in 58,480 person-years of observation in five other rural populations of Papua New Guinea, the annual rate being 8.5 per 100,000 (7). In 1981 Smith (9) reported a very interesting study from a remote society in the Highlands of Papua New Guinea and concluded that: "Twenty-six cases occurred over an eight year period (17 cases per 100,000 population per year) and 23 of these were female. The method chosen by all females was hanging and in 16 cases interpersonal conflicts appeared to have been the precipitating factor". Murphy (10) in an epidemiological study reported a suicide rate of 10.7 per 100,000 in the National Capital District and for the rest of Papua New Guinea the suicide rate of 2.4 per 100,000 population. This reported suicide rate of 2.4 per 100,000 for the rural areas of Papua New Guinea is very low compared with the rate of 17 per 100,000 reported by Smith (9). Sainsbury (12) reported high rates of suicide in areas of London in which there were many inhabitants of boarding houses, many immigrants and divorced people. He found the common factor to be social isolation. Sainsbury's work on social isolation followed directly from the original reports of Durkheim (13) in 1897. In his study from France in 1897 Durkheim (13) found a relationship between suicide and social conditions. He divided suicide cases into three categories: 1) egoistic suicide occurred in individuals who had lost their sense of integration with their social group, so that they no longer felt subject to its family, social and religious groups, 2) anomic suicide occurred in individuals who lived in a society that lacked collective order because it was in the midst of a major social or political change, 3) altruistic suicide occurred in individuals who sacrificed their lives for the good of the social groups, thus reflecting the influence of group identity. Durkheim's theories emphasized social factors at the expense of personality and cognitive factors. In his paper from Papua New Guinea Pataki-Schweizer (6) commented that PNG is a country where traditional, transitional and modern life styles are simultaneously present, thus experiencing the acceleration and stress of rapid acculturation and social change.

There are differences within and between countries in their suicide rates. In interpreting these differences, many workers have given attention to the possibility that such differences are the result of artifacts in recording and reporting of death by suicide (14,15). "Although such artifacts undoubtedly play some part, there are almost certainly real differences between geographical areas and between countries" (16). Barraclough (17) stated that: "The independence of the rank order from the effects of ascertainment procedures is strong evidence that differences in national official suicide rates truthfully reflect that countries do differ in their incidence of suicide." Odejide et al. (18) reported a study from Ibadan (Nigeria) in which they found that disturbed interpersonal relationships, especially with parents, motivated acts of deliberate self-harm (DSH). They further stated that: "From the few reports on DSH in Nigeria, the prevalence rate ranged from 1 to 7 per 100,000; males predominated and major psychiatric disorders were found to be associated with the act (Asuni 1967; Eferakeya 1984). Regarding the methods used for DSH, Asuni (1967) found physical self-harm (slashing of the throat etc.) to be more common, although a more recent report showed that the ingestion of psychiotropic drugs and chemicals was more prevalent" (18). Daradkeh (21) reported a study of suicide in Jordan in which he found that the problems of suicide was small (2.1 cases per 100,000 population) and limited to the younger age groups. He gave two possible explanations for his findings, namely: "First the majority of the mentally ill people committing suicide, who accounted for 63% of the total suicides were in the younger age groups. Second, young adults are thought to be less religious than the elderly, thus making them more vulnerable to stress" (21).

The literature on suicidology shows a dichotomous development, with preliteracy related by different investigators to both higher and lower frequencies of suicide. On the one hand, "reports claiming a low incidence of suicide in preliterate cultures go back to the observation of kraepelin made during his tour of southeast Asia and Java in 1903" (22). On the other hand, "reports that the incidence of suicide in preliterate cultures is not low also have an ancient and respectable lineage, traceable to Steinmetz (23), who in 1894 examined the topic of suicide among primitive peoples. Zilboorg, (24) in a review of suicide among 'civilized' and 'primitive' races, reached similar conclusions, as did Dublin (25) in his sociological and statistical study of suicide and Bohannan (26) and his co-workers in a study of suicide and homicide in Africa" (22). In a survey of suicide rates in the Kandrian District of southwest New Britain in Papua New Guinea, Hoskin et al. (22) concluded as follows: "The suicide rate of 23 per 100,000 per annum in the indigenous population of the Kandrian area of southwest New Britain appears to be greater than that of most Western societies. The finding runs counter to the belief that suicide is rare amongst preliterate cultures. Other New Guinea populations - as yet uninvestigated - are also reported to have high suicide rates."

The study reported in the present paper is limited to completed suicide cases reported in the two years 1986 and 1987 in the National Capital District and the adjacent Central Province of Papua New Guinea. This is a retrospective study.

MATERIALS AND METHOD

Data on completed suicide cases in the National Capital District (NC) and Central Province of Papua New Guinea were collected from two main sources. The first source was the Port Moresby General Hospital (PMGH) Mortuary Department in consultation with the Senior Specialist Pathologist in-charge. The author consulted the Senior Specialist Pathologist who made the register of all medico-legal post mortem examinations available to him. Relevant data were collected from the register and recorded on purpose prepared questionnaires. The collected data on patients who died in hospital were cross-checked by looking up their clinical casenotes with the help of the Medical Records Department. The second source of data collection was the coroner's office. After obtaining the permission of the Chief Magistrate in-charge, three final-year medical students assisted the author by collecting all relevant data from the register and files of the coroner's office. The data were collected by completing purpose prepared questionnaires as mentioned earlier. All the data collected on officially reported completed suicide cases in the two years 1986 and 1987 were subjected to statistical analysis.

RESULTS

The findings and results of the study are shown in tables 1 to 6. The incidence rate of completed suicide for the National Capital District in 1986 is 12.6 per 100,000 based on the officially estimated population of 142,497. The comparable incidence rate of suicide for 1987 is 14.18 per 100,000 based on an estimated population of 148,054. Therefore the mean annual incidence rate of completed suicide in the whole study is 13.4 per 100,000 population. The following is a description of the results:

Age and Sex Distribution:

In 1986, the age range was 15 to 45 years and the mean age was 26.3 $\pm$ 8.6 years. The ratio of male to female cases was 1.2. The comparative figures for 1987 were age range 13 to 46 years and mean age was 26.8 $\pm$ 9.3 years. The ratio of male to female cases was 2.25:1. In 1986, the peak age group for committing suicide was 30-34 years for both males and females. In 1987, the peak age group for committing suicide was 20-24 years for both males and females followed by 25-29 years for males only. The most interesting finding in this table is that in 1986 twice as many females as males committed suicide whilst in 1987 the reverse is the case - twice as many males as females committed suicide.

TABLE 1: Age and Sex Distribution

1986

Age (in years)	Male No	Male %	Female No	Female %	Total No	Total %
10 - 14	0	0.0	0	0.0	0	0.0
15 - 19	1	5.55	3	16.66	4	22.2
20 - 24	1	5.55	3	16.66	4	22.2
25 - 29	0	0.0	1	5.55	1	5.55
30 - 34	3	16.66	3	16.66	6	33.3
35 - 39	1	5.55	0	0.00	1	5.55
40 - 44	0	0.0	1	5.55	1	5.55
45 - 49	0	0.0	1	5.55	1	5.55
50 - 54	0	0.0	0	0.0	0	0.0
TOTAL	**6**	**33.31**	**12**	**66.7**	**18**	**100.0**

Age Range: 15 to 45 years
Mean Age : 26.3 ± 8.6 years
Ratio of Male to Female = 1 : 2

1987

Age (in years)	Male No	Male %	Female No	Female %	Total No	Total %
10 - 14	1	3.8	0	0.0	1	3.8
15 - 19	2	7.7	1	3.8	3	11.5
20 - 24	5	19.2	6	23.1	11	42.3
25 - 29	5	19.2	0	0.0	5	19.2
30 - 34	1	3.8	0	0.0	1	3.8
35 - 39	0	0.0	0	0.0	0	0.0
40 - 44	1	3.8	1	3.8	2	7.6
45 - 49	3	11.5	0	0.0	3	11.5
50 - 54	0	0.0	0	0.0	0	0.0
Total	**18**	**69.2**	**8**	**30.8**	**26**	**100.0**

Age Range: 13 to 46 years
Mean Age : 26.8 ± 9.3 years
Ratio of Male to Female = 2.25:1

Distribution according to Nationality: National/Expatriate

In 1986 all the 18 reported suicide cases were Papua New Guinean nationals. There was no case of suicide reported from the expatriate community. The comparable figures for 1987 were: 14 (53.8%) males and 7 (26.9%) female suicide cases were reported for Papua New Guinean nationals; 4 (15.4%) male and 1 (3.85%) female cases of suicide reported were expatriate.

TABLE 2: Distribution according to Nationality: National/Expatriate

1986

PNG NATIONAL				EXPATRIATE				TOTAL	
Male		Female		Male		Female		No	%
No	%	No	%	No	%	No	%		
6	33.3	12	66.7	0	0.0	0	0.0	18	100

1987

PNG NATIONAL				EXPATRIATE				TOTAL	
Male		Female		Male		Female		No	%
No	%	No	%	No	%	No	%		
14	53.8	7	26.9	4	15.4	1	3.85	26	100

Methods of Suicide: In both 1986 and 1987 the two main methods for committing suicide were intentional drug overdose and deliberate physical self-injury. In 1986 four females took chloroquine overdose, one male took chloroquine plus ethanol overdose and one male took an unknown liquor, making a total of six cases. The comparable figures for 1987 were: five females (all PNG nationals) and three males (one PNG national and two expatriates) took chloroquine overdose; seven PNG nationals took overdose of ethanol only and another PNG national took Amodiaquine overdose. A total of 17 (11 males and 6 females) people committed suicide by taking overdose in 1987, that is more than two times the number in 1986.

TABLE 3:

1986

(PNG Nationals only)

Method	Male No	Male %	Female No	Female %	Total No	Total %
Drug Overdose:						
Chloroquine only	0	0.0	4	22.2	4	22.2
Chloroquine+Ethanol	1	5.55	0	0.0	1	5.55
Unknown liquor	1	5.55	0	0.0	1	5.55
Sub-Total:	**2**	**11.1**	**4**	**22.2**	**6**	**33.3**
Physical Injury:						
Hanging	1	5.55	7	38.9	8	44.4
Cut-throat	0	0.0	2	11.1	2	11.1
Jumped off moving	0	0.0	1	5.55	1	5.55
Gunshot by self	0	0.0	1	5.55	1	5.55
Sub-Total:	**1**	**5.5**	**11**	**61.1**	**12**	**66.6**
Total:	**3**	**16.65**	**15**	**83.3**	**18**	**100**

1987

Method	MALE PNG No	%	EXPAT. No	%	FEMALE PNG No	%	EXPAT No	%	TOTAL No	%
Drug Overdose:										
Chloroquine only	1	3.8	2	7.7	5	19.2	0	0.0	8	30.8
Chloroquine + Ethanol	0	0.0	0	0.0	0	0.0	1	3.85	1	3.85
Ethanol only	7	26.9	0	0.0	0	0.0	0	0.0	7	26.9
Amodiaquine	1	3.85	0	0.0	0	0.0	0	0.0	1	3.85
Sub Total:	**5**	**34.6**	**2**	**7.7**	**5**	**19.2**	**1**	**3.85**	**17**	**65.4**
Physical Injury:										
Hanging	4	5.4	2	7.7	1	3.85	0	0.0	7	26.9
Jumped off moving vehicle	0	0.0	0	0.0	1	3.85	0	0.0	1	3.85
Gunshot by self	**1**	**3.85**	**0**	**0.0**	**0**	**0.0**	**0**	**0.0**	**1**	**3.85**
Sub Total:	**5**	**19.25**	**2**	**7.7**	**2**	**7.7**	**0**	**0.0**	**9**	**34.6**
TOTAL:	**14**	**53.8**	**4**	**15.4**	**7**	**26.9**	**1**	**3.85**	**26**	**100**

The most common methods of physical self-injury in both 1986 and 1987 were hanging, gunshot by self and jumping off a moving motor vehicle. In 1986, a total of 8 people (7 females and 1 male) hanged themselves, one female shot hereself and one female jumped off a moving motor vehicle. Also in 1986, two females committed suicide by using the cut-throat method. In 1987 a total of 7 people (6 males and 1 female) hanged themselves, one male shot himself and one female jumped off a moving motor vehicle. The most typical suicide case in this study is a young adult female who has taken chloroquine overdose or caused herself physical injury (hanging, cut-throat, jumping off a moving vehicle or gunshot wound).

Past History of Psychiatric or Physical Illness :

In 1986 only 4 (22.2%) out of 18 cases suffered from a psychiatric illness prior to committing suicide. In 1987 only one (3.9%) case suffered from psychiatric illness before committing suicide. No physical illness was diagnosed before the act of suicide in both 1986 and 1987.

TABLE 4

1986

	No	%
Psychiatric Illness	4	22.2
Physical Illness	0	0.0
No History of any Illness	14	77.0
Total:	**18**	**100.0**

1987	No	%
Psychiatric Illness	1	3.9
Phsyical Illness	0	0.0
No History of any Illness	25	96.1
	26	**100.0**

Severe Social Distress: All the 18 suicide cases reported in 1986 and all the 26 suicide cases reported in 1987 gave a history of severe social distress preceding the act of suicide. The most common forms of severe social distress in 1986 were due to interpersonal conflict (quarrel with husband 6 cases; quarrel with parents 5 cases; quarrel with wife 1 case). The most common forms of severe social distress in 1987 were also due to interpersonal conflict (quarrel with husband 7 cases; quarrel with wife 6 cases; quarrel with parents 6 cases). Acute alcohol intoxication and sudden collapse which claimed 7 lives was a significant cause of suicide in 1987.

TABLE 5:

1986

Social Distress	No. of Cases
1) Quarrel with husband	6
2) Quarrel with parents in adolescents	5
3) Non-specific social distress in pschiatric patient	2
4) A student from a vocational centre who had serious problems with her studies	1
5) Unemployment. This patient recorded a suicide message on a casette recorder	1
6) Abnormal offender admitted to a psychiatric hospital	1
7) Acute alcohol intoxication with sudden collapse	1
8) Quarrel with wife	1
Total number of cases:	**18**

1987

Social Distress	No. of Cases
1) Quarrel with husband	6
2) Quarrel with parents in adolescents	6
3) Acute alcohol intoxication with sudden collapse (including one known psychiatric patient	7
4) Quarrel with wife	6
5) Jumped off a moving motor vehicle after quarrel with her husband	1
Total number of cases:	**26**

Monthly Distribution of Completed Suicide Cases:

In 1986 the peak months for committing the act of suicide were January (4 cases, 22.2%), April (4 cases, 22.2%), February (3 cases, 16.7%) and June (2 cases, 11.1%). The comparable peak months in 1987 were December (6 cases, 23.1%), July (5 cases, 19.2%), April (4 cases, 15.4%) and February (2 cases, 7.7%). When the reported suicide cases for both 1986 and 1987 are added up the most popular months for committing the act are April (8 cases), December (7 cases) and January (7 cases); followed by July (6 cases) and February (5 cases). Therefore, the three-month period December, January and February accounted for 19 (47.5%) cases out of the total number of 40 cases of suicide among Papua New Guinean nationals reported in the two years, 1986 and 1987.

TABLE 6:

Month	1986 No	1986 %	1987 No	1987 %	Remarks
January	4	22.2	3	11.5	New Year
February	3	16.7	2	7.7	-
March	1	5.55	1	3.85	-
April	4	22.2	4	15.4	-
May	1	5.55	4	15.4	-
June	2	11.1	1	3.85	-
July	1	5.55	5	19.2	National General Elections in July 1987
August	0	0.0	0	0.0	
September	0	0.0	1	3.85	-
October	0	0.0	1	3.85	-
November	1	5.55	1	3.85	-
December	1	5.55	6	23.1	Christmas Season
Total:	**18**	**100.0**	**26**	**100.0**	

DISCUSSION

Discussion of the results and findings of the study will be based on (1) socio-demographic characteristics and annual incidence rates of suicide, (2) methods of suicide, (3) past history of psychiatric illness, (4) presence of severe social distress and (5) months distribution of suicide cases.

Sociodemographic Characteristics and Annual Incidence Rates of Suicide: One of the high-lights of the results is that in 1986 the ratio of male to female cases was 1:2, but in 1987 the male to female ratio was 2.25:1. It is difficult to explain this reversal of male to female ratio over the two years, 1986/1987. The male to female ratio for both years are both different from the findings of Parker and Burton-Bradley (5), who found 13 males to 14 females (giving a ratio of 1:1.1) out of 41 suicide cases. The male to female ratio of 2.25:1 found in 1987 is similar to those reported by Odejide (18) from Ibadan (Nigeria) and by Darakeh (21) from Jordan. When the figures for 1986 and 1987 are combined the peak age group for committing suicide is higher than that of Odejide who reported a peak age group of 15-19 years. It is slightly different from the peak age group of 15-24 years reported by Daradkeh (21).

The incidence rate of completed suicide for the National Capital District in 1986 is 12.6 per 100,000. The comparable incidence rate of suicide for 1987 is 14.18 per 100,000. The mean annual incidence rate of completed suicide is 13.4 100,000 for the whole study. This suicide incidence of 13.4 per 100,000 is considerably higher than the figure of 2.5 per 100,000 reported by Odejide (18) from Ibadan (Nigeria). The suicide incidence of 13.4 per 100,000 is also higher than the figure of 10.7 per 100,000 reported by Murphy (10) in an epidemiological study in the National Capital District four years ago in 1983. This finding is probably an indication of a real increase in the incidence of suicide cases in the National Capital District over the four year period (1983 to 1987). The finding of a high suicide incidence of 13.4 per 100,000 in the National Capital District also compares favourably with the finding of Smith (9) from a remote society in the Highlands of Papua New Guinea. According to Smith (9): "Twenty-six cases occurred over an eight year period (17 cases per 100,000 population per year) and 23 of these were female. The method chosen by all females was hanging and in 16 cases interpersonal conflicts appeared to have been the precipitating factor."

Methods of Suicide

The results of the study showed that the methods of committing suicide fall into two main groups namely, drug over-dose and physical self-injury. This is similar to the report by Odejide (18), who found that the methods used were mainly ingestion of chemicals or psychotropic drugs and physical self-harm. In 1986, two (11.1%) Papua New Guinean males and four (22.2%) females committed suicide by taking drug overdose. The most common drug ingested were Chloroquine tablets only or Chloroquine tablets plus

ethanol (see Table 3). Also in 1986, seven (38.9%) Papua New Guinean (PNG) females and one (5.6%) male hanged themselves. In addition, two (11.1%) PNG females out their throats, one (5.6%) female jumped off a moving motor vehicle and one (5.6%) also shot herself (see Table 3). In 1987, seven (26.9%) PNG males poisoned themselves with ethanol, one (3.85%) took Chloroquine overdose and another one (3.85%) took Amodiaquine overdose (see Table 3). On the other hand five (19.2%) PNG females took Chloroquine overdose. In the same year four (15.4%) PNG males hanged themselves and one (3.85%) male shot himself. One (3.85%) female hanged herself and another female jumped off a moving vehicle. In both 1986 and 1987, the most common methods used by Papua New Guineans (male and female) for committing suicide were hanging 33.3% (13 out of 39 cases), Chloroquine overdose 30.8% (12 out of 39 cases) and ethanol poisoning 17.95% (7 out of 39 cases). These latter results are similar to those of Smith (9) in 1981 and Burton-Bradley (11) in 1973 which were reported from Papua New Guinea.

Past History of Psychiatric Illness:

In 1986, four (22.2%) cases were reported to have had a past history of psychiatric illness before the act of suicide. In 1987, only one (3.9%) patient had a past history of psychiatric illness before the act. All five patients were reported to have had chronic psychiatric illnesses, most probably chronic schizophrenia. The majority of the cases in both 1986 and 1987 did not have past history of any illness (physical or psychiatric). These results are different from those reported by Daradkeh (21), who found "nearly two-thirds of the total population that committed suicide had previous psychiatric illness", and Odejide (18) who found five cases of mental illness and one case of unresolved physical illness.

Severe Social Distress

Interpersonal conflict was the most common cause of severe social distress and consequently of suicide in both 1986 and 1987 (see Table 5). Specifically, quarrel with one or both parents in adolescents (five cases in 1986, six cases in 1987), quarrel with wife (one case in 1986, six cases in 1987). These results are in agreement with those of Odejide (18) who found disturbed relationship with parents, interpersonal discord with significant others, marital discord and frustration or shame due to failure in examination as common reasons for deliberate self-harm in his study from Ibadan (Nigeria). Another significant cause of suicide in the present study is acute alcohol intoxication (alcohol poisoning) resulting in sudden collapse (one case in 1986, seven cases in 1987).

Substance abuse (especially alcohol and cannabis abuse) is rapidly emerging as a common cause of psychopathology and 'social pathology' in Papua New Guinea.

Monthly Distribution of Cases:

Cases of completed suicide were reported in all the months of the year except August, September and October in 1986 and August only in 1987 (see Table 6). In 1986 most of the cases were reported in January (four cases), February (three cases) and April (four cases). In 1987, on the other hand, most of the cases were reported in December (six cases), January (three cases), April (four cases) and July (five cases). In contrast to reports based on studies from some other countries, there is no clear-cut seasonal distribution of suicide cases in this study.

CONCLUSION

The main conclusions which can be reached from the study, on the basis of the results, are (1) completed suicides are remarkably common among Papua New Guinean nationals (incidence rate is 13.4 cases per 100,000 population per annum) compared with other developing countries; (2) the major precipitating factor for carrying out the lethal act is interpersonal conflict with significant family members (eg. parents and spouses) and (3) the most common methods of self-destruction are hanging by the neck in both males and females followed by drug overdose (mainly chloroquine and ethanol). The author would like to suggest further studies on completed suicide in both urban and rural areas of Papua New Guinea and other South-Western Pacific countries.

ACKNOWLEDGEMENTS:

The author would like to thank Drs Geetha Ranmuthugala, Sammy Thomas and Kilagi Vanuga for their assistance with the collection of data from the coroner's office. My sincere gratitude is due to Mrs Annelise T. Johnson for typing the manuscript.

REFERENCES

1. Duncan A S., Dunstan G. R and Welbourn R B (Editors); Dictionary of Medical Ethics. Published by Darton, Longman and Todd. London. 1981: 424-425

2. Camus A. The myth of Sisyphus. London: Hamish Hamilton; Harmondsworth: Penguin Books. 1955

3. Criminal Code of Papua New Guinea. Ch. No 262: Attempting Suicide and Aiding Suicide. Port Moresby.

4. Gelder M., Gath D, Mayou R. Oxford Textbook of Psychiatry Suicide and Deliberate Self-Harm. Published by Oxford University Press/ELBS. Oxford. 1985: 398-421

5. Parker N, Burton-Bradley B G. Suicide in Papua New Guinea. Medical J. of Australia, 1966, 2: 1125-1129.

6. Pataki-Schweizer K J. Suicide in Contemporary Papua New Guinea. An attempt at an Overview. Working Paper Series, Pacific Islands Studies Programme. University of Hawaii and East West Centre, Hawaii. 1985

7. Stanhope J M. Suicide in Papua New Guinea (letter). Med. J. of Australia 1967, 1: 140-141.

8. Wilkey E S. Chloroquine Suicide. Med. J. Australia, Case Reports 1973, 1: 396-397. Case reports.

9. Smith D. Suicide in a Remote Preliterate Society in the Highlands of Papua New Guinea. PNG Med. J. 1981, 24:242-246.

10. Murphy HMB. Mental Health Trends in the Pacific Islands Noumea: South Pacific Commission. 1983

11. Burton-Bradley B G. "Longlong": Transcultural Psychiatry in Papua New Guinea. Published by Public Health Department, Port Moresby 1973: 82-94

12. Sainsbury P. Suicide in London: An Ecological Study Basic Books, New York, 1956

13. Durkheim E. Suicide: A Study in Sociology. Translated by Spalding J A and Simpson G. New York. Free Press, 1951

14. Barraclough B M. The effect that coroners have on the suicide rate and the open verdict rate. In: Hare E R, Wing J K ed. Psychiatric Epidemiology. Oxford University Press. Oxford, 1969: 361-365

15. Sainsbury P. Epidemiology of Suicide. In: Roy E, ed. Suicide. Williams and Wilkins, Baltimore. USA, 1986: 17-40

16. Henderson A S. Suicide and Parasuicide. In Introduction to Social Psychiatry. Oxford Medical Publications. Oxford University Press. Oxford, 1988:57

17. Barraclough B M. Differences between national suicide rates. Br J. Psychiatry 1973, 122: 95-96.

18. Odejide A O. Williams A O. Ohaeri J U and Ikusesan B A. The Epidemiology of Deliberate Self Harm. The Ibadan Experience. Br J. Psychiatry 1986, 149: 734-737.

19. Asuni T. Attempted suicide in Western Nigeria. West African Med. Journal 1967, 13(2): 51-54.

20. Eferakeya A E. Drugs and Suicide attempts in Benin-City, Nigeria, Br. J. Psychiatry 1984, 145: 70-73.

21. Daradkeh T K. Suicide in Jordan 1980-1985. Acta Psychiatr. Scand. 1989, 79: 241-244.

22. Hoskin J O, Friedman M I and Cawte J E. "A high incidence of suicide in a preliterate primitive society." Psychiatry, 1969; Vol. 32: 200-210.

23. Steinmetz S R. "Suicide among primitive peoples." Amer. Anthropologist, 1894, Vol. 7: 53-60.

24. Zilboorg G. "Suicide among civilized and primitive races." Amer. J. Psychiatry, 1936, Vol. 92: 1347-1369.

25. Dublin L I. "Suicide: A Sociological and Statistical Study." 1963; Ronald Press.

26. Bohannan P. Editor. "African Homicide and Suicide." Princeton Univ. Press, 1960.

CIGARETTE SMOKING IN A PERI-URBAN VILLAGE IN PAPUA NEW GUINEA

P. FREEMAN & K. PATAKI-SCHWEIZER[1]

INTRODUCTION

Cigarette smoking is an outstanding example of a preventable behaviour that is implicated in multiple pathology, both for the smoker and those who live or work in close proximity. Of patricular note are the effects of passive smoking on children. For example, lower respiratory tract illness is significantly more common amongst children whose parents smoke and where household members other than the parents smoke(1) . Children with long term exposure to passive smoking may also be at an elevated risk of developing premature coronary heart disease(2) and lung cancer in later life.(3)

Papua New Guinea is a country with a high rate of smoking prevalence, up to 85% in men and 80% in women in some populations according to one WHO source(4). Respiratory disease, especially pneumonia, is the major cause of death and admission - excepting normal childbirth-in health institutions in Papua New Guinea(5). How much passive smoking contributes to this mortality and morbidity, especially in young children, has not been established in Papua New Guinea but demands scrutiny in the light of studies elsewhere.

Although cancer is not a major cause of morbidity and mortality compared to infectious disease in Papua New Guinea, from 1977 to 1988 there has been a marked increase in the seven common cancers. Considering those common cancers known to be associated with cigarette smoking, there has been a 60% increase in oral cancer, a 64% increase in lung cancer, a 75% increase in oesophageal cancer and a 64% increase in cervical cancer over this eleven year period(6). This increase in these cancers is paralleled by a great increase in the consumption of commercial cigarettes - more than ten-fold in the twenty years to 1979(7). It would be incorrect to attribute the increase in these cancers to smoking commercial cigarettes alone, for example the contribution of a better reporting system, the prevalence of betel nut chewing, especially with lime, in mouth cancer, and the role of increasing promiscuity associated with cervical cancer must be also considered. However, their increase in association with

1 Department of Community Medicine
University of Papua New Guinea

the increased consumption of commercial cigarettes in Papua New Guinea cannot be ignored in the light of overseas evidence. Given these concerns we undertook this study of smoking-related knowledge and behaviour, with particular interest in passive smoking effects on children and in knowledge and practice concerning this topic.

METHODS

The head of each household or the most senior authority figure present in that household in a long-established village outside Port Moresby was identified and interviewed for two sets of data: age, sex, domestic relationship, highest level of education reached, current employment status, and cigarette usage of all members of their household; and their personal cigarette-related practices and beliefs about illnesses caused by smoking for the smoker and for children passively inhaling cigarette smoke. Interviewees were also asked in what rooms they smoked at home and specifically if they smoked in the room where their children slept. Other questions covered beliefs about the benefits of cigarette smoking, attempts to give up cigarette smoking and their tolerance of others smoking in their house. Reliability of answers given was checked by subsequent repetition of one in ten of the interviews; 150 persons were interviewed out of a total village population of 1544. The average household size was 10 persons, ±4.43% of males and 10% of females was employed.

RESULTS

Respondents identified 246 smokers out of the total population of 1544, or 26% of the 943 people aged 15 or more. There were fewer smokers among those who worked in non-clerical positions than among manual labourers or members of the forces. Labourers had the highest proportion of smokers (50%) whilst clerical staff had the lowest (24%). Levels of education did not appear to have any association with presence or absence of smoking.

40% of men and 12% of women over 15 years of age were smokers; 78% of all smokers were male and 24% of all smokers smoked 20 or more cigarettes a day. 60% of smokers used commercial brands, 31% commercial and local, and 9% local brands only. Selected smoking data for households follow:

<u>**Of 150 Households**</u>:

79% had 1 or more smokers resident
43% had 2 or more smokers resident
21% had 3 or more smokers resident

<u>**Of Children aged 14 or under**</u>:

81% lived with 1 or more smokers
45% lived with 2 or more smokers

Of Children aged 4 years or under:

80% lived with 1 or more smokers
46% lived with 2 or more smokers

Of the 150 persons interviewed, 77 (51%) were smokers. 77% of the 150 and 51% of interviewed smokers said that smoking caused illness in children, and smokers were as likely to associate passive smoking with disease in children as non-smokers. They were also more likely to associate smoking with illness than non-smokers. 97% of smokers smoked inside their houses, and 61% reported smoking where their children slept.

Smokers identified four main benefits from smoking: it made them feel good (26%), it was an aid to socializing (18%), it kept them awake (10%) and it gave a feeling of confidence (9%); 21% said there was no benefit, it was only a habit. 61% had tried to stop smoking in the past three years.

25% (18) of the 73 non-smokers interviewed were ex-smokers. Of these, the commonest reasons given for stopping smoking were bad health (33%), expense (17%), the smell (3%) and pressure from their spouse (3%). 77% of all interviewees said that smoking causes sickness in smokers, and 69% sickness in children. The two commonest diseases associated with smoking were cancer (49%) and chest infections (5%), while the commonest associated diseases for children were chest infections (57%) and cancer (32%).

SUMMARY OF RESULTS

1. Cigarette smoking is relatively prevalent.

2. Children begin at age 15 if not younger.

3. Over 80% of children are exposed to passive smoking in the home from birth.

4. There are subgroups within the smoking population with a higher rate of smoking than other subgroups.

5. Knowledge about the negative effects of smoking and passive smoking is relatively common.

6. A majority of smokers (61%) tried to stop smoking or at least identified cessation as a desirable behaviour. That 25% of non smokers are ex-smokers suggests that there are those that succeed.

IMPLICATIONS OF FINDINGS AND COMMENTS

Because of the differences in demography and media access in PNG, our findings are only referable to populations around Port Moresby. They do however raise some issues for wider consideration. Overall the findings are supported by a similar study conducted for the Department of Health in 1989(8). In that study 1200 individuals were interviewed in Port Moresby, Lae, Rabaul, Mt Hagen and adjacent rural areas. It determined an overall prevalence of smoking of 37%, with a prevalence of 34% in that population most similar to ours, the rural areas adjacent to Port Moresby, and a prevalence of 14% in the 10-16 year age group. It is possible that our figures underestimate the real prevalence of smoking. In any case several recommendations can be made:

1. There is a need for specific education programmes aimed at school children, beginning at latest in the fourth grade, and for teenagers.

2. There is a need for specific education about the effects of passive smoking.

3. There is a need for education campaigns aimed at specific subgroups where smoking is more common.

4. Since knowledge about smoking does not of itself lead to cessation of smoking, special education campigns are needed to meet the needs of the potential ex-smoker moving through the stages towards cessation.

Overall, Department of Health funds available for health education campaigns about substance abuse are minimal, compared to that spent by tobacco companies who can, for example, run full page advertisements in local newspapers every week. Therefore maximum use needs to be made of such potential tools as legislation and education for the control of this widespread health problem. Papua New Guinea has most of the components of a tobacco control programme in place, including legislation in the Tobacco Products (Health Control) Act of 1987 (9).

However, within the Tobacco Act itself (Section 8) there are exemptions which allow the use of the brand names of cigarettes in the mass media. It would appear, given the level of current usage of commercial brands and the saturation of advertising campaigns, that the brand name itself is a powerful behavioural cue. A number of studies have shown that desire to smoke is more dependent on such cues and the circumstances associated with previous smoking, than blood nicotine levels(10). In Papua New Guinea, cigarette hoardings are ubiquitous and through sponsorship, sports champions are associated with promotion of cigarette brands thus linking cigarettes with sport. That eighty percent of those who smoked predominantly commercial brands of cigarettes smoked the two brands most prominently associated with sport in PNG is an indication of the efficacy of this advertising approach.

In a 1983 seminar on cigarette smoking in PNG, it was said of developing antismoking campaigns for children, that to reach children, it is necessary to know what things interest them currently, including their heroes to "sell your product".[10] Cigarette companies appear to have followed this premise well, and the need for health education on the dangers of cigarette smoking is now extensive. This is a need which cannot be met unless it is given a priority as high as the seriousness of its health implications.

REFERENCES

1. Woodward A. Passive smoking and acute respiratory illness in children. Ph.D. Thesis University of Adelaide 1988.

2. Moskowitz. W B., Mosteller M., Schieken R M. et al. Lipoprotein and Oxygen Transport Alterations in Passive Smoking Preadolescent Children. Circulation 1990 81:(2) 586-592.

3. Janerich D T., Thomason W D, Varela L R. et al. Lung Cancer and exposure to tobacco smoke in the household. New Eng J. Med. 1990 323 (10) :632-6.

4. World Health Organisation Smoking Prevalence in 30 countries. Results of surveys 1975-86. quoted in Kenneth S, Stjernsward J. Lung Cancer-A worldwide Health Problem Chest 96(1): 58 July Supplement 1989.

5. Department of Health Papua New Guinea National Health Plan 1991-1995. 1991 P22-23.

6. Department of Health. National Health Plan 1991-1995. Pp 185.

7. Brott K. Tobacco Smoking in Papua New Guinea. P.N.G Med.J 1981; 24(4): 229.

8. First Marketsearch (PNG) Omnibus survey. Health Department Research Report 1989-1990. P.O. Box 7164 Boroko PNG 1990.

9. Tobacco Products (Health Control) Act of 1987. Parliament House Port Moresby.

10. Chapman S. The Place of Education in Smoking Control: An Overview of Issues in Programme Planning. In: Smith D E, Alpers M P ed. Cigarette Smoking in Papua New Guinea PNG Institute of Medical Research Monograph 1984 No. 7:65-68.

STRENGTHENING THE HEALTH COMPETENCIES OF HOME ECONOMICS TEACHERS IN THE PROVINCIAL HIGH SCHOOLS OF PAPUA NEW GUINEA

NORMA L SIMPSON[1]

INTRODUCTION

During the past few years UNICEF, WHO and UNESCO experts have begun to recognize once again that the need for more knowledge about health issues on the part of ordinary people is so great that it cannot be provided only by health professionals. This paper addresses the role in this respect of Home Economics teachers.*

In 1987 I was hired by the University of Papua New Guinea to develop the Advanced Diploma in Teaching Home Economics at Goroka Teachers College. The Advanced Diploma was a five year World Bank project administered initially by the National Department of Education but since 1989 also funded by the Department. It is designed to up-grade secondary school teachers in all subject areas taught in provincial high schools (lower secondary system).

INITIAL STAGES

In order to prepare the course, consideration was given to the pre-service teacher training curriculum and to the proposed changes to the home economics secondary curriculum as proposed by the Home Economics Advisory Committee to the Provincial High School Board of Studies. From here a list of course titles and possible contents was selected for inclusion in the new advanced diploma course. At the same time, a series of interviews and a survey were conducted with home economics teachers, headmasters and secondary inspectors in all provincial education offices and high schools of the country. The survey consisted of marking eight topics from a list of 26 that were considered in need of in-service training. The top two choices were 'Family Health' and 'Nutrition and Social Development'.

1 Goroka Teachers College, of the University of Papua New Guinea

---

* Details of syllabus and materials used in the ADT course are available from the author at Goroka Teachers College, PO Box 1078, Goroka

One of the reasons for interest in family health for schools in Papua New Guinea, is that these seldom have a school nurse. Students, therefore, tend to seek health information from home economics teachers or school administrators. Teachers, in turn, with little specific training to provide the assistance required, feel that they are being asked to perform above their training. Until recently home economics teachers had not been trained sufficiently in family health and nutrition subjects, but the present three year curriculum is now including more relevant scientific concepts along with their application to Papua New Guinea conditions. Such is the case, for example, with the 'Science in Home Economics' and the 'Personal and Family Health' courses. The science course allows first year pre-service students to refresh the science knowledge received at high school. They are also able to apply scientific concepts to areas such as agriculture plates, growing bacteria from unsanitary food preparation, hands, hair and rotting foods, and food science principles related to the preparation of foods, such as preventing ropy bread due to spore forming bacillus and the food additives used to prevent ropy bread. Students learn about preparing emulsions for children and adults who are ill with diarrhoea. The 'Personal and Family Health' course is taught in cooperation with the Health Trainers' programme.

Given the current and future needs of the provincial high school curriculum, there is the need to upgrade the preparation of home economics teachers and such is, as explained earlier, the role of the Advanced Diploma programme.

CONTENTS, MATERIALS AND PROCEDURES OF THE HOME ECONOMICS ADVANCED DIPLOMA PROGRAMME

Family Health is the course that forms the basis of the Advanced Diploma. Its main topics were selected with the assistance of Goroka Teachers' College staff in the Home Economics and Science Education departments, health trainers, students and a nutritionist with long-standing experience in Papua New Guinea. The topics are the following:

-- Review of systems of the body;

-- Major health problems in Papua New Guinea and home care for them;

-- Remedial actions related to health problems that can be undertaken by families to increase their well-being, including acting against substance abuse;

-- Good and harmful patterns of traditional health care, to help people build on the strengths of their customs and beliefs;

-- Symptoms of eight communicable diseases and home care that families can perform in relation to these;

-- Symptoms of food-borne illness in Papua New Guinea;

-- Health care concerns of girls and women;

-- Health care concerns of boys and men;

-- Symptoms and treatments for common sexually transmitted diseases;

-- Family planning and contraceptive techniques;

-- Minor health problems that can be altered by changes in family living patterns, including skin, ear and eye problems;

-- Demonstration of first aid, CPR and ABC techniques;

-- Bodily responses to stress in a Papua New Guinea context;

-- Case studies based on local experience to dramatize health care measures that families can do before health officials are involved;

-- Planning and reporting of a community or school health activity in coordination with a health official.

Prior to taking the Family Health and Nutrition courses, Advanced Diploma students are pretested to determine their knowledge status. In teaching the course, lecturers attempt to review the participants' misunderstandings and correct these with new information. Discussions are held with teachers and students in other disciplines to see if there is a difference between home economics teaching and the others regarding the nature of these misunderstandings. It appears from these informal conversations that some of the misunderstandings are shared by all types of teachers and students.

To assist the course, great effort has been made to find locally relevant research and materials to use in the course. For example, Nutrition in Papua New Guinea by Badcock (1983) and Child Health for Extension Officers and Nurses in Papua New Guinea by Biddulph and Stace (1986) are two texts frequently referred to. The Child Health text has been abridged to exclude pharmaceutical information contained in it.

Because of the limited nature of the scientific background of home economics teachers, a first task in the course is to review student knowledge of the human body. Thus a special 'aunty body' kit was developed (Simpson, 1989) of 33 separate parts of the body, including also a set of 30 A3-size human biology and other charts for use in the classroom. Texts by Anthony and Thibodeau (1980), Marks (1980), Coonan, Wolsey and Maynard, 1977, Hughes and

Marshal (1974) provided background material to complete the anatomy review.

The body kit was made of paper to facilitate replacement of possible missing parts by simply photocopying and coloring the parts.

In relation to the content of the course, information from the Papua New Guinea Institute of Medical Research has been useful, for example results of the 1982-83 National Nutrition Survey. Also from the Institute is the 1985 Food Composition Table which is used and preferred to a more recent version.

In the past home economics teachers spent more time learning about basic food groups and little about specific nutrients in food. The Advanced Diploma now includes:

-- Recording three days of 24 hour food consumption and nutritional analysis of nutrients in foods;

-- Comparative analysis of nutrients in food in regional diets;

-- Use of the Diet Mannual for Papua New Guinea by Copeman and Earland (1988).

The Institute of Medical Research has been helpful also through providing insights about local views of health care, developing information about viruses, and especially useful by explaining differences between viral and bacterial infections and explaining why antibiotics or 'suts' should be used only at certain times. Former staff from the Institute have provided videos, slides and lectures about measles, typhoid fever and diarrhoea. Librarians have been helpful in locating copies of Papua New Guinea medical research articles for the course. For example, Jenkin's (1987) article on 'Beliefs and behaviours concerning water in Papua New Guinea' is an ADT required reading as is Kanawi and Bradley's (1986) article on 'Wife beating'. This article is used in conjunction with the video 'Stap Isi'. Other materials used include: Aitken, 1985; Alto and Cutts, 1991; Brand, Thomas and Hyndman, 1991; Biddulph, 1983; Bukenya and Freeman, 1991; Chandra, 1987; Charlwood and Dagoro, 1987; Frankel, 1985; Green, Woolcock and Dowse, 1982; Heywood, 1985; Heywood, Singleton and Ross, 1988; Jeliffe, Derrick and Jelliffe, 1987; Kanawi and Bradley, 1986; Lawrence, Walker, Freestone and Shann, 1979; Marks, 1980; Mola, 1989; Pataki-Schweizer and Tabua, 1980; Poschl, 1989; Ree, 1982; Schumacher, 1987; Shann, 1987; Smith, 1978; Wohlfahrt, 1981; Smith and Alpers, 1984; Temu, 1991; and the PNG medical journal 1988 Special Issue on Nutrition. Facts from Joy Gillet's (1990) book on The Health of Women in Papua New Guinea have been incorporated in the Family Health Course and used for the option on Women in Development. With the rapid cultural changes, economic tension and family disruptions more attention needs to be directed to understanding stress. Materials from the University of Idaho Extension Service on stress are being made available to students.

The Helen Keller Foundation, the Mt. Sion Centre for the Blind and Lorengau Hospital provided lectures on eye diseases, prevention and treatment of eye injuries, reading and writing by braille and integration of visually impaired students into the public school system.

One of the assignments of the Advance Diploma Home Economics students consists in conducting a Health Event in cooperation with Provincial Health officials either in their villages or at the provincial high school where they teach. Some of these Events have centred on malaria control, AIDS, hygiene in provincial high school dormitories, understanding the human body, typhoid fever, learning what villagers want to know followed by instruction on preventing and controlling diarrhoea, making oral re-hydration salts in ORT, understanding the Child's Record Book, and cooperating in health checks of students. Aid post orderlies, students and staff from schools of nursing, provincial departments of health and trainees from Goroka Teachers College have been invited into the schools with much success.

Population Education is usually included in the home economics curriculum primarily along the lines of family planning information. There is need, however, for more training to understand terminology used in the Population Bureau demographic charts. More effort is needed to cover spacing of children and opening communication with spouse and clan about smaller family size. The Working with Villagers kit has guidelines and teaching aids for these topics.

Substance abuse is included in home economics courses - especially of alcohol, tobacco and betel nut. Most teachers in Papua New Guinea are aware of alcohol problems, but do not understand the effects of alcohol on the body nor the extent of its consumption in the country. Perhaps the Papua New Guinea syllabus should also include narcotic drugs as some headmasters have indicated that marijuana or cannabis is already a problem in school dormitories.

Food borne illness is a topic covered in food courses, mostly from the standpoint of avoiding illness through sanitary practices in food preparation and safe selection of tinned and storage food. Especially important in the past few years has been instruction on the transmission of typhoid fever. One of the best explanatory materials on this came from a book called 'The New Putting Food By', about food preservation. This material is used supplemented by sections from Black's Medical Dictionary and current journal articles and newspaper clippings.

Home Economics courses cover sanitary treatment of human waste, construction of latrines such as VIP toilets, septic tanks and problems with their placement near homes, schools and water supplies. More needs to be done on the testing of water and use of the information to teach village people how to protect their water supplies. More could also be taught about water-borne illness.

Diseases related to nutritional deficiencies or excesses are covered in the Nutrition and Social Development course: protein energy malnutrition, kwashiorkor, marasmus, goiter, diabetes, obesity, heart attacks, and food needs during illness such as diarrhoea and measles. Weight charts of children and immunization record health books are explained in detail. Visits to malnutrition wards re-emphasize the importance that grade 7-10 students be able to explain the chart to mothers in their villages.

Physical fitness is a an important aspect of good health. ADT students coach girls in sports, learn the importance of stretching exercises, aerobics and how to treat people who injure themselves during sports or a cultural day. Usually an aerobics instructor or physiotherapist from the hospital works with the home economics teachers to introduce students to the topics and also to become acquainted with personnel who could be invited to the school for a health event.

Emergency first aid and coronary pulmonary resuscitation are part of the training that the home economics teacher takes back to the school to assist both students and staff there. The video 'Save a Life' explains in detail steps for first care and this is followed by the use of dummies for practice, loaned by the provincial Red Cross Officers.

Given the fact that in August 1990 the Vocational Subjects Advisory Committee of the National Department of Education recommended teaching Home Economics to boys as well as girls, home economics teachers are having ad hoc sessions in which they teach boys about hygiene, nutrition, skin diseases, pregnancy, child birth, sexually transmitted diseases and family violence.

The Advanced Diploma course also includes a seminar choice on Food Habits. Clark's (1976) book on Food Habits of the People of Papua New Guinea provides a good starting point for work in the seminar, but the book has gaps that need to be filled in. Issues relating to nutritional adequacy of food habits could be included. The concern continues to be about changes in food habits that may be detrimental to health, especially in the light of the increase in nutritionally related diseases in Papua New Guinea.

CONCLUSION

Provincial high school home economics teachers take seriously their job of teaching about family well-being. They appreciate the cooperation of health care professionals in this task. The health components of the school curriculum will greatly benefit from the instruction patterns and teaching aids developed during the Advanced Diploma in Teaching Home Economics.

Of concern is the impact that budget cuts may have on the distribution of aids and training for home economics teachers in the country. It is hoped that this paper will serve to stimulate sponsorship for the production of aids, and for training in their use.

REFERENCES

Advanced Diploma Unit (nd) "Home Economics Programme," Advanced Diploma in Teaching Student Guide, Goroka Teachers College, pp.48-55.

Aarons, Audrey and Hugh Hawes (1979) Child to child. London and Basingstoke: MacMillan Press, Ltd. p.104. ISBN 0-333-26137-2 Pbk.

Aitken, Iain W. (1985) "Scientific Medicine and Traditional Healing in Papua New Guinea: Pragmatic Perspectives, "Chapter 6 in Traditional Medicine and Primary Health Care in Papua New Guinea, edited by Wolfgang G. Jilek, World Health Organization and the University of Papua New Guinea, pp. 44-56.

Allen, William A., Nicholas L Piccone and Christopher D'Amanda (1987) How Drugs Can Affect Your Life: The effects of Drugs on Safety and Well-Being - with Special Emphasis on Prevention of Drug Use., second edition. Springfield, III. USA: Charles C. Thomas Publishers, pp. 50-58/83-89. ISBN 0-398-05370-7.

Alto, W and Cutts D (1989). "Measles Immunization and its Effectiveness in the Southern Highlands" in the Papua New Guinea Medical Journal, 32:1, pp.45-49.

American Home Economics Association (1981) "Spacing Children" from Working with Villagers: Prototype Lessons: Trainers' Manual; Media Resources Manual. Alexandria V A, USA: American Home Economics Association, pp. 64-104.

Anthony Catherine Parker and Gary A Thibodeau (1980) Structure and Function of the Body, sixth edition St. Louis: C V Mosby Company, p. 286. ISBN 0-80016-02887-4 pbk.

Badcock, Jacquie (1983) Nutrition in Papua New Guinea, Konedobu: Papua New Guinea: Nutrition Section, Department of Health, p. 420.

Benenson, Abram S., editor (1980) Control of Communicable Diseases in Man: Thirteenth Edition, Washinton, D.C.: The American Public Health Association, p. 443.
ISBN 0-87553-077-X

Biddulph, John (1983) "Legislation to Protect Breast Feeding:, Papua New Guinea Medical Journal, 22:1, pp. 9-12.

Biddulph, John and John Stace (1986) Child Health for Health Extension Officers and Nurses in Papua New Guinea, 6th ed. PNG Government Printing Office, p.261.

Bothwell, T H and Charlton R W (1891) Iron Deficiency in Women: A Report of the International Nutritional Anemia Consultative Group. US Agency for International Development, p.68 ISBN 0-935368-25-6.

Brand, Janette C, Diana E Thomas, and David Hyndman (1991). Composition of the Subsistence Foods of the Wopkaimin People of Papua New Guinea" Papua New Guinea Medical Journal, 34:1, pp. 35-48.

Burton-Bradley, B G (1973). "Suicide" and "Amok" Stone Age Crisis Nashville, Tennessee USA: Vanderbilt University Press 129 p. ISBN 0-8265-1199-6.

Burton-Bradley, B G (1990) "Traditional Medicine" in History of Medicine in Papua New Guinea: Vignettes of an Earlier Period Kingston, Australia: Australasian Medical Publishing Company Ltd., pp. 1-13. ISBN 0-85557-027-X.

Bukenya, G W and Freeman P A (1991). "Possible Reasons for Non-Completion of Immunization in an Urban Settlement in Papua New Guinea" Papua New Guinea Medical Journal 34:1, pp.22-25.

Buttfield I H and Hetzel B S (1971) "Endemic Cretinism in Eastern New Guinea: Its Relation to Goitre and Iodine Deficiency" in Endemic Cretinism Proceedings of a Symposium at the Institute of Human Biology, Goroka, Jan. 27-29, pp. 55-69.

Calder, Peter "Smoking - The Killer Habit" in Exchange of Gases, Biology 4. Goroka Teachers College Advanced Diploma Unit. p. 47-55.

Chandra, R K (1987) "Nutrition and Immunity," Papua New Guinea Medical JOurnal, 30:2, pp 97-104.

Charlwood, J D and Dagoro J (1987). "Impregnated Bed Nets for the Control of Filariasis Transmitted by Anopheles Punctulatus in Rural Papua New Guinea". Papua New Guinea Medical Journal, 30:3, pp.199-202.

Clark, Diane (1978) Food Habits of the People of Papua New Guinea: A Handbook for Field Workers. Nutrition Section, Department of Health, p. 389.

Cluney, Sue (1988) "Injury: Understanding the Cause, Prevention and Management of Injuries." from the Physiotherapy Centre of the Goroka Base Hospital, Goroka: Papua New Guinea, p.2.

Coakley, K J, Coakley C A, Spooner V, Smith T A, Javati A and Kajoi M (1991). "A Review of Measles Admissions and Deaths in the Paediatric Ward of Goroka Base Hospital during 1989". Papua New Guinea Medical Journal. 34:1, pp.6-11.

Coonan, Wayne, Anthony Wolsey and Edward Maynard, 1977. "Your Body Systems", in Body Owner's Manual an Easy to Follow Plan Covering Fitness, Nutrition and Relaxation: Life Be in It, CO.

Copeman J P and Jane Earland (1988). "Supplimentary Fluid Feeding in Cases of Malnutrition, Especially in Children" and "Diet for the Treatment of Anaemia", in the Diet Manual for Papua New Guinea Department of Health Papua New Guinea, p. 18-23 and 33-34. ISBN 9980-85-089-2.

Cox, Elizabeth and Molly Daure (1991) Changes, Challenges and Choices: Women in Development in Papua New Guinea. Women's Division of the Department of Home Affairs and Youth of Papua New Guinea, p.256.

Department of Home Affairs and Youth (1991) "A Women's Training and Awareness Program on Women's Health, Women's Participation in Developing and Networking and Communication." A paper distributed at the UPNG-Waigani Seminar, Port Moresby, Papua New Guinea, June 15-19, 1991, p.17.

Dickson, Murray (1985) Where There is No Dentist. Palo Alto, California, USA: Hesperian Foundation, p. 188. ISBN 0-942364-05-8 Pbk.

Ebrahim G J (1983) Nutrition in Mother and Child Health. London and Basingstoke: The MacMillan Press, p. 201. ISBN 0-333-26966-7 pbk.

Edwards, Keith (1982). Diagnosis and Treatment of Sick Children for A.P.Os, Wewak, PNG: Christian Books Melanesia, Inc. p.69.

Erasmus R T, Sinha A K, Gena M, Betuelai, Muthaiah and Nathaniel K (1991) "Serum Lipid Levels in Diabetic in Papua New Guineans", Papua New Guinea Medical Journal, 34:1, pp.17-21.

Fitness/Wellness Center (ND) "Stretching for the Health of It: The Standing Routine." p.4.

Frankel, Stephen (1985). "Social and Cultural Aspects of Family Planning Programmes," Papua New Guinea Medical Journal, 28:3 pp. 155-162.

Gabr. M. (1987). "Managing the Child with Ear Infections: Otitis Media." in ARI News Issue 8, Appropriate Health Resources and Technologies Action Group Ltd. ISSN 0296-1493.

Gardner, Ward A and Roylance Peter J (1984). New Essential First Aid London and Sydney: Bay Books, p.192. ISBN 0-330-26363-3.

Gillet Joy E. (1990) Health of Women in Papua New Guinea, Papua New Guinea Institute of Medical Research, p.180. ISBN 990-71-008-X.

Green W, Woolcock A J and Dowse G (1982) "House Mites in Blankets and Houses in the Highlands of Papua New Guinea," Papua New Guinea Medical Journal. 25:4, pp.219-222.

Griffen, Vanessa (1983) Caring For Ourselves: A Health Handbook for Pacific Women. Suva, Fiji: Fiji Times and Herald Limited, p.215.

Groos, Anita D. and Garner Peter (1988) "Nutrition, Health and Education of Women in Papua New Guinea. Papua New Guinea Medical Journal 31:2, pp.117-123.

Hale, Glorya, editor (1979) "Personal Needs" and "The Disablers" in the Source Book for The Disabled, New York and London: Paddington Press. pp. 134-149 and 258-263. ISBN 0-448-22429-1(pbk)

Henty, E E (1980) Harmful Plants in Papua New Guinea, Botany Bulletin No.12, Department of Forests, p.153.

Hertzberg, Ruth, Vaughan Beatrice and Greene Janet (1982) "Why Put-By Foods Spoil" in The New Putting Food By, Brattleboro, VT, USA: Stephen Greene Press, pp.5-12. ISBN 0-8289-0469-3 (pbk)

Heywood P (1985). "1983 National Nutrition Survey - Preliminary District-Level Analysis of Length and Weight Data," internal report for the PNG Institute of Medical Research, Goroka p.18.

Heywood, Peter (1988) "Editorial: Focus on Nutrition," Papua New Guinea Medical Journal, 31:2, pp.87-89.

Heywood, Peter, Singleton Nicola and Roos Jay (1988) "Nutritional Status of Young Children - The 1982/3 National Nutrition Survey" Papua New Guinea Medical Journal, 31:2, pp.91-101.

Horton, Kirk J (1986). "Part I: The Eye" and "Part III: Activities of Daily Living" in Community Based Rehabilitation of the Rural Blind. p.1-8 and p.61-94, Helen Keller International Foundation. ISBN 0-915173-04-2.

Hipsley, Eben H. and Kirk (Nancy E) (1965) Studies of Dietary Intake and the Expenditure of Energy by New Guineans, South Pacific Commission Technical Paper No. 147, p.158.

Hovey, Bette (1986) "Survival Skills: Understanding Stress in our Lives," University of Idaho Extension Service, p.2.

Hughes D T D and Marshall P T (1974) Tropical Health Science:
Human and Social Biology, 2nd edition. London: Cambridge Press, p.192.

Hymovich, Debra P. and Martha Underwood Barnard, 1973: Family Health Care. New York, Sydney et al: McGraw-Hill Book Company, p.462. ISBN 0-07-031656-2.

Ida, Sr Mary (1975) "Family Planning A Natural Way: The Ovulation Method of Family Planning". Kokopo: St. Mary's Hospital, Vunapope, p.28.

International Planned Parenthood Federation (1987) "Aids and the Family" IPPF Review of Population and Development. 4:4, p.7-8 and 14.

Jelliffe, Derrick B and E F Patrice Jellife (1987). "Nutritional Assessment in Early Childhood (Newer Perspectives)," Papua New Guinea Medical Journal, 30:2, pp91-96.

Jenkins, Carol (1987) "Beliefs and Behaviours Concerning Water in Papua New Guinea," Village Water Supplies in Papua New Guinea, Proceedings of a workshop sponsored by the Papua New Guinea Institute of Medical Research and the Eastern Highlands Province Division of Health, July 19-20, 1984, pp.61-63.

Jilek, Wolfgang, editor (1985) Traditional Medicine and Primary Health Care in Papua New Guinea, World Health Organization and University of Papua New Guinea, p.160. ISBN 9980-84-012-9.

Journal of Home Economics (1981) "Stress Special Issue" Washington D C: Amerilican Home Economics Association, Fall.

Kaiser, Martin and Hiltraut Kaiser (ND) Daunim Sik Long Ples, Madang: Kristen Press, p.30 chapters, ISBN 9980-74-125-2.

Kanawi, Josepha and Bradley Christine (1986) "Wife-Beating in PNG - Is it a problem? a paper presented at the Medical Society of Papua New Guinea, 22nd Annual Symposium p.8.

Koblinsky, Sally A., Weeks John R, and Cooke Gwen C (1985) "Preparation and Practices of Secondary Family Life Education Teachers in Home Economics and Other Disciplines" in Home Economics Research Journal, 13:3 pp. 334-344.

Lawrence, Gregor (1984) "The Pathogenesis of Pigbel in Papua New Guinea" in Pigbel Necrotising Enteritis in Papua New Guinea edited by Michael W Davis. Goroka: Papua New Guinea Institute of Medical Research, Monograph Series No. 6. p.17-27. ISBN 9980-71-005-5.

Lawrence, Gregor, Walker P D, Freestone D S, and Shann Frank (1979) "The Prevention of Pig-Bel in Papua New Guinea," in Papua New Guinea Medical Journal, 22:1, pp.30-34.

Lehman, Deborah, Howard Peter and Heywood Peter (1988) "Nutrition and Morbidity: Acute Lower Respiratory Tract infections Diarrhoea and Malaria" in Papua New Guinea Medical Journal, 31:2, pp.109-116.

Llewellyn, Joan (1986) Children's Illnesses in Warm Climates: A Guide for Teachers and Parents and Health Workers, London and Melbourne: Macmilan Publishers, p. 179. ISBN 0-333-42344-5.

Malcomb, L.A.(1970) Growth and Development in New Guinea: A study of The Bundi People of the Madang District Institute of Human Biology - Monograph Series 1, p. 103.

Malhan, Surjeet (1988) "Water Storage in Rural Households" in the proceedings of the Resource Management: Environmental Issues for Home Economics: the Proceedings of An IFHE Training Program for Technology for Improving Family Economic Well-Being, 17-21 July, 1988 at the University of Minnesota, St. Paul, Minnesota, USA, edited by Catherine R. Mumaw p.47-48.

Marks, G. (1980) "North Solomons Provincial Nutrition Survey 1980: A Report of Findings, "Nutrition Section, Division of Health, North Solomons Provincial Government.

Marks Harriet (1972) Nutrition and Elementary Food Science. Brisbane, Australia: Watson and Ferguson Co., p. 200. ISBN 0-7016-1616-4.

Marshall, Mac, editor (1982) Through A Glass Darkly: Beer and Modernization in Papua New Guinea. Port Moresby, IASER, p. 482.

McElroy, Ann and Townsend Patricia K. (1985) "Stress and Disease" in Medical Anthropology in Ecological Perspective. Boulder, CO, USA and London: Westview Press, 482 p. ISBN 0-8133-0176-9 pbk.

Montgomery, Edward and Bennett John (1979) "Anthropological Studies of Food and Nutrition: The 1940s and the 1970s" in The Uses Anthropology edited by W. Goldschmidt. Washington, D. C.: Special Publication No. 11 of the American Association of Anthropologists, pp. 124-144.

Mola, G. (1989) "Maternal Deaths in Papua New guinea, 1984 -1986" in Papua Mew Guinea Medical Journal, 32:1, pp. 27 -31.

Morley, David (1973) Paediatric Priorities in the Developing World. London: Butterworth & Co., p. 470. ISBN 0-407-35110-8 pbk.

Nilsson, Lennart (1979) A Child is Born London: Farber/Farber Ltd. p. 160. ISBN 0-571-11139-4.

Papua New Guinea Institute of Medical Research (1989) 1982-83 National Nutrition Survey: Provincial Tabulations, separate booklets for 17 provinces (excluding North Solomons and Simbu Provinces studied previously) from 31-34 pages.

Pataki-Schweizer, K J and Tabua T W (1980) "Psychosomatics of Venereal Disease: Toward a Programme for the 1980s," in Papua New Guinea Medical Journal, 23:1, pp.46-50.

Poschl, Rupert and Poschl, Ulrike (1985) "Children on Kiriwina, Trobriand Islands, Milne Bay Province" in Papua New Guinea Journal, 28:3 pp137-145.

Post Courier (1989) "Dengue: Beware and Stay Healthy", June 14, 1989.

Ree, G H (1982) "Knowledge and Attitudes of Young People regarding Sexually Transmitted Diseases", Papua New Guinea Medical Journal, 25:1, pp.33-36.

Ripa, Paulas and Harari Michael (1988) "Viewpoint: Papua New Guinea" in Dialogue on Diarrhoea, the international newsletter on the control of diarrhoeal disease. London: AHRTAG Ltd., p.5.

Ritchie, Jean (1983) Nutrition and Families. London and Basingstoke: The MacMillan Press Ltd., p.171. ISBN 0-333-35767-1 (pbk).

Rodgers, Jenny and Julian Stenhouse (1986) "Airways, The Recovery Position and Mouth-to-Mouth" in the video Save a Life plus Save a Life Instructors Guide. London: B.B.C. Education and Training.

Ross, Jay and Enoch Posanai (1988) "Activities of the Nutrition Section: Alternatives to Intersectoral Nutrition Planning." Papua New Guinea Medical Journal, 31:2 pp.141-145.

Rubenson, Birgitta (1988) What is AIDS: A Manual for Health Workers in Papua New Guinea, Disease Control Unit of the Department of Health, p.32.

Schieffelin, Edward L. (1982) Cultural Dimensions of Alcohol Abuse" in Through a Glass Darkly: Beer and Modernization in Papua New Guinea, Port Moresby, IASER, pp 49-55.

Schumacher, Ernst (1987) "Village Midwife Training on the Huon Peninsula," Papua New Guinea Medical Journal, 30:3 pp.213-219.

Schull, C R (1980) Diagnosis and Treatment of Common Health Problems of Adults in Papua New Guinea, Madang, PNG: Kristen Press Inc. p.275. ISBN 0 85804 187 1.

Senturia, Yvonne D (1987) AIDS ACTION. The International Newsletter.

Shann, Frank (1987) "Pneumonia in Children in Papua New Guinea", Papua New Guinea Medical Journal, 30:2 pp.143-149.

Simpson, Norma L (1988) "Evolution of the Advanced Diploma in Home Economics: Advantages and Constraints" and "The Experimental Model for the Advanced Diploma at Goroka Teachers College," in a Report of a Second Workshop to Plot the Future Directions of the Advanced Diploma in Teaching into the 1990s, April 1988, p.24-29 and p.134-164.

Simpson, Norma L (1989) "Aunty Body Bit-by-Bit: A Kit of the Human Body Parts for Assembly" Goroka, Papua New Guinea: Goroka Teachers College, p.50.

Simpson N L (1991) "Dynamics of Population Growth: How does your village grow?" Goroka, Papua New Guinea: Goroka Teachers College, p.5.

Simpson, Norma L. (in progress) Family Health for Home Economics Teachers in Papua New Guinea: a Distance Education Text for the Advanced Diploma in Teaching Home Economics, Goroka: Papua New Guinea: Goroka Teachers College Advanced Diploma Unit.

Simpson, Norma L. (in progress) Nutrition and Social Development for Home Economics Teachers in Papua New Guinea: a Distance Education Text for the Advanced Diploma in Teaching Home Economics, Goroka: Papua New Guinea: Goroka Teachers College Advanced Diploma Unit.

Smith, Clifford (1978) Problem with Drink: A Resource Book for Teachers, Health Personnel and other Community Workers, Institute of Health Education, p.32, ISBN 0-7247-0433-7.

Smith, David and Alpers Michael (1984) Cigarette Smoking in Papua New Guinea, Monograph No. 7 Papua New Guinea Institute of Medical Research, p.83. ISBN 9980-71-006-3.

Smith, David (1981) "Otitis Media in the Highlands of Papua New Guinea," in Papua New Guinea Medical Journal, 24:4 pp214-216.

Standard Treatment for common illnesses of children in Papua New Guinea: A Manual for Nurses, Health Extension Officers and Doctors. (No date or publisher mentioned but believe it to be the Department of Health) p.88.

Smith, Tom and Heywood Peter (1991) Mid Upper Arm Circumference (MUAC) in Relation to Other Indices of Nutritional Status in Papua New Guinea" Papua New Guinea Medical Journal, 34, pp.26-33.

South Pacific Commission (1989) "The Sinister Threat of Urban Lifestyle Diseases." Information Circular Serial No. 133, South Pacific Commission: Noumea, p.1-4.

Spooner, Veronica (1989) "Hepatitis B." p.3 Mimeograph, Goroka, Papua New Guinea.

Strathern, Andrew (1987) "Problems of Health and Development Strategy in the Western Highlands, Papua New Guinea," in Human Ecology of Health and Survival in Asia and South Pacific, edited by Tsuguyashi Suzuki and Ryntaro Ohtsuka, Tokyo: University of Tokyo Press, pp. 133-147.

Temu, Puka I. (1991) "Adult Medicine and 'New Killer Diseases' in PNG and Urgent Need for Prevention" in Papua New Guinea Medical Journal, 34:1, pp.1-5.

Townsend, Patricia K (1984) "Family Planning in Goroka District 1976-1981". IASER Discussion Paper No 46, p.1-33.

Townsend, Patricia K (1985) "The Needs of Infants" in the Situation of Children in Papua New Guinea: Boroko, NCD, Papua New Guinea: IASER and the Department of Finance and Planning, p.90. ISBN 9980-75-002-2.

Thompson, William A R (1984) Black's Medical Dictionary, 34th edition. London: Adam and Charles Black, p.997. ISBN 0-7136-2367-5.

UNESCO (1990) "Timing Births and Saving Lives" in The State of the Worlds Children 1990. Oxfordshire, UK: Oxford Press, p.27.

United Nations Food and Agriculture Organization (1974) Population, Family Life Resources: A population education curriculum guide: Rome: Food and Agriculture Organization, p.102.

United Nations Food and Agriculture Organization and the U.S. Department of Health, Education and Welfare (1972) Food Composition Table for Use in East Asia. Rome, Italy and Bethseda, Maryland, USA, p.334.

UNICEF, WHO and UNESCO (1989) Facts for Life: A Communications Challenge, Oxfordshire, UK: P&LA, p.84.

Washi, Sidiga (1988) Water Issues in Rural Sudan" in the Resource Management: Environmental Issues for Home Economics: the Proceedings of An IFHE Training Program for Technology for Improving Family Economic Well-Being, 17-21 July, 1988 at the University of Minnesota, St. Paul, MN, USA, p.48-74.

Watt, Philip (1988) "Anaemia in Children", in the Papua New Guinea Medical Journal, 31:2, pp.147-148.

Werner, David (1980) Where There is No Doctor, Melbourne: MacMillan Publishers, p.403. ISBN 0-333-26258-1 Pbk.

Werner, David and Bower Bill (1982) "Learning to Use the Book, Where There Is No Doctor" Part Three in Helping Health Workers Learn and Chapter 7 "Looking at Customs and Beliefs." Palo Alto, CA, USA: The Hesperian Foundation, p.632. ISBN 0-9442364-10-4.

Werner, David and Friends (1987) Disabled Village Children: A Guide for Community Health Workers Rehabilitation Workers and Families, Palo Alto, CA, USA: The Hesperian Foundation, p.672. ISBN 0-942364-06-6.

White, Gilbert F, Bradley D J and White Anne U (1972) Drawers of Water: Domestic Water Use in East Africa. Chicago: The University of Chicago Press, p.306.

Wheeler, Erica (1985) Types of Malnutrition. London: Hygower Ltd. London School of Hygiene and Tropical Medicine. pp.2-17

Williams, Sue Rodwell (1985) "Drug Use and the Outcome of Pregnancy" in Nutrition and Diet Therapy. St. Louis: Times Mirror/Mosby Publishing, pp.383-384. ISBN 0-8016-5566-8.

Wilson, Christine E (1979) "Food-Custom and Nurture: An Annotated Bibliography on Soiocultural and Biocultural Aspects of Nutrition. Journal of Nutrition Education Supplement 1, 11:4, pp.211-264.

World Neighbours (nd) "Home Remedies: Health Care at the Doorstep" in World Neighbors in Action. World Neighbours International Press: Oklahoma City, OK, USA. 18: 2E, p.4.

World Neighbours (1991) "Training Materials Catalogue: Development Communications Materials for Participatory Education in Health and Nutrition, Family Planning, Community Development and Agriculture", Oklahoma City, OK, USA, p.31.

Wohlfahrt, Damien J (1981) "Paraquat Poisoning in Papua New Guinea," in Papua New Guinea Medical Journal, 24:3, pp.164-168.

Wimin na Lo Komiti o Lo Riform Comisen (1988) "Stap Isi" (Take It Easy) video and brochures produced by the Women's Law Committee of the Law Reform Commission, P.O. Box 3439, Boroko, Papua New Guinea.

Young, Beverly and Durston Susan (1987) "Diseases, Diseases" in Primary Health Education, Essex: Longman, p.208. ISBN 0-582-77924-3.

INTERRELATIONS BETWEEN POPULATION, FERTILITY, FAMILY HEALTH AND DEVELOPMENT: GLOBAL EVIDENCE

JOHN C CALDWELL AND PAT CALDWELL[1]

Interrelations in the population and health field are important but complex and inadequately understood. For most of the world's history the great majority of mankind has lived in rural areas as farmers, food gatherers or hunters. Children, like parents, were productive, and family size was uncontrolled partly for this reason and partly because mortality was very high. The first sustained fall in fertility resulting from the deliberate attempt to control family size started in France around two hundred years ago. Fertility decline began more generally in northern Europe, North America and Australasia during the last quarter of the nineteenth century. Only since the 1940s has it been generally accepted that both fertility and mortality would eventually fall to low levels in all parts of the world. The first declines in Third World fertility date back to the 1960s when birth rates began to fall in much of Latin America and parts of East and Southeast Asia. Even now the fertility transition has hardly begun in sub-Saharan Africa, the Middle East and Melanesia.

The first national family planning programme was established by India in 1952. Subsequently, national family planning programmes spread widely through the Third World and have clearly accelerated, and possibly initiated, fertility transitions.

The present situation is that all industrialized countries are characterized by low mortality and low fertility. Nearly all poor countries with annual per capita incomes under US$1500 have high fertility and mortality. However, this is not universally true as some societies with smaller per capita incomes than Papua New Guinea now have life expectancies at birth close to 70 years and crude birth rates around 25 per thousand population (ie half the

1 Health Transition Centre
Australian National University, Canberra

fertility level once found generally in the Third World). Some of these societies, such as Sri Lanka and the Indian state of Kerala, have achieved this because of the independence of their women and high levels of education. In these radical and democratic societies people in every village demand educational and health services and insist by popular pressures that these services should be run efficiently, should be adequately supplied by the central or state government, and that the personnel should work hard and serve everyone. China, and possibly Vietnam, have achieved the same ends by more revolutionary means.

The thinking of international agencies in the economic demographic field was strongly influenced by a book written thirty three years ago by Coale and Hoover [1]. The authors argued that high rates of population growth prevented per capita incomes from rising as much as they might by necessitating the expenditure of savings on economic and social infrastructure duplicating the existing roads, schools, hospitals and work places so as to provide the population increments with the same facilities as the pre-existing population had possessed. Thus, savings could not be invested in improving the ratio of capital to labour and so increasing productivity. In addition, per capita income remained low because working adults were saddled with large numbers of unproductive child dependants. The assumptions were probably too simple. The building of new work places may well have made possible more advanced equipment. In poor societies children can be very productive.

Somewhat unexpectedly, empirical data on real populations have failed to support the Coale and Hoover thesis. Simon Kuznets [2] [3] showed that during the late nineteenth century and the early twentieth century per capita income had risen at least as rapidly in populations with high rates of demographic growth as those with lower rates. It can be argued that the problem here is that the world did not experience really high rates of population growth, namely levels above 2 percent per annum, until after the Second World War when mortality fell steeply in many Third World countries. However, both Richard Easterlin [4] and J C Chesnais and Alfred Sauvy [5] have come to the same conclusion from an analysis of recent trends. Caldwell [6] analyzed the experience of all sub-Saharan African countries over the last quarter of a century and was unable to show that the more slowly growing populations had economically benefited. The problem may have been the fact that these societies have not controlled fertility and that the more prosperous had achieved both lower-mortality levels and net immigration, both tending to make the population growth rate relatively high. Julian Simon[7] has argued that some of the gains shown by Coale and Hoover as accruing to societies which controlled their fertility were transitional ones which would pass as populations stabilized again. This is not a very damaging charge as the respite during this transitional period might be sufficient to lift economic levels and growth rates to a point where continued economic growth was ensured.

Is there any point, then in adopting policies and attempting to curtail high levels of fertility? Almost certainly there are gains to be made for the following reasons.

(1) The right to control fertility or to determine family size should be regarded as a basic human right and all women should be able to determine whether they become pregnant or not. This is particularly the case with such minorities as sexually active adolescent girls who might otherwise be forced into unwanted marriage, to drop out of school, or to procure life-threatening abortions. Fertility control may also be needed by many older women to protect their health or the living standards of their families. They may also wish to be free to work or to be allowed the option of dissolving an unsatisfactory marriage.

(2) Population momentum is so great, and family planning provision takes so long to reach the whole population that a desired future curb on population growth can be ensured only by action now. With an immediate start to a national family planning programme it is unlikely that Papua New Guinea's population can be stabilized under nine million. A delay in real efforts for another decade would probably make that figure twelve million or higher.

(3) It is possible that the scenario forecast by Coale and Hoover (1) will prove to be closer to the mark than has been the historical experience to date. The factor rendering this more likely will be the increasing withdrawal of children from the workforce as education levels rise.

(4) There may well prove to be increasing problems with regard to population density and available per capita resources.

(5) Family Planning programmes and the control of fertility probably induce emotional and economic changes within the family, both between spouses and between parents and children, of a kind that is most compatible with economic development.

(6) Smaller families and the deliberate planning of family size almost certainly lead to lower levels of both maternal and child mortality (see appended paper by Pat Caldwell).

(7) If an AIDS epidemic develops, much will be gained by having a family planning programme already in place. Firstly, there will be greater familiarity with condoms and greater availability. Secondly, it will be necessary to try to contain a greater proportion of sexual relations within marriage without shortening birth intervals. This can be done only if contraception is substituted for post-partum sexual abstinence.

An important question is whether family planning programmes cause or hasten fertility declines in contrast merely to providing easier means once social change has induced such a decline. There is increasing evidence that they play a distinct role in accelerating fertility decline both because of the information they provide and the legitimation their arguments offer and because of the services they provide. Without them, demographic transition would take a much longer time. Absolute programmes are absolutely successful as has been proved in China and in India during the Emergency. However they are an affront to civil rights and take the society in a direction that most of its citizens do not want to go. In addition, in much of the world - certainly in Africa, and probably in Papua New Guinea - they would lead to the downfall of governments long before they were fully executed.

Asia has more successful family planning programmes than sub-Saharan Africa for a number of reasons. One reason is the ancient concept in Asia of the nation state and the development of elites who take on the role of moral and political guidance. In Africa the nations are new, and fertility has been so central to the traditional religious belief system that every citizen feels that he or she knows as much as the government about what should be done with regard to fertility. In addition, the African family structure, especially in West Africa, means that husbands and their families of origin make the fertility decisions while wives bear much of the economic burden of raising children. Fathers later secure returns in security and income from children so that they are unlikely to see benefits in low fertility. The position is rendered more complex by existence of polygny and by the widespread fostering of children, institutions which make nonsense of simpler economic-demographic household models. When fertility decline occurs in Africa it may happen because women have been successfully encouraged by family planning programmes to assume the responsibility for decision-making with regard to fertility.

Special projects have increased our knowledge about successful family planning approaches in poor countries. The experimental approaches in the Matlab area of rural Bangladesh have shown that, even in one of the poorest populations in the world, fertility can be brought down if services are taken to the household and if they include methods particularly suited to women such as injectibles, the pill and the IUD. The availability of Depo Provera injections at the door has been of critical importance and accounts for about half of all fertility control. The experience has been similar in Africa both in Botswana and in the Chogoria area of Kenya where the Church of Scotland has provided special services. Success has been gained by providing dense health services for mothers and children and contraception suited to women. In Africa some female sterilization is now being accepted, although the same is not true with regard to male sterilization.

There seems no reason to doubt the official estimates of population growth rates in Papua New Guinea in the 2-2 $^1/_2$ per cent per annum range. These are low by some Third World comparison but may be high enough to give rise to economic disadvantage.

REFERENCES

1. Coale AJ, and Hoover EM, Population Growth and Economic Development in Low-Income Countries: A Case Study of India's Prospects, Princeton University Press, Princeton NJ, 1958.

2. Kuznets S, "Quantitative Aspects of the Economic Growth of Nations, Part 1: Levels and Variability of Rates of Growth", Economic Development and Cultural Change, 1956 5(1):94.

3. Kuznets S, "Population and Economic Growth", Proceedings of the American Philosophical Society 11, 1967: 179-193.

4. Easterlin RA, "Effects of Population Growth on the Economic Development of Developing Countries", In: Durand JD ed. World Population. Special Issue of Annals of the American Academy of Political and Social Sciences, 369, 1967: 98-108.

5. Chesnais J C, and Sauvy A, "Progrès Economique et Accroissement de la Population: Une Expérience Commentée," Population 1973; 28, 2: 843-857

6. Caldwell JC, "The Soft Underbelly of Development: Demographic Transition in Conditions of Limited Economic Change". In: Fischer S, de Tray D and Shah S, eds., Proceedings of the World Bank Annual Conference on Development Economics 1990, Supplement to the World Bank Economic Review and the World Bank, Research Observer, The World Bank, Washington, 1991 207-253.

7. Simon JL, The Ultimate Resource, Martin Robertson, Oxford, 1981.

POPULATION POLICIES AND WOMEN'S HEALTH

PAT CALDWELL[1]

When countries adopt population policies they make a commitment to furthering health services for two reasons. First, women cannot be expected to reduce their family size unless they are guaranteed that there will be a reduction in the risk of children dying. Secondly, the fertility control programme is likely to prove successful only if child mortality is falling.

From the experience of such Asian Countries as Sri Lanka and such African countries as Botswana, we now know at least one successful formula for improving the health of countries. In each case an educated young woman is selected from each village and trained by the Department of Health as a health visitor.

She is sent back to her own village and paid a modest salary. Her most important task is to identify pregnant women and to follow them through until after the infancy of the child. The health visitor encourages the woman to have antenatal check-ups and arranges where and when this is to be done. She books the woman into a health facility for the birth and make sure she gets there. She helps the mother to identify any sickness in the infant or herself and encourages any advisable visits to the health centre. More generally, she keeps an eye on the woman's general needs and those of her other children as well.

Population programmes have to ensure that the smaller families will survivie. Fortunately, there is evidence that they are much more likely to do so because of the concern that both parents feel about families that have been deliberately kept small. In the West steep infant mortality decline followed close behind the first falls in fertility. We found in a research project in Ibadan city, Nigeria that there was much lower mortality among planned small families. This also appears to be the case among China's one-child families.

[1] Health Transition Centre, Australian National University

Population programmes also have to ensure that contraception is safe. In fact, most modern contraception contraceptives is much lower than the risk of maternal mortality in childbirth.

There is little double that more slowly growing populations find it easier to provide adequate education and health services.

There is no doubt that women's empowerment plays a major role in promoting both fertility and mortality declines. Child mortality is so low in both Sri Lanka and the Indian state of Kerala because women there are sufficiently independent and health conscious to decide, immediately upon identifying the problem, that a sick child needs treatment. In both societies they are completely prepared to set off immediately with the child to a health centre without waiting for their husbands or mothers-in-law to come home and endorse the decision. There is another side to this picture. Where women are poor or have little control over the family finances such actions can be carried out only if health services are free or very, very cheap. This means that continued government subsidization of health services is of great value not only in ensuring society equity but also in improving the chances of success of the family planning programme.

THE STATUS OF WOMEN IN PAPUA NEW GUINEA

MARIA KOPKOP[1]

INTRODUCTION

Following Independence Papua New Guinea's policy towards women was identified clearly and succinctly in the National Development Strategy of 1976. It was Item number 7 in the famous Eight Point Plan, first developed in December 1972 as the Eight Point Improvement Programme. Recognising that the women of Papua New Guinea were at a disadvantage, and I stress at a disadvantage, it advocated "a rapid increase in the equal and active participation of women in all forms of economic and social activity".

The First Principle of the Constitution of Papua New Guinea declares 'for every person to be dynamically involved in the process of freeing himself or herself from every form of domination and oppression'. The Second Principle of the Constitution declares, amongst other things, a goal for all citizens to have equal opportunities 'to take part in the political, economic, social, religious and cultural life of the country'.

Fifteen years after Independence there has definitely NOT been a rapid increase in equal and active participation of women in the economic, social and political life of the Nation.

Little over 10% of female urban dwellers are wage earners, and most of these are in the low level clerical workers activities. Only 18% of the Public Service is composed of women, whereas only 8% of urban non-government workers are women. Only one head of a Public Service Department is a woman. In public life the record is even more discouraging. The numbers of women in Local Government are extremely few. In 1978 only 7 women councillors stood amongst a total of 4313 (1). In Provincial Government few women are elected. Only five Provinces have nominated women members. The PNG National Government is probably one of the few democratically elected Governments in the world where in the last National Elections no woman was elected to represent her people.

1 President, Papua New Guinea National Council of Women

So poor has been the participation of women in the development of Papua New Guinea that following the recent 17th Waigani Seminar, which had as its subject 'The Ethics of Development', the third volume of papers printed was entitled 'Women as Unequal Partners in Development'.

It is quite evident that there must be a radical and dramatic effort on the part of the PNG Government to redress the serious imbalance in women's participation in national affairs. Otherwise the advance of Papua New Guinea in the economic and social sector will be much slower than it should be.

FACTORS CONSTRAINING WOMEN'S PARTICIPATION IN NATIONAL AFFAIRS

This Paper will discuss some of the major constraints affecting the status of women in Papua New Guinea. It will also outline some of the measures currently being undertaken to overcome these obstacles.

Perhaps the main constraint facing women in Papua New Guinea is the lack of training and educational opportunities (2). This is compounded by the persistent and unproductive social attitude of males towards females. Firstly, the status of women has traditionally been subservient. But also, in the colonial era, most administrative, educational and employment opportunities were oriented to males. This attitude still exists.

In the cities there are few unskilled jobs available. Generally speaking, in urban areas, laws prohibit and certainly inhibit the informal sector. Women rely heavily on their husbands' income. Their capacity to supplement the family income is hampered by the inability to obtain small loans to set up mini-self-employment ventures. In rural areas women, traditionally, are the main workers in the subsistence sector. Yet it is a fact that government Department of Primary Industry field extension workers, called didimen, are primarily concerned with the male population. There are very few female agricultural extension officers. While the country's economy is agricultural in nature the importance of the women's role is grossly underrated.

Another major constraint is not only the attitude of males to females but also the self-perception of women themselves. Papua New Guinean men continue to hold the traditional view that women should only be wives and mothers. Unfortunately many women unconsciously support this attitude by maintaining a profile which is riddled with low esteem and low aspirations. In addition women are constrained because they lack basic information on social and political issues. And finally, women's organisations themselves often lack co-ordination, duplicate each other in some instances, and in some cases are debilitated by constant in-fighting.

Many of these constraints will inevitably be overcome by education. It is most unfortunate that in Papua New Guinea, although much progress has been made, girls continue to be disadvantaged in terms of access to education. The primary system is now 44 percent female. And nation-wide there are now 38 percent females in Grades 7 to 10 (3). Although there is no universal education in Papua New Guinea the Government is moving positively towards this. Universal primary education is planned in the immediate future, with a consequent expansion of enrolment in high schools. It is planned in this year's budget that by the year 2000 50 pecent of Grade 6 leavers will be able to pass on to secondary education, and 75 percent of these will be able to go beyond Grade 8. Twenty five out of every 100 of those who leave Grade 10 will be able to pass on to National High Schools.

GOVERNMENTAL REACTIONS

Faced with this multitude of women's problems it is small wonder that the male-dominated infrastructure of government has at times felt powerless to overcome them. Women's activities and programmes since the 1970's were mostly initiated by the church missions. More recently, it can be said that the Government of Papua New Guinea has emphasised the building up of women's confidence and participation by trying to strengthen women's institutions.

In pre-Independence days a Woman's Adviser was appointed to the Chief Minister, Michael Somare. At the national level, a "Women's Section" has existed since the mid '70s, though it has experienced frequent organisational changes. It was initially part of the Department of Social Development and Home Affairs. In 1983 it was upgraded to divisional status within the Office of Youth, Women, Religion and Recreation, in the Department of Community and Family Services.

In 1984, the government introduced the National Women's Development Programme (NWDP). It was an effort to stimulate policy and programme developments for women. It had two main objectives:

* to mobilise women into the development of the country in accordance with the National Goals and Directive Principles;

* to build up a strong network of women's organisations from the district levels to the national level to encourage greater participation by women and also to implement programmes for women.

In addition to the government structure, the National Council of Women was established in 1975 as a complementary body outside the government. It is subjective to an Act, and because of this suffers from a certain amount of inflexibility. Nevertheless, it is currently the means of galvanising the women of the Nation.

The Women's Division of the Department of Home Affairs and Youth and the National Council of Women together constitute Papua New Guinea's national machinery of women's affairs. Parallel structures have been established at the provincial level.

Women's functions are still a concurrent activity of the national government. Through the process of decentralisation, provincial governments have taken responsibility to support women's activities and programmes. The implementation of the NWDP has provided the overall guidelines for provincial governments to follow in the development and implementation of women's programmes in the provinces. In addition, some provinces have developed and funded new initiatives of their own.

There has been expressed, on a number of occasions, dissatisfaction with the way services are being provided to women at the grass-roots. Similarly there does not seem to be a smooth information flow reaching policy-makers from the village level.

There are many reasons for this. But one of the prime causes seems to be in the current structuring of women's support groups. There are two distinct groups dealing specifically with women. They are the Women's Division of the Department of Home Affairs, which reports to a Minister. And there is the National Council of Women which also reports to the same Minister. The nexus between both is unclear, confused, and, despite the best of good-will between both organizations, fails to react in the most efficient manner to the betterment of women.

There needs to be a reorganising of the whole system. What is envisaged is basically an Office of the Status of Women which reports to a Minister specifically dealing with Women's Affairs, (for example, a Minister Assisting the Prime Minister). This Ministry should have the closest access to the Prime Minister, and the Council of Women should be a consultative body properly representative of all the Nation's women, and have a policy advising role to the Office of the Status of Women.

ACCOMPLISHMENTS

Despite the problems of organisation affecting women's groups the existing national machinery and programmes have been successful in the following areas:

* in mobilising women at the grassroot, district and national level in increasing consciousness of their rights and in raising their living standards;

* in identifying the need to build a strong network of women's organisations from the district and provincial level to the national level;

* in improving communication and dialogue with non-government organisations;

* in recognising the roles of non-government women's organisations and assisting them in obtaining greater support from the government;

* in training provincial women's officers and Provincial Councils of Women in leadership and management skills, which had been identified as a priority for effective programme implementation;

* in developing a formal avenue for co-ordination of women's issues with government;

* in facilitating the establishment of small-scale business by women;

* in improving the conditions of female public servants;

* in stimulating and supporting informal mutually supportive networks of women;

* in beginning and maintaining a dialogue with international agencies.

A MAJOR RECENT PROBLEM

Despite a decade of government initiatives to improve the status of women, the process of policy development and the integration of women's issues in the <u>mainstream</u> of development planning has been slow. While there was progress in mobilising women and in developing some programmes targetted to women, women's issues remained isolated from general development strategies or were dominated by other interests.

Policy and programme planners failed to see women as productive agents contributing to national development. **Women and children were and still are seen as welfare problems who are dependent on the economy.** As a result they were given little budgetary consideration. Specific policies and programmes for women were developed outside the development planning guidelines for the government. Policies and programmes reflected a perception of women as primarily concerned with reproduction and household maintenance, and have overlooked their role in economic production.

The National Women's machinery has realised that for women to be physically fit to participate in development activities specific emphasis must be placed on a programme called the Family Life Development Programme. A systematic training package has been developed for women's organisers, educators and trainers all over Papua New Guinea. It provides the details of the most important issues and information they need to be aware of to improve women's health, family life, and participation in development. The Programme will be the subject of a later address in this Seminar (see 'Changes, Challenges and Choices: Women and Development in Papua New Guinea').

The instability caused by frequent re-organisations of the department in which the Women's Division has been located has also contributed to a lack of continuity and clear policy direction. In addition, both the national machinery and sectoral departments have been hampered by the absence of an overall policy to guide their activities with respect to women and development. In 1986 and 1987 great efforts were made in every quarter to produce a Papua New Guinea Women's Policy. This was finally endorsed by the National Executive Council on 11 January 1990.

In addition the Papua New Guinea government has at last recognised as a critical issue the problem of the isolation of women from the mainstream of development planning. An important recent initiative, funded by UNIFEM, is to Mainstream Women in National Development Plans and Programmes. It aims to promote greater participation of women by the incorporation of women's issues and concerns in national planning processes and mainstream programmes.

This naturally requires serious input by women to vocalise their concerns. It also requires greater receptivity of government planners to such input. The main tasks of the Project are therefore to include the strengthening of the

Councils of Women, national and provincial, as well as Government Women's Offices so that they can make effective input. It also means making government planners more sensitive to gender-sensitive planning.

The series of project activities in the Mainstreaming Programme will be carried out as follows:

* in country-wide workshops on sectoral and national planning with both government planners and women leaders.

* in country-wide hands-on-training assistance from project consultants to National Councils of Women, Government Women's Offices, and Development Planners;

* in the production of a draft gender-sensitive development plan and in the formulation of strategies for follow-up action.

Another major recent initiative concerns women's contribution in the Agriculture Sector. Following research to determine the need to set up facilities for women to engage directly in the formal sector in the form of self-employment, it was revealed that there is a grave need for women to have better access to credit and all that goes with it. This includes the smallness of capital inputs needed by women, the high interest rates charged by banks, high illiteracy rates amongst village women, and the tedious bureaucratic procedural requirements of banks. In addition, many women are afraid to approach banks, either due to lack of knowledge or just mere apprehension. To overcome this a feasibility study has been conducted recently by the Women's Division of Home Affairs together with the Department of Trade and Industry, and with technical assistance from ILO, and resources from the UN Development Fund for Women. It is hoped to introduce a scheme for credit assistance to self-employed women.

On the legal front the Department of Labour has just drafted a Bill, yet to be introduced in Parliament, entitled <u>Being an Act for Respecting and Improving the Welfare of Women Workers, including the Guarantee of Equal Opportunity and treatment between Men and Women in Employment.</u> So you can see, in Papua New Guinea we feel that while progress has been slow, there has been definite progress. We believe that as more women are drawn into the development process through understanding and training and knowledge the impetus for equal opportunity will grow.

The National Council of Women in PNG is placing strong emphasis on strengthening its networks so that a greater awareness can be instilled in women. Workshops, in conjunction with the Women's Division, are being conducted in each Province in leadership training, and political education awareness. The Council believes that by strengthening Provincial Women's groups the particular needs of an area will be better catered for in our own planning process.

REFERENCES

1. Stratigos S and Hughes P. Ethics in Development: Women as Unequal Partners in Development, UPNG Press, 1988.

2. Wormald S. and Crossley M. Women in Education, UPNG Press, 1988.

3. Weeks S. Times of PNG, Thursday 01 February 1990.

WOMEN IN HEALTH AND DEVELOPMENT - AUPIK VILLAGE, EAST SEPIK PROVINCE

JOHN SAIRERE[1]

INTRODUCTION

Recently, a participatory health research project was introduced to women in remote and isolated areas in Asia and the Pacific. Aupik village in the Maprik District, East Sepik Province was selected as one of the project villages. The women were encouraged to take the initiative in extricating and addressing their own health needs through communal deliberation and action. The eventual goal was self reliance and sustainability of health programmes developed by the women themselves in their community. Through the process documentation approach the mechanism by which women's participation in the formulation and implementation of the health plans were to be extricated. The initial stage of dialogue to evoke women's opinions and the selection of viable health projects were to be followed by a training programme that would utilize available resources in the community geared towards the needs to be addressed. Programme implementation, monitoring and evaluation would be undertaken by the women themselves.

Aupik village was selected because of its history as a cooperative, development minded village and its progress in women's activities. The role of women in Aupik Village in the last decade has changed drastically as the women organised themselves, created new roles and responsibilities and showed their desire and ability to be active in village development. Apart from that, Aupik village is a patrineal society whereby men still play a dominant role in the village and dominate all the functions of the community. The women do all the gardening, cooking, cleaning, wood gathering and child rearing.

OBJECTIVES

1. The objective of this research was to assess and field test the capability of women in isolated rural communities to formulate and implement a self-reliant and sustainable health programme.

[1] Assistant Secretary for Health, Wewak, East Sepik Province

METHODOLOGY

The primary data for this project was collected by a survey carried out through personal interviews and observations. The survey was carried out on a random sampling of the families of 36 hamlets within Aupik village. Interviews were conducted with heads of households, with equal interview of men and women and young and old.

The collection of this data was to assist the underserved women to improve their capabilities, broadening their opportunities and strengthening their motivation through involvement in health projects by:-

a) Increasing their awareness of health problems and their appreciation of their role in health service delivery;

b) Developing their skills in management of health projects;

c) Fostering self confidence and self reliance in the identification of their health needs and the formulation of solutions and;

d) Strengthening or creating linkages between the community's organisation and health agencies.

In the initial phase of this project a dialogue was established by the field assistant researcher, the principal investigator and a consultant with the community to discuss the health research. Various community leaders such as the councillor, village court magistrate, youth leader, women's leader, pastor etc were consulted and after lengthy discussion they agreed that their women would participate in this research.

A meeting was then organised for women, and approximately sixty women turned up. They were told to discuss health problems as well as other problems, and the possible solutions to them. The ensuing dialogues were aimed at identifying some general perception about health status and village needs, and to get the women together to co-ordinate their activities and encourage cooperation.

Later, the women were divided into four groups to discuss two questions:-

1. What are the health problems or any other problems in the village?

2. What is needed to solve those problems?

After forty five minutes the women reconvened and reviewed their findings.

RESULTS

In response to question one the following problems were identified:-

1. No clean water source ****
2. Inadequate medical supplies at the aidpost ****
3. The MCH clinic house needed repair *
4. No electricity ****
5. Aidpost served too many people *

* represents a group

In response to question two there was very little variation. The overall consensus was to raise funds in order to facilitate changes.

On the following day ten women were chosen by a woman leader, were assembled and trained in the use of survey techniques, their purpose, and the proper manner in which to collect data. A questionnaire was designed by the women themselves to identify health problems in families, especially those with children under the age of five years. During the training session the women went through the questionnaire making sure they knew each question, making revisions and basically altering questions to suit their own situation. Each woman was given the task of interviewing five families with children under five years. A total of fifty families were surveyed, evenly distributed throughout Aupik.

After a couple of months a workshop was arranged to analyse the survey results.

During the workshop the ten women, together with some observers, met the health team and together they analysed the questionnaires. Problems identified were discussed and the goals and the purpose of the survey were reviewed. The women were shown how to extricate health problems, and they prioritised them as follows:-

(1) No safe water source in the village.
(2) Lack of cooperation in the village, especially in health related matters and emergencies.
(3) Diarrhoea, malaria and respiratory diseases were very common in the village.
(4) Lack of knowledge on nutrition.
(5) Lack of understanding on the causes of diseases.
(6) Lack of family planning.

The women acknowledged that after the survey they were able to identify health problems better, compared to their first meeting. Possible solutions to solve problems were identified, and it was decided that priority number one needed financial assistance, whilst the other five problems could be solved using other resources.

The results of the survey were presented to the community leaders and the people in a meeting held on a Sunday after church.

The following strategies were then considered:-

1. There is an urgent need to improve their water supply.
2. There is a need to arrange a village workshop to teach women and men on the causation of diseases and how to treat, control and prevent them.
3. There is a need to train a village health aide (marasin meri) to dispense and treat common illnesses.

After these strategies were selected the following resources were identified:-

a) <u>Fund Raising for Water Supply</u>

Fund raising activities were commenced with individual contributions from families, labour fees for collecting coffee beans from coffee growers and doing other village chores. The fund raising activity was resented by the men simply because of their lack of involvement in the initial phase of this project. These differences were solved in an urgent meeting emphasising the importance of this community project which required support from the menfolk. The men eventually agreed and supported the women by raising K1,020.00 within two weeks. A 6000 gallon water tank was purchased immediately and installed by the Division of Health. A second tank was purchased and installed as a contribution from this project. With those two tanks installed the people were happy with their improved water supply and thus encouraged to continue their fund raising to purchase four more tanks.

b) A three day village workshop was also organized to teach women and men about health and health related problems and diseases and how to treat, control and prevent them. Resource health personnel were notified to participate. Stationary and textbooks were also provided. A total of 20 participants attended this workshop, (15 women and 5 men).

Topics that were presented and discussed were dental and diarrhoeal diseases, leadership and management, germ theory, waste disposal, malaria, skin diseases, immunization, TB and Leprosy, sexually transmitted diseases and Aids, malnutrition, water supply, primary health care and sores and ulcers.

At the end of the workshop the participants expressed their satisfaction and understanding of different diseases, how to treat, control and prevent them and most importantly, how to stay healthy.

There were other topics raised which the women had requested, but due to the time limit of this project, they were not organized. They include cooking demonstrations, book keeping, training of a village health aide and management and monitoring of projects.

EVALUATION OF THE PROJECT

Due to limited time the Aupik women concentrated mainly on health issues and only three goals were achieved:-

1. Improved water supply by purchasing and installing two 6000 gallon tanks.

2. Educating women on health and health related problems, diseases and the causation of diseases and how to treat, control and prevent them.

3. The training of women to conduct a simple survey, prepare a questionnaire, identify health problems, prioritise them and to work out possible solutions.

DISCUSSION

The position of women as an essential element in the health development process is considered important. Two facets in health can be recognised for women. One is to enable them to contribute more effectively to the satisfaction of their families basic health needs within the framework of their traditional responsibilities. The other is the fundamental need for women themselves to further their social independence and their integration into the community beyond the narrow circle of their families.

For instance, after the implementation of this research project, women are now cooperating and coordinating their activities. They are able to constructively identify problems and solve them. Some of the activities successfully implemented were the installation of two water tanks and continued fund raising for four more tanks. The understanding of health problems through health education has improved the knowledge and understanding amongst women on the causation of common diseases, and how to control and prevent them. They also realised the importance of pregnant mothers attending regular antenatal clinics as well as the children under five years attending regular clinics to assess their nutritional status, and for immunisation and the treatment of common ailments. Other activities such as the promotion of personal hygiene, sanitation and general cleanliness of the village were also implemented.

Unfortunately, the successful implementation of the project was short lived after the election of the new local government councillor. The new councillor assumed that his position had been threatened by the woman leader and he promptly prevented any further activities carried out by women. He even went as far as accusing the woman leaders of misappropriating the water supply fund collected. Consequently, the women split into two groups and even into nuclear families.

CONCLUSION

My personal view is that for the successful implementation of this project it should have been organised through the primary health care approach. Primary health care, as you all know, involves the delivery of health services to communities with their full participation and at a cost they can afford. For example, in my primary health care project villages, the woman leader is a member of the Village Development Committee. Any project suggested by women is discussed by the VDC and put into the village development programme. The community participate in implementing those projects, including projects initiated by women. There is therefore no argument as to whether a project belongs to this group or that group.

A WOMENS TRAINING AND AWARENESS PROGRAMME ON WOMENS HEALTH, WOMENS PARTICIPATION IN DEVELOPMENT AND NETWORKING AND COMMUNICATION

JOSEPHINE GENA[1]

INTRODUCTION

Development, in simple terms, connotes the achievement of better social and economic standards. The ultimate object of development is to bring about sustained improvement in the well-being of individuals and the nation as a whole. The need for approaches that will contribute to 'human development', taking into account both the potential contribution's of women to development as well as the potential effects of development on the role and status of women, has gained increasing recognition. It is heartening to note our Honourable Prime Minister at this Waigani Seminar address issues relating to Women in Development.

The Women's Division of the Department of Home Affairs and Youth has been vested with the responsibility of promoting and sustaining programmes for the advancement of women and to build up a strong network of women's organisations in order to encourage greater participation by women.

It is significant to note that the activities of the Division have gained momentum by implementation from May 1990 of the project - "Population and Family Life Education and Skill Training Programme for Women's Organisers and Community Leaders in Papua New Guinea". The project is technically assisted by the International Labour Organisation (ILO) and funded by the United Nations Population Fund (UNFPA). The project seeks to:

(a) strengthen the organisational structure of the Women's Division of the Department through a programme of management and administrative training

(b) expand and administer a network of women's organisations and groups that will foster and facilitate the active participation of women in the social and economic development of Papua New Guinea.

(c) provide a programme of population and family life education for improved family welfare and planned parenthood

[1] Assistant Secretary, Women's Division, Department of Home Affairs and Youth

(d) improve the quality of life of women and enhance their status and literacy

(e) encourage women to participate in income generation activities and

(f) involve men as well in the programme so as to change male attitude towards women

A National Women's Training Package has been developed by the Women's Division with the assistance of a local Training Advisor, Ms. Elizabeth Cox to facilitate the activities envisaged under the project.

BACKGROUND

The initiative to develop a nationwide training programme emerged in 1988 during the review of the National Women's Development Programme. The need for the Government to strengthen its commitment and to develop concrete plans or projects in aspects of Family Life Education was clearly eminent during the period of the review (1974 - 1978).

The Division saw the need to resource and strengthen the existing Family Life programme especially those initiated by the Churches and other Non-Government Organisations through the introduction of a comprehensive Training Package focusing specifically on issues that would strengthen the roles of women as well as enhance the status of Family Life in Papua New Guinea.

Furthermore, having experienced past developments of women's programmes and efforts at different levels and by various agencies in the country, the Division saw the need to develop a programme that would create linkages and integrate developmental issues within existing programmes targetted at the women's population.

The programme is also targetted at sensitising change agents, educators, leaders and trainers to realise the need to incorporate and broaden their perspectives to ensure that they respond appropriately to the issues affecting the lives of women. At the same time to ensure they deliver appropriate educational awareness programme to women so that women are well-informed and able to make necessary adjustments in a rapidly changing society and at the same time are able to participate and contribute meaningfully towards the process of development.

PART 2: PROCESS OF MATERIALS DEVELOPMENT

A loose framework was developed by setting out the critical issues and information in three parts;

- Women's Health
- Participation in Development and
- Communication and Networking

The work was benefitted greatly from the recent UNICEF/IMR publication on The Health of Women in Papua New Guinea. This book compiled by Joy Gillett for health workers in Papua New Guinea provided the facts - the results of extensive medical research and the statistics collected from hospitals and health centres all over the country. The basic information was derived from and integrated with local, provincial and national, social, political and economic issues. The intention was to present the material in a popular and easy to use form for grassroots leaders and trainers.

It was quite clear that the training materials should not be presented in the form of a standard imported style adult education training manual. On the other hand, the materials were not to be made exclusive to women only. There was a feeling that the package could have wider application and should, therefore, not be prepared with rigid prescriptions for running training sessions only.

There was great inspiration from UNICEF's twin publications - Facts For Life and All For Health which present the main information in a learning and teaching format in one booklet, and the ideas, innnovations and inspiration for communicating those methods in another. It was decided that the training package would also separate the main issues and information from the suggested training methods and techniques.

An Inter-Sectoral Advisory Committee was set up to guide the material production process. The committee discussed each aspect of content and presentation style, and helped us to link the training package to their ongoing efforts and complementary materials. The Committee consisted of people from the Department of Health, Lifeline, Law Reform Commission, Family Planning Association, UNDP, YWCA.

All main issues and information were written up in the same format. The information is factual in so far as it is based on national health research and statistics. The presentation of issues is frank in that it deals in very straight forward and direct terms with the social, political and economic influences on womens lives in PNG today. The style of writing reflects collective understanding and experience based on women's own stories about their health, their family life and the possibilities and problems associated with their increased participation in development.

Once the first draft of the issues and information text was completed, it was circulated widely throughout the country. This extensive consultation process called for corrections, comments, criticisms, additions, deletions etc., from all women's workers, leaders and planners who saw it. Every verbal or written response received was taken into consideration when the material was revised. The material went through several draft and revision phases before it was finally printed earlier this year, 1991.

A set of posters which summarize and simplify all material presented in the issues and information text was then prepared. This was done to address the low levels of literacy, the multiple languages and the limited range of support training materials available for village level education and information programmes.

A draft handbook has been developed to assist the wide range of trainers who might use the package. This is supported by a back-up kit for all provinces stocked with a variety of teaching aids and resources kits for all provinces. These items of the training package are currently in use in draft form. They are being developed and improved by the first trainers who have already begun to use the materials out in the provinces. They are open to change and improvement. By early 1992 we hope to have a more permanent form of the trainer's handbook.

PART 3: THE PACKAGE

The new National Womens Training Package is made up of 4 main parts or items, namely:-

1. THE ISSUES AND INFORMATION BOOK
2. THE TRAINERS HANDBOOK
3. THE POSTER SET (24)
4. THE PROVINCIAL RESOURCE KIT

1. <u>THE ISSUES AND INFORMATION BOOK</u>

The Book is a simple written text or reference book. It is titled "CHANGES, CHALLENGES AND CHOICES: WOMEN IN DEVELOPMENT IN PAPUA NEW GUINEA".

The Book is 256 pages long, and illustrated with more than 400 photographs. Currently, 2000 copies have been printed for the 20 provinces.

The Trainers are encouraged to introduce the book as a background reader for key political and administrative decision-makers, as well as heads of government divisions involved in development project planning and implementation.

The book will also serve as the central reference book for all literate trainers of women.

The material covered in the ISSUES AND INFORMATION BOOK is set out under 24 Topics, broken down into 3 main parts:

1A **<u>PART A: WOMENS HEALTH</u>**

This part deals with the physical, social, political, and economic factors which currently affect womens health in Papua New Guinea. It stresses the fundamental importance of good health among women for viable development. It explains that womens' health is shaped by physical living conditions, social status, roles and responsibilities, the nature of family life and the levels of respect for women, their workloads and the way in which development projects and activities disrupt or otherwise determine their family life.

The section points out how easily women can be affected by national, local and even family decisions about participation in development.

1B **PART B: WOMENS PARTICIPATION IN DEVELOPMENT PROGRAMMES AND PROJECTS**

This section helps women's trainers and leaders as well as local planners to develop a more conscious and critical approach to planning or promoting certain kinds of development projects for women.

The basic theory and documentation on Women in Development, developed over the last two decades, is presented here in very simple English and with direct application to the PNG context.

Issues of gender-sensitivity, environment and sustainability, good management and administration and the right of women to challenge and choose are highlighted in this section.

Basically, this section is concerned with broadening women's horizons and helping them to understand that they can participate in both large scale (macro) and small scale (micro) developments.

This section warns women against being so preoccupied with small projects that they do not see and understand what is really happening to their nation, province, community or family.

Furthermore, it encourages women to be much more cautious, critical and careful in planning for or participating in, even the smallest development activities.

1C **PART C: NETWORKING AND COMMUNICATION**

The third part is devoted to Communications and networking.

It starts by spelling out how important communication skills are for women. Women who can communicate effectively about themselves and for themselves will have far greater chance of making sure that their health and well-being is considered, and that the planning and implementation of development projects allows women to participate, contribute and benefit.

Improved communications skills will also enable women to educate their own families, communities and local leaders about development in general, and women's role in development, in particular.

Better communication will enable women to elicit husbands, children and community leaders support. It will enable women to work more effectively together, and, to be educators and advocates of better development in the wider world.

Networking is partly an outcome of better communication, but it is also a way for women to build bridges of common understanding, cooperation and solidarity among womens groups and organisations throughout the world.

2. THE TRAINERS HANDBOOK

The Trainers' Handbook is the tool for translating the Issues and Information into practical education and development programmes and projects. It is a resource guide for organisation and action by women on the main theme raised in the Text.

The Handbook is really an introduction to particular strategies for adult education, awareness raising and action. It encourages trainers to make the most of available opportunities and different methods to educate, inform, organise, mobilise and to build better development for PNG.

The Handbook is intended specifically for people who will play an active role as Trainers in the new National Womens Training and Awareness Programme. While the Issues and Information book can be used as a general reader, it can also be seen as a key textbook for our trainers.

The Handbook helps the trainer to understand issues and build them into programmes and activities to educate and involve women in development.

The Handbook has several main sections:

- <u>Introduction</u>:

  Linking the National Womens Training and Awareness Programme to the National Womens Policy and the programmes of other government departments.

- <u>Workshops:</u>

  This part spells out why women need to do much more than simply rely on 'on-off' Workshops, as a tool for training and mobilising the nation's women. Workshops have often become the means and the end in adult education in Papua New Guinea.

Workshops are looked at in terms of the context, by looking at their positive aspects as well as their limitations. The message that trainers are encouraged to learn is that they should do much more than just workshops.

Other methods of training women and maximising the opportunity to inform the community and to really challenge and change entrenched ideas, customs and approaches to development are also explained in detail.

- Using International and National days of Observance:

  A Calendar of 15 important days relevant to key women in development issues is provided as well as numerous programme ideas for organising events and activities on these days.

- Videos:

  There is a detailed section on the use of videos for education. Approximately 15 videos are discussed in detail - emphasising their use as tools for education rather than entertainment. Trainers are encouraged to provide useful introductions and lead follow-up discussions on documentaries which help women to develop a critical view on development themes, while others are more straight forward videos on Reproduction, STD, AIDS..etc. supplied by the Department of Health and W.H.O.

  This section recognises that there is much valuable video material available in the country. The problem is simply to ensure that it is used effectively for education and awareness raising.

- Songs/Stories/Drama:

  Trainers are encouraged to develop some more active and creative methods of educating and communicating the themes in the Issues and Information Text.

  The production and use of Songs, Stories and Community Theatre is also presented with numerous local examples.

- Campaigns

  The final section in the Trainers' manual is concerned with Campaigns. Campaigns are introduced as a way of informing, educating, challenging and changing behaviour and attitudes, policies and projects, in a cooperative and ongoing manner. Campaigns provide an opportunity to use many different methods of creating awareness and building constructive action to bring about better development.

A number of very successful local-led women and development campaigns are presented and analysed in detail to enable women to better understand what campaigning involves and what it can achieve.

3. POSTER SET

A Set of 25 Posters has been produced. The Set corresponds directly with the 24 sub-topics in the ISSUES and INFORMATION BOOK. In fact, the Posters provide the same information in visual and summary form. In addition, they are written in Tok Pisin and are currently being translated into the Motu language.

The Posters are intended as a simple format for the presentation of the ISSUES and INFORMATION BOOK. They can be used by literate trainers who can refer back to the Book, as well as by semi-literate trainers, who can learn about the main issues and information through workshops, videos, songs, theatre, campaigns, etc.

4. THE PROVINCIAL RESOURCE KITS

Provincial Resource Kits are currently being prepared for each Province. Ideally, each Province will hold a Kit which can be used by their provincial and district trainers, and which can be used for local events, video screenings, workshops, campaigns, seminars, school programmes etc.

The Kit will be built over the next 3 years, and, will contain:

- important and relevant documentary and educational videos and posters;
- relevant handbooks and manuals on different development issues and different methods of training;
- relevant booklets/training modules produced by different government departments on topics covered in the entire package;
- relevant magazines and newsletters related to women and development programmes worldwide;
- book of songs, stories, poems, plays and photos produced by women in Papua New Guinea, who participate in the National Womens Training/Awareness Programme;
- Cassettes of songs, stories etc., produced by women in PNG, on topics covered in the entire package.

PART 4: IMPLEMENTATION PROCESS

The implementation of this National Womens Training and Awareness Programme, is being supported by I.L.O's Labour and Population Team for Asia and the Pacific (LAPTAP) with the financial support of the United Nations Family and Population Agency.

There are three (3) Mobile Trainers who have been appointed, and, will work under the supervision of a Coordinator from the Women's Division Training Unit.

The Trainers are responsible for introducing the Training and Awareness package to the nation, and, in particular with facilitating and resourcing the establishment of specific training programmes in all Provinces of the country.

There have already been two (2) Regional Workshops conducted for the Momase, Highlands and Papuan provinces. These involved working with two (2) Trainers from each Province to introduce the package, involve them in it's ongoing development and assist them to plan a three year programme of implementation in their respective provinces.

In each of the Provinces, the trainers are drawn from different departments and non-government agencies, and are fitted in to the current structure of womens organisations and activities as well as the nature of the provincial development context.

Training teams and committees in each Province are being encouraged to maximize the involvement of all relevant government departments, churches, other non-government organisations and community groups in their programmes.

In every province, the package is being introduced to the provincial political and administrative leaders, as well as heads of relevant departments and non-government agencies and organisations.

In most cases this will be in 1-2 day workshops. Participants will be provided with an Issues and Information Book. They will be encouraged to read and inform themselves on the issues in general. They will also be asked to suggest ways in which these issues can be addressed in their own plans, policies, programmes and projects, and how their personnel could collaborate with the national mobile training team.

The next step is for all Trainers to begin building a training network and structure which best suits their Province, and builds on locally available resources, resource people and ongoing activities of different divisions and agencies. This process will vary from province to province and in some cases the national Trainers' will provide more assistance than others.

Certain specific aspects will be discussed in close consultation with the Department of Personnel Management, with regards to specialised training for women.

There is obviously an awakening in the womens network about acquiring skills and knowledge and information for personal betterment and work improvement.

The National Trainers will be travelling extensively and will be evaluating and improving the National Training and Awareness Package at regular intervals. They will also be collecting Poems, Songs, Case Studies, new Articles....etc., from programmes and activities conducted under the Programme. These will be used in the ongoing revisions of the parts of the package, as well as in the production of new support handbooks.

To date, the response to the materials has been overwhelming. Even male counterparts have expressed high hopes for a breakthrough in the attitudes, behaviour and approaches to development.

The content of the Training materials is likely to be well-used in many places, such as the adult literacy programmes initiated at provincial levels.

Current Expansions:

Further development and applications will be translated and done by UNICEF in its current provincial programmes in the Southern Highlands and the Milne Bay Provinces.

The Goroka YWCA Womens Kisim Save Skul have initiated ways in which the Training Package can be effectively integrated into Womens Literacy Programmes.

The East Sepik Women and the Eastern Highlands women are already implementing and carrying out provincial awareness meetings with their politicians and departmental heads/divisional heads.

The Non-Formal Education Officers who are men have conducted awareness activities at marketing outlets in Wabag.

The Milne Bay Province has a major provincial training and awareness programme for all its districts, as far as the islands of Misima and the Trobriand Islands. A major provincial Literacy Training and Awareness Workshop on the Trobriand Islands is using the Package themes as well as translating Posters into their different languages.

The Kiunga District of the North-fly area and the Balimo Districts have developed their awareness programmes with the Posters.

Women are taking the initiative on their own. The applications are endless and the Trainers hope to build gender-sensitivity into development among the grassroots - from the bottom up.

A FINAL WORD ON POPULATION ISSUES IN RELATION TO WOMEN'S HEALTH, CHANGING FAMILY LIFE AND PARTICIPATION IN DEVELOPMENT

Population is one of the key issues which inspired the production of the National Women's Training Package. Population awareness is one of the intended aims of the long term National Women's Training Programme. However, the usual simplistic discussion and superficial proposal of solutions (Papua New Guinea's population is growing too fast, therefore more women should use contraceptives) is not spelt out in our materials.

Instead we have attempted to raise the population issue in a total social, political and economic context, and from the perspective of women. Programmes built on top-down national policies and externally funded programmes for the provision of condoms, pills and shots will not necessarily improve the quality of life for women or the quality of development for the nation.

The National Women's Training Programme is built instead on a belief in our people, and their capacity, once informed, involved and educated, to make the right choices about family life and family size. It is also built on the belief in their right to challenge development projects which destroy and erode resources and undermine sustainable livelihoods.

Too often conventional economic development projects lead to resource loss and cash dependency which in turn create a false picture of development. The people are unjustly blamed for the destruction of the environment, then population control and even more top-down economic development projects are proposed as a solution.

Our people must be informed of the whole picture. They must know of all options and be given the right to make their own choices. We believe that if our women are given more information and opportunities, and are encouraged to make their own choices, this will provide the most just, equitable, and sustainable basis for national development.

STATUS REPORT ON POPULATION POLICY

JENNIFER LITAU[1]

INTRODUCTION

My topic, the "Status Report on Population Policy" is the subject of an ongoing research project which the Department of Finance and Planning has engaged the National Research Institute (NRI) to undertake.

My presentation is divided into: an overview of past and previous attempts at the formulation of a population policy (or programmes and strategies); Second, briefly discuss the recently adopted population policy and outline some potential problems associated with implementation of selected policy objectives; and finally, present my concluding remarks. The views I will present are my personal ones and not those of NRI or the Department of Finance and Planning.

BACKGROUND

Population policy has been a concern for the Papua New Guinea government since the 1970s, although it was more or less thought of in terms of population control. Debates concerning birth control or contraceptive adoption for Papua New Guinea have not been uncommon between parliamentarians and the Catholic Church. Later issues added to the birth control concern were calls to improve the status of women and reduce the negative impacts of rural-urban migration. Sharpless (1988) presents an excellent review of the background to population policy, why population control or family planning became the major population policy issue and why it still is. Hayes (1990) presents other significant considerations necessary for the development of a sound integrative population - development policy.

The first explicit attempt at drawing up a population policy was in 1978 and resulted in a joint submission to the Cabinet of a draft policy, by the Ministers for Environment and Conservation, and Health.

[1] National Research Institute, for the Department of Finance and Planning

The draft policy asserted that Papua New Guinea was experiencing a rapid population growth rate (3.5%) which needed to be curbed or lowered to three percent (3%) by 1980, predominantly through the use of family planning, and to be complemented by improvement in the status of women. If family planning and contraceptive use was not fostered at a rapid pace, it argued, the perceived growth rate, estimated at three percent (3%) for 1980, would cause regional land pressure in many provinces beyond 1986, and a shortage of or pressure upon the provision of health and education services.

The National Executive Council (NEC) did not ratify the draft population policy, primarily because of the overemphasis on population growth and control. The feeling was that Papua New Guinea was in no danger of overpopulation and that a land mass of 460,000 square kilometres could still sustain further growth. Socio-cultural attitudes and values favoured large family sizes in terms of the economic and social security that children would provide for their elders. Hence, the call to reduce fertility was obviously impractical. It appeared that the impetus to the development of a population policy was being manipulated by expatriates or externally (Warom 1990). The draft policy was shelved. By 1980, census data showed that the growth rate was lower than expected (2.3%) so there was no serious attempt to review the policy again.

The next attempt was in 1987 following a submission to the NEC, by the Minister for Health, Micah Wes, in which he expressed concern about the long-term, socio-economic impact of Papua New Guinea's high population growth rate. NEC Decision 3/87 directed the Department of Finance and Planning to convene a Population Advisory Committee. The Department of Finance and Planning acted by establishing the National Advisory Committee on Population Policy (NACPP) and the Population Planning and Coordination Unit (PPCU) within its jurisdiction, in the same year.

By May, 1988, NACPP had formally determined topics covering a wide range of areas which would be guidelines towards the formulation of a National Population Policy. The guidelines presented:

- Bases and Principles for a National Population Policy
- Population Trends and Implications
- Goals and Objectives
- Population Distribution, Migration and Urbanisation
- Population Density, Land Tenure, Rural Development and Food Production

- Population and Education
- Employment and Human Resources
- Family Health, Family Planning and Family Welfare
- Children and Youth

Principles which necessitated the formulation of a National Population Policy were identified:

1. Concern that the present growth of 2.3 percent would threaten the attainment of any development objectives in terms of ensuring the quality of life.
2. Alarm that a considerable decline in infant and child mortality, with an associated increase in life expectancy, coupled with the current growth rate would continue to result in higher future growth rates.
3. Concern about the socio-economic impacts of migration and urbanisation on living standards and employment.
4. Sustainable development goal.
5. Need to explicitly address the rights of couples with regard to fertility and reproductive behaviour.
6. Compliance with international awareness calls by the World Population Plan of Action of Bucharest (1974); Asia-Pacific Call for Action on Population, of Colombo (1982); and International Conference on Population, of Mexico (1984), for explicit actions on population and development.

These principles are reiterated and further elaborated as the bases for the formulation of the 1991 National Population Policy. Integrative population and development planning is explicitly advocated as fundamental to achieving the goals and objectives of the policy.

An Integrated National Population Policy for Progress and Development

The 1991 National Population Policy has been approved by the National Executive Council, has been adopted, and is into its early stages of implementation. Most of the participants at this seminar have seen a copy or can get one, as it is in circulation already. This is a major step forward for Papua New Guinea, in terms of the existence now of explicit policy guidelines towards development planning for the country's population needs.

This policy has passed through several drafts which were reviewed by both government departments and technical personnel. Although it has taken two years to finalise, it has received broad support by Cabinet. The policy is now in place. However, serious thought should be given to the mode of implementation because if this is not handled well, there may be a serious setback for the policy.

POLICY GOALS

The ultimate goal of the policy is to limit population growth as much as possible in order to ensure that all citizens attain an acceptable standard of living and improve the quality of their lives through social and economic progress.

The main explicit goals of the National Population Policy are to:

(1) improve the standard of living and the quality of life of the citizens of Papua New Guinea;

(2) improve health and welfare of the population through preventing premature deaths and illness among high risk groups, especially mothers and children;

(3) achieve a population growth rate which will not threaten future development prospects; and

(4) achieve universal primary education and expand secondary education enrolment to 70 percent of the population by the year 2000.

All these goals are essential and should complement each other to achieve goal (1). Goal (1) calls for improvement in the `standard of living' and the `quality of life' for the citizens of Papua New Guinea. `Standard of living' is a crude measure of the quality and quantity of goods and services enjoyed by a person, group or nation (Webster's II Dictionary). In order to attain 'quality of life', the population must be kept in check and marked regional variations in the distribution of services should be reduced. The achievement of goal (1) depends a great deal upon the adequate government supply of basic services such as health and education when needed. Health and Education departments however get less funds to cope with present demands for these services, to maintain existing levels of services or to deal with increases in population size.

Goals (2) and (3) indirectly refer to family planning and population control, respectively, which suggests that these goals receive major consideration in the policy.

Goal (4) calls for both an achievement of universal primary education (UPE) and an expansion of secondary school enrolment to 70 percent by the year 2000. The achievement of UPE has been a target for the Education Department for some time now. The current education strategy has not permitted its attainement. It seems feasible if planned and accomplished in stages. Part two of goal (4) is a call to expand secondary school enrolment to 70 percent by the year 2000. Secondary school enrolments may have or have attained the target. Weeks (1990) shows that national secondary school enrolments had improved over the decade 1980-89 to 35 percent and 66 percent increases in Grades 7 and 10 respectively. Blocking up and the expansion and growth of high schools are responsible for the increases seen in Grade 10. Increases in Grade 7 enrolments have only kept pace with population growth. National retention rates also increased between 1980 and 1986 to 65 percent (Weeks and Gibson, 1990). Educationally disadvantaged groups like female students and those from isolated rural areas need to given more places in high schools if goal (1) is to be achieved.

POLICY OBJECTIVES

Policy objectives to achieve these goals are to:

(1) promote awareness among the citizens of Papua New Guinea of population problems and the effects of population growth on future development;

(2) sensitise planners, decision makers and opinion leaders at all levels and the general public at large to the implications of population dynamics in social and economic planning, at both the national and provincial levels;

(3) provide necessary information and education on the value of reasonable family size to both the individual family and the future of the nation;

(4) raise the living conditions in rural areas and provide objective information on living conditions in urban areas to prospective migrants;

(5) promote and expand primary health care services, especially maternal and child care;

(6) make family planning means and services available to all couples and individuals willing to regulate childbirth;

(7) improve demographic data collection, analysis and dissemination for use in social and economic development planning; and

(8) enhance integrated rural and urban development in order to improve living conditions in rural areas and to promote an equitable distribution of socio-economic services.

OBSTACLES TO THE IMPLEMENTATION OF THE POLICY

Major obstacles which could inhibit or prevent the implementation of any part of the policy objectives are institutional factors, economic factors, cultural values; unavailability of appropriately trained manpower, the time factor, and the lack of community, family or individual level support by the populace.

Institutional obstacles relate to organisational capacity in terms of defining plans or programmes, coordination between national and provincial departments and with sectoral ministries, implementation of plans and projects, and their consistent management and evaluation. Economic obstacles refer primarily to inadequate, lack or shortage of revenue and funds needed to finance approved programmes and projects. Cultural values favour larger completed family sizes, are suspicious of modern forms of contraception, prohibit open discussions of fertility behaviour, and impose upon a couple desires for the family type in terms of family size, number of children and genders of children 'required'. These are all potential hindrances to a successful implementation of family planning programmes. The lack of appropriately trained reliable personnel, sensitive to linkages between population issues, implies a potential lack of proper coordination and integrative implementation of the policy objectives. Targets which have been set to be achieved within a given time period may fall short due to limited time as determined by the allocated funding, manpower and resources indispensable to project completions. Finally, lack of community and family support of programmes, especially family planning, for whatever reasons, could hinder progress towards the achievement of targets. These obstacles will be further discussed in term of the proposed goals and objectives.

Of the four main goals of the National Population Policy, Goals (2) and (3) directly propose family planning and population control. Policy Objectives (3), (5), and (6) deal with the two areas also. Some questions that policy planners and implementers will need to have considered, although it is not too late now are: what target group is family planning directed at and who will administer or implement the policy. The important, although indirect emphasis accorded family planning here, poses the question, 'are Papua New Guinean families unplanned?' and 'does the population majority, which is in the rural villages, perceive family planning as we do?' Obviously the answer is **NO** to the latter question. Cultural and economic values favour having more children and larger (completed) family sizes.

Likely problems therefore that will be encountered are resistance to adopting contraceptive practices or low levels of acceptance in adopting or using modern contraceptives. Should we then be pushing for contraceptive use to limit family sizes and growth or providing incentives such as improving living conditions, which would indirectly ensure more surviving children and ultimately contribute to desired smaller (completed) family sizes? These considerations need to the borne in the minds of policy planners and implementers for future review of the policy.

Another problem is that in most of Papua New Guinea where male or cultural values dictate much of what goes on within the household, particularly in relation to child-bearing and related matters, the call to reduce or limit family sizes is one that indirectly advocates change in cultural values or men's dominance in decision-making. Both large and small-scale awareness campaigns utilising all available forms of the media will need to precede any serious attempts directed at curbing fertility.

Policy objective (8) calls for integrated rural and urban development in order to improve living conditions in rural areas and promote the equitable distribution of services. Integrating population and development planning appears to be the way to go. Thus, teaching people to be literate should include providing a situation to which the skill can be meaningfully employed to improve the quality of life.

It is important to note that two different types of population policy associated with integrated population-development planning exist. On the one hand are policies which aim to directly influence demographic variables **(or "population-influencing policies")**. For example, up to the mid-1970s, population policy was understood to mean "population-influencing" policy or population "control". It is still the concept in the minds of many planners in Papua New Guinea. On the other hand are policies aimed at the socio-economic system as responding to expected future demographic conditions **(or "population-responsive" policies)**. The call for an integrative approach means that equal emphasis is placed on reactive policies or the reciprocal effects of population change on development and vice versa, in terms of consideration of other variables such as housing, health, agriculture, transportation, employment creation policies, and environmental effects. In this view, population growth may sometimes provide opportunities rather than only creating problems (Hayes 1990) as it is perceived in this policy.

Hayes (1990) also points out that the full integration of population factors into development planning may be limited or prevented to some extent by (any of) these factors:

- scarcity of appropriately trained planning staff with technical knowledge of population development linkages, and the lack of funds to appoint and train such staff;
- low priority placed by the government on population issues relative to other development issues such as fiscal and monetary policy, trade, foreign investment, aid and so on;
- absence of or insufficient, reliable demographic data to incorporate into plans and planning process; and
- lack of detailed, scientific knowledge of economic-demographic linkages within Papua New Guinea.

The lack of or insufficient political will-power can also affect priorities goals and objectives and hence negatively affect planning.

Objective (7) aims to improve data collection, analysis and dissemination for use in planning. Indirectly, this is a call to devise new data collection systems or revise existing ones. Insufficient data or unreliable data negatively affect sound planning because research which is not corroborated by adequate or appropriate data lacks the stamina needed to improve its attractiveness for use in planning. Furthermore, instead of only seeking to improve data collection systems we could also attempt to create systems which would provide the needed data on a regular basis. Civil or vital registration systems are virtually lacking in Papua New Guinea, and may not be instituted yet for quite some time. There should be interdepartmental cooperation in dispensing relevant data to other departments, particularly those data based on current research.

Implementation: Phase I

Initial implementation of the policy is going to occur in two main phases. Phase 1 objectives are to:

1. establish a Population Planning and Coordination Unit (PPCU) within the Department of Finance and Planning in order to coordinate policy formulation, and to develop, monitor and review projects;
2. identify and appoint a resource person to coordinate activities between departments;

3. establish a National Advisory Committee on Population Policy (already in place);

4. establish a database; and

5. establish relations with (outside) potential donor agencies.

A National Population Council has been established to monitor and coordinate overall implementation of policy. A Population Planning and Coordination Unit now exists as its secretariat whose responsibility is to ensure that population and development are integrated, consistent activities. Functions of such a unit must be explicitly determined in order to have a better sense of direction. Hayes (1990:5) lists the following as some possible functions of the unit:

1. To act as a catalyst for population policy, training, and research;

2. To facilitate information exchange between government, research and training institutions, and between ministries within government;

3. To coordinate and collaborate in the activities of other planning units within sectoral ministries to ensure consistency between population and development goals;

4. To provide technical inputs to the work of other planning sections where required;

5. To identify data requirements and data gaps and promote the collection of relevant information and statistical data;

6. To construct an inventory of existing population-development research and summarise its policy implications;

7. To commission relevant policy studies where required;

8. To provide population data and other relevant information to other planning units and ensure consistency between sectoral plans with regard to the information used; and

9. To formulate training programmes in the field of population and development for staff of the planning unit itself and for other staff of sectoral ministries.

Some of these functions are already being performed by the Unit, but it may not be as effective due to "obstacles" already listed and its newness.

Problems associated with a lack of commitment, interest and collaboration could also hamper the efficiency of these agencies in implementing policy. Continued planning in isolation by key departments such as Health and Education (as occurs now) would act as barriers to implementation. As most functions associated with the delivery of health care and education services are decentralised, planning at provincial level or lack of corresponding provincial policies and/or integration of national policies into provincial programmes could seriously cause set-backs to the policy PPCU should work towards coordinated and collaborative planning with provincial planners and devise strategies through which national goals and objectives could materialise into action plans at provincial levels.

Implementation: Phase II

In Phase II, the following targets or specific objectives will be achieved:

1. Increase in family planning prevalence from the existing three percent (3%) to about 22 percent by 1995 and 63 percent by the year 2000.

2. Increase the percentage coverage of family planning services or information to **all** couples by 2000.

3. Expand birth-spacing knowledge and increase birth-spacing to at least two-year intervals to more than 50 percent of couples.

4. Reduce Total Fertility Rate (TFR) from 5.4 per woman to 4.4 by 1995 and 3.2 by 2000.

5. Reduce Infant Mortality Rate (IMR) from 72 to 50 per thousand by 2000.

6. Reduce Crude Birth Rate (CBR) currently 35 per thousand to 30 per thousand by year 1995 and reduce overall growth rate.

7. Reduce the number of people entering the labour market through the increase in qualification levels and prolonging education, especially of women.

8. Expand secondary education to at least 50 percent by 1995 and achieve Universal Primary Education by year 2000.

9. Promote relevance of education for rural areas, and better incentives to reduce attrition rates especially among females.

10. Increase adult literacy from the present 32 percent to 50 percent by 1995 and 80 percent by 2000.

11. Promote the positive use of elements of Papua New Guinea traditions and cultures to encourage better understanding and use of family planning practices.

Essentially, Phase II of the implementation plan calls for such drastic measures as increases to adoption of family planning practices by:

- coverage;
- birth spacing intervals;
- reductions in TFR, IMR, CBR, and rural-urban migration;
- expansion of education opportunities and achievement of UPE;
- promoting better incentives to retain female students in school;
- increases in the adult literacy rate; and
- promoting the use of positive traditional means to complement the effectiveness of modern family planning practices.

Imagine what Papua New Guinea would become at the turn of the century if all of these objectives were materialised into actions. We would be a perfect country, whatever that means. At least for the rural majority, it would be the first time that some could enjoy the benefits of modernisation, not to mention that while we congratulate Papua New Guinea for its adoption of the population policy, the majority of our people are unaware that the government has just launched such a policy which aims to drastically change their behaviour for better or for worse, over the next nine years. Has the government actually placed funding aside to implement the population policy? What programme has been laid down? Is it possible that the government may only be paying lip service to concerns of the World Bank and other agencies such as the Australian government? Essentially, how serious is the government in implementing the policy after having launched it?

I suspect, therefore, that many of these objectives will be unattainable by the turn of the century, but not in the long-term. The policy objectives already listed particularly in Phase II, are overambitious. No empirical justification is provided as to why such achievements must be effected by 2000. Practical situations today do suggest the need to plan in these identified areas but there is a want of empirical evidence to guide in the determination of a set of criteria which could assist to prioritise the targets according to population need. Alternatively, other projections in health care or education may be tied to the proposed targets in crude birth rate, crude death rate and total fertility rate, hence it is possible to estimate financial or resource needs for UPE by 2000.

It is obvious that real obstacles to implementation do exist. First, think of research and data-related problems associated with gathering information on reproductive behaviour which is taboo in Papua New Guinea. Pre-conditions of a successful implementation of the policy involve such things also as basic changes in attitudes, traditional values and behaviour, not to mention that what the policy proposes seeks to undermine basic social, traditional, cultural and economic systems that are inherent in attitudes and behaviour. These have inevitable implications on the need for awareness programmes. I do not have an answer to this scenario except to say that while some factors contribute to hindering the implementation of the population policy, other factors supplement or complement a successful implementation of the policy.

I do not suggest that all the objectives (and thus goals) are unattainable in the long-term. On the contrary, action plans must be developed within frameworks based on empirical evidence. Priorities should be determined according to needs and problem areas as identified by research. Projects need to be planned and funds sought for their establishment and future appraisals. Collaborative and cooperative complementary action and planning is a must between national departments, sectoral ministries, provincial departments and non-government organisations (NGOs). Interest, political willpower and consistency are important considerations as well in terms of coordinating the successful implementation of the policy objectives.

On the other hand, the population, both at the national and provincial levels, needs to be positively receptive to the adoption of the fertility control measures required of them. Cultural values, behaviour and taboos will inevitably be challenged or violated. Positive stimuli to change ought to be the foci. Thus, the quality of life and the equal right of every citizen to services such as education or health care, whose access would be restricted by more population pressure should be stressed as fundamental rationales in reducing population growth rates, lowering family size, encouraging population control through family planning and contraceptive use, encouraging more female participation in the education system and work-force, and so on. Political will, institutional collaboration and cooperation, explicitly stated strategies or action plans of implementation (which are feasible as supported by data and economically viable or affordable), awareness on the part of the population in terms of voluntary acceptance and actions, monitoring and evaluation of feedback on the linkages between population and development planning, and sensitivity to inevitable outcomes, need to be noted as factors contributing to a successful achievement of objectives.

CONCLUSION

Papua New Guinea is well endowed with natural resources, has a relatively low population growth rate of 2.3 percent compared to 3.5 percent for the Solomon Islands, has a lower total fertility rate of 5.4 percent compared with 6.4 percent for the Solomon Islands, has a considerable land area of more than 460,000 square kilometres and an average density of about eight persons per square kilometre, and thus could still sustain further growth. It is not simply a question of sufficient land and so on but the quality of life and standard of life that matters. This depends a great deal on the supply of services such as health and education which are getting less funds to deal with increasing population. It also depends on the capacity of the country to use the population or manpower productively. For instance, countries with high population densities, like Singapore and Thailand, can comfortably sustain their populations, while a country like Papua New Guinea with a low density still finds its population too much in terms of high unemployment, and health and education services cannot be made accessible to all at a reasonable cost. The need to have children for economic and cultural reasons will still for some time override basic concerns embraced within the policy. While it is true that a country's population is its most valuable resource, the experience of countries such as India, also indicate that beyond a certain limit, this 'valuable resource' becomes a liability. Thus, the beginning of explicit planning now is to be commended and consistently supported in order to achieve the 'desired' outcomes over the long-term.

REFERENCES

Hayes, G. 1990. 'Integrated population and development planning in Papua New Guinea', Paper presented at the South Pacific Commission high level seminar on Population and Development for Government Ministers (Planning) and Heads of Planning Departments, Noumea, 20-22 August 1990.

Minister for Environment/Office of the Environment, 1978. A Population Policy for Papua New Guinea. (Draft only).

Minister for Health, 1987. Population Policy for Papua New Guinea.

Ministry of Health and Medical Services, Government of the Solomon Islands. Solomon Islands Population Policy.

Sharpless, J B. 1988. The troubled history of Population Policy Initiatives in Papua New Guinea 1968-1988. Paper prepared for Yagl-Ambu issue on Population Problems in Papua New Guinea.

The National Advisory Committee on Population Policy, 1988. Guidelines Towards a National Population Policy for Papua New Guinea.

Warom, Homolpi, 1990. 'Population Policy in Papua New Guinea: Background Information', in The Morobe Population and Development Workshop (Report), 14-16, May 1990, Morobe.

Webster's Dictionary II: New Riverside Dictionary. 1984. Berkley Books: New York.

Weeks, Sheldon. 1990.

CLOSING SPEECH BY UTULA SAMANA, M.P.

Ladies and Gentlemen, I believe that in a democratic environment we hope that the policy-making process is one where the basic needs of the electorate are channelled through to the authorities for decision, and eventually influence the manner in which resources and services are delivered. However, effective policy-making cannot be accomplished without analysis of social and economic factors and without thorough discussion and debate. I believe this is the over-all purpose of Waigani Seminars.

Whilst there are indeed positive merits to the great Waigani tradition, we hope that the process does not become a digression producing more paralysis by analysis without offering practical solutions to solving basic human problems; water, food and shelter. Hence, the selection of the theme, Population, Family Health and Development by this year's Waigani Seminar Organisers is most appropriate.

After having eighteen such seminars in the past, what has become of the health of our population within the development syndrome after so many decades of political ineptness in Papua New Guinea and the Pacific. Much of what has been said and deliberated on has been based upon thorough research, and assessments and recommendations that have been made add in-put to the formulation of policies at a later stage. For many years since independence basic data on population and it's wide ranging implications for development affecting basic services such as health, education, transport, communication and food production has been critically lacking.

No effective planning for human development can realistically be established without basic data on population and the physical environment, providing the socio-economic indicators that should serve as a guide to policy decisions governing resource allocations.

Generally speaking, significant numbers of departments both at national and provincial level either lack basic statistical data or the skills required for developmental planning. For example, if you ask the Department of Primary Industry and Livestock as to how many kilograms of traditional food crops are produced, kaukaus, bananas and taro grown mostly by women in the rural villages for example, and the quality of these food crops in terms of nutritional and commercial value, they may have problems in answering these questions. If you ask the Department of Transport for the facts about the percentage of population nearest to vehicular transport per district or province in the country, to determine the transport needs and priorities of an area, you probably will not get a satisfactory answer. Going on to the Health Ministry, we do not really know which villages require better water systems. Due to population growth, in terms of doctors per head of population and general accessibility to basic primary health care services, this country's primary health delivery system is far from being adequate.

Turning to my own Ministry of Education, priorities for establishing educational services seem to be dictated more by political pressures than planning in relation to population need. Within over-all governmental decision-making the budget process seems to be dictated more by priorities for balancing the books as seen through the eyes of the Finance Department rather than determined by socio-economic objectives. This indicates the incapacity of our bureaucratic institutions and decision-making processes to respond effectively to the rising socio-economic demands of our people.

Population, family health and development issues as discussed with wide ranging perspectives relating to women's health, environment, socio-economic development, family care and family health, are not only essential to the general welfare and well being of society, but as demands for improved adequacy and quality by the citizens of our respective countries in the Pacific increase, are becoming a potential political issue. It is therefore politically pragmatic that we manage our own population well through effective and realistic planning in accordance with our population needs. Otherwise we will be moving from crisis to crisis, and instead of managing crisis we will be prompted to management by crisis, moving here and there and getting nowhere.

So much has been said and written and deliberated upon in the past Waigani Seminars on a number of important issues such as Land, Politics, Education, Rural Development, Environment, Agriculture, Urbanisation, Pacific Vision, Trade, The Eight Point Aims, The Role of Science and Technology, Ethics of Development and the last one on the State-of-the-Arts in the Pacific. What has happened to the findings and the recommendations derived from this intellectual labour? Have they resulted in some tangible benefit to society? I would say some have and many are collecting dust in academic libraries and old files. For example, what has happened since the great constitutional debates on decentralisation, rural development, pacific vision, the Eight Aims? So far decentralisation and the concept of power-sharing has led to the creation of provincial political elites and the emergence of political factionalism, resulting more in national discord than providing a forum for building national cohesion and national concensus through complimentary development.

Since Independence, successive governments have produced verbal platitudes rather than developing a comprehensive policy on rural development. The Eight Point Aims which were introduced in December of 1973 were thrown into the gutter in October of 1975, and since then no one has made any reference to the infamous Eight Aims. Self reliance and self sufficiency in terms of developing our human and material productive potentials has been re-interpreted to mean fiscal self reliance through resources exploitation in order to balance the books of an inefficient and ineffective state apparatus.

Today state micro-management is dictated more by the World Bank and IMF and big resource investors than the basic conditions and needs of our population. On the domestic scene, rumblings of urban based unions and the dictates of pressure groups are twisting and turning decision makers to meet their demands, rather than establishing national purpose and coordination to achieve greater goals of self sufficiency and equal and fair distribution of goods and services to meet the needs of the wider population of our society.

Given this contextual reality in our political process the challenge to all of us is to work much harder. Given the will we can forge national concensus and purpose, which is so lacking in our society today. Where do we go from here? Will the findings and recommendations of this Seminar end as yet another academic exercise by the intelligentsia providing some resource material for yet another academic thesis, or will they form the basis for policy options upon which political commitments and decisions can be made and implemented effectively for the benefit of the majority of our population. I am here not to close and bury the 19th Waigani Seminar, but rather throw it open to the next stage for policy-makers, administrators, you and I, to make some real deliberate effort to implement some of the findings most appropriate to the needs of our countries and our populations.

As politicians our job is to direct the politics of the budgetary process on an annual basis, and also from the medium and long term perspective, in order that adequate resources are allocated to improve the basic quality of life of our people.

Let me assure you that your participation and contribution in this seminar will not be a waste. We, as your ministers of government will study carefully your findings derived from your analysis of factors affecting our society and citizens. We will endeavour as a matter of duty to initiate policy discussions on the basis of your findings and recommendations, and I urge and encourage all of us to work towards this end. Through public awareness of issues raised we all can help to shape public opinion and in turn assist the computerised Waigani budget process to see some meaning and purpose in human terms.

At this juncture, I wish to thank the donors for their generous donations that made the seminar possible and indeed a success. To our distinguished guests and speakers from overseas, we offer our thanks for your participation, for your time and for your efforts.

May I also extend our appreciation to all the participants from Papua New Guinea from within Port Moresby and particularly from the provinces. On behalf of all the participants, let me also thank the Chairman of this seminar and our Patron, and all the hard working organisers for work well done, despite problems within the university. I believe this is the first time ever for a Waigani Seminar to be held outside of the university campus. So, the population is really increasing.

Finally, ladies and gentlemen with much pleasure and gratitude I now officially declare the discussion part of the Nineteenth Waigani Seminar closed, and initiate the next phase, action and the implementation of the resolutions passed. Thank you.

www.ingramcontent.com/pod-product-compliance
Lightning Source LLC
Jackson TN
JSHW050737140926
108091JS00023B/22